DIVIDED LEGACY

A HISTORY OF THE SCHISM IN MEDICAL THOUGHT

Volume II

DIVIDED LEGACY
A HISTORY OF THE SCHISM IN MEDICAL THOUGHT

Volume II

THE ORIGINS OF MODERN WESTERN MEDICINE: J.B. VAN HELMONT TO CLAUDE BERNARD

Harris L. Coulter

Wehawken Book Co.
Washington, D.C.

North Atlantic Books
Berkeley, California

1988

Passages from Erwin H. Ackerknecht, *Medicine at the Paris Hospital* (copyright 1967 by The Johns Hopkins Press), Paul Talalay, ed., *Drugs in Our Society* (copyright 1964 by The Johns Hopkins Press), and from articles appearing in the *Bulletin of the History of Medicine* used by permission of The Johns Hopkins Press.

Passages from Owsei Temkin, *Galenism: Rise and Decline of a Medical Philosophy* (copyright 1973 by Cornell University) used by permission of the Cornell University Press.

Passages from Kenneth Dewhurst, *Dr. Thomas Sydenham (1624-1689). His Life and Original Writings* (copyright 1966 by Kenneth Dewhurst) used by permission of the author and the University of California Press.

Passages from R. Virchow, *Post-Mortem Examinations and the Position of Pathology among Biological Studies* (copyright 1973 by the New York Academy of Medicine) and J. B. Morgagni, *The Seats and Causes of Diseases Investigated by Anatomy* (copyright 1960 Preface, Introduction, and Translation by the New York Academy of Medicine) used by permission of the New York Academy of Medicine Library.

Passages from R. Virchow, *Disease, Life, and Man* (copyright 1958 by the Board of Trustees of the Leland Stanford Junior University) used by permission of the Stanford University Press.

Passages from L. S. King, *The Medical World of the 18th Century* (copyright 1958 by the University of Chicago) used by permission of the University of Chicago Press.

Passages from Allen Debus, ed., *Science, Medicine, and Society in the Renaissance: Essays to Honor Walter Pagel* (copyright 1972 by Science History Publications) used by permission of Watson Neale Academic Publications.

Passages from Thomas S. Hall, *Rene Descartes: Treatise of Man* (copyright 1972 by the President and Fellows of Harvard College) used by permission of the Harvard University Press.

Passage from J. R. Partington, *History of Chemistry* (copyright 1961 by J. R. Partington) used by permission of the Macmillan Publishing Co.

Passages from H. Isler, *Thomas Willis, 1621-1675* (copyright 1968 by the Hafner Publishing Co.) used by permission of the Hafner Publishing Co.

Passages from Friedrich Hoffmann, *Fundamenta Medicinae:* translated and introduced by Lester S. King (copyright 1971 by Lester S. King) used by permission of Lester S. King.

Library of Congress Catalogue Card Number
73-75718

Second printing, 1988.
ISBN 1-55643-035-3

To my wife

INTRODUCTION

This second volume of my history of Western medical philosophy analyzes the dispute in the seventeenth, eighteenth, and nineteenth centuries over the criterion of reliability of medical thought and practice. As was pointed out in Volume I,[a] this controversy polarizes the medical profession into Empirics, who invoke therapeutic observation and experience, and Rationalists, who seek their criterion of reliability in some discipline external to the therapeutic process.

The earlier volume discussed this conflict in ancient Greece and Rome, showing that it extends to every area of medical thought and activity, generating opposite interpretations of the symptom, different therapeutic procedures, and conflicting views of the relationship between theory and practice.

The writings of Galen were the culmination of ancient Rationalism and the vehicle conveying this tradition through the Dark Ages to the Renaissance and early modern period.

The *De Medicina* of Celsus, and some Empirical fragments incorporated in the writings of other authors, did the same for Empiricism. The sixteenth-century heir to this tradition was Theophrastus Paracelsus (1493-1541).

The present volume traces the history of the Galenic and Paracelsan legacies in the seventeenth, eighteenth, and nineteenth centuries.

[a]*Divided Legacy: A History of the Schism in Medical Thought. Volume I. The Patterns Emerge: Hippocrates to Paracelsus* (Washington, D.C.: Wehawken Book Co., 1975).

The differing attitudes of Empiricism and Rationalism to the problem of reliability and certainty in therapeutics reflect their differing physiological assumptions. Empiricism, both ancient and modern, has regarded the human organism as a vital entity subject only to its own laws, while Rationalism has held the organism to be determinate, not spontaneous or autonomous, in its behavior.

The ancient Empirics rejected the possibility of *a priori* or analytical knowledge of the living organism, demanding that medicine be based on *a posteriori* observation and experience. The Rationalists professed the contrary: knowledge of the living organism must be *a priori.* Since the impressions made by phenomena on the senses of the observer are fleeting and evanescent, reliable knowledge requires a coherent analytical structure to which sensory data must be subservient.

Hence ancient Rationalism sought medical certainty in the rules of formal logic.

These differing attitudes toward the organism generated differing interpretations of the symptom. The Empirics saw the organism as continually reacting to morbific stimuli, thus maintaining equilibrium with the environment: the reaction took the form of "coction"—the "cooking" of the morbific cause or principle by the organism, rendering it inoffensive. Symptoms were interpreted as signs of the coction process, of the body's own healing effort, hence beneficial. They indicated to the physician the course he should follow in assisting the organism to heal itself. Rationalism, on the contrary, viewed the symptoms as morbific, reflecting the impact of the morbific cause on the organism's humoral balance.

The Rationalists called this altered humoral balance the "proximate cause" of the disease. They considered it to be the principal object of the physician's attention and developed diagnostic techniques to ascertain its nature. The Empirics followed a different course: rejecting diagnosis as passing beyond the limits of sensory observation, they employed prognosis instead. To the Rationalist stress on the "proximate cause" the Empirics opposed their interpretation of disease as a process, with its stages of buildup, crisis, and resolution. The physician obtained guidance not from diagnosing the "proximate cause" but from predicting these disease stages.

Rationalist therapeutics proceeded on the assumption that cure comes about through "opposition" between disease and remedy, i.e., through "contraries"—an idea originating in Aristotle's "principle of contradiction": "It is impossible for anyone to believe the same thing to be and not to be."[b] The disease "proximate cause" and the curative principle of the remedy were defined in logical language as "hot," "cold," "wet," "dry," or a combination of these. It followed of necessity that a "cold" remedy cured a "hot" disease, a "hot and wet" remedy a "cold and dry" disease, etc. An analytical relationship obtained between the disease and its treatment.

The Empirics rejected this line of reasoning and considered logical categories inappropriate to medicine. Instead, they held each remedy and each disease process to be unique and irreducible. The impact of a medicine on the organism could only be determined *a posteriori,* and its utility in disease could thus be learned only through trial and error—i.e., through experience. The body of pharmacological knowledge did not arise analytically but historically, by gradual accretions, being contained in the records of successful cures.

Furthermore, since they administered remedies to further the process of coction, they viewed them as "similars" (Celsus' *secunda remedia)* and not as "contraries."

The interpretation of the symptom in the two schools diverged in yet another way. Since the Rationalists were concerned with abstractly conceived humoral imbalances, they looked for guidance to the gross and striking symptoms, those which many somewhat similar cases of disease had in

[b]*Metaphysics* 1005b 23.

common. To the Empirics, however, these *communia* were less interesting than the *propria*—the symptoms unique to a given patient which distinguished him from all others with a somewhat similar affliction. Since to them all diseases were variations of the fundamental process of coction, the symptoms *always* present were of little value, and they sought instead the symptoms differentiating one coction process from another.

The division of symptoms into *propria* and *communia* throws a clear light on the distinction between the Empirical and Rationalist thought structures. An abstractly conceived analytical doctrine could not make allowance for the true variety of nature. But the non-reductive and infinitely expandable Empirical doctrine could find in itself unlimited space for the natural variety of diseases and states of health.

This leads to the final conflict between the two traditions: the relative primacy of theory and practice.

The Rationalists in the ancient world assimilated medical theory to formal logic and deduced practice from it *via* the principle of contradiction.

The opposite relationship obtained in Empiricism, all its doctrinal threads converging on the principle that theory is derived from practice.

The organism is a vital reactive entity which is itself the first physician of disease. The organism's therapeutic effort, its "practice," is the process of coction which is at the same time its "theory." The physician's practice can only copy that of the organism, since he can heal only by following and assisting the latter. Hence his own "theory" is only a crystallization of his practice and the "practice" of the organism.

But the "practice" of the organism is its "experience," and the physician's experience thus reflects that of the organism. Hence the primacy of experience as a source of knowledge in Empiricism. This pure and immediate experience was unknown to Rationalism which interposed a web of speculative categories between the physician's senses and the object of investigation.

In the seventeenth, eighteenth, and nineteenth centuries Empirical physicians accepted the principle of the immediacy of therapeutic experience and sought ways to structure it intrinsically—ordering the phenomena without doing them violence. Rationalism sought its rules and principles outside the living body, oscillating back and forth among chemistry, physics, mathematics, and mechanics—finally settling on physiology.

Modes of treatment remained relatively stable in Empiricism, reflecting the stability of its doctrinal basis. In Rationalism they varied according to the new field of knowledge which was temporarily accepted as the criterion of reliability.

The principal defect of ancient Empiricism was the absence of a precise relationship between the medicine and the morbific process which it cured. Paracelsus attempted to rectify this by fusing medicine with chemistry. He held that the organism (microcosm) and its environment (macrocosm) interact, since both are formed of the same minerals; disease arises when the external mineral ignites its twin in the organism, and cure results from administering as medicine the mineral which lies at the root of the disease process. Treatment by "similars" was strengthened by endowing "similarity" with a chemical content.

Paracelsus' attempt, while a rich and stimulating source of ideas, was ultimately a failure, as his writings did not indicate how the disease was to be identified with its mineral root. Jan Baptista Van Helmont (1577-1644) attempted to hold the Paracelsan system together by developing its chemical side but foundered on the same reef as his master—the problem of a precise technique for matching remedies with diseases. Hence the system disintegrated: the mineral remedies became staples of practice but lost their connection with the cosmology.

The Rationalist tradition, severely shaken by Paracelsus' diatribes against formal logic and the four Galenic qualities, was for a while in a quandary while researchers cast about for a new unifying principle. Recovery came through adoption of the enemy's weapons: Paracelsus' salt, sulphur, and mercury were accepted as the elemental components of natural objects but integrated in a way different from that proposed by Paracelsus himself.

The Iatrochemical school, based upon Van Helmont's researches, came into being in the sixteenth and seventeenth centuries led by Franciscus de le Boe Sylvius (1614-1672) and Thomas Willis (1621-1675) who reformulated the Galenic contraries in chemical terms, hypothesizing as the fundamental physiological principle an opposition between "acids" and "alkalis."

The discovery of the circulation by William Harvey (1578-1657) and the development of mechanics and hydraulics by Pierre Gassendi (1592-1655) and Giovanni Borelli (1608-1679) issued in a school of Iatromechanists. The circulation of the blood—which Harvey had posited as autonomous and anterior to the movement of the heart and other organs—was interpreted by this school as a problem of hydraulic engineering.

The infinitesimal calculus of Isaac Newton (1642-1727) and the analytical geometry of Rene Descartes (1596-1650) inspired a school of Iatromathematicians.

And all these various schools drew support from the physiological and anatomical discoveries of this period. The *Fabrica Corporis Humani* of Andreas Vesalius (1514-1564) appeared in 1543, two years after the death of Paracelsus. Presenting the *summum* of all anatomical knowledge together with many new observations, it was the indispensable foundation for further research in this field. Marcello Malpighi (1628-1694) discovered the capillary circulation: by showing how the blood passed from the arteries to the veins he put the coping stone on man's knowledge of the circulation. And this was made possible by the microscope, discovered and improved by Athanasius Kircher (1602-1680), Robert Hooke (1635-1703), Jan Swammerdam (1637-1680), and Anton Van Leeuwenhoek (1632-1723).

Others of importance to anatomy and physiology were Gasparo Aselli (1581-1626), Jean Pecquet (1622-1674), Conrad Peyer (1653-1712), and Olaus Rudbeck (1630-1702) who worked on the intestinal lymphatic system; Nicolaus Steno (1638-1686) who discovered the parotid duct; Thomas Wharton (1614-1673) who discovered the submaxillary; Johann Georg Wirsung (1600-1643) and Regnier de Graaf (1641-1673) who worked on the pancreas; and Rene de Reaumur (1683-1757) who discovered the gastric juice.

Eighteenth-century Rationalism found a new starting-point for speculation in the muscular and neurological investigations of Albert von Haller (1708-1777), Luigi Galvani (1737-1798), and Alessandro Volta (1745-1827).

The list of these various discoveries could be extended indefinitely (as is usually done in histories of medicine), but we relegate them to a secondary position, since they could not determine the form and shape of therapeutic practice. Anatomical, physiological, and chemical knowledge is only the raw material of therapeutics and is employed quite differently by Rationalist and Empirical physicians.

The Rationalists took this information to reveal proximate causes, and they replaced Galen's logical categories with new ones drawn from chemistry and physics. Causal relations within the organism were seen as identical to those presented in the particular science accepted for the time being as a medical guide.

Empirical physicians often ignored this new knowledge and, when accepting it, subordinated it to their sense-based epistemology and vitalistic physiological assumptions.

Another philosophical current in medicine during this period was Methodism.

In the ancient world Methodism represented the introduction into medicine of the atomic hypothesis of Democritus, Epicurus, and Lucretius. It was an offshoot of Rationalism, a tracking down of proximate causes to their ultimate refuge in the atoms of the body. Emerging in the first century B.C., this school interpreted health and disease in terms of the flow of atoms or corpuscles through a porous solid. One class of diseases was caused by an excessive flow and another by blocked or constricted flow, treatment being reduced to nothing more than adjustment of these two irregular forms of flow.

Modern Methodism appeared initially in the *Treatise of Man* (1662) of Descartes. This first textbook of physiology accepted a corpuscular interpretation of the organism identical with that of the ancients, and Descartes' doctrine of blocked or superabundant flow had a powerful impact on Rationalism generally. The corpuscles or atoms were thought to obey the laws of physics and hydraulics, and in this way all vital spontaneity of the organism was abolished.

The Methodist idea that diseases fall normally into only two or three classes emerged a second time in the thought of William Cullen (1712-1790) and John Brown (1735-1788), and a third time in the doctrines of F. J. V. Broussais (1772-1838) and Francois Magendie (1782-1855).

Empiricism in these centuries was drawing inspiration from other sources and following a different course of development.

A major stimulus was the revival of Hippocratic medicine by Byzantine scholars who fled west in 1453 after the fall of Constantinople. They brought to Europe the older Greek manuscripts which threw a quite different light on teachings hitherto preserved mainly in perverted Arabic translations and commentaries. Niccolo Leoniceno (1428-1524), professor of medicine at Padua, Bologna, and Ferrara, translated the *Aphorisms* into Latin. Thomas Linacre (1460-1524), who had studied with Greek scholars in Italy, translated into Latin the *Oath*. Jacques Houllier (1498-1562) and Francois Rabelais (1490-1553) translated the *Aphorisms* and *Coan Prognosis*.[c] Anutius Foesius (1528-1595) issued an edition of the

[c]Rabelais was one of the first to lecture to medical students (at Montpellier) from the Greek text of the *Aphorisms.* He probably used the 1526 edition of Aldus and Asulanus in Venice. The Basel edition of Froben appeared in 1538.

Hippocratic writings which remained standard until the great nineteenth-century compilations of Emile Littre (1801-1881) and F. Z. Ermerins (1808-1871). Louis Duret (1527-1586) and his son produced annotated translations of *Coan Prognosis* and *Regimen in Acute Diseases.*

German mysticism was another intellectual current influencing Empirical medicine. The formalization of theology and its rationalization evoked a reaction among those who sought another path to the discovery of religious truth, one separate and apart from the manipulation of logical categories. Meister Johannes Eckhart (died 1329) and his followers held that knowledge was disclosed through the religious experience of the faithful (exercising a faculty of the soul different from the intellect) and their practical works. The conviction that knowledge could be attained through experience and practice was an important stimulus to Van Helmont and others who contributed to the latter-day emergence of a scientific outlook.

In its search for a new avenue to knowledge mysticism was allied with neo-Platonism, which held the object of investigation to be the "form" beneath the visible surface. Such "forms"—equivalent to the Platonic Ideas and the Aristotelian "formal causes"—also played a major role in the philosophy of Francis Bacon (1561-1626).

Empirical physicians in the seventeenth, eighteenth, and nineteenth centuries espoused different combinations of all of the above themes.

After Van Helmont's failure Empiricism abandoned the chemical side of medicine and concentrated on the theory of vitalism. Prominent here was Georg Ernst Stahl (1660-1734) who ignored the investigation of remedies and worked instead to elaborate the doctrine of the Hippocratic *physis* (vital force) which he called the *Anima sensitiva.* Thomas Sydenham (1624-1689) also accepted a purely Hippocratic medicine. Giorgio Baglivi (1668-1707) combined Hippocratic precepts with the doctrines of Bacon, the teachings of the ancient Empirics, and the Iatromechanism of his Italian contemporaries.

Stahl's *Anima sensitiva* passed to Montpellier in the early eighteenth century where it was elaborated by Francois Boissier de Sauvages (1706-1767), Theophile Bordeu (1722-1776), and Paul-Joseph Barthez (1734-1806). In the nineteenth century, however, this vitalism underwent a Rationalist metamorphosis into the doctrine of "morbid elements."

Montpellier Empiricism was extended to Paris after the 1789 Revolution, replacing the Galenic and Boerhaavian doctrines of the Faculté. This crossing of strains was very fruitful, generating the succession of therapeutic systems known as the Paris School.

Like the Montpellier Empiricism on which it was based, however, Paris Empiricism suffered from the absence of a valid theory of drug action.

This lacuna in Empiricism was filled in the most dramatic fashion by the homoeopathic doctrine of Samuel Hahnemann (1755-1843). Like Stahl, Hahnemann foreswore a chemical explanation of the action of remedies and announced a wholly new technique for elucidating their therapeutic powers—trials or "provings" on the healthy. He held that substances act curatively only by virtue of the capacity to make healthy persons sick and thus provided one more interpretation of the concept of "similarity." Medicines were henceforth to be administered to sick persons manifesting the same symptoms as those which the substance produced when taken by the healthy.

Hahnemann's new interpretation of "similarity" yielded an analytical relationship between the medicine and the disease process and thus filled the gap in Empiricism which had bedeviled the ancient Empirical School, Paracelsus, Van Helmont, Stahl, and the School of Montpellier. Thereafter homoeopathy was a completed system which could be developed along existing lines but not altered in its fundamental principles. It has remained a force in medicine, unchanged in its essentials, down to the present day.

Being a radical criticism of all existing therapeutic modes, homoeopathy was bitterly resisted by the prevailing Rationalism and Methodism—and even by Paris Empiricism—which in time attempted to neutralize it by borrowing its weapons. Just as the Iatrochemists had reacted to Paracelsus, so these nineteenth-century orthodoxies reacted to homoeopathy—adopting many of its medicines while ignoring its doctrinal basis. This is seen most clearly in the system of Armand Trousseau (1801-1867).[d]

While Volume I of this history covered what is usually considered the "pre-scientific" stage of Western medical thought, this second volume treats the figures who are viewed as the founders of "scientific" medicine. Hence a major issue in the following pages is the relationship between these thinkers and a scientific method in medicine.

As we maintained in the earlier volume, however, the distinction between an earlier "pre-scientific" and a later "scientific" period in medicine (wherever the line may be drawn) is incorrect. An essentially scientific approach to therapeutic problems has been present in medicine since the dawn of western civilization and did not emerge suddenly in the seventeenth, eighteenth, nineteenth, or twentieth century. The clash between a scientific and an unscientific therapeutics is identical with that between the Empirical and the Rationalist traditions and is thus perennial. It permeates all of the controversies recorded in the following pages.[e]

[d]This process is discussed in detail in *Divided Legacy: A History of the Schism in Medical Thought. Volume III. Science and Ethics in American Medicine, 1800-1914* (Washington, D.C.: Wehawken Book Co., 1973). See, also, Harris L. Coulter, *Homoeopathic Influences in Nineteenth-Century Allopathic Therapeutics* (Washington, D.C.: American Institute of Homeopathy, 1973).

[e]In medical literature since at least the seventeenth century one finds the recurring theme that medical practice became "scientific" at a time which is seen to be coterminous with the given author's period of medical study. This phenomenon is so pervasive as almost to deserve qualification as a law of medical thought.

It is not the dearth of anatomical, chemical, or even pharmacological knowledge which inhibits the scientific practice of medicine but the inability and unwillingness of physicians to make scientific use of the knowledge which *is* available.

Their inability and unwillingness are compounded and reinforced by the social and professional organization of medicine.[f]

The medicine of the future will not become increasingly "scientific" by amassing a larger body of data, as the problem of ensuring scientific use of these data will remain. Only by overcoming professional constraints on a scientific practice of medicine will true progress in therapeutics be achieved.

This volume concludes with the Methodist reaction to Trousseau's Empiricism. Originating in the thought of F. J. V. Broussais, Francois Magendie, and Rudolf Virchow (1821-1902), this reaction culminated in the reductionist physiology of Claude Bernard (1813-1878) whose conviction that therapeutics rests on an intimate knowledge of proximate causes, interpreted in physiological terms, sets the stage for twentieth-century medicine.

[f]This is discussed comprehensively in *Divided Legacy,* Volume III.

Note: In the following pages the vital force or vital power of the body is designated by the words, *physis* (Greek), *natura* (Latin), *la nature* (French), *la naturaleza* (Spanish), *die Natur* (German), and Nature or "the nature," without any difference in meaning.

PROGRESS AND REGRESS: J. B. VAN HELMONT TO CLAUDE BERNARD

TABLE OF CONTENTS

But it is particularly necessary, in my opinion, for one who discusses this art to discuss things familiar to ordinary folk. For the subject of inquiry and discussion is simply and solely the sufferings of these same ordinary folk when they are sick or in pain.

Ancient Medicine

CHAPTER I

THE ROOTS OF MODERN EMPIRICISM: ECKHART, PARACELSUS, VAN HELMONT, BACON

When Paracelsus created modern medicine by proposing a substitute for the Galenism of the schools, he sought inspiration in the Hippocratic Corpus and probably in Celsus. But he was also influenced by a mighty current in the theological and popular thought of his times—the fusion of mysticism and neo-Platonism.

This current was important for medical Empiricism, and thus for the scientific outlook, in urging the possibility and necessity of a new path to knowledge. Its impact was especially strong on Jan Baptista Van Helmont (1578-1644), one of the most powerful intellects in the history of medicine, who sought to give form and dimension to the cosmological insights of Paracelsus.

Francis Bacon (1561-1626), however different in other respects from his contemporary, was equally desirous of establishing an alternative path to knowledge of nature. He also turned to neo-Platonism, specifically to the doctrine of "forms," for a principal component of his philosophy of investigation.

Mysticism and Neo-Platonism

By prescribing the intellectual forms in which religious feelings may be expressed, churches bring these feelings under organized control. But this mapping and grading of religious experience provokes the emergence of more spontaneous modes of worship and belief outside sanctioned channels. Medieval mysticism was such an irregular mode of religious observance, representing the will of the pious to find a way back to God—"not to the Church's God, hidden under a thousand outward ceremonies and obscured by a mass of intricate syllogisms, but to the deep pure serene source itself from which all life flows."[a]

Mysticism thus arose in opposition to formal church doctrines. In the thirteenth century, after the ultimate rationalization of the content of Christian belief by the Dominican monk, St. Thomas Aquinas (1225-1274), it enveloped wide areas of public opinion. It was preached, in particular, by Meister Johannes Eckhart (d. 1329), also of the Dominican order, who reacted to the formalization and increasing remoteness of Christian doctrine by attempting to democratize the form and content of belief, to make it accessible to all.

Eckhart preached "sermons to the common people" which urged the virtuous life as a way to attain knowledge of God. Since priestly and episcopal authority was based on the knowledge possessed by priests and bishops, "knowledge" had to be reinterpreted in such a way as to undermine this authority. Hence Eckhart equated "knowledge" with the moral and spiritual development attainable by everyone, with or without book-learning. The simple man is capable of "inner experience of the truth." The believing Christian leading a life in the imitation of Christ is, in the sight of God, equal to the Pope. His *experience* is more significant than any formal knowledge, vow, or ritual: "If [anyone] find that his vow hinders him and that if he were loosed from it, he could draw nearer to God, let him boldly quit his vow . . . To take a vow with the good intention of binding oneself to God is the best one can do at any time. If, however, a man knows a

[a]Egon Friedell, *A Cultural History of the Modern Age* (New York: Knopf, 1953), I, 136.

better way, one that experience has taught him is better, then the first way is at once superseded."[1] [b]

Mysticism in the German lands was thus an early form of Protestantism. To the nationalist urge of Germanic Europe to lessen the authority of Rome was added a democratic belief in the equality of the virtuous and the conviction that experiencing the virtuous life generates the necessary knowledge of God.

The Spiritualization of Knowledge

Since rational knowledge was a Church monopoly, the knowledge generated by the life of virtue was spiritual—just as God, the object of this knowledge, was spiritual.

The division of knowledge into rational and spiritual presupposed the existence of two separate faculties in the mind or soul, and belief in the duality or dichotomy of the intellectual faculty is a hallmark of all mystical and neo-Platonic thought. The founders of neo-Platonism, in the third century A.D., divided the soul *(anima, psyche)* into a physiological part (governing the physical functions) and a psychological or spiritual part concerned with the higher intellect and also representing the divine essence which survives after death.[2] [c] This latter part is not bound to matter and not dependent on the senses for its information; partaking of divinity, it cognizes the world by its reception of Ideas or "forms" which are simultaneously the thoughts of God and the modes of His actualization in nature.

Hugo and Richard of St. Victor (died 1141 and 1173), early German mystics, held that man has three eyes: the eye of the flesh to know the corporeal world, the eye of reason

[b]Eckhart was accused by the authorities of advocating doctrines "which might easily lead his listeners into error" and condemned posthumously for "sowing thorns and thistles amongst the faithful and even the simple folk," deceived by the "father of lies, who often appears as an angel of light" (R. B. Blakney, *Meister Eckhart: A Modern Translation* [New York: Harper, 1941], xxiii-xxiv).

[c]The Empirical physician, Menodotos of Nicomedea, who lived in the first century A.D., rejected "the naming which is by man and demand[ed] that things be known according to the soul" *(Divided Legacy,* I, 271).

to know his own inner nature, and the eye of contemplation to cognize the spiritual world and the Deity. This contemplation is a *visio intellectualis*—more than the mere exercise of reason.[3] Eckhart himself allowed the soul two eyes: "one looking inwards and the other outwards. It is the inner eye of the soul that looks into essence and takes being directly from God. That is its true function. The soul's outward eye is directed toward creatures and perceives their external forms [*Bilder*]."[4] The soul's "outer eye" sees by the "light of nature" (a term introduced by Albertus Magnus [1193-1280]), employing as its agents the five senses and manipulating the forms in the intellect.[5] But the "inner eye" is far more important: through it the soul sees God, not by the "light of nature" but by the "divine light."[6] Eckhart calls this the "spark"; it is eternal and uncreated, coexistent with God and thus capable of knowing Him.[7] [d]

The knowledge of God is beyond perception, beyond ideas, beyond phenomenal nature.[8] It demands the abandonment of particularity, multiplicity, and plurality. It demands rejection of false pride of knowledge (the *docta ignorantia* of Nicolas Cusanus [1401-1464]). It demands a pure heart and withdrawal of the soul from the world into itself (*Abgescheidenheit*). The soul knows God through community of life and being with that which is known.[9]

The World as Spirit

Implicit in the spiritualization of knowledge was spiritualization of the object of knowledge. The mystics and neo-Platonists proceeded from the spirituality of God to that of the created world. "For neo-Platonism the whole of nature is regarded as real only insofar as it is soul."[10] The more it possesses of divinity, the more real it is.

Here we see one of the most peculiar shifts in the history of thought—that Plato, the founder of Idealist philosophy, should have stood as a guide to nature against Aristotle who,

[d] Here he came closest to heresy, holding that part of the soul is not created by God at all.

of all ancient thinkers, was the most concerned with natural science. But as Aristotelianism became frozen into the categories of scholasticism, Plato's *Timaeus,* with its theory of the creation and emergence of the world of nature, was taken as a handbook and guide to scientific investigation.

The *Timaeus* had presented nature as a living unity: "we may say that the world became a living creature truly endowed with soul and intelligence by the providence of God."[11] This vital universe was created in imitation of an eternal pattern "which is apprehended by reason and mind and is unchangeable."[12] And this pattern, in turn, is composed of Ideas—"self-existent Ideas, unperceived by sense and apprehended only by the mind."[13]

The visible created world is only an imperfect copy of this primal pattern of Ideas, but an understanding of the Ideas yields some knowledge of it. While sense-perception has a role here, knowledge is mainly a process of recollection whereby the soul, as it were, bethinks itself of the Ideas—creating them anew out of its remembrance from former ages.

Neo-Platonism abandoned Plato's dualism of Ideas and matter in favor of a monistic view in which the whole created universe consisted of soul or life and was the emanation of God. Plato's Ideas became original thoughts of God. At the same time, however, they were spiritualized as agents or extensions of the human mind adapted to apperception of the external world.

Thus the Ideas were the point of contact and common denominator of the human mind and the mind of God.

Attempting to explain how God acts on nature, Philo of Alexandria in the first century A.D. identified the Ideas with the thoughts of God. This enabled him to fill the gulf between God and the world with a succession of intermediate stages which he called the *logos* of God: descending from unity to plurality, from unchangeability to changeability, from immaterial to material, from spiritual to sensuous, from perfect to imperfect, from good to evil, etc.

The human mind moves in the opposite direction, ascending from the imperfect and pluralistic world of the senses and sense-perception to the understanding of God.

Plotinus (204-269 A.D.), the true founder of neo-Platonism, presented these same concepts in an analogy with light shining forth from God. Whatever is close to the source of light is illuminated brightly, but further away the light becomes weaker and is finally converted into its opposite—darkness, evil, depravity.

The Western mind was preoccupied with neo-Platonism for a thousand years. This matrix of problems concerning the relations among the forms, between form and matter, between form and God, between form and man's perception of it, etc. was capable of unlimited development along a variety of different lines. The Arabs in Spain made matter metaphysically self-subsistent, thus equivalent to God, and generating the forms contained within it at all times as seeds. Duns Scotus (810-880) held that both form and the individual object possess reality. William of Occam (1300-1349) overcame this paradox by rejecting the form as a necessary intermediate between the object and man's concept of it *(entia non sunt multiplicanda praeter necessitatem).* Objects are presented in the mind intuitively. Since we are also capable of formulating ideas about objects, Occam distinguished between "real" and "rational" knowledge, the "real" being knowledge of the relations among objects and the "rational" being our ideas of these relations. Nicolas Cusanus held that objects are presented to the mind by means of signs but that such knowledge is only conjectural—reflecting the nature of the mind and not the nature of reality. The object itself is metaphysically separate.

Eckhart holds that nature is permeated by God. He transforms Plotinus' simile of light into one of water flowing from a spring: the more distant from the spring, the more polluted the water. But even though polluted, it still contains attributes of divinity: "If God were not in everything, nature would not function, nor would desire be in anything . . . secretly all nature seeks God and works toward Him."[14]

"Here is the unity of blades of grass and bits of wood and stone, together with everything else . . . all that nature tries to do is to plunge on into that unity, into the Father-nature, so that it all may be one . . . Nature, coming from God, does not seek its externals [as ends]. Indeed, nature itself, the *Ding an sich,* has nothing to do with its adornments but rather aims at nothing short of the likeness of God."[15]

Hence God is to be seen in every production of nature, although this knowledge is inferior to that of the divinity itself: "If the soul knows God in creatures, night falls. If it sees how they have their being in God, morning breaks. But if it sees that Being that is in God himself alone, it is high noon . . ."[16] The same spiritual procedure must be followed to learn about nature as to learn about God: abandonment of particularity, multiplicity, and plurality until one penetrates beneath the surface to the divine essence. "If you want to discover nature's nakedness, you must destroy its symbolism, and the farther you get in, the nearer you come to its essence."[17]

The soul apprehends the objects of nature as follows:

> When the agents of the soul contact creatures, they take and make ideas [*Bilder*] and likenesses of them and bear them back again into the self. It is by means of these ideas that the soul knows about external creatures. Creatures cannot approach the soul except in this way, and the soul cannot get at creatures except, on its own initiative, it first conceive ideas of them. Thus the soul gets at things by means of ideas, and the idea is an entity created by the soul's agents. Be it a stone or a rose or a person or whatever it is that is to be known, first an idea is taken and then absorbed, and in this way the soul connects with the phenomenal world.
>
> But an idea so received necessarily comes in from the outside, through the senses.[18]

Running through mystical and neo-Platonic thought is thus the conviction that the objects of nature are apprehended through the forms or Ideas which are, in turn, associated with man's spiritual, not his rational, dimension.[e] The relations among natural objects differ from the relations among the concepts manipulated by man's rational faculty.

After the founding of the School of Chartres in the twelfth century, whose purpose was to direct neo-Platonism to the investigation of nature, this residue was a natural stimulus to the scientific spirit. To scholasticism was left the task of working out the relationships among concepts: neo-Platonism took on itself that of determining the relations among the objects themselves.

A final aspect of mysticism and neo-Platonism which binds them to the scientific mentality is their utilitarian orientation. They found themselves allied with empirical research and practice in their mutual antagonism to logic and dialectic.[19] Windelband contrasts scholasticism, whose task was to construct a unified church doctrine, with neo-Platonism and mysticism which took the practical "direction of guiding the individual, through knowledge, to blessed oneness of life with the deity."[20]

Eckhart, to be sure, held that the most virtuous life was one of contemplation, good works being suitable only for those who are too weak for this higher pursuit. The later mystics, however, Johann Tauler (1300-1361) and his contemporary, Gerhardt Groot, stressed more the practical side of Christianity. The latter founded the Brethren of the Common Life whose aim was to encourage mystical devotion to Christ and charity toward one's fellow humans; the most famous member of this order was Thomas a Kempis (1380-1471) whose *Imitation of Christ* is the greatest and best-known guide to practical Christianity.

[e]Many of the neo-Platonist departures in thought were, of course, inherently confused, blurring real distinctions and perverting analysis. Thus Windelband: "in place of regular causal connections appears the mysterious, dreamily unconscious weaving of the world-soul, the rule of gods and demons, the spiritual sympathy of all things expressing itself in strange relations among them. All forms of divination, astrology, faith in miracles, naturally stream into this mode of regarding Nature, and man seems to be surrounded by nothing but higher and mysterious forces: this world created by spirits, full of souls, embraces him like a *magic* circle" *(History of Philosophy,* I, 249).

The Legacy of Paracelsus

Theophrastus Paracelsus had been the first to bring to medicine the insights of mysticism and neo-Platonism.[f] Within the framework of a vast analysis of the inner and outer worlds—the microcosm and the macrocosm—anatomy, pharmacology, and therapy found a starting-point and a resting place in a general theory of cure through similars. But this all-inclusiveness was achieved at the expense of the details: how precisely to diagnose diseases, and how precisely to ascertain the curative powers of medicines, were left in suspense. The exact application of the principle of similars in the day-to-day practice of medicine was unclear even to his immediate followers, and a division soon appeared in Paracelsan doctrine between the "theory" (his cosmology) and the "practice" (his mineral remedies).

The medicines he had popularized passed rapidly into general use, "begged from fugitive servants" by the Galenists (according to Van Helmont).[21] [g] Boerhaave writes that the Paracelsans "gained so much authority in a few years that the princes of Germany would hardly admit any to be their physicians who were not chemists."[22]

Thus the leading Paracelsans rose to high positions in society. Theodore Turquet de Mayerne (1573-1655), for example, was appointed physician-in-ordinary to James I of England at the unimaginable salary of 400 pounds per annum

[f]See *Divided Legacy,* I, 339-507.

[g]But over the furious opposition of the school authorities who invoked the secular arm whenever possible. At their urging the Paris Parlement in 1566 banned the use of antimony, and in 1582 the Senate of Augsburg decreed that dangerous substances such as *"labdanum minerale,* called antimony, *terpetum minerale,* and other mercurial purgative medicines" should be employed only under the supervision of a physician—not by the Paracelsan *"empirici"* or *"chymici"* (Robert Multhauf, "Medical Chemistry and 'the Paracelsans,'" *Bulletin of the History of Medicine* XXVIII [1954], 101-126, at 119).

The acceptance of Paracelsan medicines by the schools is discussed also in Allen G. Debus, "Guintherius, Libavius, and Sennert: the Chemical Compromise in Early Modern Medicine" *(Science, Medicine, and Society in the Renaissance: Essays to Honor Walter Pagel* [New York: Science History Publications, 1972], I, 151-165).

together with 200 pounds more for his wife; he was also exempted from taxation and in 1624 was knighted.[h]

Chemical practice took on a life of its own, the medicines being applied to diseases in ways which could not be justified in Paracelsan terms. Gerhard Dorn (sixteenth century), Petrus Severinus (1540-1602), Joseph du Chesne (1520-1609), Oswald Croll (1560-1609), Johann Hartmann (1568-1631), David de Planis-Campy (born 1589) and Turquet de Mayerne himself, were unable to put together the two halves of the master's doctrine: "It appears that although these Paracelsans adhered to both medical chemistry and to Paracelsus' theories of medicine and chemistry, they kept the two remarkably distinct . . . the *magna opera* of Dorn and Croll are sharply divided into two sections on theory and practice, so little related that they have the aspect of separate books. Severinus' book on Paracelsus' theoretical medicine contains no remedies, and the pharmacopoeias of Du Chesne, Hartmann, and Mayerne contain practically no theory. Planis-Campy prefaces his pharmacopoeia with a number of disconnected observations, etc."[23]

The theory of the microcosm and the macrocosm was too vague in its details to support the growing burden of practice, and as Paracelsan remedies became popular, the Paracelsan ideas fell into abeyance. He himself had been able to contain the contradictions of his cosmology and to find (perhaps *ad hoc*) solutions to pressing problems of practice, but these contradictions came immediately to the fore once his doctrines became the property of a group.

[h]The Paris Faculté in 1603, led by Jean Riolan (1538-1606) whose life work it was to contest and criticize the Paracelsan remedies, placed Turquet de Mayerne formally under the ban: "All physicians, too, who practice medicine anywhere, are admonished to banish from themselves and their households the said Turquet and all similar monsters of mankind and monstrosities of opinion and to remain true to Galen." In 1609 this decree was invoked against a certain Besnier who was deprived of all rights of professional intercourse and only received back into the bosom of the Faculté after swearing to use antimony no longer. The interdiction was removed in 1666 when the Faculté voted for chemical remedies over Galenic by a majority of 92 (J. H. Baas, *Outlines of the History of Medicine and the Medical Profession* [New York: Vail, 1889], 396, 496). The Besnier incident inspired one of Moliere's most famous scenes (see *Divided Legacy,* I, 333).

Jan Baptista Van Helmont

The final attempt to restore the unity of Paracelsan theory and practice was made by Jan Baptista Van Helmont who developed the chemical side of the system and attempted to fuse it with Paracelsus' vitalism.

Van Helmont is second only to Paracelsus himself in the depth, subtlety, and complexity of his therapeutic philosophy. And his assumptions, like those of the Swiss reformer, are Empirical: acceptance of the theory of coction, a vitalist physiology, the rejection of "proximate causes," and adherence to sense-perception as the only reliable source of medical knowledge. To this he added the Paracelsan emendations of Empiricism: the doctrine of Christian love combined with a general chemical interpretation of physiology.

He is thus a striking example of how the tenets of Empiricism perpetuate themselves and reappear in new historical periods.

Biographical

Van Helmont was born in 1578 to a noble Flemish family of Brussels. He displayed remarkable intellectual capacities from an early age and studied philosophy, logic, astrology, and mathematics with such diligence as to be offered the university degree at age seventeen.[24] But he had already resolved that no truth was to be found in these disciplines and declined the honor: "being unwilling that professors should play the fool with me, that they should declare me master of the seven arts who was not yet a scholar."[25]

He then went to study with the Jesuits, attending lectures in natural magic by the Spaniard, Martin del Rio (1551-1608). He studied the mystics, Johann Tauler and Thomas a Kempis.[26] He even took up law. But ultimately he settled on medicine, finding that he admired Hippocrates as much as he disliked Galen and the Arabs.

He obtained the medical degree in 1599 at Louvain and for a while lectured in surgery. But he was still haunted by feelings of inadequacy and lack of confidence in what he had learned. "In the multitude of books there was nowhere comfort or knowledge; but vain promises, abuses, and very many errors."[27] "Physicians are made the comedy of stages because they have scarce done anything worthy of thanks."[28] "I had known indeed . . . to dispute of any disease, but I knew not how to cure the very pain of the teeth."[29] School medicine has "brought no light into the art of healing."[30]

The dominant traits of Van Helmont's character and intellect were already manifest. The love of learning: "I even from my tender bones or years, have esteemed knowledge before riches."[31] And a powerful current of sympathy and obligation toward his fellow-humans, which he intellectualized and fused with the former after the fashion of the mystics: "Most of the moderns suppose the end of wisdom to be the knowing of one's self. I call the ultimate end of wisdom, and the reward of the whole course of life, charity or dear love, which accompanieth us after other things have forsaken us."[32]

Hence he disapproved of his colleagues who practiced medicine purely for money: "a cruel thing to heap up money by others' miseries . . . an unseemly thing to translate an art founded in charity and bestowed under the condition of exercising mercy, into gain."[33] [i]

He looked into herbal medicine but found this knowledge also unreliable: "for although there be no field more spacious, plentiful, and delightful in the face of the whole

[i] Owsei Temkin writes that the covetousness of physicians was a favorite theme of popular culture at this time: *Dat Galenus opes, dat Justinianus honores* (Galen gives riches, Justinian gives honors). Jacopus Sylvius (1478-1555) was so avaricious that the following epitaph sprang up after his death (translated by Lilian Temkin):

> Here lies Sylvius, who never alive
> From *gratis* giving could pleasure derive.
> Now that he's dead and worms on him feed,
> He's still vexed that for free these lines you may read.

(*Galenism: Rise and Decline of a Medical Philosophy* [Ithaca and London: Cornell University Press, 1973], 131).

earth, and where the mind is more delighted than in herbarism, yet there hath scarce been a less progress made in any other thing. For truly the Arabians, Greeks, or Gentiles, barbarians, wild country people, and Indians have observed their own simples more diligently than all the Europeans. For even from the days of Plato (wherein Dioscorides, a man of war, lived) nothing almost hath been added to herbarism, but much diminished."[34]

From 1600 to 1602 he traveled in Switzerland and Italy. Returning to Brussels he had an experience which finally made clear to him the gap between medical theory and its practice. After a social visit to "a certain gentlewoman," and, on parting, holding "her hand and glove for some little while," he contracted the itch (scabies) and thereupon called in "two of the more famous physicians of our city, almost rejoicing that I might now understand in myself whether their studies might answer to their practice":

> But the physicians, having seen the mattery scab, presently judged that a dust or burnt choler did abound in me, together with salt phlegm, and so that the faculty of making blood in the liver was distempered. I rejoiced presently because those things which authors had sung unto me were confirmed by most expert masters, because I who had learned that in science mathematical all speculations were most exceeding true, did believe that thing to be likewise common and unseparable to the rules or maxims of healing . . . And presently, according to my ancient credulity, I asked what that distemper of the liver should be, which at one and the same act should enflame yellow choler more unjustly than was meet, and also engender more phlegm than was meet, seeing an act of the same root, or of the same sanguinification, could not be at the same time, and in the same bowel, a two-forked or double generation, and so unlike, to wit, that which should abundantly send forth a fiery choler, and also a cold and watery phlegm. The most expert masters doubted, and being amazed with their eyebrows bent,

they long beheld themselves, and at length the junior of them answered that the same distemper of an inflamed liver did not therefore afford true phlegm, but an abounding salt phlegm, but that the temperature of salt was hot and dry . . . [the physicians prescribed purgatives] . . . on the sixth day I had at least fifteen stools; in the meantime they praised my providence, whereby I had made or prepared my body so fluid. Presently after two days from thence, because the scab had not laid aside any of its cruelty, I took the same medicine, with a notable loathing of my stomach, and the like stools succeeded. They said that the flourishing age of eighteen years was apt for the breeding of choler. And when they saw that for all that the itching and wheals were nothing diminished, they decreed that two days after I should take the purging medicine the third time. But then a little before evening, my veins were now exhausted, my cheeks had fallen, my voice was hoarse, the whole habit of my body going to ruin, had waxed lean; also it was difficult for me to descend from my chamber and to go, because my knees did scarce support me . . . But I considered too late that before the purging medicines I was well in health in my bowels; but now that through a dejected appetite and digestion, I had contracted much leanness, but that the scabbedness remained safe or firm . . .[35]

He now left Brussels for the second time. After taking a vow of poverty and conveying all his property to his sister, he travelled to Spain, France, and England to find medical wisdom and understanding.[36]

He continued to study the mystics and concluded (like Paracelsus) that the ancient medical doctrines had to be reformed on Christian lines: "I long considered with myself that the art of healing was a mere juggle, brought in by the Greeks; till at length the Holy Scriptures better instructed me."[37] He also looked into alchemy, meeting a spagyric who knew "the art of the fire."[38] "And I myself, being fraught with hope, persuaded myself that by the mere free gift of

God I should at some time obtain the science of the adeptist."[39]

On the way home in 1605 he encountered an epidemic of malignant fever which he combated as best he could, saving many lives and becoming reinforced in his contempt for the standard medical practices:

> I considered that the plague was a most miserable disease in which everyone forsook the sick, and unfaithful helpers, distrusting their own art, more swiftly fled than the unlearned common people and the homely curers of the plague. Therefore I proposed to myself to dedicate one salutation to the miserable infected. Although then no medicine was made known to me but trivial ones, yet God preserved my innocence from so cruel an enemy. For though I was not sent for, I went of my own accord to see them, not so much to help them, as being desirous to learn. Yet all that saw me seemed to be refreshed with hope and joy.[40]

In 1609 he married an heiress who bore him a number of children, among them Franciscus Mercurius Van Helmont (1618-1699), a medical philosopher in his own right and the editor of his father's posthumous works. The family settled in the town of Vilvorde, withdrawing from the world just as Eckhart had urged the Christian to withdraw into his own soul: "that being the less troubled I might proceed diligently to view the kingdoms of vegetables, animals, and minerals by a curious analysis or unfolding, by opening bodies and separating all things. I went about the search for full seven years. I searched into the books of Paracelsus, filled in all parts with a mocking obscurity or difficulty, and I admired that man, and too much honored him, till at length understanding was given of his works and errors."[41] "An earnest desire of knowing and operating daily increased in me. For not much above two years later I had gotten such household stuff to myself whereby I was, though absent, in great esteem among the sick . . . Wherefore I presently resigned up all books, and I perceived myself more to profit by the fire, in conceptions attained by praying, than in any kind of books, which sing always the same cuckoo's note."[42]

Charity and devotion to learning remained his guides. He refused offers from many of the courts of Europe and stayed in Vilvorde, dividing his time between his chemical laboratory and an extensive free practice among the poor: "I willingly cured the poor and those of mean fortune . . . being stirred up by human compassion."[43]

For such a retiring scholar his declining years were eventful. His alchemical leanings and criticism of the medical profession had aroused hostility. He was "an apostate from Galen; I exposed myself willingly unto the vile esteem of physicians . . . by haters I am called a Paracelsian and a forsaker of the schools."[44] A treatise which explained animal magnetism in natural terms rather than divine, published without his consent in 1621, was seized upon by his enemies as evidence of heresy and taken to the Inquisition. Thereafter Van Helmont was prosecuted by this body, although slowly and reluctantly.[j] His writings were condemned in 1625, and he himself was arrested in 1634 and confined to house arrest for two years. He continued to write and practice after his release, dying in 1644.[k]

Perception and Understanding

The philosophical and medical views which Van Helmont acquired during his education were shaken by his initial attempts at healing. He turned away from Aristotelian orthodoxy to Empiricism and mysticism, fusing the Empiri-

[j]The Inquisition was not very zealous in the matter and moved only at the incessant urging of Van Helmont's (presumably medical) enemies (Willem Rommelaere, *Etudes sur J. B. Van Helmont* [Bruxelles: Manceaux, 1868], 38). However, the works of Franciscus Mercurius Van Helmont are still on the *Index Librorum Prohibitorum.*

[k]Guy Patin (1601-1672), dean of the Paris Faculté, wrote in 1645: "Van Helmont was a nasty Flemish rascal who died some months ago. He never accomplished anything worthwhile. I have seen everything he wrote: he dreamed only of a medicine made up entirely of chemical and empirical secrets. And to turn things upside down more quickly, he strongly opposed bloodletting—as a result of which he died frenetic" (quoted in Paul Neve de Mevergnies, *Jean-Paptiste Van Helmont: Philosophe par le Feu* [Liege: E. Droz, 1935], 3).

cal postulate that knowledge is from observation and experience, with mystical, neo-Platonic, and Paracelsan doctrines.

Thus he rejects scholastic logic as a path to truth: "logic is unprofitable," "syllogisms do not bring forth knowledge,"[45] "the knowledge which we have by demonstration was already before in us and only is made a little more distinct by a syllogism."[46]

He accepts the Paracelsan view that reason and logic are pagan and must be superseded by the new Christian dispensation. "Reason doth on every side bring forth only a thinking instead of faith; but faith is of grace, not of thee, subtle reason, who doth delude and miserably lead astray the most witty or quick-sighted man, that trust in thee, unto a hell of miseries."[47] Reason and logic are taught through the agency of the devil and lead only to the "heathenish theorems" which block medical progress.[48] Just as logic has led to discord within Christianity itself: "for thy flexible juggling deceit hath brought forward a hundred sections or divisions and clefts in faith, even in the more refined men. But every section hath its rational induction, or bringing in of sophistry."[49]

Logic does not yield knowledge of nature. "Let the schools know that the rules of mathematics, or learning by demonstration, do ill square to nature, for man does not measure nature, but she him."[50] "Truly reason is by no means a cause, part, or essence of the thing caused, much less doth the rational faculty in man reach unto things. For a thing is that in itself which it is, without the reflection on it of any discourse and invention of human reason."[51]

Thus Van Helmont accepted the mystical and neo-Platonic dichotomy between the relationships obtaining in nature and the ideas or concepts manipulated by man's rational faculty. The former he calls the "premises," and they are not known through reason which "more wearieth the addicted or readily following soul . . . and covers the skull with dog's hairs, than it is able to produce within us a true knowledge of the truth."[52] Instead, they are known through the "intellectual light," the "understanding": "the discourse of reason doth extenuate or lessen, overshadow, hinder, and cloak that noble act of the understanding whereby the knowledges of the premises are implanted in us."[53] "The knowledges of the truth of things and premises do proceed, not indeed from reason, but from a far different beginning, to wit, the intellectual light of the lamp or candle."[54][l]

Reason, the pagan inheritance, must be overcome by the Christian dispensation of "understanding," just as the Christian religion prevailed over the idols of Greece and Rome.[m]

Van Helmont's doctrine of "understanding" is basic to his philosophy, as it is to the emergence of the modern scientific mentality. Since this area of the history of thought is confused, and, in particular, since Van Helmont's theory of perception is still regarded by some as relying on the "magical" power possessed by the select or elect person to penetrate to the heart of things, it must be examined in detail.

The "magical" interpretation of Van Helmont's theory of perception seems at first plausible in the light of his own statements, e.g., "the things themselves seem to talk to us without words, and the understanding pierceth them being shut up, no otherwise than as if they were dissected and laid open."[55] But he refers here only to the *outcome* of a complex process; it is the ultimate result of a laborious method.

For the ability to see into the heart of things directly was possessed by Adam alone: he was able to give names to things because he knew their "innermost properties."[56] *After the Fall, this power was lost.* Once God had introduced the soul between the mind and the body, "Adam afterwards lived in the soul and middle life, that is, after a modern or mean manner; and his mind (for the support of the sensitive soul)

[l]Cf. with Eckhart's "spark" and Plotinus' "light" simile (above, pp. 6 and 8).

[m]Paracelsus also distinguished the pagan sensual "reason" from the Christian "soul" (*Divided Legacy,* I, 402).

dispersed from itself only a darksome light through the mists of the flesh upon the life of a new and impure generation."[57]

Modern man learns only through observation and experience, but "experience" also encompasses the life of Christian virtue. When these preconditions have been met, God *may* vouchsafe to man the knowledge which he desires.

Van Helmont epitomizes his rejection of occult (magical) perception by a dream in which he stands in a palace where a spirit hands him a bottle containing medicine. The bottle symbolizes the inaccessibility of medicine to direct perception and the need to ascertain the properties of medicines through experience. He "endeavored diversely to experience [*experiri*] what the bottle might contain,"[58] and after a long discussion of various medicines whose properties are revealed through experience, i.e., through observation of their effects, he concludes: "These things I have spoken concerning occult or hidden properties out of a dream, that we may *cease to be occult philosophers* and may follow the manifest doctrine of the more tractable ones" [*ut occulti philosophi esse desinamus, et manifestam doctrinam mitiorum sequamur*].[59]

Thus man learns not through magic but through his senses: "I am not wont to call to me any other judge concerning contingent things known by sense, besides touching. For I am so stupid that I stand to nought but the judgment of the senses concerning sensible objects."[60] It is the school physicians who pretend otherwise, who "privily escape into lurking places that they may defend those things which are perceived by Galen."[61]

The conquest of knowledge by sense-perception is through experience, meaning working, suffering, searching, and struggling for it. "A crown presupposes a striving merit and a victory; for we cannot bring back an increase of grace for victory but by fighting."[62] "The means of obtaining sciences are only to pray, seek, and knock."[63] "All its clearness, nobleness, fullness, light, and truth do come to [the understanding] by receiving and suffering . . . it is so much the more ennobled by how much the more it suffers by the light which is beyond all nature."[64] "Ye that will give a wished peace to your studies and to the complaints of the sick, seek and ye shall find."[65] "For the awakening of [the schools] I wish God might take His honor and mortals the benefit [*usumfructum*] which I wish from my labors."[66]

But all of this striving is pointless unless the striver possesses faith in God and moral virtue: "The first thing, therefore, is in the simplicity of an operative faith [*fides operativa*] to have lived in abstinency from evils and to have done good. And then, that they worship God in the spirit of naked truth and that through an operative faith they proceed through an attainment of fatherly love, worthy deed, or merit in charity . . . helping to be more and more illustrated in their understanding."[67] He must admit his inability to acquire knowledge through his own efforts alone, that his "understanding is vain, empty, poor, and dark."[68] He must beg God "that He may vouchsafe to open the eyes of the mind, who to Adam and to Solomon demonstrated the properties of things at the first sight."[69]

> Good God, the comforter of the poor in spirit, who are nearer to none than to him who with a full freedom resigns up himself and his endowments into Thy most pleasing will, and seeing Thou enlightenest none more bountifully . . . than him who acknowledges the lowliness of his own nothingness . . . Grant thou, O Thou profound master of sciences, that I may rather be poor in spirit than great with child or swollen through knowledge. Grant me freely an understanding that may purely seek Thee and a will that may purely adhere unto thee. Enlighten Thou my nothing-darkness as much as Thou wilt.[70]

Then God may accord the researcher that knowledge which he desires: "A man did watch and build in vain unless the Lord did cooperate."[71] "I conclude that as we are constituted in the middle and sensitive life, we know, have, are, or are able to do nothing but only by grace, merit [*meritum*] cooperating, and it is to be supposed that the degrees of this merit in the adoring understanding are confirmed by God."[72] "For as we Christians are constrained to believe that our intellect or understanding is an immortal spirit, light, and image of the almighty whose beginning, as it exceeds nature, so it cannot be fitted or squared to its rules . . . without particular or special grace it cannot understand anything, because the object of understanding is truth itself."[73]

Understanding, when accorded by God, is of the essence of things: "the truth of essence and the truth of understanding are one and the same thing."[74] It is quite different from the knowledge given by the reason which is a "certain crooked manner of understanding, proceeding by reasons and discourses . . . therefore that rational manner is an abusive and deceitful understanding."[75] "Truth is a real true being, but reason is a mental, problematical, or intricate being, only appearing."[76] "The understanding knows things as they are; and therefore likewise the understanding is made true concerning the things themselves by the things themselves; forasmuch as the being of things from themselves is always true, and their essence is truth itself."[77]

Van Helmont accepts the basic postulate of the mystics and Paracelsus—that charity or Christian love is the absolute precondition of understanding:

> And although He hath not restored unto us the ancient clearness of [Adam's] understanding, and exquisite speculative knowledge of the mind, yet He hath raised up our dignity far higher. For truly the understanding being reduced by grace unto the obedience of faith proceedeth in a humble resignation unto the victorious reward of love whereby we are supported and constrained. And the least abiding of that love is far more glorious than the whole unoccupied life of Adam in Paradise.[78]

Hence the Galenists, who heal only for financial reward, *cannot attain true knowledge:* "seek and ye shall find, so that medicine be not for gain. For if your intention be mercy, from charity—truth and light descending from the Father of Lights shall meet you in the journey."[79]

And when God does vouchsafe knowledge to man, He does so in the way prescribed by Plato and Meister Eckhart: man finds the truth in his own soul, or, alternatively, remembers that which was in his mind before the Fall. "Our soul, understanding itself, doth after a sort understand all other things, because all other things are in an intellectual manner in the soul, as in the image of God."[80] "And so, at length, the mind is loosed in that dark prison of bloods and intellectually beholds itself, and with humility admires the not before seen light."[81] When Adam and Eve started to propagate like animals, "all his knowledge, as well former as latter, of Good and Evil, to wit, the remembrance of the same, were obliterated, and man thereby was born a vain or empty table."[82] And yet "the former knowledges which he had before the Fall were in the sensitive life laid up through remembrance: yet overclouded with the dim and wretched discourse of reason."[83] And the former knowledge again comes to the fore once man has renounced the use of reason as a means of acquiring it:

> Then indeed the image of God shines all over within and becomes glorious. Good God, whitherto dost Thou bring mortals? But surely such an intellectual thought is not made with a distinction of words or properties of speech; neither with the girding of the fences of reason; neither with a certain more swift conception of a whole discourse abundantly drawn in; nor with a dependence and sequel of things before thought of . . . But one is not in the understanding without the other . . . In that state, now, here, *sense, reason, imagination, memory and will are at once melted into a mere understanding* . . . Then, then, I say, a certain light falls upon the soul. And that, in my judgment, is all of whatsoever could ever be declared by word, thought, speech, and writing. But whether that light be altogether supernatural, or that the understand-

> ing be of its own nature thus enkindled or enflamed, *I had rather experience than determine.* One thing at leastwise I know is that it doth not happen without grace. Wherefore, whether the understanding be transformed, or whether it doth transform itself into the image of the thing understood, surely it had need of help from God . . . and in that its glass it beholds itself intellectually . . . and so it conceiveth a knowable thing, together with all its properties.[84]

Van Helmont's ideas about perception and understanding are a key not only to the history of medicine but to the history of science. Like his contemporary, Francis Bacon (with whom he had no contact), he was trying to define the nature of the new knowledge emerging in the embryonic scientific disciplines of his time. Researchers in various areas were perceiving new relationships in nature and trying to determine the precise character of this new knowledge. Van Helmont (again like Bacon) did define it—in Platonic or neo-Platonic terms.

He realized, first of all, that this "understanding" of the "premises" or "truth" was of ultimate importance: "understanding . . . is a certain immortal thing, far removed from frail or mortal things,"[85] all truth issues from "one only and primitive truth" and all understanding from "one only and infinite understanding."[86] He knew, furthermore, that this is a process of discovery, "knowledge of that which before there was ignorance of."[87] He realized that it emerges from a mixture of memory, reason, imagination, and will which he would "rather experience than determine." But his great contribution was to cast this new knowledge in the Platonic form of recollection of preexisting ideas—thus according the new scientific knowledge a privileged position in the world of discourse. In so doing he expanded the Empirical definition of knowledge as observation and experience preserved in the memory. While accepting this definition,[n] he extrapolated

[n]The old fox is more intelligent than the younger one "by the remembrance of experience" (*Oriatrike,* 20).

from it, using it as a vehicle to justify the emergence of a new form of knowledge by fusing it with the Platonic recollection (memory) of eternal Ideas.

An example of how this process worked is his discovery of the origin of urinary calculi—which Galenic doctrine attributed to overlong retention of urine in the kidneys and bladder causing the contained phlegm to be heated and cooked into stone:

> We do teach anyone in vain unless the Master of all truth shall also teach us . . . Therefore I long and seriously searched after what manner I might attain the knowledge of the stone from this Master. For truly I most perfectly knew that authors had not so much as the least light, and that therefore neither could they give me that knowledge. But I confessed myself to be a great sea of ignorance and an abyss of manifold darkness and to want all light . . . And so, although I frequently prayed, yet I despaired in my mind. At length, after making a thorough search of my own self, I found that I was myself free from the stone. For I had never felt any pain of my reines [kidneys] or had taken notice of one only sand therein. Yet I had now and then beheld that sand adhering in the urinal, yet without any sliminess or disturbance of heat or local pain . . .
>
> It once happened that I was conversant with some noble women, the wives of noblemen, and so also with the Queen herself from the third hour after noon even to the third hour after midnight, at London in the court of Whitehall . . . But I made water when those women first drew me along with them to the King's Palace; wherefore, for civility's sake I withheld my urine for at least twelve hours space. And then, having returned home, I could not, even by the most exact viewing, find so much as the least mote of sand in my urine. For I feared lest my urine having been long detained and cocted beyond measure would now be of a sandy grain. Wherefore I made water the more curiously through a napkin; but my urine was

> free from all sand. Therefore, the next day after, in the morning, I pissed new urine through a towel and detained it in a glass urinal as many hours (to wit: 12). And at length I manifestly saw the adhering sand to be equally dispersed round about where the urine had stood. Lastly, pouring forth the urine, I touched the sand with my finger. And being perfectly instructed by my own experience I concluded with myself that forasmuch as the urine was by me, the pisser, detained for twelve hours space, and yet it contained no sand, neither that I had cast it forth, and that otherwise in the lesser space of a day, sand had been condensed in my urine . . . I knew more certainly than certainty itself that a sliminess of matter was no way required for that sand, and that the heat of the member did in no wise effect the coagulation of the stone. I thereupon, taking my progress home, cast from me the doctrine of the Schools, and presently the truth took hold of me. For I being confirmed, and no longer staggering by reason of doubt, believed as being certainly confirmed, that the internal and seminal cause of the stones in men was unknown to mortals. With a great courage, therefore, I again disdaining all the books of writers, cast them away and expelled them far from me. Neither determined I to expect the aid of my calling from any other way than from the Father of Lights, the one only Master of Truth.[88]

Since a twelve-hour retention of urine in the bladder produced less sand than Van Helmont had in a normal day, he realized the Galenic theory of the stone to be untrue. Like the mystics, he attained this knowledge by first admitting his own ignorance and unworthiness, praying, and despairing of enlightenment. Then he looked into himself. Finally, he was instructed by experience, and his soul was filled with the truth.

The Physis and the Archeus

The neo-Platonic assumption that nature is a vital entity, functioning as a whole and subject to laws unknown to man but reflecting the will of God,[o] is, clearly enough, peculiarly suited to the biological and physiological study of man—a vital entity which also functions in ways unknown *a priori* to the observer but possibly reflecting the will of God.

The ambiguity of the word, "nature" *(physis)*, which since ancient times had also denoted the vital force of the organism, contributed to the transferability of neo-Platonism into medicine.

Van Helmont accepted the *physis* as an agent of cure: "truly the natures themselves have been known of old to be the physiciannesses of diseases."[89] But the *physis* is part of the pagan dispensation and thus can no longer remain the sole instrument available to the body. So he hypothesized a second, Christian, vital force which, although parallel to the *physis* and often indistinguishable from it, was nonetheless different.

Adam in Paradise possessed only a body and a mind, the former being governed directly by the latter.[90] After the Fall the "sensitive soul" *(anima sensitiva)* was introduced between the body and the mind as the "principle of life" and located at the pyloric valve between the stomach and the intestine.[91] [p] Subject to it is the *Archeus* (one of the names devised by Paracelsus for the *physis*) located in the spleen.[92] Together they form the "duumvirate" which controls the functioning of the organism.[93]

Another reason for hypothesizing the existence of the *Archeus* in addition to the *physis* was the existence of two

[o]"I believe that nature is the command of God whereby a thing is that which it is and doth that which it is commanded to do or act" (*Oriatrike,* 42).

[p]Van Helmont decided on this location after taking a small dose of *Aconitum napellus* (wolfsbane) and finding that his thoughts seemed to emanate from the stomach: "the whole faculty of discourses was remarkably and sensibly in the midriff, with an excluding of the head" (*Oriatrike,* 274). This sensation is a common symptom of aconite poisoning, as was shown later by the homoeopathic school (see C. Hering, *Guiding Symptoms of Our Materia Medica* [Philadelphia: American Homoeopathic Publishing Society, 1879], I, 17: "ideas seem to come from the stomach"). Van Helmont also felt a constrictive headache, as though a cord were tied around the outside of his head (*loc. cit.* Cf. Hering, *Guiding Symptoms,* I, 19: "headache, as if a hot iron was bound around the head").

classes of remedies: the traditional ones acting to promote coction and the new group of Paracelsan remedies which cured without coction.[q] For all practical purposes the *physis* and the "sensitive soul" are assimilated to the *Archeus.*[94]

Van Helmont sought authority for the *Archeus* in the pneumatic writings of the Hippocratic Corpus (*Breaths, The Sacred Disease*), holding that it governs the body through its "Blas"–i.e., "blast," a translation of *pneuma* or *physa:*

> The *Archeus* is a fountainous being which by its own Blas doth stir up every assault or violation in us, according to Hippocrates . . . the *Archeus* himself, according to the diversity of his motions, doth stir up a various household stuff of symptoms. The spirit (saith Hippocrates) hath made three motions in us: within, without, and into a circuit, and he moveth and transchangeth all things with himself, even when he is orderly. But in his irregularity, whatsoever he shall perform, he shall also utter memorable effects of his disorder.[95]

He is quite categorical that this Blas is non-material and not to be confused with gas in the intestines.[96] [r]

The vitality of the external world, as of man, is represented chemically by fermentation–a concept first introduced into medicine by Paracelsus.[s]

The external world is not composed of the four Aristotelian elements, since God created only the earth (out of earth) and heaven (out of air and water).[97] But fermentation reduces all matter, including earth, to air and water: "earth is, as it were, born of water."[98] Hence air and water are the only elements.[99] And these have been suffused with life by God in the form of ferments which yield seeds: "the ferment

[q]See below, pp. 38-44.

[r]Here he is arguing against the equation (in *Breaths*) of *pneuma* with the environmental air (see *Divided Legacy,* I, 55-56).

[s]In Basel Paracelsus started a lecture on putrefactive fermentation by uncovering a pan of human excrement. When the invited physicians hurriedly left the room, he called after them, "If you will not hear the mysteries of putrefactive fermentation, you are unworthy of the name of physicians" (Partington, *History of Chemistry,* II, 118).

is often before the seed and doth generate this from itself."[100] All living matter arises out of ferments and seeds.

The vitality of man is also represented by fermentation: one such process takes place in the stomach, a second and third in the liver, a fourth in the heart, a fifth in the arteries, and a sixth in each individual member of the body, enabling it to assimilate nutriment.[101]

The "sensitive soul" in the stomach (the site of the first digestion) and the *Archeus* in the spleen control all the physiological processes of sickness and health.

By this doctrine of the sixfold digestion Van Helmont assimilated the principle of coction to new chemical research and at the same time broadened the application of this principle. He called this fermentation process *concoctio.*[102] The *Archeus* is the principle of coction, and it governs the functioning of the body through subsidiary processes of coction.[103]

We have discussed the confusion in ancient medicine between "coction" in its two senses.[t] Originally denoting the process by which the organism overcomes a morbific cause, in the second or first century B.C. it came to be identified as well with the digestion of food. This same confusion can be seen in Van Helmont,[104] but it is now a distinction without a difference, for Van Helmont's sixfold digestive process performs both functions, converting food into the body's sustenance and also warding off morbific causes. Van Helmont does not distinguish between physiological and pathological processes: "whatsoever utters healthy actions in healthy bodies, that very thing utters vitiated ones in diseases. For that spirit heats man naturally in health, it being the same which in fevers rageth with heat."[105]

Van Helmont's stress on the digestion showed great physiological understanding, as this was a neglected area in the sixteenth century.[u]

[t]*Divided Legacy*, I, 141, 240-247.

[u]Michael Foster notes with surprise that the *Fabrica Corporis Humani* (1543) of Vesalius devotes hardly more than a sentence to the whole subject of nutrition

He sides with the Empirical Hippocrates against the Rationalist Galen. Hippocrates was a "partaker with the adeptists" and "first laid up his observations into a written style or method," putting medicine on the correct basis.[106] But Aristotle showed man a false way in trying to subject nature to logic, and his errors were compounded by Galen who promised "in an easy method, mathematical demonstrations of those things which nature only is able to measure."[107]

> Truly I find Galen diligent in opinions and a boasting writer, without judgment or discretion. For neither hath he better perceived of nature, diseases, causes, and effects, than of the decrees of Hippocrates and Plato.[v] For I profess I have twice read over those volumes of Galen with attention, but I have found the poverty and undistinct ignorance of Galen to fight with his rashness. For truly those books do touch at nothing less than the doctrine of Hippocrates or Plato. Neither also hath Hippocrates anything common with Plato.[108]

Hippocrates rightly stated that "the nature alone (which is only one) is the physicianness of diseases, but the physician the minister or servant."[109] The *physis* is also the physician of wounds.[110]

While studying medicine Van Helmont virtually memorized the *Aphorisms.*[111] His writings make especially laudatory reference to *Ancient Medicine,* the capstone of the Hippocratic Empirical doctrine.[112] He regarded the proto-Rationalist writing, *Nature of Man,* as spurious—"a little book (feigned on Hippocrates) concerning human nature."[113] And in one of the few works published in his lifetime he called himself a "Hippocratic and Hermetic physician."[114]

and digestion (Michael Foster, *Lectures on the History of Physiology* [Cambridge: at the University Press, 1901], 122). Hunger pangs in these times were confused with disease symptoms, and Van Helmont has to argue that hunger is not a disease "because the *Archeus* is in no wise diseasy in hunger" (*Oriatrike,* 495).

[v]*De Placitis Hippocratis et Platonis,* an Aristotelian treatment of Hippocrates and Plato which is a caricature of the views of both.

As a Hippocratic and an Empiric Van Helmont makes the *physis/Archeus* the starting-point of his medical philosophy. He complains that this subject is neglected in the schools.[115] And knowledge of the *physis/Archeus* is obtained only from sense-perception: "we do not know other natures *a priori*, but only by naked observation, and the alterations of the *Archeus* in the same way."[w] Its internal mechanisms are concealed from the physician who can only make conjectures, judging their correctness by the outcome of his practice:

> I cannot meetly explain the means whereby the *Archeus* doth make his own voluntary eccentricities nor decypher the ideas of these by a proper etymology, if they are invisible, unperceivable, and made in the withdrawing of the *Archeus* from corporeal edifices. For I have not known the manner or means whereby seminal beginnings do express their natural endowments, the which is plainly unknown unto me from a former thing or cause: for I counterfeit it by conjectures only attained from a similitude or like thing. Indeed, by things regular in man I have made conjectures which another more judicious than myself may explain; but it hath seemed to me that it would not be worth my labor for these things to be now wholly searched into according to individuals; but that it is sufficient as well in knowing as in healing to have withstood generated ideas and to have taken away all disorder from the *Archeus*.[116]

Pathology: Disease Causes

Just as neo-Platonism held the world of nature to be a vital entity upon which the Ideas of God are stamped, so Van Helmont regards "disease" as a stamp, seal, or impression upon the *physis* or *Archeus*, an "idea" or image in its mind.

[w]*Oriatrike*, 459: *"neque enim alias de cetero cognoscimus naturas a priori neque Archei alteritates modo scimus, nisi per nudam observationem."*

The *Archeus* "frames erroneous images to himself which should be unto him as it were for a poison . . . Which images or likenesses, indeed, as being the seeds of disease beings, should be thenceforth wholly marriageable unto him in the innermost bride-bed of life. This indeed is an hard saying, in the ears which are not accustomed to hear beyond trifles, heats, and dirt."[117] "I do not name a disease a diathesis or disposition, but the very wandering or erring being which is stamped by the vital *Archeus* himself."[118] "A strange image or seminal idea of the corrupt nature."[119] "And so every disease is caused from the violent assaulting spirit, by ideas conceived in the proper subject of the *Archeus,* by whose fault alone a live body, but not a dead carcase, suffers all diseases."[120]

And the morbific influence affecting the *Archeus* in this way is from a disease "seed." As already noted, "seeds" and "ferments" are at the origin of all life, hence of diseases as well. Seeds are not material, but "ideal".[121] They are subject to astrological influence.[122] [x] The power of the disease, like that of a plant, resides in its seed.[123] Certain disease seeds (epilepsy, gout) can become rooted in the body and pass on to the next generation.[124]

But the disease seed affects the body only through the *Archeus:* "the matter of a disease is Archeal, and its efficient cause is vital . . . every disease is of necessity an ideal efficient act of the vital power, clothing itself with a garment of Archeal matter and attaining a vital and substantial form according to a difference of the slowness and swiftness of ideal seeds."[125] Since the *physis,* according to Hippocrates, is the physician of disease, the *physis* must also be its cause.[126] The ideal cause in the seed compels the *Archeus* to act in a certain way, just as an idea in the mother's mind can have a physical effect on the fetus, and this action by the *Archeus* is the actual disease.[127] Thus the disease proceeds from spirit to matter, from non-being to being.[128]

[x] Fracastorius in 1530 had published his *Syphilis, sive Morbus Gallicus* ascribing this disease to seeds governed by astrological influences (see below, pp. 405-406).

Later Empirics were to wonder how the *physis,* if it indeed possesses curative power, can let itself be impaired by disease causes.[y] Van Helmont's answer is that only a part of the *Archeus* is affected, and is thereupon separated from the rest—"for the banishment whereof the remaining part of the *Archeus* doth collaborate and is earnestly careful that it may not be pierced by the symbol or impression and perish . . . For truly the life is not immediately hurt but by a certain poison of its own, and proper to it, which it hath suffered to be applied unto itself."[129]

The Galenic materialist disease theory is erroneous: "I have long since admired that no physician hath hitherto known in what the essence of disease should shine: but that they have wandered about elementary qualities, humors, complexions, contrarieties, and dispositions. Neither have they once observed that as filths are not diseases, so neither are diseases in filths, but that they live only in the life itself."[130]

Like Paracelsus, therefore, Van Helmont rearranged the Galenic (Aristotelian) theory of disease causes. The "idea" is the efficient cause of disease, the *Archeus* is the material and formal cause, while the humors, elements, and qualities are disease *effects:*[131]

> The stone is not the disease but the primary lithiasis or stony affect, and the true disease duelech is the idea itself radically implanted in the powers of the *Archeus* of the kidneys or bladder, the which indeed is wanting in healthy persons . . . that idea, I say, inhabiting in the implanted *Archeus* of those parts, is the disease separator and workman, commanding the implanted faculty of that organ, and which leads it bound at its own erroneous pleasure.[132]

"Heat in the reins is not the parent of the stones, but a symptom, but an effect following upon the placing of the hateful guest, the stone, in the bowel. For as a thorn being

[y] See below, pp. 247, 405-406, 410.

thrust into the finger is neither hot nor hardened by heat, nor by reason of heat thrust into the flesh, yet heat follows the hurt as a companion."[133] "Every man hath a potential stone in his urine (for that thing the condition of the microcosm or little world did require if it ought on every side to express the macrocosm or great world) but he is only miserable, to wit, in whose urine a power of stonifying lying hid, is actually unfolded within his skin."[134]

Thus the Galenists steadily confuse disease causes and disease products.[135] In pleurisy, for example, they regard its effect, "the bloody apostheme wherein the pleura or coat which girdeth the ribs is plucked from the ribs with a continual fever and pain of the place," as its cause, while actually the cause of pleurisy is spiritual.[136] For this reason their claim to discover causes through anatomical investigation is false: "anatomy, being founded on bad principles, is oft-times childish or a mockery."[137] "After a thousand years' anatomy the moderns do scarce either the better know diseases or the more successfully expel them."[138] "[The schools] do measure him to be a true physician who shall point out most in the filths of dead carcases, and who shall certainly find by his own knife those things which are published by predecessors in this respect, even unto superstition."[139]

He tells of a friend who died complaining of pain around the liver and the spleen; but an autopsy could find no pathological changes in these areas.[140]

In support of his position Van Helmont invokes Hippocrates who understood that "heats" and "colds" are the effects of diseases, not their causes.[141] In *Ancient Medicine* a dynamic theory of disease causation had been set out,[z] and this is the work to which Van Helmont refers:

[z]In cap. XIV: "there is in man salt and bitter, sweet and acid, astringent and insipid, and a vast number of other things, possessing powers [*dynameis*] of all sorts, both in number and in strength" (W. H. S. Jones, *Hippocrates* [Loeb Classical Library, 1962], I, 39). This passage is discussed in *Divided Legacy,* I, 74.

> It was rightly decreed by Hippocrates, to the carelessness of the Schools, that hot, cold, moist, or dry . . . are not diseases or the causes of them, but sharp, bitter, salt, brackish, etc. . . . But it is a matter of amazement that he whom the schools do boast of to follow as their captain they have skipped over this his text, through sluggishness.[142]

> Yea truly Hippocrates first insinuated that diseases are to be distinguished by their inns and savours [tastes]; and I wish his successors had kept this tenor. But that old man, being as it were swollen with fury, presaged of the future rashnesses of the succeeding schools, and precisely admonished them, that they should not believe that heats, colds, moistures, sharpnesses, or bitternesses were diseases but bitter, sharp, salt, brackish, etc. itself. But he sung these things before deaf or bored ears: for truly the long since forepast ages, being inclined unto a sluggishness of enquiring, and an easy credulity, snatched up the scabbed theorems of heats and colds, and subscribed unto them by reason of a plausible easiness, and bid adieu to their master.[143]

The physician must also consider occasional and exciting causes: "a disease is a real being having its causes, the material and efficient, stirred up by occasional causes."[144] Such can be within the body or outside it: poisons, unhealthy food, witches' spells, epidemic and astrological influences ("the Blas of the stars"), undigested food remnents, products of previous diseases still unexpelled from the body, an organic weakness of some sort, etc.[145] He attributes to Hippocrates the idea of a divine cause of all diseases:

> For so, wheresoever Hippocrates hath not found any visible matter as the occasion of a disease, he accuseth a divine beginning in diseases, because it is invisible from the hidden storehouse of seeds, from the invisible world, or out of Pluto's river of hell, or from the chaos of successive changes; therefore I do in all things wholly

> admire at this Divine Beginning (be it spoken by the liberty of Hippocrates) in diseases, as the judge of a broken purity . . . lurking in the flesh of sin and therefore also persevering in the radical disorder of a vital principle.[146]

Ultimately, all disease springs from original sin.[147]

In his treatment the physician should avoid confusing the occasional cause with the disease itself: "though I name an occasional cause for disease, yet I will not have it to be understood as if the occasional cause were the disease itself; but rather that a disease, as an invisible being, may be understood to be occasionally stamped by an external matter."[148]

Therapeutics

Van Helmont proposed two methods of cure, through coction and by specific medicines, although the distinction between them is not always maintained.

The Hippocratic Empirical writings, and the Empirical School itself, had seen cure as consisting in the coction or maturation of the "crudeness" at the origin of the disease; the process passes through a "crisis" with ultimate resolution and expulsion of the concocted matter in the form of urine, sweat, hemorrhage, stool, or a skin rash. This was all accepted by Van Helmont. He discusses a child with quartan ague who recovered "through a crisis or judicial expulsion and many stools."[149] Skin disorders such as measles or erysipelas represent the ultimate stage of cure by the *Archeus,* since "health, for the most part, accompanies a motion to without."[150] Each ferment in the body is a kind of coction: "for truly three concoctions are completed in man: to wit, the first in the stomach, another in the liver, but a third in all particular members."[151]

Fever is a sign of the curative process: "for, indeed, the *Archeus* inflames himself in his endeavor whereby he could earnestly desire to expel the occasional matter, as it were a thorn thrust into himself."[152] The physician should stimulate it: for instance, he can prescribe hot water, wine, and *aqua regis* in fevers, allowing the patient to take as much as he wants.[153]

> If therefore the motion of heat be that of the *Archeus* himself, for the expelling of the enemy, and wine add heat; therefore, he who proceeds by wine heals according to the conformity of nature.[154]

In the same way, "the sharp distillation of sulphur (which in itself is most dry and corrosive) is wont to mitigate that deceitful thirst [of fever] no otherwise than as water quencheth fire."[155]

Sudorific medicines, which draw matter from the inside of the body to the outside, are very suitable in fevers.[156] Laxative medicines should be used only sparingly and after the crisis; otherwise they will draw off crude humors, and this is not beneficial. The Galenists err by giving them too early, "before the maturity and coction of the peccant matter."[157] "From which surely an honest physician doth then also more justly abstain, because it then disturbs the crisis, induceth the danger of confusion and of a relapse. For a loosening medicine doth always and by itself draw out things not cocted, no otherwise than those which are afterwards called cocted ones."[158]

There are other remedies, the "specifics,"[a] which operate on the *Archeus* directly and allow the physician to bypass the crisis.[159] These "do not draw out the disease by sweat, vomit, or stool, but do unsensibly resolve, in whatsoever part the disease is entertained, the nature being busied about the rest."[160] "For the nature causeth not a crisis or time of judgment unless when she alone carried the whole burden, on set days. A true physician, therefore, ought to overcome the disease before a crisis, and therefore neither doth he wait nor wish for a crisis."[161]

[a]The word, "specific," had been introduced by Paracelsus (*Divided Legacy,* I, 405).

When the correct medicine is prescribed, the "stirred up confusion of the *Archeus*" is reduced, and the fever ceases: "those things which do there materially offend are easily tamed by the nature and retire themselves as rightly subdued. This way indeed: fevers do presently depart at the arrival of some one *arcanum,* but the remainder of expulsion is committed to the shoulders of the nature that Hippocrates, his dignity, may be preserved: that the natures themselves are the physiciannesses of diseases."[162] "Seeing that the fever being well nigh overcome, the *Archeus* composeth himself to tranquillity or rest, as by crises, sweats, or by bleeding at the nose, or also by hemorrhoids or piles, as it were the remaining wrestling of furies, he hath ofttimes brought quietness and health."[163]

Thus there are medicines which "pacify the tumult stirred up in the life; those which follow are such as overcome the poison of a fever. But those are more famous which contain both together. Lastly there are some which are serviceable expulsively, to wit, by a plausible cleaning and resolving; wherein the liberality of the Almighty is wonderful which hath directed crude simples for fevers, and the which being moderately prepared, do mow down a fever like a scythe."[164]

The specific remedy assists the healthy part of the *Archeus* in its battle with the diseased part: "by appeasing his griefs, disturbances, and a continual and successive substituting of nourishing ideas."[165] "Cures, as well by medicines as by the nature, are made by an appeasing of the disturbed *Archeus,*"[166]

The problem of how specifics can possess this power over disease was solved by Van Helmont along neo-Platonic lines. In general, medicines possessing a "specific quality" or "specific gift" act "by an overflowing of goodness . . . because they are so commanded to act by the Lord of things who alone hath given knowledges, bounds, or ends to seeds, known to Himself alone . . . for Christian philosophy doth dictate this thing, but the heathenish school is ignorant of it."[167] And the vehicle of God's will is the specific stamp, seal, form, or idea imprinted on each such medicine. Just as disordered health arises from poisonous "ideas" implanted in the *Archeus,* so "suitable helps or remedies have ideas which are chiefly the extinguishers of the poisoned ideas."[168] The powers or formal properties of these medicines are from the "forms of the three principles, salt, sulphur, and mercury, or salt, fat, and liquor, from whence every body is composed, and again resolved into the same; and the mercury or liquor is so often diverse as there are species or particular kinds of things, let the same judgment be of the salt and sulphur."[169] From the "fantasy or the forms of the mixed body, and those of this sort are in the whole composed body by reason of its form . . . [or] by reason of the whole homogeneal mixture."[170]

The Empirics had held that each remedy acts by its "whole substance," and Galen himself had put into this category snake poisons and other substances whose powerful effect on the body seemed unrelated to their qualities of taste or smell.[b] Van Helmont's mention of the "whole composed body" or the "whole homogeneal mixture" shows his awareness of this tradition. And regardless of the word he used, whether "whole mixture," "occult quality,"[171] "form,"[172] "specific quality," or "gift,"[173] he meant precisely what was always postulated in the Empirical tradition—that medicinal substances cannot be analyzed *a priori* (in the Galenic fashion, into hot, cold, wet, and dry) but are known only from their effects: "the searching after hidden or secret things is not but from the effect to the cause, according to the Gospel."[174] Just as the configuration and fruit of a plant permit recognition of the seed:

> [Remedies] become fruits or effects in us, as they do fructify in our tree, and so they are not only the fruits of their own native tree, whence in the nature of things they are derived; but rather they are new fruits, from an ingrafting of a product, and so are plainly promiscuous of

[b]See *Divided Legacy,* I, 259, 314-315.

a branch or fruit of the tree implanted, and of the vital power of the stock whereunto it is ingrafted.[175]

Although he likens the medicine's effect to "magnetism," this is only to symbolize its unknowability.[176] He also ascribes it to "magic": "the whole action is magical; neither hath a thing any power of acting which is not produced from the fantasy of its form, and that indeed magically."[177] "Every agent acts on its proper object, to wit, by a fore-feeling of that object whereby it disperseth its activity, not rashly, but on that object only; to wit, the fantasy being stirred after a sense of the object, by dispersing of an ideal entity, and coupling it with a ray of the passive entity. This indeed hath been the magical action of natural things."[178] "Magic" and "magnetism" here mean only that man cannot understand how medicines produce their effects—not that the physician can cure by incantations, spells, or the like.

He has other metaphorical ways of describing the action of the specific medicine. "I perceived that the *Liquor alkahest* did cleanse the nature by the virtue of its own fire. For as fire destroyeth all insects, so the *alkahest* consumeth diseases."[179] *Mercurius vivus* "doth clarify the organs no otherwise than as stibium clarifies gold."[180] "All renewing remedies do operate by refining, and in this respect by exhilarating."[181] Some minerals affect the body through their "smoke" just as mercury miners contract the mercurial disease from the smoke of the mine.[182] Others act by their "odor."[183]

To cure, the physician brings together the formal property of the medicine and the "form" or "idea" of the disease.[c] Both disease and remedy are "wholes" and act on each other as whole entities: "The *Archeus* doth conclude in him a unity and identity; hereafter from hence also we must teach that curing and restoring from all diseases doth consist

[c]Francis Bacon at this time was writing: "Man whilst operating can only apply or withdraw natural bodies, nature internally performs the rest" (*Novum Organum* I: V).

in the unity of a remedy. But the schools of the humoralists will argue to the contrary."[184] Thus plant remedies affect the *Archeus* by virtue of their own *Archei,* while mineral remedies act by "aspect" alone.[185] Some metals affect the *Archeus* by their "alterative Blas."[186]

While the wholeness of the remedy is contained in its "form," that of the disease is centered in the stomach—the locus of the *Archeus.*[187] The remedy acts on the *Archeus* in the stomach, through "an unfolding of [its] native endowment into the very middle life of the *Archeus,*"[188] and not through the digestion.[d]

> I consider the whole disease itself and its remedies to be in the *Archeus,* to wit, altered or appeased. And so with the least touching at, shaking, darting, yea, only by radiation or beaming, or illumination (so that they shall in the seat of the soul touch at the sensitive life) cures are perfected and completed, no regard being had into occasional causes.[189]

> [The *arcana*] begin in the stomach (the which I have professly elsewhere demonstrated to be the seat of the soul) to unfold or expose the direct beam of their own faculties, and their endowed virtue, and to which end they were ordained of God. Whence, at length, the bedewed beaming virtue being drawn in by the *Archeus,* is dispersed into the whole body, and health thereupon succeeding is greedily received.[190]

> Every remedy doth immediately and principally act only into the *Archeus* of the stomach . . . but this *Archeus* afterwards acts according to a disposition, drawn and generated to himself from the endowed gift of the

[d]Vegetables are not good remedies because they are subject to the digestion; *Mercurius diaphoreticus* is powerful precisely because it lies in the stomach undigested (*Oriatrike,* 579, 584). While some metallic and mineral salts act similarly to foods, passing through the six digestions and affecting the organism by stimulating certain processes there, these are inferior to remedies which act directly upon the *Archeus* (*ibid.,* 473, 477). Passage through the digestions alters their medicinal properties (*ibid.,* 473).

> remedies. It also further follows that every remedy exceeding the limits of food doth act by its touching in manner of a glass. For truly it acts only by touching at the *Archeus,* without a material commixture of itself. Indeed, the *Archeus* himself doth first feel the endowment drawn from the remedy, but in that act of perceivance he fashions to himself an idea of things to be done by him, by following the dispositions of that endowment, from whence he consequently stirring up peace, rest, or anger to himself, and assuming the gotten ideas of these, doth presently sealingly disperse the same into the bowels, hearkening to the action of government, performing prosperous or opposite offices, according to the command of the vital *Archeus.*[191]

Hence medicines do not act through contrariety: "nature is ignorant of contraries."[192] "Qualities are and do operate in the elements without respect to contrariety."[193]

> Galen being instructed by his elders, observing that fire was quenched by water, and that water being heated by fire did vanish away, supposing that he held the hare by the ears, boldly constituted almost all diseases and their remedies in those first bodies and their qualities. For he said: the fire was at enemy with the water and this with it, whence he established it by a general decree that there is in us the combat of four elements . . . and that there doth skirmish in us a continual and unexcusable strife of contraries . . . Therefore all the Schools do determine that only contraries should be the remedies of contraries; to wit, whereby every excess (being notably marked with the name of a disease) might be reduced into a mediocrity or mean . . . for he would have necessities to be subservient to his own maxims; but he erected not maxims conformable to necessities.[194]

But he also denies that they act as similars: "not by contraries, nor by alike things, but only by things that are endowed and appropriated."[195]

> For it is not requisite that the remedy and external cause of a disease should have a coresemblance, however notwithstanding Paracelsus hath so commanded, whereby he might oppose the maxim of Galen: contraries are cured by contraries. For poisons are not overcome by a coresemblance of the venom, but by that which conquers the venom. For those medicinal powers are the gifts of God, which do neither bear a contrariety, or character of hostility, mutually towards themselves nor towards diseases. But everything acteth from a gift, that which it is commanded to act.[196]

The Paracelsan *arcana* themselves heal without any "likeness or contrariety."[197 e]

He had unremitting contempt for the school physicians who thought to cure by "contraries." The body's reactive power does not obey the laws of contrariety but does whatever is necessary at the time: "for truly our nature doth always work a univocal or single thing, whether it resolveth coagulated things or at length coagulateth resolved things. For it doth no otherwise than as gold-finer's powder which giveth a hardness to lead, a difficult melting to quicksilver and tin, both which qualities it taketh away from iron."[198] The doctrine of contraries is a scholastic mode of thinking, alien to medicine: "as if medicine did not work naturally, but stood by learning by demonstration alone."[199]

These physicians are mistaken in thinking they can dispatch the remedy to some particular part of the body: "diuretics themselves do not indeed materially descend into

[e]He hedges somewhat on this, however, making a small concession in the direction of similarity: "Though likeness doth involve a familiarity and easy receiving of a remedy, its union, entrance, and piercing by reason of an agreement or coresemblance; yet that good man was ignorant that those are not agents sufficiently requisite to healing but are only occasional external means or reconcilors of healing; such is also the purity and subtility of a medicine" (*Oriatrike,* 171). He even mentions isopathic treatment favorably: a patient with *zinzilla* is cured by applying to his skin the blood of another sufferer from the same disease (*ibid.,* 769). For more on isopathy and on the relationship between the "similar" and the "specific" see below, pp. 387, 413-416.

the bladder, as neither vulnerary drinks into a remote wound, but all the aid of diuretics or urine-provokers, and wound potions, is framed in the stomach itself."[200] They attempt to cure asthma by applying substances to the head in order to prevent matter from moving down into the lungs, but "truly . . . the asthma stands in a poisonous seed which hath gotten the spirit of some bowel for its root and inn. But the property of that seed is to contract the pores of the lungs whereby it gives passage for breath into the breast . . . it affecteth the whole body because it is dispersed into the common *Archeus,* the instrument to the whole body."[201]

Galenic medicines are directed against disease products, not their causes. "The composition, connexion, qualities, effects of humors, and the diseases that are dreamed to arise from thence are mere fictions . . . bloodletting never helps unless it be by accident . . . cuttings of a vein do always take away long life."[202] "The repetitions of purges are vain and hurtful in these effects because they are those things which are appointed only about the products, but not about the causes . . . the former causes or roots they are not able to touch."[203] "He therefore labors for the most part in vain who . . . doth place his endeavor in the brushing away of occasional causes, the *Archeus* being not first appeased . . . for it happens unto him no otherwise than as he who having not first stopped up the spring head presumes by exhausting of water to dry up the brook."[204] "The *Archeus* is a fountainous being . . . how neatly soever disease products are taken away."[205]

The schools cannot seem to understand that medicines act spiritually on diseases and not materially. When the wrath of the *Archeus* has been appeased, the material disease products will disappear as well.[206] "I have oft-times perfectly taken away the colic, choler, flux, bloody flux, and other diseases by a true *laudanum* without opium, although the residing mass or lump were as yet entertained within."[207] Medicines do not act through quantity but by their specific quality: "erring life would not be conquered and subdued by the quantity of a remedy."[208] This quality can even be transferred to another medium. Thus *Argentum vivum* can transfer its quality to water "so that one only ounce of quicksilver shall be able a thousand times to infect a measure of water, and yet remain in its ancient weight and property. For so the Schools also do against their wills perfectly learn that some agents do freely, always, and with unwearied forces, act without a passion or reaction of their patients, and the same weight of themselves always remaining. For *argent-vive* doth act on the water and imprint its own character on it, yet it doth not likewise resuffer any thing from the water. It is manifest, therefore, that a certain medicinal virtue is transferred and doth change its natural subject, and departeth into a foreign object, as it were only by its beam or aspect."[209]

The best example is Butler's Stone–which the (otherwise unidentified) Irish physician, Butler, who visited Van Helmont in Vilvorde, could immerse in a barrel of oil and convert it into medicine, with one drop curing the migraine of a female patient.[210]

School medicine is thus unnatural and harmful to the patient rather than beneficial. Purges and solutive medicines "change the blood into a mortal poison,"[211] while the *arcanum,* on the contrary, "doth not only change the venous blood into a medicine like a balsam, but the very excrements of man themselves (to wit, his urine) do remain tinged with its supereminent goodness . . . even as the urine smells of eaten asparagus. So also the urine by its own washing or anointing doth cure every disease residing in the habit of the body."[212] In gout, when a "hurtful solutive medicine" is taken, the *Archeus* is "defiled, rageth, and is obedient to the drunk contagion of the venom."[213]

> For seeing that besides cutting of a vein and the shop of laxatives, the Schools as yet to this day do scarce acknowledge other remedies, and all their endeavor is that by blood, dung, bath, a cautery, sweat, and so not but by the diminishing of the body and its strength, and

> likewise by the corrupting of the blood (which they call a purge) and by miserable butchery they do presume to take away all griefs of the body. Hence it comes to pass that . . . the admirers of those frail effects have erected a plenteous company of incurable diseases . . . and have brought in a dissembling kind of cure, full of calamity and despair.[214]

These doctrines are "fictions . . . commanded to work ruin."[215] "For that reason miserable mortals have hitherto groaned under this burden of blindness, expecting cure from those who were fully ignorant of the constitutive causes of diseases."[216] "There is no medicine to be found in dispensatories which may not contain more hurt than profit."[217] "Little pains hath been taken, nothing known, but much promised, and very much neglected, long expectations, and everywhere error."[218] Their "helps for the sick are so uncertain and of so little credit . . . an art filled with conjectures and uncertainty."[219]

He particularly criticized them for rejecting the one course which promises results, that is, the search for specifics:

> When the ancients saw any disease to be cured by a specifical and appropriated remedy, they were amazed, as it were, at the miracle of an unwonted thing: but afterwards the Schools thought it satisfaction enough to have banished their blockishness into a general ignorance.[220]

Since these procedures harm the patient instead of benefiting him, Van Helmont resolved to reconstruct medical philosophy, "to destroy the whole natural philosophy of the Ancients and to make new the doctrines of the Schools."[221] "That physicians may repent and may learn those things which they know not; may enter on a safer way and may cease from badly handling the life of their neighbors; that they may cease, I say, to destroy widows, orphans, and their own souls."[222]

The Search for Remedies

Van Helmont's reconstruction aimed to offset the neglect of pharmacology by the schools. He investigated: (1) the various possible sources of remedies, and (2) ways of ascertaining the specific effect of a remedy on the patient.

He accepted four sources of medicines: (1) herbal and folk remedies, (2) the new chemical remedies, (3) the Paracelsan *arcana,* and (4) the specifics.

The herbal simples used traditionally in folk medicine were an important component of Van Helmont's pharmacopoeia. When he lost interest in school medicine, he undertook to collect "all the usual plants of our country."[223] "[God] himself hath made and endowed simples for the appointed ends of all necessities. Therefore I believe that the simples, in their own simplicity, are sufficient for the healing of all diseases. Therefore we must more study about the searching into the virtues than about disputing any hard questions, seeing that in simples there is a perfect cure and healing of all diseases."[224] "In truth the knowing and philosophical preparation of simples requires almost the whole life of the whole man to themselves."[225] However, their powers have remained unknown.[226]

Even poisons are valuable remedies, since nothing has been made by God in vain.[227]

His writings extoll many herbal simples: *Agnus castus* as a diuretic, *Helleborus niger* for coughs and catarrhs, *Bryonia alba* in dropsy, *Symphytum* for broken bones, etc.[228]

His second major source is the world of minerals and metals, particularly as improved by chemical manipulation.[229] Alchemy has "long since indeed observed a noble treasure of healing to lay hid in minerals, but it long doubted in what respect they might most fully derive themselves into the inward buttery of the similar parts."[230] "In stones a great virtue is declared to be by the Holy Scriptures, which is hitherto hidden as well in the university as in the chymical schools, until kings and commonwealths shall look into the reformation of Schools."[231] Since minerals take longer to form than plants, their powers are that much greater.[232] And metals, especially, are "the most rich and constant offspring and chief treasure of nature [and] do exceed plants and minerals in healing by long stades or distances."[233]

Chemical processing of metals and minerals will bring forth new remedies not previously known to man.[224] [f] The Paracelsan purification of medicines enables them to communicate more freely with the *Archeus.*[235] The salts of minerals, for example, are an intensification of their powers.[236]

The Paracelsan *arcana* constitute his third source of remedies. Many of these are capable of curing all diseases.[237] He used *Elixir proprietatis* (saffron, myrrh, and aloes) for long life, since these same substances prevent corpses from decomposing.[238] Also *Mercurius vivus* "which wholly sups up every sinew of a disease," tincture of antimony, *Mercurius diaphoreticus, Liquor alkahest,* fire of copper, milk of pearls, corollate, the volatile salts of various herbs and stones, etc.[239]

His final group of remedies, the specifics which operate through their formal properties, sympathy, magic, "fantasy," "fore-feeling," etc., to some extent include all the others. A scrofulous tumor is healed by placing on it the hand of a dead man, so that the cold of the hand pierces the tumor; if this is done several times, there will be a cure.[240] The moss from a dead man's skull possesses "mumial virtue, that is, the implanted and cofermented spirit which surviveth in bodies slain by violence" and which contributes vitality to the person receiving it.[241] "A slow and more stubborn fever is frequently loosed by the appetite of unwonted things (to wit, of a herring and smoked things), it hoping by such an unthought-of matter to subdue the guest, its enemy . . . because they blot out the impressional idea of the *Archeus* and feverish seal."[242] The remedy for kidney stone is not to remove the stone, since another would grow in its place,

[f] Van Helmont himself developed many new remedies in this way (W. Rommelaere, *Etudes sur J. B. Van Helmont* [Bruxelles: Manceaux, 1868], 24).

but the medicine by which "the over-exquisite separating faculty [in the urine] is to be laid asleep."[243] A bloody dysentery, caused by the enraged *Archeus,* is cured by frightening the *Archeus* into submission: a rabbit (the most timid creature) is killed by a pack of dogs and given the patient to eat, curing the dysentery.[244] "For I have noted in things loves, hatreds, terrors, and the seminal products, seals, ideas, and characters of these: whence I have found out the immediate causes of many hidden remedies."[245]

He supports the magnetic healing of wounds: the sword is anointed with an unguent, or blood from the wound is allowed to dry on the sword and then anointed.[246] Or a towel may be dipped in the blood and the remedy applied to the towel.[247] Such sympathetic remedies have been revealed by God that we may be led "from external and the more appearing diseases unto the reliefs of internal and the more abstruse diseases."[248]

But how does the physician ascertain these and other specific properties of medicines?

The traditional Galenic technique of determining the medicinal (secondary) qualities of a medicine from its primary qualities of taste and smell is erroneous: "the natural endowed virtues or faculties of things, which the divine goodness hath given from a gift for the sick, for the most part want the testimony of taste,"[249] and even poisons do not reveal their lethal qualities by taste, as there is one taste in the mouth but quite another in the stomach.[250]

The doctrine of signatures is equally unhelpful: "there is in the *Archeus* of vegetables no anatomical alliance or affinity with us, whether we regard the whole or at length their parts; for the endowments of simples are by creation."[251]

Paracelsus' quintessence is an error as well. Many substances such as mercury, crystals, and stones have no essence at all. Some herbs acquire an essence when dried, while others lose it.[252]

Astrological concordance provides no guidance.[253]

And the techniques of the chemists, who have attempted to substitute salt, sulphur, and mercury for the Galenic qualities, reveal no truth.[254] Noting that vegetation does not grow in sulphurous ground, they mistakenly conclude that sulphurous remedies will dry up the mucous in a sick person.[255] Chemistry, indeed, "hath its principles not gotten by discourses, but those which are known by nature and evident by the fire; it prepares the understanding to pierce the secrets of nature and causeth a further searching out in nature than all other sciences put together; and it pierceth even unto the utmost depths of real truth."[256] But it still does not reveal the powers of medicines. When Joseph du Chesne (Quercetanus) invokes "divination by fire" to elucidate the powers of herbs—burning them to ashes and then observing the crystal patterns when the ashes are mixed with water and frozen, "that good man declareth his ignorance of principles, not knowing, first of all, that . . . the *Archeus* is the figurer of the thing to be generated, which is burnt up by the fire long before a coal or ashes is made."[257]

In short, the powers of remedies cannot be perceived directly "by mortal eyes" *(cum oculis carneis)*. While God may have revealed these to Adam and Solomon, "it is to be feared lest He who hath suffered the Books of Solomon to perish may reserve this knowledge of simples for the age of Elias the Artist."[258]

The only way which remains is to observe the effects of remedies and from these deduce their powers: "the knowledge of specifical properties is drawn from the effect of the cause . . . we thereby by the effects come to the causes . . . being led by the hand from one knowledge to another."[259] Furthermore, this is the way prescribed in the Holy Scriptures:

> Truly in this were the Schools blinded, because they have proceeded against the doctrine of the Gospel; for primitive truth willeth that we know the tree by its fruits, but the Schools will that the fruit ought to be known by the tree. I will therefore show by the fruits in what

> manner we must come unto the knowledge of the tree.[260]

By observing their effect on the sick the physician learns how to employ medicines properly: "by observation, no otherwise than as a boy who sounds or sings the music doth notwithstanding not compose it, as neither hath he known the first grounds of harmony by means whereof the tunes or notes were so to be disposed. If this thus happens in sensible things which are to be known by sense, the reason whereof the hearing measureth, what shall not be done in medicinal affairs wherein the virtues of simples are not penetrable by any sense?"[261] While the mineral world will, in future, supply "almost an infinite virtue of remedies," this must be "often and diversely drawn under experience [*postquam . . . subter experentiam tracta fuisset*]"[262] The things which Hippocrates set forth were from "his own experience [*experientia*], without any false paint."[263] Hence the ancient remedies are not to be derided but regarded as "some experiments [*experimenta*]."[264] And his own remedies (he observes) "are not so new that there are only the thousandth of experiences in them [*ut millesima tantum sint in se experiente*], the which have been made consonant with truth by a hundred thousand experiences [*quae centies millies veritate experientiis sunt facta consona*]."[265]

He does not invoke experience only in general terms but employs particular experiments to prove particular points. He tested Galen's hypothesis that kidney stone arises from phlegm heated in urine by boiling some phlegm in urine and saw that it did not calcify but was "resolved like glue."[266] Other chemical experiments proved to him that "the matter of gas was water."[267] "Practical experience" has confirmed that the moss from the skulls of men broken on the wheel is no less effective a remedy than that from the skulls of men hanged.[268] To test whether the state of the health can be determined from the blood he in one day examined the blood of two hundred healthy peasants from his district, finding that the samples differed widely from one to another but that all the donors were equally healthy: "therefore I have laughed at the table of judgments from the beholding of blood let out of the veins."[269]

He refuted the Galenic postulate that mucus is excreted by the brain in observing that he blew his nose more often in winter than in summer: "notwithstanding in either station I, through the grace of God, do enjoy a brain and its fruitfulness or operations alike strong at both seasons."[270] Furthermore, the nose does not run during sleep, and Van Helmont concluded that mucus is designed to protect the windpipe from cold air.[271] By the same token, coughing protects the respiratory passages from impure air.[272]

He tells of a wounded friend who did not believe in magnetic cures, but "on the other hand he had seen some experiences made by honest men. Therefore . . . he made trial of the thing in this manner, to wit, he sprinkled the powder of the best vitriol on a bloody towel with the express protestation that he was unwilling to experience any thing, or to be hereafter cured, if there were even the least cooperation of a contract, or of the evil spirit; yet he saw the wound to be healed sooner than was wont, and the blood also to be presently allayed. And, therefore, afterwards he believed that natural causes, although unknown to us, did operate in the aforesaid sympathetical cure."[273]

He urged the Galenists to compete with him in a trial of remedies on 200 or 500 patients, casting lots to ensure random allocation: "I will cure them without bloodletting and sensible evacuation . . . let us act friendly and by mutual experiences [*per experientias mutuas*], that it may be known henceforward which of our two methods are true . . . We shall see how many funerals both of us shall have."[274]

Van Helmont looked to experience alone as the ultimate test of scientific knowledge of remedies: "It is not suitable to the custom of naturalists to dispute from naked authorities; we must come up to handy blows with those that contend with us, to wit, unto experience. Make trial, therefore, and convince us of a lie; if thou canst not, at least believe us."[275]

On the other hand, he was contemptuous of the random trials of the Galenists and *their* invocation of "experience" in support of their results. They have "subjoined some additions from their own or the gathered experiences [*experientiis*] of others, but as yet plainly confused, uncertain, and badly distinct."[276] "Some of them confess their own and their author's weaknesses, and many do unwillingly flee unto chemical unknown remedies, most of them abounding with their adultery and ravishment. They fly back to books, not likewise to furnaces, for their unexperiences do promise most ample fruits [*tyrocinia enim pollicentur amplissimos fructus*]."[277]

The difference between Van Helmont's "experience" and the "unexperience" of the Galenist tyros is that the former is based upon *scientia* while the latter is not: "because they have not written from knowledge [*scientia*], but either from the noted revelations of the vulgar, or they being things drawn from a casual experiment [*casuali experimento*]."[278] "For the knowledge of diseases containeth the knowledge [*scientiam*] of the causes, the dependence and appropriating the same to our defensive faculties . . . But the finding out [*inventio*] of the remedy doth presuppose the aforesaid knowledges [*cognitiones*] and, moreover, of the faculties and powers, I say, the manner and means of acting."[279]

Paracelsus had introduced the concept of *scientia,* meaning the body of laws governing the functioning of natural objects.[g] He also held that true experience had to be based on *scientia* while, at the same time, *scientia* is generated by experience. While in a sense contradicting himself, Paracelsus merely meant that experimentation must be based upon a hypothesis.

Van Helmont accepted Paracelsus' *scientia,* appreciating that investigation of a drug must proceed from some *a priori* idea of its functioning—this *a priori* idea, in turn, being derived from previous experimentation. The whole problem "hath not yet been treated of by the Schools" with their

[g]*Divided Legacy,* I, 466-470.

"ridiculous lessons of complexions and degrees."[280] Hence the "powers of simples and their immediate subjects have remained unknown."

> For those, besides a clear and visual knowledge of them, do require a desired preparation and appropriation. First of all, the knowledge of science [*scientiam*]; but that doth not presuppose traditions declared at pleasure and transcribed one to another. For preparation doth not only require the boilings and bruisings of the shop, but the whole art of the fire. At length, a fitting or suiting, applying or appropriating, requires a speculation founded in the light of nature, of man, diseases, and effects, and then their dependencies, changes, and interchangeable courses.[281]

Van Helmont's method of trial-and-error and successive approximations is identical with that used by the Empirical School to ascertain the curative powers of remedies.[h] As such it is a proto-scientific procedure, reinforced by his acceptance of Paracelsus' *scientia* which plays the role of hypothesis.

While not a fully scientific method, its intent is scientific, and its rejection of Rationalist causal metaphysics is an important step in that direction.

Van Helmont as an Empiric

Van Helmont's philosophy is the fourth stage in the Empirical tradition—after Hippocrates, the Empirical School, and Paracelsus. His aim was to complete the unfinished business of these thinkers, specifically, to find a precise relationship between remedies and diseases.

His philosophy is vitalistic and holistic: the *physis,* the *Archeus,* and the "sensitive soul" are not clearly distinguished from one another and, indeed, represent three aspects of the organism's vitality. Since the vital force is unitary, the organism must be considered an individual, unanalyzable,

[h]*Ibid.,* I, 265-270.

whole: "nature doth nowhere exist, nor is seen, but in individuals."[282] The stomach is the locus of this holism, of the "feelings [and] faintings of the whole body."[283]

Disease is also a whole and unique to the individual sick person. "The sealing notes and impressions of diseases do not cohere with species but with individuals only."[284] Asthma, although contracting the pores of the lungs, nonetheless "affecteth the whole body because it is dispersed into the common *Archeus,* the instrument to the whole body."[285] The line is blurred between somatic and mental diseases: "a fear of the plague creates the plague; a sudden fear of death hath oftentimes killed the gout. Likewise, the fear of honor lost, or to be lost, if it hath endured for the space of one day, hath now and then caused the falling sickness [epilepsy]."[286]

The number of diseases in the world is infinite, being equivalent to the "diversities of filth in us" or to the number of ideas that could influence the *Archeus.*[287] Van Helmont uses the accepted disease names in his writings only for the sake of convenience.[288]

Medicines are equally to be considered wholes. Their powers come from "the whole composed body by reason of its form, as the magnetism of the lodestone, the virtue of tinctures, likewise all specifical and appropriated things or medicines which happen by reason of the whole homogeneal mixture or of the form of any one entire part, but not of some one principle alone."[289] Even though composed of salt, sulphur, and mercury, medicines are infinite in their variety because salt, sulphur, and mercury themselves come in an infinite variety—being as "diverse as there are species or particular kinds of things."[290]

Because each medicine is a unique whole, Van Helmont opposed polypharmacy. God has placed in each substance that which is necessary, and this power is impaired when other substances are added to it.[291] "In nature everything is singular, lives in its own healing family-administration, nor rejoiceth it in wedlock."[292] The Rationalists of the schools substitute their own ideas for those of God and nature when they add sugar and honey to make medicines more palatable: to many patients "the taste of aloes is more grateful than that of honey."[293] To *Symphytum* (comfrey) they add vinegar, bole, and other condiments "when as God hath composed this simple as altogether sufficient against the ruptures of bones."[294]

This procedure of the Rationalists stems from their erroneous belief that the proximate causes of diseases and medicines can be known: "in respect of the causes [medicine] is wholly invisible and unpassable . . . the most difficult of sciences by reason of the invisibility of diseases and deceit much increased by heathenish theorems."[295]

The disease whole can be known only from its symptoms, and Van Helmont emphasizes symptomatic description.[i] Like Paracelsus, he considered this to be knowledge of the formal cause of the disease, but where the former had identified the formal cause with the mineral at the disease root, Van Helmont identified it with the *Archeus*, which is "a certain natural and formal act."[296]

The formal cause residing in the medicine is the "seal" or "imprint" it has received from God, and Van Helmont devoted much thought to the problem of how the formal causes of diseases and remedies are related.

He rejected outright the fundamental principle of the Iatrochemical school[j] (of which he is reputed one of the founders) that salt, sulphur, and mercury within the body are identical to these substances outside it—hence that the relations between diseases and remedies can be elucidated by an understanding of the relations among chemicals. These three substances (he observes) have been "falsely intruded" into medicine as "essential causes."[297] Physicians are

[i]See his accounts of patients with asthma (*Oriatrike*, 356-372). The symptomatic descriptions go on for thousands of words, and Van Helmont concludes: "I thus draw out things at length whereby the seeds of an asthma may be the more manifest."

[j]On the Iatrochemists see below, pp. 110 ff.

tempted to take this path precisely because salt, sulphur and mercury are visible, palpable, and demonstrable, thus possessing an advantage over the Galenic humors or qualities which are "undemonstrable" and "arisen from feigned beginnings."[298] He even attributes this later Iatrochemical view to Paracelsus himself:

> For he had learned that from Galen, thinking that the blood did consist of as many simples as it was resolved into. I wonder, therefore, at the unconsiderateness of Paracelsus, that he did not know that the three first things are never separated but by fire . . . neither hath that man ever seen the three first things of any composed body to have appeared in living creatures . . . I am also angry that it is not known that the same first things remaining, they are nevertheless materially subject to the divers transmutations of seeds . . . He hath after a sort relapsed into the errors of Galen who thinks that the elements do essentially remain in mixed bodies. For thus was he deluded in his three principles. For there is everywhere the same defect of both in the principles of philosophy: which teach that the life alone doth operate in a living body and into a body.[299]

As already noted,[k] Paracelsus' cosmology, his microcosm and macrocosm, provided a system of correspondences between diseases and remedies which none of his disciples could comprehend or employ. Hence his salt, sulphur, and mercury became hypostatized and identified with the chemicals of the same name. Van Helmont was not sympathetic to the Paracelsan cosmology (the above passage indicates that he perhaps misunderstood it) and was equally unwilling to accept the Iatrochemical formulations. He sought a middle way.

Like all Empirical thinkers, he saw great promise in pharmacology. He criticized the schools for ignoring herbal remedies[300] and ridiculed their dietary prescriptions of

[k]See above, p. 11. Also, *Divided Legacy,* I, 339-481.

pheasants, partridges, blackbirds, capons, starlings, etc. "as if meats and drinks should be the medicines of the more grievous diseases . . . cures [are] the effects of medicines, but not of meats."[301]

And he felt, like all other Empirics, that knowledge of these medicines is given by experience—experience which will yield an "almost infinite virtue of remedies for the future."[302] "More heretics are converted by the examples of a Christian life than by the discourses of disputations."[303]

But he hoped to go beyond mere trial-and-error and establish a system of analytical relationships between medicines and sick persons based on an understanding of how objects act on each other from a distance, their "forefeeling," their "formal" qualities. It is this kind of language which has led historians to regard him as relying on magic or "occult" knowledge,[l] even though he called the cabala and natural magic he studied under Martin del Rio "only empty stubbles and most poor patcheries, void of judgment."[304]

Van Helmont was convinced that a way could be found, better than mere empirical trials, to associate remedies with diseases, one which did not involve magic or supernatural forces but only the natural power possessed by all bodies to act on other bodies and interact with them. He followed certain suggestions made by Paracelsus, and at the same time foreshadowed discoveries later made by Samuel Hahnemann,[m] in claiming that poisons would be excellent remedies if we only knew how to use them, in tasting *Aconitum napellus* and finding that it generates certain specific symptoms, and in suggesting that diseases can be classified in function of the effects which certain herbal simples have on the orga-

[l]Thus Michael Foster: "as we read Van Helmont we seem to see two men, two intellects of very different kinds. On the one hand, we see a patient, careful, exact observer, a child of the new philosophy . . . On the other hand we see a mystic, speculative dreamer . . . weaving a fantastic scheme of the powers and forces ruling the universe, calling in the aid of invisible supernatural agencies to explain the occurrence of natural phenomena," etc. (*Lectures on the History of Physiology,* 129-130).

[m]See below, pp. 351 ff.

nism.[305] But he was not able to carry these fruitful ideas further and thus failed to reconstruct the Paracelsan cosmology.

The latter divided in two: its chemical side issued in the Iatrochemical school, while its vitalistic dimension was reformulated in the *Anima* of Georg Ernst Stahl.[n]

Van Helmont made gigantic contributions to chemistry (of which he is one of the pioneers) and physiology (where he was one of the first to use quantitative methods), and these are the discoveries for which he is most praised by historians.[o] But this was not what interested him. His own life was spent largely in seeking an answer to the riddle of the sphinx: how to establish an *a priori* relationship between the sick person and the medicine which will cure him.

His Critique of the Medical Profession

Van Helmont, like Paracelsus, carried his ideological critique into the social realm, relating the incorrect theory and practice of his colleagues to the social and economic conditions of their professional life.

To the Empirical principles of observation and experience Paracelsus had added Christian love: genuine observation and experience are possible only through empathy with the object observed and experienced. Van Helmont accepts this, and his critique of physicians is oriented around (1) their failure to respect experience and (2) their lack of Christian love for their patients.

Since God loved all men equally, he gave to each the ability to observe, make discoveries, and acquire experience. Laymen treat as well as physicians in many cases.[306] "God gives knowledge to rustics and little ones which he denies to

[n]See Chapter IV.

[o]See Partington, *History of Chemistry,* II, 209-243. This side of Van Helmont's life is discussed very comprehensively in Walter Pagel's two books: *J. B. Van Helmont; Einfuehrung in die Philosophische Medizin des Barock* (Berlin: Springer, 1930) and *The Religious and Philosophical Aspects of Van Helmont's Science and Medicine* (Baltimore: Johns Hopkins, 1944: Supplement No. 2 to the *Bulletin of the History of Medicine*).

those that are blown up with heathenish learning."[307] "Every maker or seller of oils and ointments, and old women, do thrust themselves into medicine, scoffing at physicians because they do oft-times excell them in many things."[308] "Hence it comes to pass that many an old woman is in many places far more successful in curing some defects than is the whole School of medicine, with all their discursive speculations, speculative prescriptions, and kitchen precepts of diet confirmed by long experience of the destruction of their neighbors."[309]

Many of the physician's best medicines, when not discovered by accident, have come from folk practice: "they have learned some remedies from old women or countryfolk which . . . might cure disease ideas by a specific gift."[310]

Hence the first duty of the physician is to be aware of these sources of medical experience and make use of them.

But physicians refuse to learn from therapeutic experience:

> I would to God [that physicians] were mindful of their own maxim wherein their chief curative indication or betokening sign is to be taken from things profitable and hurtful. Which rule, although it be shameful and only that of Empirics, I would that at least, by the same, they would now skip back from their committed errors.[311]

They reject knowledge which comes from laymen: they "esteem it to be a thing full of disgrace that himself being a doctor or teacher ought as yet to learn of others. A nourishing clyster, therefore, is an old-wives' invention."[312]

Instead of holding themselves open to new experience, maintaining an open mind to new discoveries, they follow the teachings of Galen, not drawn from nature and experience but cut to the measure of the human mind:

> That plausible and stupid doctrine easily pleased all that were inclined to a sluggishness of subscribing. Because it was that which might easily be conceived by a rustical sense, a great compendium, and in all places by any one;

> and hence, therefore, it was most greedily drunk in . . . Galen [took all things] from their due order as though they were contraries, that he might make an establishment of his foolish rule . . . the natural indications or betokenings of diseases to be made only by the oppositions of contraries. For he would have necessities to be subservient to his own maxims; but he erected not maxims conformable to necessities . . . Therefore that maxim hitherto remains adored by the Schools.[313]

> Physicians will not be wise but according to the custom of the Schools. For what they read they believe, and what they believe they deliver to the trust of the apothecary, his wife, and servant or family to be put in execution.[314]

They will not and cannot be wise beyond heats and colds.[315] Because lay knowledge is of effects, physicians insist that their own knowledge is of proximate causes. They will not admit to ignorance: "the modern Schools had rather to commit the essences of diseases unto discords of the elements than that they would confess the bodies of nature to bespeak nothing else besides a connexion of constitutive causes to them unknown."[316]

Hence they disregard experience which does not support their preconceived notions about proximate causes. For example, they hold that a red-hot iron promotes the healing of wounds: "what if, on the contrary, the histories of many are compared whereunto cauteries have proved ill?"

> They presently say, "We are not Empirics, nor are we moved by examples. For the Schools are rational and are supported, moreover, by the authorities of the ancients." And that thing they thus loftily thunder out as oft as they, being destitute of reasons and convicted by experiences [*convictae experientiis*] do cease to be most expert masters, neither will they be bowed down by experiences contrary to their own [*per contrarias experientias*]. But they flee with one accord into the reasons of

> predecessors, the which I have shown to be wan, sluggish, and stumbling in their first entrance.[317]

When they encounter an effect to which they cannot ascribe a cause, they either deny its existence altogether:

> It is an action of insolent malapartness for any one to deny the being of that fact which is everywhere frequent because he hath not searched out the truth thereof nor hath endeavored so to search . . . and that indeed for one only fault, to wit, because the manner of its operation by its cause cannot be understood by our censurer, by a censurer who by the sharpness of his own understanding and the study of Aristotle's *Physics* presumes that he hath on every side exactly viewed the whole circle of nature.[318]

Or they hold that such knowledge is inaccessible to the mind of man:

> The Schools are amazed when they come unto occult qualities, as they do therefore call them. For when they cannot ascribe their trifles to heats, colds, and the begged complexions of these, writers indeed do lay aside their pen, and physicians do lift up their shoulders and eyebrows because they accuse that property to be known to them in the effect but unknown in the cause. And they excuse themselves of this ignorance because the searching into those properties is impossible for man's understanding, the which they else had already long since inquired into. As if they should say: "We Schools are able to determine as much as the mind of man can search. We therefore decree that no powers of things can be understood or searched into by man but those which are the first qualities of the elements, or to arise from these."[319]

Or they invoke divine or diabolical influence: they ascribe the magnetic cure of wounds to the devil "not because it consists from an unlawful end, and of unlawful means, but because it proceeds after a manner unknown to [them]."[320]

This is all paganism, not Christianity. Instead of humbly subordinating themselves to nature, the command of God, these physicians assert themselves against nature. Their pride of knowledge cuts them off from nature: "Unto these men Seneca saith: many have not attained unto wisdom because they thought they had attained it."[321]

The physician's second duty is to love his patient. By his practice, his dispensing of curative medicines, he acts as the agent of God on earth, conveying His love to mortals. "These *arcana* do testify that they are akin to the infinite goodness, while as they do by degrees disperse their almost and, as it were, infinite virtues."[322] The physician shows his love not only by his willingness to absorb experience but also by his actual medical practice.

But to the school physicians medicine is only an economic activity. They practice in the pagan spirit—not for charity but for gain:

> Surely the ignorant flatterer is a slavish kind of cattle acting the part of a physician, yet not having any thing besides the diminishments of the body and strength, refusing to learn because he hath grown old in ill-doing, neither hath he ever diligently searched into anything worthy of praise, as being wholly intent upon gain.[323]

> For as soon as they are dismissed from the schools with the title of doctor, they enquire through the streets and inns, with the eyes of a lamprey, whether there are not sick folks which may entrust them with their life. But stop your proceedings, medicine is not to be exercised after the manner of mechanic arts . . . Possess ye charity, and gain will voluntarily follow you with honor and glory, the which take hold of a physician that shuns them, whom the most high hath commanded to be honored.[324]

Christian love requires that treatment be mild. Medicines affect the *Archeus* only by their "aspect," from afar, "without their dissolution or destruction, without their penetration, inward admission, commixture, and changing

. . . as it were only by their aspect, in beaming or darting forth of their virtues produced in a mean."[325] "Truly it acts only by touching at the *Archeus,* without a material commixture of itself. Indeed, the *Archeus* himself doth first feel the endowment drawn from the remedy, but in that act of perceivance he fashions to himself an idea of the things to be done by him, by following the dispositions of that endowment."[326] Butler cured the woman's migraine with only one drop of oil applied to her forehead.[327]

Van Helmont reduced his doses to a half-grain or less, and he opposed bloodletting, the cautery, and other violent measures of the Galenists. He urged that the patient's diet not be changed often or greatly.[328]

The physician must allow the patient to eat and drink what he wants, because his appetite represents the curative instinct of the *Archeus.*[329]

But the physicians of the schools violate all these principles, and their treatment is not only ineffectual but actually harmful to the patient: "they conspire for the destruction of mortals, likewise the destruction of the Commonwealth and families; it hath been my part utterly to destroy this execrable heresy of the doctrine of medicine."[330] Van Helmont's colleagues from time to time admitted to him that their procedures were unavailing even in acute conditions (they had long since lost hope of curing chronic ones).[331] "No wonder that the common people, heeding the vanity of these cures, have took an occasion to say: that it is the best medicine not to use medicine."[332]

Typical is their insistence on the most expensive remedies, designed only to make the patient pay more, while God has placed in each country the remedies which are needed there.[333] Medicines, in any case, need not be expensive, since the spirit of a remedy can be transferred to another medium (like Butler's stone): "for why shall the little stone touching at the tongue less cure than wolfsbane doth cause the tongue to swell by its co-touching? God hath made benefits in respect of diseases at least equal in authority, if not much more famous and more. So far is it that I should consecrate these kind of effects to the devil that I am the more powerfully moved in admiring of the divine goodness, to adore the most ready mercies of Jesus Christ my lord whereby without the labor of physicians, apothecaries, and others, who like lice are fatted only by others' miseries, to wit, whereby the miserable sick are the more safely and speedily helped."[334] "Physicians shall not remain unpunished while as the poor shall at some time mournfully complain at the Last Judgment that they were neglected, who might easily and by the way have been cured without any charges."[335]

If they had used the correct medicines in the correct small doses, they could have treated many more patients at much lower cost. "I desist not to cure some ten thousands of sick persons every year by my remedies, neither are my medicines therefore diminished."[336]

The hostility and antagonism of physician to patient is symbolized by the doctrine of contraries: "they know no other action than that which from a superiority of the agent rules over the patient. But surely those things do not savor of an help."[337] And this doctrine by the same token reflects the physician's opposition to the patient's intrinsic healing capacity:

> Hippocrates will have a physician to be only the minister or servant of the nature; but the natures themselves to be their only physiciannesses . . . otherwise a physician is the patron and master of the nature being prostrated.[338]

> From the first time wherein the Schools placed contraries in nature they presently universally established that nothing acted without strifes, war, and discords . . . Likewise, they have determined that in the whole sublunary frame or stage nothing is done or generated but by a relation of the superiority of an agent unto a patient. So, indeed, that the patient is with violence compelled, tamed, altered, destroyed, and is wholly translated into the nature of the agent only by the relation of a stronger on a weaker.[339]

The *Archeus* is "trodden under foot" by the "assumed destructive power of purging medicines and poisons."[340] Laxatives operate against "us, rather than against diseases."[341] "Neither is the law of Christ (by whom all things were made) conformable to those laws of the Schools; and so, either Christ is not the parent of the nature or an adversary to himself in the nature, or such heathen speculations of healing are rotten."[342]

If a healing power has been placed in the organism by God, the physician who employs contraries works against God as well—further proof of the pagan origin of school doctrine.

Van Helmont concludes that the school teachings only institutionalize the physician's domination of the patient, justifying all procedures which enhance this domination and furnishing convenient excuses for failure. The aim of anatomy, for example, is to find *post facto* evidence justifying the physician's diagnosis:

> For anatomists, when as they nowhere find feigned humors, yet they promise to prostitute every cause of death by the knife; first of all, they admire, then also they are earnestly angry that death should happen without their leave. For as if they had their hope and remedy in their knife, they rejoice that they have found a part in a dead carcase whereto they may attribute death.
>
> And then they dry out, "Behold a noble bowel hath long since failed by putrefying. Neither is it in the power of the physician that the sick may always find relief." And so physicians do for the most part cover their errors and comfort heirs by trifles; kinsmen are amazed and do conceive a comfort from the necessity of death. As though the putrefaction of a bowel had forexisted many months before, which a gangrene in the outward parts killeth in a few days.[343]

When the patient dies, they blame it on his intrinsic inability to be cured or his failure to follow instructions.[344] "Physicians, joining compositions to compositions, give sometimes the hodge-podge of a thousand simples to the sick to drink, that if one thing help not, at least wise another may help, or at least that they may excuse themselves that they have managed the cure of the sick according to the common rule."[345] "Excusing the deaths of men because he hath cured according to art, as having followed the flock of predecessors."[346] Thus they "never dismiss the sick out of their hand but detain them for perpetual clients, as it were, gotten bondslaves."[347]

The physician claims knowledge he does not possess. He scorns experience, the true source of wisdom. He blames failures on God or the patient. He should act as the instrument of God's mercy but is concerned only for his own advancement. He does not search humbly to improve himself but is barred by personal and professional pride.

These were the factors which drove Van Helmont into opposition:

> Truly it shamed me, even from a young man, that a workman, being called to a work, should promise that work and stand to his promises; but that I, being called to a sick man at the beginning of the disease, and his strength as yet remaining, should suffer the same man to die. For I being full of fear, believed that it was not enough to say: "It is not in the physician that the sick party always be eased." And by a liberty springing from thence rashly to proceed and continue in the work of a physician by saying, "I shall be excused because I have done what I could according to the maxims of art," if I know myself in every way defective, and that the suppositions of art themselves are rotten in their root. For indeed the ignorance of physicians proceeding ill in healing is almost capital because it is not to be blotted out with God, where a man will give skin for skin. For it is a sign that such a physician entered not in by the doors but by the windows, and attributed a false name to himself.[348]

Francis Bacon

Francis Bacon is considered the founder of British Empirical philosophy, but scholars have ignored his ties with the Empirical tradition in medicine; thereby they have underestimated the medical contribution to scientific method.

Bacon's philosophy of science seeks solutions to the same problems as those confronting the Empirical physicians: (1) the meaning of experience, (2) the strengths and limitations of sense-perception, and (3) the relations between reason and nature. Furthermore, he may well have been influenced by Paracelsus' injection of "Christian charity" into therapeutic speculation, and, although unacquainted with the writings of Van Helmont, Bacon was oriented toward the same problems and came to similar conclusions.

Reason and Nature

Like other Empirical philosophers in history, Bacon proceeded from an awareness that relations among natural objects differ from the relations among man's ideas of these objects. He was stirred by the thought that a world of knowledge lay waiting to be discovered, one alien to the interpretation of nature accepted by the dominant scholasticism:

> Men have withdrawn themselves from the contemplation of nature and experience, and sported with their own reason and the fictions of fancy. These intellectualists, though commonly taken for the most sublime and divine philosophers, are censured by Heracleitus when he says: "Men seek the truth in their own little worlds, and not in the great world about them."[349]

This new province of knowledge must be investigated in the way suited to it, according to its own rules: "the thing we mean is a kind of logic, by us called the art of interpreting nature, as differing widely from the common logic."[350]

"The specious meditations, speculations, and theories of mankind are but a kind of insanity, only there is no one to stand by and observe it."[351]

All existing philosophies are inadequate, as modern logic and philosophy yield only "arguments and discourses,"[352] "anticipations of nature" and not "interpretations of nature."[353] "The art of inventing and discovering the sciences remains hitherto unknown."[354]

"It is vain to expect any great progress in the sciences by the superinducing or engrafting new matters upon old. An instauration must be made from the very foundations."[355] Man must return to the original sources of knowledge: sense-perception and experience:

> Man as the minister and interpreter of nature, does and understands as much as his observations on the order of nature, either with regard to things or the mind, permit him, and neither knows nor is capable of more.[356]
>
> Men have hitherto dwelt but little, or rather only slightly touched upon experience, whilst they have wasted much time on theories and figments of the imagination.[357]
>
> The subtlety of things . . . is manifested by experience.[358]
>
> The foundations of experience (our sole resource) have hitherto failed completely or have been very weak.[359]

Bacon's problem was thus identical with that of the Empirical medical tradition: how man, through his senses and experience, can understand the "subtlety of nature [which] is far beyond that of sense or of the understanding."[360]

Here the scholastic invocation of sense-perception and experience is a false trail:

> Aristotle . . . corrupted natural philosophy by logic . . . being everywhere more anxious as to definitions in teaching and the accuracy of the wording of his propositions than the internal truth of things . . . Nor is much stress to be laid on his frequent recourse to experiment in

> his books on animals, his problems, and other treatises; for he had already decided, without having properly consulted experience as the basis of his decisions and axioms, and after having so decided, he drags experiment along as a captive constrained to accomodate herself to his decisions.[361]

The categories of scholastic logic distort experience and bend it to the contours of the human mind. They are too general, whereas nature is made up of particulars:

> We have but one simple method of delivering our sentiments, namely, we must bring men to particulars and their regular series and order, and they must for a while renounce their notions, and begin to form an acquaintance with things.[362]

> Men commonly take a view of nature as from a remote eminence, and are too much amused with generalities: whereas, if they would descend and approach nearer to particulars, and more exactly and considerately examine into things themselves, they might make more solid and useful discoveries.[363]

Hence a method is needed which can grasp the particulars of nature and from them develop true categories of increasing generality.

The Forms

Rejecting the scholastic method of analysis, Bacon invokes the Platonic and neo-Platonic doctrine of "forms" as a holistic technique which will do justice to the multiplicity and variety of natural objects:

> It appears to us that scarce anything in nature can be fundamentally discovered, either by accident, experimental attempts, or the light of physical causes, but only by the discovery of forms.[364]

> It is manifest that Plato, a man of sublime genius who took a view of everything as from a high rock, saw in his

> doctrine of Ideas that "forms were the true object of knowledge"; though he lost the advantage of this just opinion by contemplating and grasping at forms totally abstracted from matter, and not as determined in it; whence he turned aside to theological speculations and therewith infected all his natural philosophy. But if with diligence, seriousness, and sincerity we turn our eyes to action and use, we may find and become acquainted with those forms, the knowledge whereof will wonderfully enrich and prosper human affairs.[365]

But Bacon completely transvalued and renovated the concept of "form." It no longer meant the (non-material or material) abiding essence of an object or phenomenon, but rather the law governing the behavior of the object or phenomenon—the *formal cause.*

> When we speak of forms we mean nothing else than those laws and regulations of simple action which arrange and constitute any simple nature, such as heat, light, weight, in every species of matter, and in a susceptible subject.[366]

> This law, therefore, and its parallel in each science, is what we understand by the term, form, adopting that word because it has grown into common use and is of familiar occurrence.[367]

The discovery of forms, however, presents difficulty, since they are distorted by the objects which they rule. Furthermore, they lie beneath the surface and are thus beyond sense-perception: "It is only for God (the bestower and creator of forms), and perhaps for angels and intelligences, at once to recognize forms affirmatively at the first glance of contemplation: man, at least, is unable to do so."[368] [p]

[p]In contrast to Van Helmont, Bacon does not allow Adam and Solomon to have perceived the forms directly (see above, pp. 20, 51).

The task of philosophy is hence to give help to the senses (and also, by the way, to the understanding):

> We are not to deny the authority of the human senses and understanding, although weak, but rather to furnish them with assistance.[369]

> The unassisted hand and the understanding left to itself possess but little power. Effects are produced by the means of instruments and helps, which the understanding requires no less than the hand; and as instruments either promote or regulate the motion of the hand, so those that are applied to the mind prompt or protect the understanding.[370]

This is done by applying a suitable *method,* one which compensates for the weakness of the senses and understanding: "our only remaining hope and salvation is to begin the whole labor of the mind again; not leaving it to itself but directing it perpetually from the very first, and attaining our end, as it were, by mechanical aid."[371]

Bacon, like other Empirics, was striving to master experience and reduce it to a method. "For vague and arbitrary experience is (as we have observed) mere groping in the dark, and rather astonishes than instructs. But when experience shall proceed regularly and uninterruptedly by a determined rule, we may entertain better hopes of the sciences."[372] "A system has been pursued in philosophy with regard to experience resembling that of a kingdom or state which would direct its councils and affairs according to the gossip of city and street politicians, instead of the letters and reports of ambassadors and messengers worthy of credit. Nothing is rightly inquired into, or verified, noted, weighed, or measured, in natural history; indefinite and vague observation produces fallacious and uncertain information."[373]

In proclaiming that experience must be reduced to a method Bacon went beyond the mystics (who had not imposed rules on their experience). He was also in advance of Van Helmont whose method of investigation was unclear in its details and shrouded in religious exhortation. But Bacon's method has much in common with that proposed earlier by the Empirical School.

The Idols

The first labor of the mind is a negative one—clearing away the "idols"—tissues of speculation, prejudice, and received opinion which beset man's understanding and block his view of nature.[q] These are the idols of the tribe, idols of the den, idols of the market place, and idols of the theater. All existing philosophies are vitiated by one or another of these idols.

The idols of the tribe are the misconceptions inherent in human nature, man's propensity to accept his sensory and intellectual perceptions as the measure of the universe, whereas they refer only to his own mind: "the human mind resembles those uneven mirrors which impart their own properties to different objects, from which rays are emitted and distort and disfigure them."[374]

The idols of the den are those peculiar to the individual, for each has his own "individual den or cavern which intercepts and corrupts the light of nature, either from his own peculiar and singular disposition, or from his education and intercourse with others, or from his reading."[375]

The idols of the market-place arise from the "commerce and association of men with each other; for men converse by means of language, but words are formed at the will of the generality, and there arises from a bad and unapt formation of words a wonderful obstruction to the mind."[376]

The idols of the theater "have crept into men's minds from the various dogmas of peculiar systems of philosophy."[377] They usually involve assuming the order of nature to be simpler and more regular than it actually is, "and

[q]Bacon draws a parallel between these idols of the human mind and the "forms" which are "idols of the divine mind." The former, however, are "certain idle dogmas," while the latter are "the real stamp and impression of created objects, as they are found in nature" (*Novum Organum,* I, Aph. XXIII and CXXIV).

although many things in nature be *sui generis* and most irregular, will yet invent parallels and conjugates and relatives where no such thing is."[378]

This is precisely the criticism to be made of scholasticism —that it fails to do justice to the variety of nature: "for the subtlety of nature is vastly superior to that of argument."[379]

> But [scholastic method] was of such a nature that they immediately flew from a few instances and particulars (after adding some common notions and a few generally received opinions most in vogue) to the most general conclusions or the principles of the sciences, and then by their intermediate propositions deduced their inferior conclusions, and tried them by the test of the immovable and settled truth of the first, and so constructed their art. Lastly, if some new particulars and instances were brought forward which contradicted their dogmas, they either with great subtlety reduced them to one system, by distinctions or explanations of their own rules, or got rid of them clumsily as exceptions, laboring most pertinaciously in the mean time to accomodate the causes of such as were not contradictory to their own principles. Their natural history and their experience were both far from being what they ought to have been, and their flying off to generalities ruined everything.[380]

In this they were simply yielding to an inherent weakness of the human mind:

> The human understanding, when any proposition has been once laid down . . . forces everything else to add fresh support and confirmation; and although most cogent and abundant instances may exist to the contrary, yet either does not observe or despises them, or gets rid of and rejects them by some distinction, with violent and injurious prejudice, rather than sacrifice the authority of its first conclusions.[381]

But the consequence of this philosophy's love for generalities and scorn for particulars is its omission from consideration of those rare and *negative instances* which might vitiate its conclusions.

Bacon is therefore concerned with incorporating into his philosophy of nature the rare and *negative instances* which are ignored by the schools.

The Inductive Method

As a cure for weakness of observation and understanding, a technique for preventing the idols from contaminating thought, and an instrument for obtaining knowledge of nature, Bacon proposed the inductive method.

The existing inductive mode of the scholastics is only by simple enumeration and is thus "puerile, leads to uncertain conclusions, and is exposed to danger from one contradictory instance, deciding generally from too small a number of facts, and those only the most obvious."[382] The true inductive method "should separate nature by proper rejections and exclusions, and then conclude for the affirmative after collecting a sufficient number of negatives."[383]

In contrast to the scholastic mode of flying from particulars to very general propositions, and thence deducing the intermediate ones, the true inductive method proceeds from particulars to intermediate propositions and from there to the most general ones.[384] Of these the "lowest axioms differ but little from bare experiment; the highest and most general (as they are esteemed at present) are notional, abstract, and of no real weight. The intermediate are true, solid, full of life, and upon them depend the business and fortune of mankind."[385]

In this way abstract knowledge will develop like the mechanical arts which, "founded on nature and the light of experience .... seem full of life and uninterruptedly thrive and grow."[386]

Up until now man has allowed experience to happen *to him,* in the form of chance events, and at most has sought out the occasions of such chance happenings: "but this kind of experience is nothing but a loose faggot and mere groping in the dark, as men at night try all means of discovering the right road."[387] Although such chance happenings are extremely valuable, and in the past have been man's only means of discovery, in themselves they are insufficient.[388] Man must, as it were, force nature and compel her to reveal her secrets: "for as a man's temper is never well known until he is crossed, in like manner the turns and changes of nature cannot appear so fully, when she is left at her liberty, as in the trials and tortures of art."[389] [r]

Experience must be multiplied, converted into experiments: "We must not only search for and procure a greater number of experiments, but also introduce a completely different method, order, and progress of continuing and promoting experience."[390] "Experience is by far the best demonstration, provided it adhere to the experiment actually made."[391] [s]

But experiments are not performed at random. The investigator must proceed step by step in a settled way, systematically bringing to light various aspects of natural processes: "our hope of further progress in the sciences will then only be well founded, when numerous experiments shall be received and collected into natural history, which, though of no use in themselves, assist materially in the discovery of causes and axioms."[392] As a guide to the performance of experiments Bacon proposes a "certain art of indication or direction, to disclose and bring other arts to light, together with their axioms and effects."[393] This art of indication has two parts: indications proceed (1) from experiment to experiment and (2) from experiments to axioms which point the way to new experiments.[394]

This variation in the production of experiments Bacon calls "learned" or "literate" experience: "so when a man tries all kinds of experiments without method or order, this is

[r]Cf. Paracelsus: "*in extremis* things reveal their nature and become visible" (*Divided Legacy*, I, 459).

[s]Cf. the transition from "experience" to "experiment" in the Empirical School (*Divided Legacy*, I, 264).

mere groping in the dark; but when he proceeds with some direction and order in his experiments, it is as if he were led by the hand; and this we understand by learned experience."[395] It is a technique or techniques for extending the results obtained in one set of circumstances to a slightly different set: "the variation, production, translation, inversion, compulsion, application, conjunction, or any other manner of diversifying or making chance experiments."[396]

An experiment may be varied in its subject: as, attempting to make paper out of silk instead of linen.[397] It may be varied in its efficient cause: the sun's rays, when focussed by a magnifying glass, are hot enough to burn paper, and Bacon suggests that the same be attempted with the rays of the moon "so as to show whether all the heavenly bodies are potentially hot."[398] It may be varied in quantity: "for men imagine that upon increasing the quantity the virtue should increase proportionately; and this they commonly postulate as a mathematical certainty, and yet it is utterly false."[399] A lead ball weighing two pounds will not fall to the ground twice as fast as one weighing one pound: "no, they will fall almost in equal times, and not be accelerated according to quantity."[400] "Men should therefore remember how Aesop's housewife was deceived, who expected that by doubling her feed her hen should lay two eggs a day; but the hen grew fat and laid none. It is absolutely unsafe to rely on any natural experiment before proof be made of it, both in a less and a larger quantity."[401]

Not only may experiments be "varied," they may be "transferred: (1) by nature or chance into an art, (2) from one art or practice to another, and (3) from one part of an art to another."[402]

The first is so common that "nearly all the mechanical arts owe their origins to slender beginnings afforded by nature or accident." For example, a proverb holds that grapes among grapes ripen sooner, and cider-makers, therefore, do not press their apples without laying them on heaps for a time to ripen by mutual contact. Hence mankind should continue to observe particular operations of nature "and be continually examining and casting about which of them may be transferred to arts; for nature is the mirror of art."[403] [t]

Transferring experiments from one art or practice to another is more rare, since "particular arts are only known to particular artists," but it is in principle possible. Spectacles aid the sight, and something similar for the hearing could also be devised. Embalming preserves dead bodies: "could not, therefore, something of like kind be transferred to medicine, for the preservation of live ones?"[404]

Similar is the transfer of experiments from one part of the art to another. "It greatly contributes to enlarge the art of medicine to have the experiments of that part which treats of the cures of diseases transferred to those parts which relate to the preservation of health and the prolongation of life."[405]

Experiments may be inverted, in this way demonstrating the contrary: "heat is increased by a burning-glass, but may cold be so too?"[406]

Experiments may be "compelled, i.e., forced to their farthest limits: thus, the lodestone attracts iron, but will it continue to attract when melted or dissolved in acid?"[407]

Even the failure of an experiment yields information, "for though success be indeed more pleasing, yet failure, frequently, is no less informing."[408]

The second category of experiments are those inspired by axioms. Hence we must see how the axioms themselves come into being.

The discovery of axioms—the whole purpose of Bacon's philosophy—is based on man's knowledge of the "forms" inherent in physical reality. All observed phenomena, whether spontaneous or induced, are functions of the movement of forms under the surface of matter (which Bacon calls "nature"). The investigator's task is to compare

[t]Cf. the "passage-from-like-to-like" of the Empirical School (*Divided Legacy,* I, 268 ff.). The Empirics held that discoveries came from "nature or chance" (*ibid.,* 266).

and contrast with one another the various "natures" in which forms appear, so as to isolate and define the pure form.[409] The natures must thus be separated and dissolved, "not by fire but by the mind, that divine fire."[410]

While knowledge of the phenomena is initially stored in the memory,[u] memory alone is not sufficient for this purpose, any more than a "person would be of retaining and achieving, by memory, the computation of an almanac."[411] For this reason the natures must be arranged in tables:

> There is such a multitude and host, as it were, of particular objects, and lying so widely dispersed, as to distract and confuse the understanding; and we can, therefore, hope for no advantage from its skirmishing and quick movements and incursions unless we put its forces in due order and array by means of proper and well arranged and, as it were, living tables of discovery of these matters which are the subject of investigation, and the mind then apply itself to the ready prepared and digested aid which such tables afford.[412]

The first—the "table of existence and presence"—is a table of instances whose natures agree, "although the subject matter be considerably diversified."[413] The second is one of "instances which do not admit of the given nature, for form (as we have observed) ought no less to be absent where the given nature is absent than to be present where it is present."[414] Since there would be no point in amassing all instances in which the given nature is absent, only those which are very similar to the ones in the first table are presented: "which have a very close connection with those others in which it is present and manifest." The aim is to distinguish them from the above, and this is called a "table of deviation or of absence in proximity."[415]

The third table is of instances in which forms appear to increase or decrease with increase or decrease in natures, since "no nature can be considered a real form which does

[u]On Bacon's doctrine of memory see below, p. 88.

not uniformly diminish and increase with the given nature."[416] This table is one of "degrees or comparative instances."[417]

These three tables are combined into a fourth, called an "exclusive table," which serves for the "exclusion or rejection" of natures found by the tables of review not to be of the form for whose elucidation the investigation is made.[418] "After an exclusion correctly effected, an affirmative form will remain as the residuum, solid, true, and well-defined, whilst all volatile opinions go off in smoke."[419]

This last table is the foundation of a true induction: "for on an individual review of all the instances a nature [i.e., a form] is to be found such as always to be present and absent with the given nature, to increase and decrease with it, and, as we have said, to form a more common limit of the nature."[420]

The induction which emerges from this process is the axiom which is the basic building-block of the new science. It is not merely accepted as such but must continually be polished and retested to ascertain its limits. Such axioms, furthermore, *suggest new experiments.*[421] "Axioms properly and regularly abstracted from particulars easily point out and define new particulars, and therefore impart activity to the sciences."[422]

These axioms are quite different from those now in use, which are "derived from a scanty handful, as it were, of experience, and a few particulars of frequent occurrence . . . And if any neglected or unknown instance occurs, the axiom is saved by some frivolous distinction, when it would be more consistent with truth to amend it."[423]

Bacon's method thus yields a science consisting of a structure of axioms, ranging from the lowest (which are accurate reflections of particulars) to axioms of the most comprehensive scope.[424]

Bacon and the Empirical and Scientific Tradition

Bacon's relations with the Empirical tradition may be examined in terms of the latter's three stages: (a) the

Sceptical philosophers, (b) the Empirical School, and (c) Paracelsus and his followers.

(a) *Bacon and the Sceptical philosophers.* The Sceptics aided the development of Empiricism through their critique of Rationalism and their proposal of a probabilistic basis of conduct.[v] Pyrrho of Elis (c. 360-270 B.C.) and his followers argued against the reliability of sensory data, consequently against the Stoic doctrine of the "irresistible impression" (an idea or judgment based on observation) as a reliable guide to action. They held no opinion to be so irresistible as to compel assent to a given course of action and hence opted for passivity. But the later members of this school, in particular Carneades of Cyrene (c. 213-129 B.C.) and Aenesidemos (first century, B.C.) advanced from this position of passivity to develop a probabilistic basis for conduct. While all sense-impressions are unreliable, and consequently do not compel assent, some are less unreliable than others: hence judgments can be classified according to degrees of certainty, and conduct can be based upon the probability of success.

Bacon admired the Sceptics and their critique of Rationalism:

> There were some few, both in the old and new academies, but more among the Sceptics, who held this principle of doubting in simplicity and sincerity of heart.[425]

> It was not, therefore, without cause, that many of the ancient philosophers, and some of them eminent in their way, became academics and Sceptics who denied all certainty of human knowledge and held that the understanding went no further than appearance and probability.[426]

> They who have asserted that nothing whatever can be known, whether they have fallen into this opinion from their hatred of the ancient sophists, or from the hesitation of their minds, or from an exuberance of

[v]See *Divided Legacy,* I, 184-194.

> learning, have certainly adduced reasons for it which are by no means contemptible.[427]

But he felt that they went too far in rejecting for all time the possibility of reliable sensory knowledge: "their chief error lay in accusing the perceptions of the senses, and thus plucked up the sciences by their roots."[428] "Hence arose the New Academy, which openly professed Scepticism and consigned mankind to eternal darkness; hence the notion that forms, or the true differences of things (which are in fact the laws of simple action), are beyond man's reach and cannot possibly be discovered . . ."[429]

He agreed with their urge to find a reliable guide to action but held probability to be an insufficient basis:

> Although this method [of the New Academy] be more honest than arbitrary decision (for its followers allege that they by no means confound all inquiry, like Pyrrho and his disciples, but hold doctrines which they can follow as probable, though they cannot maintain them to be true), yet when the human mind has once despaired of discovering truth, everything begins to languish.[430]

Instead, he proposed the formal cause as the true basis for action, the key to the mastery of nature. "That which in contemplative philosophy corresponds with the [formal] cause in practical science becomes the rule."[431] He who knows the formal causes "stirs the limits of things."[432]

Thus, whereas the Sceptics had rejected all four of the Aristotelian causes, Bacon accepted the formal cause and rejected the other three. The efficient and material causes apply to mechanics only and are of little use in the investigation of nature, which does not operate by mechanical laws.[433] They are of "scarcely any avail to real and active knowledge."[434] He who knows them "can induce a certain effect upon particular substances only, among those which are susceptible of it, [and] has acquired but an imperfect power."[435] As for the final cause, it is but "a barren thing, or as a virgin consecrated to God."[436]

The concern with action or practice, which in Scepticism was aimed at finding a guide to personal conduct, became, with Bacon, the desire to conquer and control the world of nature—thus contributing to the scientific outlook: "the point in view is not only the contemplative happiness, but the whole fortunes, and affairs, and powers, and works of man."[437] "For I find that even those that have sought knowledge for itself and not for benefit or ostentation or any practical enablement in the course of their life, have nevertheless propounded to themselves a wrong mark, namely, satisfaction (which men call truth) and not operation . . . as in the courts and services of princes and states it is a much easier matter to give satisfaction than to do the business."[438] "The real and legitimate goal of the sciences is the endowment of human life with new inventions and riches."[439] "Information begins from the senses, but our whole labor terminates in practice, and as the former is the beginning, so is the latter the end of our subject."[440] "Knowledge and human power are synonymous, since the ignorance of the cause frustrates the effect; for nature is only subdued by submission."[441]

Bacon's method of investigation assured the reliability of sensory observation and eliminated the need to proceed by probability: "we, as it were, restore the senses to their former rank . . . and open and establish a new and certain course for the mind from the first actual perceptions of the senses themselves."[442] "For, though the senses often deceive or fail us, yet, when industriously assisted, they may suffice for the sciences, and this not so much by the help of instruments, which also have their use, as of such experiments which may furnish more subtle objects than are perceivable by sense . . . And this we say, not to detract from the human mind, or as if the work were to be deserted, but that proper assistance may be procured and administered to the understanding, whereby to conquer the difficulties of things and the obscurities of nature. What we endeavor is that the mind, by the help of art, may become equal to things, and to find a certain art of indication or direction, to disclose and bring other arts to light, together with their axioms and effects."[443]

> Our method and that of the Sceptics agree in some respects at first setting out, but differ most widely and are completely opposed to each other in their conclusion; for they roundly assert that nothing can be known; we that but a small part of nature can be known, by the present method; their next step, however, is to destroy the authority of the senses and understanding, while we invent and supply them with assistance.[444]

(b) *Bacon and the Empirical School.* Bacon's attitude toward the ancient Empirics is ambiguous, probably because of his ignorance of the Empirical therapeutic method and his unawareness that Celsus, whom he admires and frequently cites, was the epitome of Empirical therapeutic thought.[445] Thus he criticizes the Empirics while borrowing heavily from them *via* the writings of Celsus.

Generally he reproaches this school (which he identifies with the modern "empirical" physicians, i.e., those lacking a formal education)[w] for the same failing as the Rationalists—willingness to jump from insufficient factual data to general conclusions. The difference between the two is that the Empirical factual data are the outcome of some few and unmethodical experiments:

> The empiric school produces dogmas of a more deformed and monstrous nature than the sophistic or theoretic

[w]"It is wrong to trust the natural body to empirics, who commonly have a few receipts whereon they rely, but who know neither the causes of diseases, nor the constitutions of patients, nor the danger of accidents, nor the true method of cure" (*Adv. of Learn.,* 33). This category also includes the alchemists (*Novum Organum,* I, Aph. LXIV). But he still has a lingering affection for them: "hence it chiefly proceeds that empirics and women are often more successful in their cures than learned physicians, because the former keep strictly and invariably to the use of experienced medicines, without altering their compositions" (*Adv. of Learn.,* 164).

Max Wellmann was the first to demonstrate (in 1913) that Celsus' *De Medicina* was an Empirical work or at least patterned on existing Empirical treatises (*Divided Legacy,* I, 200*t*).

> school; not being founded in the light of common notions (which, however poor and superstitious, is yet in a manner universal, and of a general tendency), but in the confined obscurity of a few experiments . . . We have a strong instance of this in the alchemists and their dogmas . . . We could not, however, neglect to caution others against this school, because we already foresee and augur that if men be hereafter induced by our exhortations to apply seriously to experiments (bidding farewell to the sophistic doctrines), there will then be imminent danger from empirics, owing to the premature and forward haste of the understanding, and its jumping or flying to generalities and the principles of things. We ought, therefore, already to meet the evil.[446]

Thus the ideas of the "empirics" also need correction from natural philosophy: "the art of medicine, without the assistance of natural philosophy, differs but little from empiricism."[447] The empirics do not understand the procedure of deducing "causes and axioms from effects and experiments, and new effects and experiments from those causes and axioms."[448] It is this philosophical expansion of empiricism which Bacon wants to provide.

He sees his philosophy as occupying the middle ground between the Empirical and Rationalist positions:

> Those who have treated of the sciences have been either empirics or dogmatical. The former, like ants, only heap up and use their store; the latter, like spiders, spin out their own webs. The bee, a mean between both, extracts matter from the flowers of the garden and the field, but works and fashions it by its own efforts. The true labor of philosophy resembles hers, for it neither relies entirely or principally on the powers of the mind, nor yet lays up in the memory the matter afforded by the experiments of natural history and mechanics in its raw state, but changes and works it in the understanding. We have good reason, therefore, to derive hope from a closer and purer

alliance of these faculties (the experimental and rational) than has yet been attempted.[449] [x]

His philosophy of investigation, however, is in no way a balance of Empiricism and Rationalism, as Bacon, in fact, leans heavily to the former.

Both his own philosophy and ancient Empiricism were reactions to Aristotle's metaphysical doctrine of causes and, specifically, to the use of this doctrine as an instrument of investigation. Bacon cites Celsus who "speaking of the empirical and dogmatical sects of physicians, gravely and ingenuously acknowledges that medicines and cures were first discovered, and the reasons and causes of them discoursed afterwards, not that causes, first derived from the nature of things, gave light to the invention of cures and remedies."[450] "It is an idle thing, and shows a narrow mind, to think that the art of discovering the sciences may be invented and proposed in perfection from the beginning, so as to be afterwards only exercised and brought into use; for men should be made sensible that the solid and real arts of invention grow up and increase along with inventions themselves; so that when any one first comes to the thorough examination of a science, he should have some useful rules of discovery; but after he hath made a considerable progress in the science itself, he may, and ought, to find out new rules of invention, the better to lead him still further."[451]

Both were therefore concerned with a method for discovering new knowledge: "the introduction of great inventions appears one of the most distinguished of human actions, and the ancients so considered it; for they assigned divine honors to the authors of inventions."[452] Scholasticism is incapable of this: "the invention of arguments is not

[x]He suggests that this was the position of "the more ancient Greeks (whose writings have perished) [who] held a more prudent mean between the arrogance of dogmatism and the despair of scepticism" (*Novum Organum,* Preface). Elsewhere in the same writing, however, he admits that this is just a flight of fancy, an "attempt" "to derive authority and honor from thence, as men of no family labor to raise and form nobility for themselves in some ancient line, by the help of genealogies" (*Ibid.,* I, Aph. CXXII).

properly an invention; for to invent is to discover things unknown before, and not to recollect or admit such as are known already."[453] "Our present sciences are nothing more than peculiar arrangements of matters already discovered, and not methods for discovery or plans for new operations."[454] Hence, knowledge must be sought in a different way—from the discovery of particulars: "and this did Celsus note wisely and truly, how that the causes which are in use and whereof the knowledges now received do consist, were in time minors and subsequent to the knowledge of the particulars out of which they were induced and collected; and that it was not the light of those causes which discovered particulars, but only the particulars being first found, men did fall on glossing and discoursing of the causes; which is the reason why the learning that now is hath the curse of barrenness and is, courtesan-like, for pleasure and not for fruit."[455]

Such discovery comes only from observation and experience, the improvement of memory, the accurate recording of history, and, finally, application of an analytical instrument to the events observed and experienced. For both Bacon and the Empirics "science" is the crystallization of experience.

Bacon's reliance on observation and experience has already been discussed, but he follows the ancient Empirics as well in stressing the importance of memory—and of history as crystallized memory—in furnishing materials for analysis. The *Advancement of Learning* has a whole chapter on the "art of memory" in which he observes: "scarce anything can be more useful in the ancient and popular sciences than a true and solid help for the memory."[456] And his writings refer repeatedly to the significance of history (the collective memory of mankind) for science:

> The sciences are like pyramids, erected upon the single basis of history and experience, and therefore a history of nature is the basis of natural philosophy.[457]

> History and experience are one and the same thing; so are philosophy and the sciences.[458]

> We must begin, therefore, to entertain hopes of natural philosophy then only, when we have a better compilation of natural history, its real basis and support.[459]

Bacon's "learned" or "literate" experience, which he calls "rather a sagacity or a scenting of nature, as in hunting, than a direct science,"[460] is identical with the Empirical "passage-from-like-to-like" *(homoiou metabasis; transitio similis)* and has the same function of enlarging the mass of experimental data to which the instrument of analysis can be applied.

And the instrument of analysis itself, Bacon's tables of instances and the inductions from them, seem clearly patterned on Carneades of Cyrene's classification of judgments as applied to medicine by Menodotos of Nicomedea and described by Sextus Empiricus and Galen.[y] The highest degree of reliability and certainty was attributed to events occurring invariably and without any contradictory instances; the second grade were those accompanied by only a few negatives; the third grade were those with a 50% probability of occurrence; and the fourth were those occurring only rarely, with negative instances predominating.[z] While Bacon's classification is an improvement over this one, and his argument that analysis reveals the underlying "form" is a new and significant element, the similarities are still great between his inductive method and that of Carneades.

In both cases the purpose of analysis was the formulation of axioms (which the Empirics called *theoremata* or *epilogis-*

[y]While many of Bacon's ideas are of course taken from Sextus Empiricus and Celsus, one is tempted to speculate that he was also familiar with Galen's *De Subfiguratione Empirica* which sets forth the Empirical method of scientific investigation in great detail (*Divided Legacy,* I, 262-274). After lying hidden for centuries this writing was discovered and issued in a Latin translation by Niccolo à Reggio in 1502 and again in 1541—twenty years before Bacon's birth.

Karl Deichgraeber, the only scholar to have discussed these matters, concludes that Bacon did not borrow from the Empirical School, despite the many parallels between them (*Die Griechische Empirikerschule* [Berlin/Zurich: Weidmann, 1965], 340-347).

[z]*Divided Legacy,* I, 189-192.

moi).[a] For both, the science consisted of such axioms. Both accepted a probabilistic definition of truth: despite his criticism of the Sceptics, Bacon admits that his own method is one of "determining the degrees of certainty."[461]

When Bacon holds that his method employs axioms to construct new experiments,[462] he is suggesting the modern procedure of investigation in the light of a hypothesis, and this seems to be an advance over the Empirical School.[b] [c]

Finally, Bacon accepts the Empirical fusion of theory and practice:

> From the discovery of forms, therefore, results genuine theory and free practice.[463]

> These two rules, the practical and theoretical, are in fact the same, and that which is most useful in practice is most correct in theory.[464]

The practical results prove the correctness of theory

> Truth, therefore, and utility are here perfectly identical, and the effects are of more value as pledges of truth than from the benefit they confer on men.[465]

[a]*Divided Legacy,* I, 271-274. Bacon is mistaken when he denies that the Empirics formulated axioms (*Novum Organum,* I, Aph. CXVII).

[b]While the surviving Empirical fragments do not specifically suggest using *theoremata* or *epilogismoi* as hypotheses for further investigation, this procedure may have been employed without being defined as such.

[c]Bacon has been criticized for alleged failure to understand the significance of the hypothesis for scientific investigation. His use of the word classifies it with the idols which inhibit true understanding (*Novum Organum,* II, Aph. VIII). A "hypothesis," in his view, is destroyed by a single contradictory instance, and he wants his axioms to be more solidly grounded (*Novum Organum,* II, Aph. XVIII). But this is merely a dispute over words. The "axiom" which points the way to further experiments serves as a "hypothesis" (in the modern sense of the word) for Bacon, as does the "experiment for light"—"the real order of experience begins by setting up a light, and then shows the road by it, commencing with a regulated and digested, not a misplaced and vague course of experiment, and thence deducing axioms, and from those axioms new experiments" (*Novum Organum,* I, Aph. LXXXII). "Hypothesis" only acquired its modern meaning in the posthumous work of Nicolaus Copernicus (1473-1543) on the heliocentric theory of the universe and in the discussion by Johannes Kepler (1571-1630) of the orbit of Mars in terms of its hypothesized ellipticity.

> Of all signs there is none more certain or worthy than that of the fruits produced, for the fruits and effects are the sureties and vouchers, as it were, for the truth of philosophy.[466]

As we have stated,[d] the Empirical and Rationalist ideologies arise spontaneously in medicine and other disciplines, being the product of social and psychological forces. Bacon did not have to inherit the Empirical outlook from some written source but could well have arrived at this standpoint himself. In any case, the parallels between his method and that of the ancient Empirics are striking.

(c) *Bacon and the Paracelsan tradition.* Bacon criticized Paracelsus' extremist view that the organism contains "definite analogies to all the variety of specific natures in the world," perverting the ancient doctrine of microcosm and macrocosm,[467] but he praised Petrus Severinus for reducing the Paracelsan theories "into a body and harmony of philosophy."[468] It seems probable that some of the Empirical themes in Bacon's philosophy came to him *via* the Paracelsan tradition.

Paracelsus had restructured Empiricism by suffusing it with Christianity; from this he developed a series of imperatives governing the relations between man and God, man and man, and man and nature.

God's love for man is manifested through medicine, which relieves some of the pain and tragedy of life. The physician is God's agent, the bearer of His love; he must be worthy of this assignment, acting responsibly (from knowledge) and not irresponsibly (from mere opinion).

The physician shows his love by his careful observation of the patient and his diligence in healing him. He should not be blinded to the patient's needs by vanity and arrogance.

The healing process is not one of domination by the physician but of equality, since all are equal in the sight of God and in the capacity to observe and experience.

[d] *Divided Legacy,* I, Introduction.

All are equal also in the obligation to work, being descended from Adam who was expelled from Paradise and condemned to seek salvation through toil.

Nature is the reflection of God's will; man can achieve salvation, coming to know God, by investigating nature.

These themes are all present in Bacon's scientific philosophy and in his comments on medicine and physicians, leading one scholar recently to suggest that he took them from Paracelsus.[469]

J. R. Ravetz poses the question why Bacon switched in his late twenties from literary-humanistic to natural-scientific interests. "The most likely source of Bacon's conversion seems to be some current of Pietistic Paracelsan philosophy; there one would find the mixture of the themes of Christian charity and manual interaction with the things of Nature. The sentiments of scepticism of official learning, pity for the sufferings of mankind, and dedication to a pure and holy reform that Van Helmont shows in his autobiography are strikingly similar to those of Bacon. This is not to assert any link of influence between the two, but to indicate that their common form of commitment may well have derived from a common source."[470] Ravetz also notes that Petrus Severinus is "one of the few 'moderns' for whom Bacon shows any respect."[471]

The themes of work, charity, sense-perception, and the pursuit of truth all figure in Bacon's prayer in *The Great Instauration,* which is remarkably like Van Helmont's prayer quoted above:[e]

> We here, at the entrance of our work, with the utmost humility and fervency, put forth our prayers to God, that remembering the miseries of mankind and the pilgrimage of this life, where we pass but few days and sorrowful, he would vouchsafe, through our hands, and the hands of others, to whom he has given the like mind, to relieve the human race by a new act of his bounty. We likewise humbly beseech him, that what is human may not clash with what is divine; and that when the ways of the senses

[e]See above, p. 22.

> are opened, and a greater natural light set up in the mind, nothing of incredulity and blindness towards divine mysteries may arise; but rather that the understanding, now cleared up and purged of all vanity and superstition, may remain entirely subject to the divine oracles and yield to faith the things that are faith's: and lastly, that expelling the poisonous knowledge infused by the serpent, which puffs up and swells the human mind, we may neither be wise beyond measure nor go beyond the bounds of sobriety, but pursue the truth in charity.[472]

Clearly charity is as important to Bacon as it was to Paracelsus—the indispensable basis of a correct scientific method; the investigator must love the objects of investigation if only because they themselves embody the will of God, and their knowledge is the path to salvation.

> The greatest error of all is mistaking the ultimate end of knowledge; for some men covet knowledge out of a natural curiosity and inquisitive temper; some to entertain the mind with variety and delight; some for ornament and reputation; some for victory and contention; many for lucre and a livelihood; and but few for employing the divine gift of reason to the use and benefit of mankind . . . a storehouse for the glory of the Creator and the endowment of human life.[473]

Ravetz observes: "Far from imagining a 'conflict between science and religion,' Bacon saw the investigation of nature as a divine work. It not only served to reveal God's works and to reform the intellect and soul of the inquirer, but also to imitate Christ in the relief of man's estate." Man's corruption is from vanity, and his salvation comes through charity.[474]

Bacon, furthermore, held that the knowledge revealed by his method was truth, not opinion: "If any individual desire . . . not in short to give elegant and specious opinions, but to know to a certainty and demonstration, let him, as a true son of science . . . join with us."[475] [f]

[f] See Paracelsus: "not to guess, but to know" (*Divided Legacy*, I, 462).

The egalitarianism which is a corollary of Christian charity is present in Bacon's writings: his method is one which "merely levels men's wits, and leaves but little to their superiority, since it achieves everything by the most certain rules and demonstrations."[476] [g] His choice of materials for investigation also betrays his democratic instincts:

> With regard to the meanness or even the filthiness of particulars, for which (as Pliny observes) an apology is requisite, such subjects are no less worthy of admission into natural history than the most magnificent and costly; nor do they at all pollute natural history, for the sun enters alike the palace and the privy, and is not thereby polluted.[477]

> The evil has been wonderfully increased by an opinion, or inveterate conceit, which is both vainglorious and prejudicial, namely, that the dignity of the human mind is lowered by long and frequent intercourse with experiments and particulars, which are the objects of sense, and confined to matter; especially since such matters generally require labor in investigation, are mean subjects for meditation, harsh in discourse, unproductive in practice, infinite in number, and delicate in their subtlety. Hence we have seen the true path not only deserted, but intercepted and blocked up, experience being rejected with disgust, and not merely neglected or improperly applied.[478]

Because men are equal in original sin they must equally work for salvation. The Fall deprived man of domination over nature, and this can be recovered only through the arts and sciences: "for creation did not become entirely and utterly rebellious by the curse, but in consequence of the Divine decree, 'in the sweat of thy brow shalt thou eat bread,' she is compelled by our labors (not assuredly by our disputes or magical ceremonies), at length, to afford mankind

[g] Anderson states that Bacon freed science from "learning and the practices and privileges of the learned" (F. H. Anderson, *The Philosophy of Francis Bacon* [Chicago: University of Chicago, 1948], 293).

to some degree his bread, that is to say, to supply man's daily wants."[479] "Not to overcome his adversaries in disputes, but nature by labor."[480]

Bacon's discussion of medicine in the *Advancement of Learning* follows similar lines.

While founded by Apollo and Aesculapius, "medicine receives far greater honor from the works of our Savior who was physician both to soul and body."[481] Since then, however, it has stagnated: "Medicine . . . has been rather professed than labored, and yet more labored than advanced, as the pains bestowed thereon were rather circular than progressive; for I find great repetition and but little new in the writers of physic."[482]

Bacon criticizes physicians for their unwillingness to labor and their excessive orientation toward generalitics.

They act in haste and without precision, hoping to accomplish quickly what must by its nature be a lengthy process:

> The methods of cure in use are too short to effect anything that is difficult or very considerable. For it is rather vain and flattering, than just and rational, to expect that any medicine should be so effectual or so successful as by the sole use thereof to work any great cure . . . Such miracles are not to be expected; but the things of greatest efficacy in nature are order, perseverence, and an artificial change of applications which, though they require exact judgment to prescribe, and precise observance to follow, yet this is amply recompensed by the great effects they produce.[483]
>
> Physicians should know, for example, that perhaps three or four remedies rightly prescribed in an inveterate disease, and taken in due order and at due distances of time, may perform a cure; and yet the same remedies taken independently of each other, in an inverted order or not at stated periods, might prove absolutely prejudicial . . . the way should be as exact as it is confined and difficult. And this part of medicine we note as deficient.[484]

> Be assured that the prolongation of life is a laborious work that requires many kinds of remedies, and a proper continuation and intermixture thereof.[485h]

Then, when their procedures fail, they blame the art and not themselves, although "to pronounce diseases incurable is to establish negligence and carelessness as it were by a law, and screen ignorance from reproach."[486] It is "to be observed in every art, namely, that its promoters convert the weakness of the art itself into a calumny upon nature: and whatever it in their hands fails to effect, they pronounce to be physically impossible. But how can the art ever be condemned whilst it acts as judge in its own case?"[487]

They are too concerned with the general and abstract at the expense of the particular and concrete: "if they would descend and approach nearer to particulars, and more exactly and considerately examine into things themselves, they might make more solid and useful discoveries . . . if physicians, leaving generalities for a while and suspending their assent, would advance towards nature, they might become masters of that art."[488] They have discontinued "that useful method of Hippocrates, in writing narratives of particular cures with diligence and exactness, containing the nature, the cure, and event of the distemper."[489]

This superficial attitude is seen in anatomy: "the general parts of the human body are diligently observed, and even to niceness, but as to the variety found in different bodies, here the diligence of physicians fails."[490]

They ignore as well the distinction between a live body and a dead one: "many subtle pores, passages, and perforations appear not upon dissection, because they are closed and concealed in dead bodies that might be open and manifest in live ones."[491] But since (as Celsus has noted) vivisection is cruel, "this anatomy of live creatures should be entirely deserted or left to the casual inspection of chirurgeons."[492]

[h]The prolongation of life is the third part of medicine after the preservation of health and the cure of diseases (*Adv. of Learning,* 166). Cf. Paracelsus on the prolongation of life (*Divided Legacy,* I, 459).

Their carelessness extends even to therapeutics: "though the present physicians tolerably pursue the general intentions of cures, yet they have no particular medicines which by a specific property regard particular diseases."[493] Their medicines "do not principally regard some one disease but have a general virtue of opening obstructions, promoting concoction, etc. . . . I remember a famous Jew physician in England would say . . . 'Our physicians were like bishops, that had the keys of binding and loosing but no more.' "[494]

The cure for this is greater openness to the variety of nature. Anatomists, for instance, know the appearance and position of the organs but "pass over the different figure and state of those parts in different persons. The reason of this defect I take to be that the former inquiry may terminate upon seeing two or three bodies dissected; but the other being comparative and casual, requires attentive and strict application to many different dissections; besides, the first is a subject wherein learned anatomists may show themselves to their audience; but the other a rigorous knowledge, to be acquired only by silent and long experience."[495] "Hearts, livers, and stomachs are as different in men as foreheads, noses, and ears. And in these differences of the internal parts are often found the immediate causes of many diseases."[496] "This variety of accidents is by anatomists either slightly touched or else passed over in silence."[497]

Recognition of the variety of nature will lead to acceptance of the variety of diseases and treatments: "As diseases vary, so we will vary the arts, with a thousand remedies for a thousand species of disease."[498] [i]

Finally, physicians must know that knowledge of remedies is acquired only by experience, not by analysis:

> It might be of great consequence if some physicians, eminent for learning and practice, would compile a work of approved and experienced medicines in particular

[i]*Et quonian variant morbi, variabimus artes; mille mali species mille salutis erint* (Ovid: *Remedia Amoris,* 525).

> diseases. For though one might speciously pretend that a learned physician should rather suit his medicines occasionally, as the constitution of the patient, his age, customs, the seasons, etc. require, than rest upon any certain prescriptions, yet this is a fallacious opinion that underrates experience and overrates human judgment.[499]

Bacon opposed the mixing and compounding of remedies:

> For they lose the benefit of traditions and approved experience by their authoritative procedure in adding, taking away, and changing the ingredients of their recipes at pleasure, after the manner of apothecaries substituting one thing for another, and thus haughtily commanding medicine so that medicine can no longer command the disease . . . if medicines require, at any time, to be qualified, this may rather be done in the vehicles than in the body of the medicine, where nothing should be altered without apparent necessity.[500]

"Witches, old women, and imposters" who "keep strictly and invariably to the use of experienced medicines without altering their compositions" are often more successful in their cures than learned physicians and are thus preferred by the public.[501]

In general, the best physicians are those "who being either learned, duly value the traditions of experience; or men of eminent practice that do not despise methods and the general principles of the art."[502]

NOTES

[1] R. B. Blakney, *Meister Eckhart: A Modern Translation* (New York: Harper, 1941), 117.

[2] William Windelband, *A History of Philosophy* (New York: Harper, 1958), I, 232.

[3] *Ibid.*, I, 306.

[4] Blakney, *Meister Eckhart,* 216.

[5] *Ibid.*, 97, 221, 248.

[6] *Ibid.*, 213.

[7] *Ibid.*, 210, 280.

[8] *Ibid.*, 216, 245.

[9] *Ibid.*, 216, 246, 247.

[10] Windelband, *History of Philosophy,* I, 249.

[11] *Timaeus* 30C.

[12] *Ibid.*, 29A.

[13] *Ibid.*, 51C.

[14] Blakney, *Meister Eckhart,* 168.

[15] *Ibid.*, 148.

[16] *Ibid.*, 172.

[17] *Ibid.*, 148.

[18] *Ibid.*, 97.

[19] Windelband, *History of Philosophy,* I, 302.

[20] *Ibid.*, I, 266.

[21] Jan Baptista Van Helmont, *Oriatrike, or Physick Refined* (London, 1662), 230. See, also, *ibid.*, 240.

[22] Hermann Boerhaave, *Academical Lectures on the Theory of Physick* (London, 1742-1746), I, 40.

[23] Robert Multhauf, "Medical Chemistry and 'the Paracelsans,' " *Bulletin of the History of Medicine* XXVIII (1954), 101-126, at 110.

[24] Extensive biographical information on Van Helmont is to be found in Willem Rommelaere, *Etudes sur J. B. Van Helmont* (Bruxelles: Manceaux, 1868), 7-46.

[25] J. B. Van Helmont, *Oriatrike,* 12.

[26] *Loc. cit.*

[27] *Ibid.*, 7.

[28] *Ibid.*, 579.

[29] *Ibid.*, 14.

[30] *Ibid.*, 204.

[31] *Ibid.*, 7.
[32] *Ibid.*, 263.
[33] *Ibid.*, 1079.
[34] *Ibid.*, 457.
[35] *Ibid.*, 317-318.
[36] *Ibid.*, 1079.
[37] *Ibid.*, 7.
[38] *Ibid.*, 1079.
[39] *Ibid.*, 7.
[40] *Loc. cit.*
[41] *Loc. cit.*
[42] *Ibid.*, 1079.
[43] *Loc. cit.*
[44] *Ibid.*, 632.
[45] *Ibid.*, 37.
[46] *Ibid.*, 39.
[47] *Ibid.*, 16.
[48] *Ibid.*, 534.
[49] *Ibid.*, 16.
[50] *Ibid.*, 34.
[51] *Ibid.*, 19.
[52] *Ibid.*, 18.
[53] *Loc. cit.*
[54] *Ibid.*, 18.
[55] *Ibid.*, 26.
[56] *Ibid.*, 711.
[57] *Loc. cit.*
[58] *Ibid.*, 470.
[59] *Ibid.*, 476.
[60] *Ibid.*, 936.
[61] *Loc. cit.*
[62] *Ibid.*, 713.
[63] *Ibid.*, 40.
[64] *Ibid.*, 27.
[65] *Ibid.*, 549.
[66] *Ibid.*, 4.
[67] *Ibid.*, 713.
[68] *Ibid.*, 27.
[69] *Ibid.*, 459.
[70] *Ibid.*, 838.
[71] *Ibid.*, 837.
[72] *Ibid.*, 713.
[73] *Ibid.*, 26.
[74] *Ibid.*, 715.
[75] *Ibid.*, 20.
[76] *Ibid.*, 19.
[77] *Ibid.*, 20.
[78] *Ibid.*, 660.
[79] *Ibid.*, 988.

[80] *Ibid.*, 25.
[81] *Ibid.*, 713.
[82] *Ibid.*, 712.
[83] *Ibid.*, 711.
[84] *Ibid.*, 23.
[85] *Ibid.*, 715.
[86] *Ibid.*, 27.
[87] *Ibid.*, 40.
[88] *Ibid.*, 837-838.
[89] *Ibid.*, 587.
[90] *Ibid.*, 1003.
[91] *Ibid.*, 284-287.
[92] *Ibid.*, 550.
[93] *Ibid.*, 33, 206, 287, 544.
[94] *Ibid.*, 285-286.
[95] *Ibid.*, 551.
[96] *Ibid.*, 81, 417-428.
[97] *Ibid.*, 47-62.
[98] *Ibid.*, 104.
[99] *Ibid.*, 104-111.
[100] *Ibid.*, 31.
[101] *Ibid.*, 206-221.
[102] *Ibid.*, 981.
[103] *Ibid.*, 33, 206, 544.
[104] *Ibid.*, 287, 702-703.
[105] *Ibid.*, 938.
[106] *Ibid.*, 2, 163.
[107] *Ibid.*, 2. See, also, *ibid.*, 33, 472, 587.
[108] *Ibid.*, 46.
[109] *Ibid.*, 524, 587, 776 (see *Epidemics* VI, cap. V: V, 315, Littre).
[110] *Ibid.*, 776.
[111] *Ibid.*, 13.
[112] *Ibid.*, 495, 530.
[113] *Ibid.*, 728.
[114] J. B. Van Helmont, *Supplementum de Spadanis Fontibus* (Leodii, 1624), title page.
[115] J. B. Van Helmont, *Oriatrike*, 472.
[116] *Ibid.*, 549.
[117] *Ibid.*, 535.
[118] *Loc. cit.*
[119] *Loc. cit.*
[120] *Ibid.*, 543.
[121] *Ibid.*, 530, 532, 535.
[122] *Ibid.*, 404.
[123] *Ibid.*, 415.
[124] *Ibid.*, 387, 533.
[125] *Ibid.*, 532.
[126] *Ibid.*, 495, 548.
[127] *Ibid.*, 540.

[128] *Ibid.*, 544.
[129] *Ibid.*, 531.
[130] *Ibid.*, 531.
[131] *Ibid.*, 492, 503, 530, 539, 566, 712.
[132] *Ibid.*, 544.
[133] *Ibid.*, 707.
[134] *Ibid.*, 709.
[135] *Ibid.*, 432, 490, 495.
[136] *Ibid.*, 392.
[137] *Ibid.*, 356.
[138] *Ibid.*, 504.
[139] *Ibid.*, 332.
[140] *Ibid.*, 485.
[141] *Ibid.*, 472.
[142] *Ibid.*, 495.
[143] *Ibid.*, 530.
[144] *Ibid.*, 492.
[145] *Ibid.*, 387, 532-533, 543, 551, 565.
[146] *Ibid.*, 543.
[147] *Ibid.*, 532.
[148] *Ibid.*, 566. See, also, *ibid.*, 534-546.
[149] *Ibid.*, 360.
[150] *Ibid.*, 940.
[151] *Ibid.*, 703.
[152] *Ibid.*, 938.
[153] *Ibid.*, 983.
[154] *Loc. cit.*
[155] *Ibid.*, 936.
[156] *Ibid.*, 940, 987.
[157] *Ibid.*, 961.
[158] *Loc. cit.*
[159] *Ibid.*, 171, 472, 476-479.
[160] *Ibid.*, 477.
[161] *Ibid.*, 981.
[162] *Ibid.*, 1008.
[163] *Ibid.*, 1010.
[164] *Loc. cit.*
[165] *Ibid.*, 583.
[166] *Ibid.*, 473.
[167] *Ibid.*, 164.
[168] *Ibid.*, 475.
[169] *Ibid.*, 788.
[170] *Loc. cit.*
[171] *Ibid.*, 474-475, 788.
[172] *Ibid.*, 474, 788.
[173] *Ibid.*, 472-478, 622.
[174] *Ibid.*, 469.
[175] *Ibid.*, 474-475.
[176] *Ibid.*, 771.

[177] *Ibid.*, 788.
[178] *Loc. cit.*
[179] *Ibid.*, 479.
[180] *Loc. cit.*
[181] *Loc. cit.*
[182] *Ibid.*, 191.
[183] *Ibid.*, 114, 115.
[184] *Ibid.*, 574.
[185] *Ibid.*, 458.
[186] *Ibid.*, 579.
[187] *Ibid.*, 287.
[188] *Ibid.*, 460. See, also, *ibid.*, 575-584.
[189] *Ibid.*, 577.
[190] *Loc. cit.*
[191] *Ibid.*, 582.
[192] *Ibid.*, 160.
[193] *Ibid.*, 170.
[194] *Ibid.*, 163.
[195] *Ibid.*, 1.
[196] *Ibid.*, 407.
[197] *Ibid.*, 164.
[198] *Ibid.*, 171.
[199] *Ibid.*, 163.
[200] *Ibid.*, 557.
[201] *Ibid.*, 360.
[202] *Ibid.*, 1.
[203] *Ibid.*, 431.
[204] *Ibid.*, 554.
[205] *Ibid.*, 551.
[206] *Ibid.*, 164.
[207] *Ibid.*, 543.
[208] *Ibid.*, 594.
[209] *Ibid.*, 576.
[210] *Ibid.*, 587.
[211] *Ibid.*, 556.
[212] *Ibid.*, 591.
[213] *Ibid.*, 533.
[214] *Ibid.*, 3.
[215] *Ibid.*, 163.
[216] *Ibid.*, 494.
[217] *Ibid.*, 461.
[218] *Ibid.*, 4.
[219] *Ibid.*, 3.
[220] *Ibid.*, 474.
[221] *Ibid.*, 1.
[222] *Ibid.*, 527.
[223] *Ibid.*, 13-14.
[224] *Ibid.*, 457. See, also, *ibid.*, 557.
[225] *Ibid.*, 332.

[226] *Ibid.,* 460.
[227] *Ibid.,* 465, 479.
[228] *Ibid.,* 368, 457, 519, 709.
[229] *Ibid.,* 527.
[230] *Ibid.,* 580.
[231] *Ibid.,* 577.
[232] *Loc. cit.*
[233] *Ibid.,* 579.
[234] *Ibid.,* 477, 481.
[235] *Ibid.,* 460, 481, 557.
[236] *Ibid.,* 478.
[237] *Ibid.,* 524.
[238] *Ibid.,* 802.
[239] *Ibid.,* 805.
[240] Robert Boyle, *On the Reconcileableness of Specific Medicines to the Corpuscular Philosophy* (London, 1685), 4.
[241] J. B. Van Helmont, *Oriatrike,* 760.
[242] *Ibid.,* 1007.
[243] *Ibid.,* 709.
[244] *Ibid.,* 475.
[245] *Ibid.,* 476.
[246] *Ibid.,* 760.
[247] *Ibid.,* 590.
[248] *Ibid.,* 593.
[249] *Ibid.,* 564.
[250] *Ibid.,* 474.
[251] *Ibid.,* 458.
[252] *Ibid.,* 414.
[253] *Ibid.,* 458.
[254] *Ibid.,* 406-407.
[255] *Ibid.,* 260.
[256] *Ibid.,* 462.
[257] *Ibid.,* 459.
[258] *Loc. cit.* On the future golden age of the prophet Elias see *Mathew* xvii:11.
[259] *Ibid.,* 476.
[260] *Ibid.,* 474. See, also, *ibid.,* 469.
[261] *Ibid.,* 459.
[262] *Ibid.,* 576.
[263] *Ibid.,* 2.
[264] *Ibid.,* 14.
[265] *Ibid.,* 527.
[266] *Ibid.,* 236.
[267] *Ibid.,* 82.
[268] *Ibid.,* 760.
[269] *Ibid.,* 942.
[270] *Ibid.,* 255.
[271] *Ibid.,* 258.
[272] *Ibid.,* 259.
[273] *Ibid.,* 590.

[274] *Ibid.*, 526.
[275] *Ibid.*, 772.
[276] *Ibid.*, 458.
[277] *Ibid.*, 579.
[278] *Ibid.*, 458.
[279] *Ibid.*, 4.
[280] *Ibid.*, 4, 578.
[281] *Ibid.*, 460.
[282] *Ibid.*, 529.
[283] *Ibid.*, 287.
[284] *Ibid.*, 709.
[285] *Ibid.*, 360.
[286] *Ibid.*, 553.
[287] *Ibid.*, 566.
[288] *Ibid.*, 625.
[289] *Ibid.*, 788.
[290] *Loc. cit.*
[291] *Ibid.*, 461, 464.
[292] *Ibid.*, 462-463.
[293] *Ibid.*, 462.
[294] *Ibid.*, 457.
[295] *Ibid.*, 534.
[296] *Ibid.*, 712.
[297] *Ibid.*, 402.
[298] *Ibid.*, 403.
[299] *Ibid.*, 406.
[300] *Ibid.*, 457.
[301] *Ibid.*, 451.
[302] *Ibid.*, 576.
[303] *Ibid.*, 19.
[304] *Ibid.*, 12.
[305] *Ibid.*, 274-275, 293.
[306] *Ibid.*, 7, 402.
[307] *Ibid.*, 956.
[308] *Ibid.*, 457.
[309] *Ibid.*, 402.
[310] *Ibid.*, 622.
[311] *Ibid.*, 431.
[312] *Ibid.*, 969.
[313] *Ibid.*, 163.
[314] *Ibid.*, 457.
[315] *Ibid.*, 537.
[316] *Ibid.*, 494.
[317] *Ibid.*, 384.
[318] *Ibid.*, 772.
[319] *Ibid.*, 474.
[320] *Ibid.*, 762.
[321] *Ibid.*, 969.
[322] *Ibid.*, 577; see, also, 591.

[323] *Ibid.*, 969.
[324] *Ibid.*, 990.
[325] *Ibid.*, 577.
[326] *Ibid.*, 582.
[327] *Ibid.*, 587.
[328] *Ibid.*, 451, 595.
[329] *Ibid.*, 450-455.
[330] *Ibid.*, 433.
[331] *Ibid.*, 403.
[332] *Ibid.*, 431.
[333] *Ibid.*, 450, 461-462.
[334] *Ibid.*, 593.
[335] *Ibid.*, 577.
[336] *Ibid.*, 1080.
[337] *Ibid.*, 494.
[338] *Ibid.*, 503.
[339] *Ibid.*, 324.
[340] *Ibid.*, 547.
[341] *Ibid.*, 477.
[342] *Ibid.*, 494.
[343] *Ibid.*, 363.
[344] *Ibid.*, 325, 451, 577, 593.
[345] *Ibid.*, 991.
[346] *Ibid.*, 969.
[347] *Ibid.*, 433.
[348] *Ibid.*, 7.
[349] *The Physical and Metaphysical Works of Lord Bacon, Including the Dignity and Advancement of Learning, in Nine Books; and his Novum Organum; or, Precepts for the Interpretation of Nature.* Translated by Joseph Devey (London: Henry G. Bohn, 1853), 51 (*Advancement of Learning,* I).
[350] *Ibid.*, 11 (*The Great Instauration*).
[351] *Ibid.*, 384 (*Novum Organum,* I, Aph. X).
[352] *Ibid.*, 183 (*Adv. of Learning,* V, cap. ii).
[353] *Ibid.*, 387 (*Novum Organum,* I, Aph. XXVI).
[354] *Ibid.*, 184 (*Adv. of Learning,* V, cap. ii).
[355] *Ibid.*, 388 (*Novum Organum,* I, Aph. XXXI).
[356] *Ibid.*, 383 (*Novum Organum,* I, Aph. I).
[357] *Ibid.*, 435 (*Novum Organum,* I, Aph. CXII).
[358] *Ibid.*, 383 (*Novum Organum,* Preface).
[359] *Ibid.*, 429 (*Novum Organum,* I, Aph. XCVIII).
[360] *Ibid.*, 384 (*Novum Organum,* I, Aph. X).
[361] *Ibid.*, 400 (*Novum Organum,* I, Aph. LXIII).
[362] *Ibid.*, 389 (*Novum Organum,* I, Aph. XXXVI).
[363] *Ibid.*, 159 (*Adv. of Learning,* IV, cap. ii).
[364] *Ibid.*, 144 (*Adv. of Learning,* III, cap. v).
[365] *Ibid.*, 138 (*Adv. of Learning,* III, cap. iv).
[366] *Ibid.*, 474 (*Novum Organum,* II, Aph. XVII).
[367] *Ibid.*, 449 (*Novum Organum,* II, Aph. II).
[368] *Ibid.*, 474 (*Novum Organum,* II, Aph. XV).

[369] *Ibid.*, 405 (*Novum Organum,* I, Aph. LXVII).
[370] *Ibid.*, 383 (*Novum Organum,* I, Aph. II).
[371] *Ibid.*, 381 (*Novum Organum,* Preface).
[372] *Ibid.*, 430 (*Novum Organum,* I, Aph. C).
[373] *Ibid.*, 429 (*Novum Organum,* I, Aph. XCVIII).
[374] *Ibid.*, 390 (*Novum Organum,* I, Aph. XLI).
[375] *Ibid.*, 390 (*Novum Organum,* I, Aph. XLII).
[376] *Ibid.*, 390 (*Novum Organum,* I, Aph. XLIII).
[377] *Ibid.*, 391 (*Novum Organum,* I, Aph. XLIV).
[378] *Ibid.*, 391 (*Novum Organum,* I, Aph. XLV).
[379] *Ibid.*, 387 (*Novum Organum,* I, Aph. XXIV).
[380] *Ibid.*, 443 (*Novum Organum,* I, Aph. CXXV).
[381] *Ibid.*, 392 (*Novum Organum,* I, Aph. XLVI).
[382] *Ibid.*, 432 (*Novum Organum,* I, Aph. CV).
[383] *Loc. cit.*
[384] *Ibid.*, 386 (*Novum Organum,* I, Aph. XIX).
[385] *Ibid.*, 431 (*Novum Organum,* I, Aph. CIV).
[386] *Ibid.*, 411 (*Novum Organum,* I, Aph. LXXIV).
[387] *Ibid.*, 417 (*Novum Organum,* I, Aph. LXXXII).
[388] *Ibid.*, 144, 384, 416, 432 (*Adv. of Learning,* III, cap. v; *Novum Organum,* I, Aph. VIII, LXXXII, CVIII).
[389] *Ibid.*, 82 (*Adv. of Learning,* II, cap. ii).
[390] *Ibid.*, 430 (*Novum Organum,* I, Aph. C).
[391] *Ibid.*, 406 (*Novum Organum,* I, Aph. LXX).
[392] *Ibid.*, 430 (*Novum Organum,* I, Aph. XCIX).
[393] *Ibid.*, 188 (*Adv. of Learning,* V, cap. ii).
[394] *Loc. cit.*
[395] *Loc. cit.* and *ibid.*, 434, 438 (*Novum Organum,* I, Aph. CX, CXVII).
[396] *Ibid.*, 189 (*Adv. of Learning,* V, cap. ii).
[397] *Loc. cit.*
[398] *Loc. cit.*
[399] *Ibid.*, 190 (*Adv. of Learning,* V, cap. ii).
[400] *Loc. cit.*
[401] *Loc. cit.*
[402] *Ibid.*, 192 (*Adv. of Learning,* V, cap. ii).
[403] *Loc. cit.*
[404] *Loc. cit.*
[405] *Ibid.*, 193 (*Adv. of Learning,* V, cap. ii).
[406] *Loc. cit.*
[407] *Ibid.*, 194 (*Adv. of Learning,* V, cap. ii).
[408] *Ibid.*, 196 (*Adv. of Learning,* V, cap. ii).
[409] *Ibid.*, 448, 473 (*Novum Organum,* II, Aph. I, XV).
[410] *Ibid.*, 474 (*Novum Organum,* II, Aph. XVI).
[411] *Ibid.*, 430 (*Novum Organum,* I, Aph. CI).
[412] *Ibid.*, 430 (*Novum Organum* I, Aph. CII).
[413] *Ibid.*, 457 (*Novum Organum,* II, Aph. XI).
[414] *Ibid.*, 458 (*Novum Organum,* II, Aph. XII).
[415] *Loc. cit.*
[416] *Ibid.*, 466 (*Novum Organum,* II, Aph. XIII).
[417] *Loc. cit.*

418 *Ibid.*, 475 (*Novum Organum*, II, Aph. XVIII).
419 *Ibid.*, 474 (*Novum Organum*, II, Aph. XVI).
420 *Ibid.*, 473 (*Novum Organum*, II, Aph. XV).
421 *Ibid.*, 188 (*Adv. of Learning*, V, cap. ii).
422 *Ibid.*, 387 (*Novum Organum*, I, Aph. XXIV).
423 *Ibid.*, 387 (*Novum Organum*, I, Aph. XXV).
424 *Ibid.*, 386 (*Novum Organum*, I, Aph. XIX).
425 *Ibid.*, 187 (*Adv. of Learning*, V, cap. ii).
426 *Loc. cit.*
427 *Ibid.*, 380 (*Novum Organum*, Preface).
428 *Ibid.*, 188 (*Adv. of Learning*, V, cap. ii).
429 *Ibid.*, 411 (*Novum Organum*, I, Aph. LXXV).
430 *Ibid.*, 405 (*Novum Organum*, I, Aph. LXVII).
431 *Ibid.*, 383 (*Novum Organum*, I, Aph. III).
432 *Ibid.*, 450 (*Novum Organum*, II, Aph. III).
433 *Ibid.*, 144 (*Adv. of Learning*, III, cap. v).
434 *Ibid.*, 448 (*Novum Organum*, II, Aph. II).
435 *Ibid.*, 450 (*Novum Organum*, II, Aph. III).
436 *Ibid.*, 144 (*Adv. of Learning*, III, cap. v).
437 *Ibid.*, 20 (*The Great Instauration*).
438 F. Bacon, *Valerius Terminus of the Interpretation of Nature*, in James Spedding, Robert Leslie Ellis, and Douglas Denon Heath, *The Works of Francis Bacon* (London: Longman et al., 1858-1874), III, 232.
439 *The Physical and Metaphysical Works of Lord Bacon*, 416 (*Novum Organum*, I, Aph. LXXXI).
440 *Ibid.*, 528 (*Novum Organum*, II, Aph. XLIV).
441 *Ibid.*, 383 (*Novum Organum*, I, Aph. III).
442 *Ibid.*, 380 (*Novum Organum*, Preface).
443 *Ibid.*, 188 (*Adv. of Learning*, V, cap. ii).
444 *Ibid.*, 389 (*Novum Organum*, I, Aph. XXXVII).
445 See, especially, *ibid.*, 184 (*Adv. of Learning*, V, cap. ii).
446 *Ibid.*, 401 (*Novum Organum*, I, Aph. LXIV).
447 *Ibid.*, 151 (*Adv. of Learning*, IV, cap. i).
448 *Ibid.*, 438 (*Novum Organum*, I, Aph. CXVII).
449 *Ibid.*, 427 (*Novum Organum*, I, Aph. XCV). See, also, *ibid.*, 8 (*The Great Instauration*).
450 *Ibid.*, 184 (*Adv. of Learning*, V, cap. ii).
451 *Ibid.*, 199-200 (*Adv. of Learning*, V, cap. iii).
452 *Ibid.*, 445 (*Novum Organum*, I, Aph. CXXIX).
453 *Ibid.*, 197 (*Adv. of Learning*, V, cap. iii).
454 *Ibid.*, 384 (*Novum Organum*, I, Aph. VIII).
455 F. Bacon, *Valerius Terminus of the Interpretation of Nature*, in Spedding and Heath, *The Works of Francis Bacon*, III, 232.
456 *The Physical and Metaphysical Works of Lord Bacon*, 212 (*Adv. of Learning*, V, cap. v).
457 *Ibid.*, 139 (*Adv. of Learning*, III, cap. iv).
458 *Ibid.*, 78 (*Adv. of Learning*, II, cap. i).
459 *Ibid.*, 429 (*Novum Organum*, I, Aph. XCVIII).
460 *Ibid.*, 196 (*Adv. of Learning*, V, cap. ii).

[461] *Ibid.*, 380, 477 (*Novum Organum,* I, Preface; II, Aph. XIX). See, also, *ibid.*, 19 (*The Great Instauration*).

[462] *Ibid.*, 438 (*Novum Organum* I, CXVII).

[463] *Ibid.*, 450 (*Novum Organum,* II, Aph. III).

[464] *Ibid.*, 451 (*Novum Organum,* II, Aph. IV).

[465] *Ibid.*, 443 (*Novum Organum,* I, Aph. CXXIV).

[466] *Ibid.*, 410 (*Novum Organum,* I, Aph. LXXIII).

[467] *Ibid.*, 157 (*Adv. of Learning,* IV, cap. ii). See, also, *ibid.*, 546, 559 (*Novum Organum,* II, Aph. XLVIII).

[468] *Ibid.*, 137-138 (*Adv. of Learning,* III, cap. iv) and especially *Temporis Partus Masculus* in Spedding and Heath, *The Works of Francis Bacon,* III, 533.

[469] J. R. Ravetz, "Francis Bacon and the Reform of Philosophy," in Allen G. Debus, ed., *Science, Medicine, and Society in the Renaissance* (New York: Science History Publications, 1972), II, 97-119.

[470] *Ibid.*, 115.

[471] *Ibid.*, 119, note 75.

[472] *The Physical and Metaphysical Works of Lord Bacon,* 9 (*The Great Instauration*).

[473] *Ibid.*, 53 (*Adv. of Learning,* I, cap. i).

[474] J. R. Ravetz, "Francis Bacon and the Reform of Philosophy," 113-114.

[475] *The Physical and Metaphysical Works of Lord Bacon,* 382 (*Novum Organum,* Preface).

[476] *Ibid.*, 442 (*Novum Organum,* I, Aph. CXXII).

[477] *Ibid.*, 439-440 (*Novum Organum,* I, Aph. CXX).

[478] *Ibid.*, 417 (*Novum Organum,* I, Aph. LXXXIII).

[479] *Ibid.*, 567 (*Novum Organum,* II, Aph. LII).

[480] *Ibid.*, 382 (*Novum Organum,* Preface).

[481] *Ibid.*, 156 (*Adv. of Learning,* IV, cap. ii).

[482] *Ibid.*, 159 (*Adv. of Learning,* IV, cap. ii).

[483] *Ibid.*, 165 (*Adv. of Learning,* IV, cap. ii).

[484] *Ibid.*, 166 (*Adv. of Learning,* IV, cap. ii).

[485] *Ibid.*, 167 (*Adv. of Learning,* IV, cap. ii).

[486] *Ibid.*, 163 (*Adv. of Learning,* IV, cap. ii).

[487] *Ibid.*, 421 (*Novum Organum,* I, Aph. LXXXVIII).

[488] *Ibid.*, 159 (*Adv. of Learning,* IV, cap. ii).

[489] *Ibid.*, 161 (*Adv. of Learning,* IV, cap. ii).

[490] *Loc. cit.*

[491] *Ibid.*, 162 (*Adv. of Learning,* IV, cap. ii).

[492] *Loc. cit.*

[493] *Ibid.*, 164 (*Adv. of Learning,* IV, cap. ii).

[494] *Loc. cit.*

[495] *Ibid.*, 161 (*Adv. of Learning,* IV, cap. ii).

[496] *Loc. cit.*

[497] *Ibid.*, 162 (*Adv. of Learning,* IV, cap. ii).

[498] *Ibid.*, 159 (*Adv. of Learning,* IV, cap. ii).

[499] *Ibid.*, 164 (*Adv. of Learning,* IV, cap. ii).

[500] *Loc. cit.*

[501] *Ibid.*, 158, 164 (*Adv. of Learning,* IV, cap. ii).

[502] *Ibid.*, 164 (*Adv. of Learning,* IV, cap. ii).

CHAPTER II

SEVENTEENTH-CENTURY RATIONALISM: IATROCHEMISTRY AND IATROMECHANISM

The six medical thinkers discussed in this chapter: Rene Descartes (1596-1650), Francois de le Boe Sylvius (1614-1672), Thomas Willis (1622-1675), George Cheyne (1671-1743), Frederick Hoffmann (1660-1742), and Hermann Boerhaave (1668-1738) were the leaders of Rationalist medicine in the late seventeenth and early eighteenth centuries.

In reaction to Paracelsus and Van Helmont they refurbished the discredited Galenic categories and filled them with the knowledge emerging in the disciplines of chemistry, mechanics, and mathematics.

The medical system of these thinkers is a paradigm of the Rationalist response to Empiricism. Paracelsus and Van Helmont had sought to derive theory from practice. The Rationalists who followed them reversed this process, drawing their theoretical categories from disciplines external to therapeutics and seeking to interpret practice in terms of these categories.

Here chemistry had to bear the major load. The salt, sulphur, and mercury, which for Paracelsus were spiritual principles, operational definitions of physiological processes, became identified with these chemical substances as produced in the laboratory and were ultimately converted into the acids and alkalis which occupy such a prominent role in the therapeutics of the period. Therapeutic practice was generated by chemical theory. Mechanics and hydraulics fulfilled similar functions.

Because the theoretical structure of twentieth-century medicine resembles seventeenth-century Rationalism, modern historians have become quite sympathetic to these thinkers.[a]

Biographical

While Descartes is not usually regarded as a medical thinker, he wrote the first textbook of physiology (his *Treatise of Man*), founded a school of Cartesian physicians, and reworked Aristotelian and Galenic thought into a theoretical guide for his Rationalist contemporaries.

His father, a landowner of Brittany, died when Descartes was a child, leaving properties which yielded the young philosopher an income of 6000-7000 francs a year. He thus never needed to work for a living, and this is perhaps why his system ignores empirical experience as a source of knowledge and favors an *a priori* analysis even more rarefied than Plato's.

From 1604 to 1612 he was educated by the Jesuits, taking particular delight in mathematics. Thereafter he "entirely quitted the study of letters. And resolving to seek no other science than that which could be found in myself, or at least in the great book of the world, I employed the rest of my youth in travel, in seeing courts and armies, in intercourse with men of diverse temperaments and conditions, in collecting various experiences . . . so that I might derive some profit from my experience."[1] But this tentative

[a]Thus,while Sprengel states: "it must be admitted that the theory of Descartes destroyed the spirit of observation and greatly contributed to the erroneous idea that calculating the movement of atoms could give medicine a truly mathematical certainty" (*Histoire de la Medecine,* V, 53), Michael Foster maintains: "indeed, a very little change in the details of Descartes' exposition, and some of that hardly more than a change in terminology, would convert that exposition into a statement of modern views" (*Lectures on the History of Physiology,* 268). Thomas S. Hall writes that physiology needed "the relentless application of the materialistic and mechanistic ideas [Descartes] espoused" (*Rene Descartes: Treatise of Man* [Cambridge: Harvard University Press, 1972], xxx).

trial of "experience," which included five years studying geometry in Paris, two years in the Netherlands army, and one in the Bavarian, proved a disappointment:

> After I had employed several years in thus studying the book of the world and trying to acquire some experience, I one day formed the resolution of also making myself an object of study and of employing all the strength of my mind in choosing the road I should follow. This succeeded much better, it appeared to me, than if I had never departed either from my country or my books.[2]

Thus Descartes' highly provisional commitment to the life of action (Holland was at peace, and he resigned from the Bavarian army in 1621, before the Thirty Years' War was properly under way) culminated in a resolve to pursue the life of contemplation. In what is almost a parody of the rejection of experience as a source of knowledge he states that he first hit on the principles of the *Discourse on Method* while dozing, of a winter's day, inside one of the large tiled stoves for which Bavaria is noted. Thereafter, "in all the nine following years I did nought but roam hither and thither, *trying to be a spectator rather than an actor* in all the comedies the world displays."[3]

The rest of his life he spent in the pursuit of knowledge, making fundamental contributions to mathematics. He discovered the infinitesimal calculus, applied algebra to geometry, and invented the method of coordinates. But unfortunately he did not limit his efforts to this area but ventured into physiology as well, adopting as his root principle a mechanical interpretation of the process of fermentation. Here his influence, although equally far-reaching, was less happy. A school of Cartesian physicians arose in the Netherlands, assimilating his corpuscular eddies to Van Helmont's ferments and for some decades dominating medical theory and practice. In Italy the more purely mathematical side of his thought helped generate the Iatromathematical and Iatromechanical movements represented later by

Alfonso Borelli (1608-1679), Lorenzo Bellini (1643-1704), George Cheyne, and Frederick Hoffmann.

Descartes was summoned to Sweden by Queen Christina in 1649 to give this monarch instruction in philosophy. The change of climate and the unusually early hours (and active life) he was compelled to maintain (she could receive him only at 5:00 A.M., whereas Descartes had been accustomed to sleeping until noon) brought on a pneumonia from which he died in 1650.

Francois de le Boe Sylvius was born in Hanau to an emigrant French noble family and studied in Paris, Sedan, Leiden, and Basel. He practiced medicine in the Netherlands and in 1658 was called to a professorship at Leiden where he remained until his death in 1672 from typhus (the epidemic also carried off his wife and daughter). He is the founder of the Iatrochemical school.[b]

His catastrophic end was beyond doubt the work of an aroused Divinity, concerned to end the havoc his medical teachings were wreaking among the populations of Northern Europe.[c] His system, which Baas calls a "systematic fantasy," vaguely resembles that of Van Helmont whose writings, although not yet published, were already circulating in manuscript and were common knowledge in the Low Countries.[4] Sylvius simplified them, rejecting the *Archeus* and the hierarchy of ferments and reducing medical theory to a clash between acids and alkalis. Therapeutics became the mere administration of the "opposite" chemical – a modern version of the Galenic "contraries."

[b]The word, "iatrochemist," first appears in the 1573 Latin translation of Paracelsus' *Grosse Wundarznei* (cf. Karl Sudhoff, ed. *Theophrastus von Hohenheim, genannt Paracelsus: Saemtliche Werke. I. Abteilung,* X, 67 with J. R. Partington, *History of Chemistry,* II, 124, 135).

[c]Sprengel states: "Any disinterested and impartial person will have to agree that this school did more harm than good, removing medicine even further from the path of observation and representing supernatural principles as sensory objects, introducing pernicious methods based only on arbitrary hypotheses. One could go so far as to say that the opinions propagated by the chemical school have been more devastating than certain wars, so far was the treatment of diseases based on these hypotheses contrary to good sense and reason" (*Histoire de la Medecine,* V, 58).

Sylvius introduced clinical instruction and by force of personality attracted more students than had ever before flocked to a single professor. He was exceeded in popularity only by Boerhaave later at the same university. According to Haeser his success as a teacher was due "as much to his physical comeliness, the amiability of his character, his modesty, his untiring zeal in the pursuit of knowledge, his brilliant eloquence, his comprehensive anatomical and chemical knowledge—as to the simplicity of his medical system."[d]

Thomas Willis was born in Wiltshire and educated at Oxford. A fervent Royalist during the Civil War, he held religious services in his lodgings while Oxford was under Parliamentary control and later served in the King's army. This paid dividends under the Restoration when he was appointed Sedleian Professor of Natural History at Christ Church.

He was also on good terms with the Puritans, Robert Hooke (1635-1703), Robert Boyle (1627-1691), Isaac Newton (1642-1727), and the other "vertuosi" who later founded the Royal Society, but is recorded as having attended only two meetings of this Society after 1660 and died owing a substantial sum in dues.[5]

He was preeminently a practitioner, despite his many publications in physiology. In his time he had the largest income in Oxford, at least 300 pounds a year (perhaps 100 times as much as was earned, for example, by a farm

[d]H. Haeser, *Lehrbuch der Geschichte der Medicin* (Jena: Mauke, 1868), 583. Michael Foster places Sylvius on a higher level than Van Helmont: "The spiritualistic fancies of Van Helmont, and still more the earlier ones of Paracelsus, had had the tendency to make men think that chemical inquiry in contrast with physical inquiry was in some way necessarily bound up with speculations about invisible agencies of a spiritual kind; and this doubtless was more or less a bar to men of sober and exact thought entering upon that line of inquiry. To Sylvius at least is due the credit of showing that there was no such necessary connection between chemistry and spiritualism; that on the contrary the newer chemistry in its attempts to solve vital problems trod the path of the most naked materialism. It is probably to his thus opening up a line of inquiry into chemical physiology free from all taint of mysticism that the great influence which as a teacher he undoubtedly exercised was largely due" (*Lectures on the History of Physiology*, 152-153).

laborer).[6] In about 1666 he settled in London, and "in a very short time after he became so noted, and so infinitely resorted to, for his practice, that never any physician before went beyond him or got more money yearly than he."[7] He was also physician-in-ordinary to Charles II, an honor doubtless forced on that monarch by Willis' high professional standing, as he once remarked that the latter "had rid him of more of his subjects than any enemy army."[8]

His physiology, like that of Sylvius, was borrowed largely from Van Helmont but made entirely incoherent through incorporation of the incompatible ideas of Descartes. He was more an organizer of the work of others than an original researcher, like the department chairman of a university who cosigns his name to articles prepared by instructors and assistant professors. Richard Lower (1631-1690), in particular, is known to have contributed greatly to Willis' book on cerebral anatomy.

While indeed a social success, Willis was not in very high esteem among his professional brethren. A contemporary, the Reverend John Ward, wrote: "Sydenham and some others in London say of Dr. Willis that he is an ingenious man but not a good physician, and that he does not understand the way of practice."[9] The Danish physiologist, Nicolaus Steno (1638-1686), accused Willis (together with his mentor, Descartes) of unsupported speculation about brain function, a "philippic" which, according to Neuburger, had a "shattering effect all over Europe."[10] [e] Steno ultimately accounted Willis one of those "positive gentlemen . . . who prefer the applause of the public to sincerity and truth."[11] An eighteenth-century biographer wrote: "Willis hath founded a body of physic chiefly on hypotheses of his own framing . . . but this foundation will not be lasting. Hence it is that,

[e] He wrote: "There abounds indeed a rich plenty of men to whom everything is clear. Such, dogmatizing with the utmost confidence, make up and publish the story of the brain and the use of its several parts with the same assuredness as if they had mastered with their actual eyes the structure of so admirable a machine and penetrated into the secrets of the great artificer" (quoted in Foster, *Lectures on the History of Physiology,* 280).

while his books show the greatest ingenuity and learning, very little knowledge is to be drawn from them . . . and perhaps no writings which are so admirably executed and prove such uncommon talents to have been in the writer, were ever so soon laid aside and neglected as the works of Willis."[12] [f]

George Cheyne is a prominent exemplar of the influence of mathematical speculation on medicine. Initially a student of this discipline, and an admirer of Descartes, he was persuaded by Archibald Pitcairn (1652-1713), himself a leading Iatromathematician, to enter medicine. In 1703 Cheyne published a work on the integral calculus which he held as applicable to medicine as to mechanics.

He brought forth in 1715 his *Philosophical Principles of Religion, Containing the Nature and Kinds of Infinities, Their Arithmetic and Uses, and the Philosophical Principles of Revealed Religion* (Cheyne had at one time been destined for the ministry), about which the *Dictionary of National Biography* observes: "the intention is excellent, but the mathematical will-o'-the-wisp once more misled Cheyne (not for the last time) into mingling theology and mathematics in a manner too fantastic to bear exposition."

Precisely the same could be said about his medical philosophy which rejected "the ridiculous cant of acids and alkalis, and the whimsical fancy of ferments" and held that the living body could be explained by the mechanical

[f]H. Isler, on the contrary, rates Willis higher than Van Helmont: "Although his attitude resembles that of Van Helmont, there is a great difference in meaning. The 'gifts and roots' of Van Helmont clearly belong to a world full of magic, whereas the 'instruments' of Willis which can be shown by distillation are parts of an environment that can be described in technical terms" (*Thomas Willis, 1621-1675* [N.Y. and London: Hafner, 1968], 51). Dewhurst writes: "[Sydenham] completely failed to realize the ultimate significance of research into the basic medical sciences undertaken by Willis and other contemporaries associated with the Royal Society. In this respect Willis was a much more scientific physician . . . It was in the sphere of *experiencal medicine* [*sic*] rather than clinical medicine that Thomas Willis reigned supreme . . . It was this propensity to seek out the hidden causes of diseases which was the mainspring of Thomas Willis's endeavor and the source of his signal achievements" (*Thomas Willis as a Physician* [Los Angeles: Univ. of California Press, 1964], 16-17).

principles of Borelli, Bellini, Boyle, and Descartes.[13] He regarded all medical history as culminating in Harvey's discovery of the circulation, a purely hydraulic process which "let more light into the theory of medicine than almost all the former [discoveries] joined together."[14]

Cheyne suffered greatly from overweight. At age fifty, finding that he weighed 450 pounds and could scarcely walk, he adopted a milk and vegetable diet to which he adhered strictly for his remaining eleven years. Many of his later writings are eulogies to this regimen: he maintained that God permits the use of meat only because—by shortening man's life and generating innumerable diseases—it thereby conduces to moral improvement.

Frederick Hoffmann, the son of a physician, was born in Halle and initially (like Cheyne) entered mathematics. He then turned to medicine and studied with the Iatrochemist, Georg Wolfgang Wedel (1645-1721).[15] He travelled to the Netherlands and England where he spent some time with Boyle and was greatly impressed by him. In 1694 he was called to the newly formed university at Halle as professor of anatomy, surgery, physics, chemistry, and medical practice; there he remained—except for a sojourn from 1709 to 1712 in Berlin as physician-in-ordinary to Frederick I—until his death.

His system was also inspired by the ideas of Van Helmont, but he materialized the *Archeus* as "tonus" or nervous force in the muscles and solid parts of the body, thus subjecting it to physical and mechanical laws. His treatment was mild, relying largely on diet.

Hoffmann's principal competitor[g] was Hermann Boerhaave—celebrated in his day as the most eminent physician in the world. The eldest son of a Dutch clergyman, he planned to follow the paternal path and studied theology, philosophy, logic, metaphysics, and mathematics, but an unwise dispute in a public place—casting him in the role of defender of Spinoza—foreclosed this career to him, and he turned to medicine instead.

[g]Aside from his fellow-professor at Halle, George Ernst Stahl (see below, pp. 228 ff).

After graduating at Leyden he became professor there of medicine, botany, chemistry, and medical practice. Like his predecessor, Sylvius, he had a talent for attracting students and was world famous during his lifetime (a letter from China reached him addressed only to "the most famous physician in Europe"). He was phenomenally successful as a practitioner and left an estate of over two million guilders.

This was largely due to his personality, which possessed great appeal. He remained humble and unpretentious, treating the poor with the same dignity and deference as the rich, and once obliging Peter the Great to wait a whole night for a consultation.

His system attracted largely by its eclecticism, incorporating elements from all previous medical thinkers and in every way violating his own maxim that "simplicity is the seal of truth."[h] He declared mathematics to be the most important of the auxiliary sciences.

But his conclusion about the medical profession was clear and simple in the extreme: "If we compare the good which a half dozen true sons of Aesculapius have accomplished since the origin of the medical art upon earth with the evil which the immense mass of doctors of this profession among the human race have done, there can be no doubt that it would have been far better if there had never been any physicians in the world."[16]

The Boerhaavian doctrine was too eclectic to lend itself to systematic development,[i] but it remained a respected monument to the author's industry throughout the eighteenth century and, in Paris at any rate, was superseded only by the new thought which entered with the Revolution.

[h] A perhaps apocryphal story holds that on his deathbed he handed a leatherbound book to his followers with the advice that it contained the *summum* of medical knowledge. When opened, its single page was found to read: "Keep the head cool, the feet warm, and the bowels open."

[i] "A learned scholar and a sound scientific thinker, he was too all round a man to be led away by any one idea however tempting; essentially eclectic in nature, he gathered truth from every source" (Foster, *Lectures in the History of Physiology*, 202).

The production of these various thinkers is gigantic, the complete writings of Hoffmann alone filling six folio volumes of 450 pages apiece.[17] We will attempt only to elucidate the guiding principles of their systems, showing how they contrast with the ideas of Van Helmont.

Reason and Experience. Theory and Practice

Van Helmont and Paracelsus held observation and experience to be the source of knowledge in medicine, with "reason" playing a secondary role. They attacked the Galenists for accepting a "theory" drawn from the categories of logic and for employing this "theory," taken from outside medicine, to integrate and elucidate the elements of practice.

Thereafter Galenism was under a cloud, and Rationalist thinkers sought a new integrating concept. In the seventeenth century they found it in the emerging disciplines of chemistry, mechanics, and hydraulics, reinforced by mathematics.

Just as Aristotle and Galen had subordinated "experience" to preconceived categories of logic, these thinkers subordinated medical experience to the auxiliary disciplines achieving prominence at this time. "Theory" was drawn from chemistry or mechanics, and practice was the reflection of this theory.

The source of this counterattack on Empiricism is found in Descartes who held that sense-perception and experience are unreliable compared to the reasoning power and that medical practice must be based upon a comprehensive theory of physical and physiological causes.

He was motivated by dissatisfaction at the multitudinous combinations of sensory data and *ratio* which marked the latter stages of scholasticism and decided to wipe the slate clean by assimilating sensory data and experience to *ratio*.

Hence he (somewhat arbitrarily) divided reality into *res extensa* and *res cogitans*. The former was the physical world considered as pure extension of space and functioning by the laws of mathematics (specifically geometry). All causes and qualities found their place in this *res extensa*. *Res cogitans* was the human mind which is perfectly adapted to understanding *res extensa*.

The physical world is composed of a series of causes, one inside the other like Russian dolls, which, while invisible to the senses, can be perceived by the mind. The object of knowledge is hence the pattern of materially conceived causes comprising *res extensa.*[18] "There must at least be as much reality in the efficient and total cause as in its effect."[19] "Whatever reality or perfection exists in a thing exists formally or else eminently in its first and adequate cause."[20]

The perceptions of the senses are unreliable and secondary to *ratio:* "I shall consider that the heavens, the earth, colors, figures, sounds, and all other external things are nought but the illusions and dreams of which God has availed himself in order to lay traps for my credulity."[21] Only spatial geometry is real, quantity and number; only arithmetic and geometry are certain, "which only treat of things that are very simple and very general, without taking great trouble to ascertain whether they are actually existent or not."[22] "The certitude obtainable by the understanding is much greater than that attaching to the senses . . . It is the understanding solely which corrects the error of sense; and no case can ever be adduced in which error results from our trusting the operations of the mind more than sense."[23]

"Experience" is denigrated by Descartes, since its primary component—sense perception—is unreliable.[24] While he defines "matter of experience" as "what we perceive by sense, what we hear from the lips of others, and generally whatever reaches our understanding either from external sources *or from that contemplation which our mind directs backwards on itself,*" the last source obviously has preference.[25] Descartes carries this mode of reasoning to ridiculous extremes: for instance, he describes his scrutiny of received philosophical doctrines as a process whereby he "made various observations and acquired many experiences."[26] [j]

[j]In the same way he calls his *Discourse*—a purely analytical exercise—a "history"!! (Adam and Tannery, *Oeuvres de Descartes,* VI, 4).

His principal technique for acquiring knowledge is the analytical deduction of causes. All particular causes are indissolubly connected with more general ones, the world is knowable *a priori,* and Descartes follows the path of scholasticism in maintaining that the grand design of the universe is revealed to anyone who can understand even a small piece of it. He urges that knowledge be constructed by starting from a few particular notions, thence proceeding to universal truths, and from these universal truths—through "experiments"—deducing the intermediate truths.[27] An example is his proposal for ascertaining the nature of the magnet:

> He will first collect all the observations with which experience can supply him about this stone, and from these he will next try to deduce the character of that intermixture of simple natures which is necessary to produce all those effects which he has seen to take place in connection with the magnet. This achieved, he can boldly assert that he has discovered the real nature of the magnet in so far as human intelligence and the given experimental observations can supply him with this knowledge.[28]

Thus, even though Descartes professes admiration for Bacon, he commits precisely the scholastic error against which Bacon most inveighed: "they immediately flew from a few instances and particulars . . . to the most general conclusions or the principles of the science, and then by their intermediate propositions deduced their interior conclusions . . . and so constructed their art."[k]

This error is seen most prominently in his use of "experiment," which was followed by all the other Rationalist medical thinkers and which differs from the function of "experiment" in Bacon's philosophy.

Bacon had employed "experiment," in the sense of "learned experience," to extend man's "experience": "There

[k]See above, p. 75.

remains but mere experience, which, when it offers itself, is called chance; when it is sought after, experiment." The "form" or axiom was obtained by induction from the mass of such collated experiments after weighing and comparing the positive and negative instances. All rare and unusual instances were useful, and even indispensible, to this process.

Descartes employs "experiment" in a quite different way—as an instrument for deducing the intermediate truths or propositions from the general principles which are obtained from comparing a few particulars. Hence the correctness and reliability of these general principles could never be disproved by experiment. The meaning of the experiment is given *a priori* by the principles which it is to exemplify. Furthermore, unusual and rare occurrences are useless, since they inhibit an understanding of general principles.[1] Descartes rejects such instances as misleading until the causes of the more common ones are known.[29]

Descartes' mathematically conceived "theory" was in principle absolutely correct and reliable; defects in its application had to be, and were, ascribed to human weakness. His confidence in his method was stupefying: he assumed that a comprehensive theory of all natural processes could be developed rapidly if only enough persons could be found to perform the experiments. Indeed, a complete knowledge of the physical universe was virtually at hand:

> For myself, if I have succeeded in discovering certain truths in the sciences . . . I may say that they are resultant from, and dependent on, five or six principal difficulties which I have surmounted, and my encounter with these I look upon as so many battles in which I have had fortune on my side. I will not even hesitate to say that I think I shall have no need to win more than two or three other victories similar in kind in order to reach the accomplishment of my plans. And my age is not so advanced but that, in the ordinary course of nature, I may still have sufficient leisure for this end.[30]

[1]As in Aristotelianism, such cases could be ascribed to the category of "chance" and thus eliminated from consideration (see *Divided Legacy,* I, 130-131).

In applying his method to physiology Descartes accepted the atom or corpuscle (*particule, petite partie*) as the ultimate causal entity in the living organism.[m]

Atomism or corpuscularism, of course, had a long history from Democritus, Epicurus, and Lucretius to the Methodist School of Rome. Among Descartes' contemporaries it was espoused by Daniel Sennert (1572-1637), Pierre Gassendi (1592-1655), and Robert Boyle.

Like the ancient Methodists Descartes maintains that these corpuscles circulate through pores (*pores, petits trous*) resembling the holes in a piece of woven cloth.[31] He does not clarify the nature of the material in which these pores are located: presumably it is composed of other corpuscles flowing through other pores, and so on *ad infinitum,* since he posits no limit of divisibility.

Of course the corpuscles are invisible, but their presence is known through *ratio:* "for no one can doubt that there are bodies so small that they cannot be perceived by any of our senses, if only one considers what is being added each moment to those bodies which increase little by little . . . We day by day see a tree grow, and it is impossible to comprehend how it becomes larger than it was before unless by conceiving that some body is added to it."[32]

The cause and effect relations among the corpuscles are governed by the laws of mechanics, since the human body is

> but a statue, an earthen machine formed intentionally by God . . . not only does He give it externally the shapes and colors of all the parts of our bodies; He also places inside it all the pieces required to make it walk, eat, breathe, and imitate whichever of our own functions can be imagined to proceed from mere matter and to depend entirely on the arrangement of our organs.
>
> We see clocks, artificial fountains, mills, and similar machines which, though made entirely by man, lack not the power to move of themselves in various ways. And I

[m]Thus Descartes falls into the Methodist subclass of Rationalism (see below, pp. 606, 653).

> think you will agree that the present machine could have even more sorts of movements than I have imagined, and more ingenuity than I have assigned, for our supposition is that it was created by God.[33]

Thus the internal movements of the corpuscles are known from the external movements of the human machine, "so that it remains only for me to explain these movements to you here in proper order and by that means to tell you which of the machine's [latent] functions these [patent] movements represent."[34]

Very probably Descartes' discovery that the laws of vision are geometrical encouraged him and his followers to assume that the remaining functions of the organism could be explained in the same way. Their self-assurance, in any case, was extreme: Cartesianism gave the theoretician absolute confidence in the results of his reasoning. And since these results were immune to correction through practical experience, physicians needed no further stimulus to plunge into far-reaching physiological speculation and medical experimentation. Theoretical knowledge was considered absolutely reliable, whatever the consequences for practice.

The other seventeenth-century Rationalists followed Descartes in elevating *ratio* and theory above experience and practice.

George Cheyne observes:

> In *medicina philosophica seu rationalis* the true natural philosophy is the stem or root, and practical medicine but a branch. From natural philosophy the physician must learn the structure and uses of the several organs of the animal body and the laws of the animal economy . . . From the same natural philosophy he must make himself acquainted with the nature, uses, and virtues of the *materia medica,* or the materials commonly used in medicine, and to the first adjust this last, in order to antidote the causes of a given distemper; and he who is

> the best natural philosopher will, *ceteris paribus,* ever be the best physician.[35]

Persons who "prescribe such remedies as they read or heard had been successful in cases which they imagine like that of their patients, but know nothing either of the cause of the distemper or of the reason of the cure" are "rather *empirics* than physicians."[36]

Medicine should follow the course of astronomy and become scientific through application of mathematics.[37] Descartes "first banished effectually the Aristotelian jargon and made men reflect upon the natural right they had to a freedom of thinking: and tho' for the most part he did substitute a bad system in its room, yet it was such a one as made men reflect more upon the necessity of applying geometry to natural philosophy . . . he was the first who explained mechanically the nature of vision and the construction of the eye."[38] If skilled geometricians would but do the needed work, "medicine in a short time might be brought to the immediate confines of demonstration."[39]

Hoffmann states that theory is general, explaining the functions of the parts and the causes of life and death, as well as of each disease and each symptom.[40] Practice descends into particulars: it is the art of applying remedies prudently, and its object is the individual.[41]

Theory is based on chemistry and physics or, more specifically, on mechanics, yielding *a priori* knowledge of the forces in natural things.[42] To the extent that theory relies on physics it is a science,[43] while practice is "the art of properly utilizing physico-chemical principles in order to conserve the health of man or to restore it if lost."[44]

Theory is a structure of causal knowledge. Everything in nature has a cause, and the task of a science is to know these causes. This is done by following the method of geometry, assuming certain principles and deducing conclusions from them: hence geometry is another model for medical reasoning.[45]

Experience is unreliable, only supplying the raw material of theory.[46] But, on the other hand, medicine relies on "experience, which is the first parent of truth" as well as upon "reason, which is the key to medical science. Experience comes first in order, and reason follows . . . in medical affairs reasons which are not founded on experience have no value."[47] Hoffmann solves this puzzle of the true relations between theory and experience by dividing the latter in twain:

> In physics [i.e., theory] experience can best be sought from mathematics and mechanics, chemistry, and anatomy; in medical practice experience derives most abundantly from the observations of disease and from more accurate histories and cures.[48]

One variety of "experience" is, thus, "experiment" in the Cartesian sense: from experiments the forces, properties, and effects of bodies are deduced following physical principles, and modern philosophy is rightly called experimental philosophy.[49] [n] The other variety of "experience" is the unstructured type which the physician accumulates at the bedside and which is useful for improving practice, i.e., for improving the art of applying the theoretical principles of medicine. But such experience alone cannot provide the art with a solid theoretical foundation, since it is impossible to make a sufficient number of observations.[50] Hence medical theory must be drawn from the experimental sciences—mechanics, chemistry, anatomy, and physics—and is the basis of a "certain, safe, and easy practice."[51]

It is not enough for the physician to know what to do: he must prove the correctness of his procedures by reasoning from definite principles.[52] A "sectarian" bases his science on

[n]He observes that, although this sort of experience should be based upon a long series of careful observations, this is difficult, and reason must be called in to help (F. Hoffmann, *Medicinae Rationalis Systematicae Tomus Prior* [Halle, 1718], 9). His treatment of these problems resembles that of his contemporary, Baglivi (see below, pp. 195-196).

indefinite, uncertain, undemonstrable principles: since the *Archeus* is just such an uncertain principle, Van Helmont was a sectarian.[53] He did not accept all that reason and experience could teach him.[54]

While many persons believe that the good theorist is necessarily a bad practitioner, this is false.[55]

Boerhaave's treatment of the relations between theory and practice, reason and experience, is eclectic and inconsistent. For he admires the method of Hippocrates, which he realizes was purely empirical, but feels that modern medicine has advanced beyond this stage and succeeded in founding practice on precise knowledge of causes.

> Though Hippocrates understood not the circulation of the blood, yet by accurately observing the effects of the disease, which he looked upon as an unknown entity, and by remarking the endeavors of the *natura,* by which the disease tended to either health or recovery, did from thence deduce a proper method of cure, namely by assisting the salutary endeavors of the *natura,* and by resisting those of the disease; and thus Hippocrates, ignorant of the causes, cured disease as well as ourselves, stocked with so many discoveries.[56]

And he criticizes Galen for confusing things "by striving to make the genuine observations of Hippocrates correspond to the false system of the Peripatetics."[57]

But this empirical approach is inadequate, for "a great many patients may be lost at the approach of any new disease, before a proper and successful course can be adjusted or assigned, as Sydenham observes."[58] [o] While in primitive times nearly all remedies were discovered by "natural instinct or promiscuous experiment," at a later date reasoning by analogy was introduced, and modern medicine based upon theory came into being.[59]

[o]See below, p. 208.

While theory in ancient times was founded on observation and experience,[60] this is a problematical procedure, "since every sect may explain the causes of particular effects upon different hypotheses."[61] To avoid this confusion in the assignation of causes to the observed phenomena "it is requisite we should fix on some principles whose certainty and effects are demonstrable to our senses, which may serve to explain the phenomena of natural bodies and account for the accidents that arise in them: such only are those which are purely material in the human body with mechanical and physical experiments . . . a physician may and ought to furnish himself with, and reason from, such things as are demonstrated to be true in anatomy, chemistry, and mechanics, with natural and experimental philosophy, provided he confines his reasoning within the bounds of truth and simple experiment."[62]

In his opinion medicine passed from its previous empirical state to its modern, more developed, form with Harvey's discovery of the circulation, proving the body to be a hydraulic mechanism subject to the laws of that science. "The immortal Harvey, by the discoveries which he demonstrated, overturned the whole theory of the ancients and founded physic upon a new and more certain basis, upon which it at present rests . . . he demonstrated the human body to be an engine, all whose offices depend upon the circulation of the blood, which alone being stopped, the whole must perish; from which thesis alone the whole theory of the Galenists and Chemists was overturned and all the learning of the Ancients; that only subsisted which was founded and approved by experiment; so that the whole progress of physick may be commodiously divided into the ancient before Harvey and the modern after his time . . . nor is the doctrine of Harvey contrary to that of Hippocrates, but rather an explanation of it."[63] [p]

[p]The discovery of the circulation of the blood by William Harvey (1578-1657) is, of course, one of the great turning-points in the history of physiology, refuting the previously accepted Galenic theory that the blood passes from the right to the

"The universal laws of nature, or affections of all bodies, depend on mechanical and physical principles, upon which

left ventricle through pores in the ventricular septum. His *De Motu Cordis,* published in 1628, sets forth this discovery, although it was prefigured in his anatomical lectures ten years earlier (C. D. O'Malley, F. N. L. Poynter, and K. F. Russell, *William Harvey: Lectures on the Whole of Anatomy* [Berkeley and Los Angeles: University of California Press, 1961], 10-11, 16-17).

Boerhaave, however, and the Rationalist tradition in medicine misunderstood the point that Harvey was making, for he did not say that the heart causes the blood to circulate but rather that the circulation of the blood causes the heart to beat. His research on the generation of chicks *in ovo,* as well as his investigation of the circulation itself, showed him that the blood, under the control of the *physis,* is present prior to the formation of the heart or any other organ. Hence he identified the blood (following the biblical injunction) with the life of man and his soul. "The blood does not seem to differ in any respect from the soul or the life itself (*anima*)..... It therefore comes to the same thing whether we say that the soul and the blood, or the blood with the soul, or the soul with the blood, performs all the acts in the animal organism" (*The Works of William Harvey* [London: The Sydenham Society, 1847], 511). "Nor is the blood to be styled the primigenial and principal portion of the body because the pulse has its commencement in it and through it; but also because animal heat originates in it, and the vital spirit is associated with it, and it constitutes the vital principle itself" (*ibid.,* 376). "The life, therefore, resides in the blood . . . because in it life and the soul first show themselves, and last become extinct" (*loc. cit.*). "So little is it true, as Aristotle and the medical writers assert, that the liver and the heart are the authors and compounders of the blood, that the contrary even appears most obviously from the formation of the chick *in ovo,* viz.: that the blood is much rather the fashioner of the heart and liver" (*ibid.,* 378). He defines the cause of the blood's motion as "an internal principle under the control of the *natura*" (*ibid.,* 137). This gives rise to the heart's diastolic motion, while the systole is the effect of the heart's "pulsific faculty": "the pulse, then, is produced by a double agent; first, the blood undergoes distension or dilatation, and secondly, the vesicular membrane of the embryo in the egg, the auricles and ventricles in the extruded chick, effect the constriction. By these alternating motions associated is the blood impelled through the whole body, and the life of animals is thereby continued" (*ibid.,* 375). Hence, although "the heart, with the veins and arteries and the blood they contain, is to be regarded as the beginning and author, the fountain and original of all things in the body, the primary cause of life," "if by the word, heart, the mere body of the heart, made up of its auricles and ventricles, be understood, then I do not believe that the heart is the fashioner of the blood; neither do I imagine that the blood has powers, properties, motion, or heat, as the gift of the heart . . . I hold that the innate heat is the first cause of dilatation, and that the primary dilatation is in the blood itself, after the manner of bodies in a state of fermentation, gradually attenuated and swelling, and that in the blood is this finally extinguished" (*ibid.,* 137).

The cast of Harvey's mind was clearly vitalist and Empirical, but he is not discussed at length in these pages because his discoveries fall in the realm of physiology, not medicine. Nothing is known of his practice.

alone their actions are explicable; the same laws are also true in the human body, for its matter appears to be universally the same with that of all other bodies, so that what may be said to be true of all bodies, may be also affirmed true in our own."[64] "The solid parts of the human body are either membraneous pipes, or vessels including the fluids, or else instruments made up of these and more solid fibres, so formed and connected that each of them is capable of performing a particular action by the structure, whenever they shall be put in motion; we find some of them resemble pillars, props, cross-beams, fences, coverings, some like axes, wedges, levers, and pullies; others like cords, presses, or bellows, and others again like sieves, strainers, pipes, conduits, and receivers; and the faculty of performing various motions by these instruments is called their functions; which are all performed by mechanical laws, and by them only are intelligible."[65] [q]

Thus Boerhaave relied on Harvey as authority for the *a priori* principle that the organism functions like a machine, greatly simplifying all problems associated with observation, reasoning, and experimentation in medicine. "Observation here is the attention of the mind to such changes as happen in human bodies, all which changes proceed from motion, which motion is produced originally in the body as a machine."[66] Knowing that the organism functions as a machine, the physician can apply the principles of mechanical reasoning to elucidate processes which are not directly observable: "the motion of our fluids through their vessels does naturally escape the notice of all our naked senses; therefore a physician ought to be acquainted as well with the objects which do not fall immediately, as with those that do; for the knowledge of the first is equally necessary to physick with the last, tho' it be only attainable by analogy, from

[q]He opposes those (*sc.* G. E. Stahl), "enemies to the very name of mechanics, who assert that our bodies are not subject to the same laws with all others" (*Dr. Boerhaave's Academical Lectures on the Theory of Physic* [London, 1742-1746], I, 75).

comparing the parts less known with those which are wholly obvious to our senses."[67] "A strict consideration and discovery of the several latent causes concealed from our naked senses in human bodies by just reasoning" is a valid way to erect medical theory.[68] "It is certain that physick may be as well supported by just reasoning as by observation and experience."[69] "Observation or experience alone will not make a physician; for any two diseases are never so much alike, but a small degree of reasoning may distinguish the difference."[70] Just reasoning is needed to discover "the great class of diseases which lie concealed from naked sense."[71]

Boerhaave rejects the argument that modes of reasoning drawn from other disciplines may not be applied to the human organism: "there is no necessity for the principles of any art to be proved in that art; it is sufficient if their certainty is by any means demonstrated in other arts."[72]

Even Hippocrates, Boerhaave concludes, operated in this same way: "he was the first that by just reasoning joined the theory to practice in physick."[73] This theory was "the philosophy of Democritus which was the purest of any system, being founded on three principles: atoms, gravity, and a vacuum, which have been in our age restored by the most solid reasonings of Sir Isaac Newton."[74]

> Hippocrates, in the same age with Democritus, being well skilled in all these particulars, and furnished with numerous wise observations of his own as well as of others, formed the best of them into a Greek system of physick; and was the first that truly deserved the title of physician: for being of incomparable reason and ample experience, supported by a sound philosophy, he laid a just and rational foundation of physick for future ages.[75]

Medical theory, "the science or knowledge of those things by whose application and effects health may be preserved when present and restored when lost," is thus made up of "facts" which are either self-evident or readily deduced from experiments in such disciplines as physics, chemistry, and mechanics.[76] "In this respect we seem to be more happy than our ancestors, in that not being seduced to errors by any authority, we only admit facts to which we are compelled by the force of truth and free consent, or else embrace such things only as are evinced by experiments, or are so apparent from them that we cannot confute their evidence."[77] "Nor are we to add any suppositions or consequences but what are deducible from them by severe and just reasoning."[78]

These "facts" are to be distinguished from the fancies of such "sectarians" as the followers of Van Helmont. A sectarian view is a "probable opinion which has been received by many people, but yet is not so evident as to compel every reasonable person, skilled in his profession, to allow it for true."[79] The difference between "real truth" and the concept of the *Archeus* or some other sectarian opinion is that the former "results from observation or . . . follows of consequence from the facts or observations, so evidently that no skilful and unprejudiced person can refuse his assent."[80]

> At present physick may be learned without adhering to any particular sect, by rejecting everything that is offered without demonstration, and by collecting and retaining only what has been offered and approved to be real truth both by the Ancients and Moderns.[81]

Thus by "fact" Boerhaave means the exemplification through experiment of the *a priori* principles of mechanics or chemistry. As in the scholastic and Cartesian tradition the purpose of "experiment" is only to make explicit certain principles already accepted as true. The Empirical idea that experiment is designed to extend the realm of knowledge, to test the truth of given principles, to make discoveries, is wholly absent.

Once the student is familiar with the "institutions of physick, which comprehend the knowledge of everything necessary for the preservation of health and the cure of diseases," he may "proceed to the practice, which is the putting those precepts, which he has before learned, in force upon his patient."[82] The first branch of medicine is physiology, "demonstrating the several parts of the human body, with their mechanisms and actions."[83] On this is based pathology, "treating of diseases, their differences, causes and effects, or symptoms"; and on pathology, semeiotics "which shews the signs distinguishing between sickness and health, diseases, and their causes in the human body . . . The objects of this branch are the non-naturals, as well as the naturals or preternaturals."[84] The fourth branch is hygiene, and the fifth branch is therapeutics.[85] The theoretical knowledge (physiology) is put into practice (therapeutics) "not by simple imitation, but by the knowledge of causes. Physicians not only know by experience that warm thin liquids abate fevers, but they also understand that they do so by relaxing the fibers and diluting the viscid blood. But the dyer is ignorant of the reason why he adds alum, tin, or gums in his art; so he also is of their action."[86] For this reason even the practical part of medicine is not so much an art as a science.[87]

Thus Boerhaave was less willing than Hoffmann to allow a role for experience in the improvement of practice. *Practice is only the crystallization of theory.* Experience and practice are entirely governed by theory and *ratio,* taking on significance only when transformed into theory:

> There are two methods which may be relied upon as certain for the attainment of our profession, which may be esteemed its solid foundations. The first is an accurate observation of all the appearances offered to our senses in the human body . . . The second is a strict consideration and discovery of the several latent causes, concealed from our naked senses in human bodies, by a just reasoning . . . Physick thus established upon judgment and observation can be only attained by a just reasoning from the several facts which have before been thoroughly considered in every respect; from comparing those reasonings with the *natura* or experience and with each other; and from diligently remarking which of them appear agree-

able or disagreeable to truth, that from the whole we may be enabled to draw just conclusions in regard to present and future events, which conclusions may then be relied upon with certainty as matter of fact.[88]

The Definition of Life

Vitalism is the fulcrum of Empirical therapeutic doctrine. Under whatever name—the Hippocratic *physis,* Paracelsus' Alchemist, Van Helmont's *Archeus*—these thinkers have recognized a vital principle in the organism representing its purposiveness and spontaneity, its reactive capacity.

Rationalism in medicine, on the contrary, is deterministic and seeks to eliminate any source of autonomy in the organism by dividing up the vitality into: 1) a physical or chemical process and 2) the immortal soul.

In the language of the eighteenth century, Rationalism rejects the existence of a "vegetative" or "sensitive" soul.[r]

Descartes is the prototype of this attack on vitalism. He identifies "life" with the immortal soul which at the same time provides the subject with rational guidance through its single point of contact with the body—the pineal gland.[89] The body otherwise functions as a machine centered on a mechanico-chemical process in the heart.

The blood entering the right ventricle is heated and evaporated, just as "the blood or milk of some animal will be dilated if you pour it drop by drop into a very hot flask."[90] The vaporization and consequent expansion of the blood cause the heartbeat and "[make] all the arteries of the body inflate at the same time as the heart."[91] From the right ventricle the blood vapor passes to the lung, where it is recondensed into liquid, and returns to the left ventricle to

[r]See Van Helmont (above, p. 28) and G. E. Stahl (below, pp. 235-236).

undergo the same heating and vaporization.[92] [s] All of the remaining motions of the organism depend on this primordial process. "It is not necessary . . . to conceive of any vegetative or sensitive soul or any other principle of movement and life than [the body's] blood and its spirits agitated by the heat of the fire which burns continually in its heart and which is of no other nature than all those fires which occur in inanimate bodies."[93] "The power of vegetation and of motion of the body which in plants and animals are called the *vegetative* and *sensitive* soul are also present in man but ought not to be called *souls* in him, since they are not the first principles of his actions and differ entirely in kind from the rational soul. Moreover, *vegetative* force in man [as in animals] is nothing other than a certain constitution of the parts of the body."[94]

When asked why the fire in the heart could not be observed, Descartes retorted that it is "one of those fires without light . . . which [is not] different from that which makes the hay heat when shut up before it is dry, and which makes new wine grow frothy when it is left to ferment over the fruit."[95]

It is worth noting that animals do not possess "life" in the Cartesian philosophy, since they lack an immortal soul. Hence, they are unable to reason or function autonomously but are mere pieces of machinery. "Life I deny to no animal . . . *except insofar as I lay it down that it consists simply of the warmth of the heart.*"[96] In fish and reptiles, which are notoriously not warm, Descartes held the heart to be still warmer than the rest of the body.[97]

But he cannot maintain with perfect consistency his likening of the organism to a machine and accepts the existence of "animal" spirits to fill some of the gaps in his physiology. The "liveliest, strongest, and most subtle parts of

[s]When someone observed that the heartbeat should then cease in a person who was standing on his head, Descartes insisted that in such a case the blood "flows" or is "inserted" into the heart "by the circulation and by the spontaneous contraction of the vessels" (T. S. Hall, *Rene Descartes: Treatise of Man,* 11, note 23).

the blood proceed to the cavities of the brain" where they "serve not only to nourish and sustain its substance but also and principally to produce there a certain very subtle wind, or rather a very lively and very pure flame, which is called the 'animal spirits'."[98]

Such "animal" or "vital" spirits had been available since Galen's time to take up the slack in Rationalist physiological theories (being related to the *pneuma* which served the same purpose).[99] They were a concession to Empirical vitalism. Descartes uses these spirits to explain the senses of sight, hearing, smell, touch, and taste, such emotions as generosity, liberality, and love, and such facets of character and intellect as confidence, courage, dreams, common sense, memory, etc. etc.[100] And when they make their way into the nervous system, they produce the movements of the body: "Now in the same measure that spirits enter the cavities of the brain they also leave them and enter the pores in its substance, and from these conduits they proceed to the nerves. And depending on their entering (or their mere tendency to enter) some nerves rather than others, they are able to change the shapes of the muscles into which these nerves are inserted and in this way to move all the members. Similarly you may have observed in the grottoes and fountains in the gardens of our kings that the force that makes the water leap from its source is able of itself to move divers machines and even to make them play certain instruments or pronounce certain words according to the various arrangements of the tubes through which the water is conducted."[101]

The fountains in the automated gardens of St. Germain-en-Laye were thus the model for the human nervous system—although Descartes admitted that the latter is more complex, being invented by God and not by the Royal Engineers.[102]

Sylvius' theory of the heartbeat is identical with that of Descartes except that he assigns the "animal spirits" a role in this function as well.[103] They are distilled from the blood in the cerebral cortex and carried through the medullary substance to the nerves and thence to the rest of the body: they are responsible for the senses, the interplay of emotion between the brain and the rest of the body, and muscular contraction.[104] "Moreover, at least in my conjecture, yea opinion, they temper any humors, choler, spittle, the pancreatical or melancholic juice, or lympha, of the conglobated glandules, and perhaps afford the primary matter to generate seed."[105] The persistence of muscular contractions in the stomach after death convinced him that, "although not perhaps seen and discerned with the eyes of the body, the animal spirits yet are demonstrated to the mind by solid reasoning."[106]

Sylvius alludes to the "so-called vital powers" (*vitales dictae vires*),[107] meaning the residual strength of the body depressed in disease, but does not mention "vital spirits."[108]

Willis builds on Descartes and Sylvius but differs from both. Humans possess a "rational soul," equivalent to the divine or immortal soul and to the intellect or reasoning power, which exercises a general supervisory function over the "corporeal soul." This latter, which man has in common with animals[t] and which is subject to chemical laws, is of more immediate interest to physiology.

Willis takes the Cartesian simile of "fire without light" (for the combustion in the left and right ventricles of the heart[u]) and elaborates it into a description of the two parts of the corporeal soul: 1) a flame continuously enkindled in the blood by the fire in the heart and 2) a nervous fluid or juice "streaming gently through the brain and its belongings

[t]Thus Willis allows animals somewhat more of life than Descartes was willing to do (*Dr. Willis's Practice of Physick* [London, 1684], Part XI, 3-4).

[u]He observes that while Descartes claims an actual fire in the heart, another authority holds that the heat there is from fermentation: "Tis almost the same thing whether it be said to be done by this or by that way" (*Dr. Willis's Practice of Physick,* Part II, 54).

. . . after the manner of light, like the rays of light emanating from that flame."[109]

"The blood is animate or hath life . . . this animation is in its accension or inkindling . . . the blood is the life or soul, which is also apparent by the observation of the most famous Harvey, for that its motion is to be observed by the eye, shows that it first lives and last dies."[110] To perpetuate the flame in the blood there must be free access of air, sulphurous combustible matter, and some provision for disposal of the products of combustion. Since, as Robert Boyle has shown, a candle cannot burn in the absence of air and animals die when deprived of air, the blood must be continually circulated through the lungs if combustion is to be maintained.[111] This circulation is done by the heart.[112] The products of combustion are removed from the blood in the form of the body's excrements and skin secretions.[113]

The "nervous fluid or juice," another aspect of the "corporeal" or "rational" soul, is distilled from the blood in the cerebral and cerebellar cortices and thence conveyed as "animal spirits" through the nervous system to all parts of the body.[114] Willis adopts Descartes' metaphor of the brain acting as "the chest of an organ which receives the wind to be blown into all the pipes" [i.e., the nerves].[115]

The precise lines of demarcation among the various spirits and parts of the "corporeal" soul in Willis' philosophy are not always clear, but his intent is perfectly so: to break down the Helmontian *Archeus* into its individual functions, subject them to physical or chemical laws, and eliminate this purposive force from medical theory.

George Cheyne rejects all speculation about animal spirits and follows Descartes to the letter, regarding the body as a mechanism actuated by a rational soul.[116] He sidesteps the problem of the vitality: "How it exerts these powers on divinely organized matter I do not here pretend to say,"[117] and merely suggests that it is through the nerves ("filled with a soft milky cellular substance") by virtue of some "infinitesimal function."[118]

Hoffman's arguments about the vitality are rather confused. He was teaching at Halle where his principal colleague was Georg Ernst Stahl, the leading vitalist of his time and one of the more important thinkers in the history of Western medicine, who proposed a theory of the organism centering on the *Anima sensitiva* ("sensitive soul").[v] Thus Hoffmann, despite his mechanistic instincts and predilections, had to make some allowance in his doctrine for a vitalist input.

The body is wholly material, being composed of "an extremely subtle matter, a subtle or ethereal matter, and a more dense or earthy and aqueous form."[119] Of these the first two are the liquids, while the last represents the solids. "Matter provides a single simple essence to things, receives various modes, and is rendered specific in various ways through motion, the most universal principle of all."[120] This matter, like all of nature, operates by the laws of mechanics.[121] "Our body is like a machine which is composed of solid and fluid particles, disposed and arranged in varying order and position."[122]

The life of the body is represented by the interaction of fluids and solids, with the former taking primacy.[123] "It is not the solid parts, considered in themselves, that can be said to be well ordered or disordered, but their due proportion depends on the proportion and motion of the fluid parts."[124] [w] "Life is achieved by causes which are wholly mechanical.[x] The mind does not bring life to the body, nor is life oriented to the mind, but rather to the body."[125] "Just

[v]See below, pp. 228 ff.

[w]Elsewhere Hoffmann states both that the state of the solids is due to the humors and that the state of the humors is due to the solids (F. Hoffmann, *A System of the Practice of Medicine* [London, 1783], I, 3, 194, 219; Sprengel, *Histoire de la Medecine,* V, 295).

[x]Hoffmann rejects all chemical interpretations of physiology. Fermentation is nothing more than the movement of the fine particles in the liquids of the body, and the body's heat itself is only the resultant of the movement of the liquids (F. Hoffmann, *Fundamenta Medicinae* [N.Y.: Elsevier, 1971], 6, 9-10).

as life consists in motion of the fluid parts, and health in well-ordered and even motion, so death is only a destruction of motion, or motion disproportionate and uneven."[126]

In this mechanical system the heart is central, "the *perpetuum mobile* which has been sought for so long; since the blood moves the heart which in turn gives movement to the blood, by this mechanism the cause produces the effect which then reproduces the cause itself."[127] "The heart is the first principle of all motion in our body and of the circulation of the blood (without which man cannot live); it is the instrument and prime force impelling the blood."[128][y]

Strong in his mechanical doctrine of life, Hoffmann attacks Stahl's theory of the *Anima.* It is too indefinite a principle to serve as a basis for demonstration.[129] One cannot explain or understand how such an entity disposes and directs the body.[130] This is akin to the "nominal" medicine of the ancients who substituted names or spiritual forces for the proximate or sense-perceptible ones which the reason can grasp.[131] The medicine of today is no longer nominal but "real"—the fruit of observation, meditation, judgment, and reasoning.[132] Stahl's *Anima* is like Van Helmont's *Archeus*—its acceptance would mean casting physics and anatomy out of medicine.[133]

But then (depending upon which book one reads) Hoffmann introduces the *Anima* at key points in the argument. "All philosophers are agreed that in our machine the first principle of motion is the *Anima* which you may, if you want, designate as the *natura,* or spirit endowed with mechanical powers, or a most subtle ethereal matter acting in an ordered and specific fashion."[134] Apart from its mechanical capacities, this principle is able to think and reason, hence is immortal.[135] "The first cause of the powers existing in the *Anima* is God Himself, on whom all things depend, including the existence and functions of our *Anima.*"[136] The *Anima* directs and guides the animal spirits: "The animal spirits are

[y]While Descartes denied life to animals, Hoffmann (a lesser thinker) denies it to plants—since plants lack a heart (Sprengel, *Histoire de la Medecine,* V, 291).

not the vital principle or the *Anima* itself, but the *Anima* uses these as instruments for achieving its functions."[137] [z] "The functions of the *Anima* are to move the spirits and to direct them to produce particular motions."[138] "The animal spirits, provided with the utmost fineness and elasticity, have a power impressed by God, not only of moving themselves mechanically, but doing so by choice, purposefully, and toward a definite goal. This power is called the *Anima sensitiva,* and it exists entirely in the most subtle fluid of the brain."[139]

Thus Hoffmann's *Anima,* like Stahl's, is able to think and reason autonomously and purposefully–consequently is not subject only to physical and mechanical laws. But this runs contrary to the major thrust of his argument. He even goes so far as to hold that "the motion of the heart is not due to any innate motor power, but to the expansive effort of the spirituous seminal fluid in the embryo itself. In adults it seems due to the expansive force of the ether and of the animal spirits and blood."[140] The ultimate cause of all motion, in the body as outside it, is "God Almighty Himself, the greatest and best mechanic and prime mover of things."[141]

As in the relationship between *ratio* and experience, in respect of the vital force Boerhaave is more rigidly rational than Hoffmann. He leaves out of consideration all "vital" or "animal spirits" and all consideration of an *Archeus* or *Anima:* "they who endeavor to persuade us into the notion of an *Archeus* or cogitative principle ought first to demonstrate the nature of that being to our senses, together with the means by which it communicates with the body."[142] [a] There is no reason to take into account this "animating principle which has been drawn into physick by some men of note."[143]

[z]He calls the "animal spirits" the "chief fluid parts of the body" (F. Hoffmann, *Fundamenta Medicinae,* 11).

[a]While he makes mention of "vital spirits," they have no doctrinal significance (*Dr. Boerhaave's Academical Lectures,* VI, 41).

Instead, his definition of "life" is on four levels: 1) the body's performance of its functions: 2) the action of the heart, as the cause of the other functions: 3) the physical properties of the body's solid parts; and 4) God Himself who conferred these properties.

On the first level, therefore, life is "the sum or aggregate of all the actions performed in the human body,"[144] "an equable distribution of all the vital humors through their respective vessels,"[145] "the determinate motion of the solids and fluids upon each other, and the change by that means made in the aliments."[146]

On the second level, since "a cause of any thing is a being whose existence gives being to some effect or other, and upon whose non-existence that being or effect must also cease to be, so long as the heart continues its motion, so long does life remain, but whenever that organ ceases to move, life itself also ceases to be; the motion of the heart is therefore the cause of life."[147]

On the third level, the movement of the heart and the solids is due to "an elastic and contractile power in the fibers, to resist their distraction or dilatation."[148] "The fluids in the human body act only by their motion, by which they dilate the vessels containing them; and the vessels exert no other action upon their contained fluids than that of resistance or reaction common to all bodies, by which the vessels endeavor to contract themselves to their smallest dimensions and resist dilatation, and which action is known either under the denomination of elasticity or the power of attraction."[149]

The proof that "life" is a property of matter is that these properties remain present even after death: "in a dead body all the actions resulting from the circulation of the blood cease, but yet this contractile force of the solids continues a long time even after death."[150] The body can live for a short time even after the heart has been removed.[151]

And ultimately "life" is due to God: "this same force or endeavor of all the parts in the same body to retain and enter more closely into their contacts with each other is an universal principle of nature, to be ascribed only to the Creator of the universe, who has determined this as a principle of uniting the parts of bodies; for the parts of matter do not cohere by any innate force of their own; but having a separate existence, it was necessary for the Creator to provide another power by which they might cohere together and resist dissolution."[152]

While these thinkers were all willing to admit that the ultimate causes of physiological and medical phenomena are unknowable,[153] their interpretation of "cause" differed from that of the Empirics who also held that causes are ultimately unknowable. Boerhaave and the other Rationalists only meant that the reasons why the liquids and solids of the body possess particular properties are unknowable. *But these reasons and causes fall outside the sphere of medical practice.* The causes with which therapeutics and pathology are concerned are those of the next higher order: the motions of the liquids and solids as determined by the ultimate properties conferred by God. And *these* causes are entirely cognizable by the physician. Indeed they are the substance of his theory and the foundation of his practice.

> There are indeed some who think that these actions ought not to be explained by mechanical laws, since the mechanical causes of them are unknown to us; but in saying this they show very little consideration; for we are not treating of the causes but the effects subject to mechanical laws. There are many, and considerable, motions performed in nature, of whose causes we are ignorant; but the motions themselves are always subject to those universal laws which appear to be true in all sensible bodies. Even the lodestone, the cause of whose action is most concealed from us, performs its motions by certain and known laws which, once observed, never fail to be true when applied to future experiments. The human body performs various motions, the causes of which are absolutely concealed from us, but the effects of those motions are the elevation of weights by fixed

> cords, the propulsion of fluids through their several vessels, etc., which effects being similar to those which are produced by mechanical causes, are not governed by any other laws.[154]

Thus, while Empiricism assumed that the ultimately unknowable vital force acts according to its own *sui generis* laws, and based therapeutics on the emerging knowledge of these laws, Rationalism assumed that the organism is explicable in terms of the laws generated in other scientific disciplines. No holistic dimension of the body or ultimate mystery of its functioning could affect Rationalist theory or practice:

> Whoever enquires further into the origin of these similar diseases will run himself into the faults of the humors or else he will fall upon some subtlety or unknown principle, neither demonstrable to the senses nor useful to the physician, and therefore the similar distempers of the temperature, of the elements, and of the *whole substance of the body,* as they are termed in the Schools, can neither take place here nor be understood; but they are to be reduced, if possible, to the compound disorders which regard both solids and fluids.[155]

Physiology. Pathology. Therapeutics

Rationalist therapeutics is derived from pathology which, in turn, is a function of physiology. Knowing the causes at work in the body in health, the physician can recognize pathological alterations. Therapy means reversing this pathology in order to restore health. "Reversing" is through application of the "contrary" medicine. Hence the logical contrariety of Galenism became chemical or mechanical contrariety in the seventeenth century.

Descartes' weak health as a child stirred him to a consuming interest in medicine. At the end of his *Discourse on Method* he suggests that it will be serviceable for medicine and "the preservation of health, which is without doubt the chief blessing and the foundation of all other blessings in this life."[156]

His *Treatise of Man,* written about 1632 but published only in 1664 after his death, had a pronounced impact on Rationalist medical thinking.

It gives a mechanical or corpuscular interpretation of the concept of "coction" or digestion—a leading problem of physiology even in ancient times[b] and one upon which Van Helmont (of whose research Descartes was unaware) and many other contemporaries were working.

The current approach, in the investigation of digestion, was to identify it with fermentation, and Descartes provides a mechanical explanation of fermentation. "The food is digested in the stomach of this machine by the force of certain liquids which, gliding among the food particles [*parties*], separate, shake, and heat them just as common water does the particles of quicklime, or *aqua fortis* those of metals."[157] [c] Moreover, food can ferment of itself, like new hay in a barn.[158] "The agitation that the food particles receive in being heated, together with the agitation of the stomach and bowels that contain them, and the arrangement of the fibers of which the bowels are composed, cause these particles—in the measure that they are digested—to descend little by little toward the [rectum]."[159] Here the "subtlest and most agitated particles" encounter "an infinity of little holes" through which they flow to a vein which takes them to the liver. But the coarser ones, which cannot pass through these holes, are excreted: "nothing but the smallness of the holes serving to separate these from the coarser particles; just as, when one shakes meal in a sack, all the purest part runs out, and only the smallness of the holes through which it passes prevents the bran from following after."[160]

The chyle elaborated in the stomach passes through the intestinal pores to the vein leading to the liver where it is converted to chyme: "the pores of the liver are so arranged

[b]See *Divided Legacy,* I, 240-247.

[c]The reactions Descartes describes are, of course, not examples of true fermentation.

that this liquid, when it enters, is subtilized and elaborated, and takes on the color and acquires the form of blood, just as the white juice of black grapes is converted into light red wine when one lets it ferment on the vine stock."[161] The chyme passes through the *vena cava* to the right cavity of the heart, thence through the lungs to the left cavity, and out through the arteries to the various parts of the body: "to replace what the continual agitation of these parts—and the divers actions of neighboring ones—detaches from them and sends away."[162] [d] Other particles of blood go to form saliva, urine, bile ("where they act like *aqua fortis* to help the digestion of food"), sweat, skin excretions, etc.[163] "And in all of these places it is only the position, or shape, or small size of the pores through which they pass that makes some go through rather than others, and keeps the rest of the blood from following, as you may have seen in divers sieves which, being differently pierced, serve to separate different grains one from the other."[164]

This physiology, with its pervasive invocation of the flow of atoms or corpuscles through holes or pores, resembles the doctrine of the ancient Methodists,[e] and, not surprisingly, the resulting therapeutics relies on a major technique of this School—the unblocking of obstructed flows. Descartes himself wrote nothing on therapeutics, but his ideas were taken up by various groups of followers who fused them with Iatrochemistry and Iatromechanism to arrive at various interpretations of "obstruction" and various recommendations for its removal.

According to Hoffmann, the Cartesian physicians aimed to establish the "acid and viscid [*viscidum*]" and the obstructions arising therefrom. Their therapeutic indication was to maintain the fluidity of the blood and the circulation by suitable remedies. They rejected plethora as a disease

[d]Here he incorporates Harvey's discovery that the blood does not pass directly from the liver to the veins (as Galen had assumed) but first to the heart and thence, *via* the arteries, to the rest of the body (Hall, *Rene Descartes: Treatise of Man,* 15, note 32).

[e]See *Divided Legacy,* I, 291-301 and below, pp. 606-645.

cause and despised bloodletting, purges, and acid medicines.[165]

A Cartesian Academy established in France combined the Master's doctrines with elements taken from Paracelsus, proving that all things come from water and salt of which several species can be distinguished: salt is volatile and consists partly of fire, while one variety of water is sulphurous and another is mercurial. The volatile salt is composed of perfectly round corpuscles, making it entirely mobile, while the fiery salt consists of elongated and square corpuscles, enabling it to act as a cohesive, etc. etc. The Netherlands school of Cartesian medicine fused it with Van Helmont's ferments and attributed all corporal functions and all diseases to the form and mixture of the humoral corpuscles—their fermentation, distillation, effervescence, precipitation, etc.[166]

A work on venereal disease by one member of this school holds that syphilis is not due to a volatile salt, excessive fluidity of the blood, or a fixed alkali. "Hence I must conclude that it consists mainly of acid." In fact, nearly all humoral diseases may be attributed to acids, and there must thus be several different kinds of acids.[167] When an acid makes contact with saliva, sperm, or menstrual blood, which are all fermentative in nature, they ferment even more violently and attach themselves to a volatile alkali which mixes with the acid to form an obstruction.[168] An alkali consists of particles like long sharp pointed scissors: when contacting the oily parts of the body, it thickens the parts which should be fluid. But the finest salt and acid particles are moved by the animal spirits and, forming a sort of fire, cut and slice as if they were several hundred knives all together—causing the ulcers and gangrene of the penis observed in this disease.[169]

In contrast to Descartes, Sylvius interpreted physiology in purely chemical terms. According to Sprengel, "he saw in the human body nothing but a magma of humors in continual fermentation, distillation, effervescence, or precipitation, and by him the physician was reduced to the level of a distiller or brewer."[170] He was mainly concerned to provide an interpretation of the problem of coction/digestion, and he did so in terms of bile, phlegm, and pancreatic juice.

The first stage of digestion is the fermentation or chylification of food in the stomach under the action of the saliva, which Sylvius regarded as acid. The second stage, chymification in the liver, spleen, and elsewhere, he attributed to a mixture of (acid) pancreatic juice and (alkaline) bile, which effervesce, release gases, and reduce the food to a state in which it can be absorbed by the body.[171] [f]

Health results from the undisturbed progress of this fermentation, while its interruption—with appearance of excess acid or alkaline "acrimony" (*acrimonia*—a word invented by Sylvius)—causes disease.[172]

By presenting coction/digestion in terms of an acid/alkaline interaction Sylvius merely repeated the analysis given earlier by Galen—expressing this physiological process in terms of contraries.[g] The consequence was a completely different practice from that of, for example, Van Helmont, who also relied on the theory of coction but did not analyze it in terms of a conflict among opposing elements.

The power of theory to mold perception and experience is seen in the fact that pancreatic juice is not acid at all but feebly alkaline. When told that bile and pancreatic juice mixed together outside the body do not ferment or effervesce, Regnier de Graaf (a disciple of Sylvius) held that the temperature present in the small intestine is needed for the process to occur successfully.[173]

In Sylvius' doctrine acids, alkalis, bile, phlegm, and pancreatic juice could combine in many ways to produce diseases.

[f]The parotid duct was discovered by Steno in 1661, and the pancreatic secretions by Regnier de Graaf in 1664. The word, "alkali," represents Paracelsus' "salt" and was introduced into medicine by him (see *Divided Legacy,* I, 413).

[g]See *Divided Legacy,* I, 307-310.

One series of illnesses are functions of the digestion, specifically, of the separation of waste liquids and solids from the chyle and their voiding *per anum* or *per urinas.*[174] The solids can degenerate in two ways, becoming a "loathsome crudity" (*nidorosa cruditas*) when fermentation is retarded by excess alkalinity, and an "acid crudity" when fermentation is accelerated by excess acidity. In both cases treatment is by contraries: "loathsome crudity" is cured by neutralizing the alkaline bile with hydrochloric acid, and "acid crudity" by medicines which "temper the acid spirit."[175]

The waste liquids can be too copious or too scanty, or the urine may be vitiated in its color, odor, taste, or consistency.[176] The first is caused by "the vicious constitution of the fleshy parts of the kidneys according to their channels or substance" and "may be cured by medicines that straighten out the slackness of their channels and amend the harm of the substance of the fleshy parts."[177] "External things applied in the form of a plaster to the region of the loins, where the kidneys are, and made of more mild corroborating and astringent things, will most opportunely straighten out the slackness of the channels in the fleshy parts of the kidneys."[178] The second comes from an unduly thick mixture of the heterogeneous parts of the blood and occurs when the acidity of the lymph is more sharp (from external cold, great sorrow, or inordinate intake of acid foods).[179] The urine is scanty and watery, "which they call crude."[180] Being attributable to deterioration of the pancreatic juice or the lymph, this is cured by bile or some other alkali; the mixture of the humors is diluted, and more urine is released.[181]

In the Hippocratic writings the progress of coction could often be read from the urine, and the physician could decide on measures to accelerate, retard, or modify the coction. But Sylvius gave chemical explanations of the state of the urine and proposed treatment through contraries.[182] "The watery urine, which is a sign of crudity, that is, of a concoction deficient in the humors of the blood, as oft as that voluntary concoction is expected in vain, or comes too late by the *natura,* so oft is it to be promoted by art, and that by medicines mildly tempering all, and chiefly the acid acrimony of the humors (whence comes to pass that more entire mixture of the humors in the mass of blood) and again a loosening the close union of the humors."[183] "A red and thick urine befalling the sick in burning fevers, as it signifies a concoction begun, so ought it not to be troubled or changed by medicines; yea rather, when this work of the *natura* goes on slowly, it is to be helped by . . . fixed sulphurs of minerals and metals [which] mildly temper all and even the acid acrimony of the humors."[184]

Sylvius triumphs in his discovery of the secret of coction: "the nature and true cause of a so much mentioned crudity in physic, yea manner whereby it is most commonly bred becomes manifest, and moreover the nature, true cause, and manner of a so much wanted concoction, how it is absolved, is not a little illustrated . . ."[185] "How true, yea most true, are these things which I have now said, daily experience confirms . . . concoction in the blood is hindered by the force of acid things, endued with an acidity exceeding; and that the same is promoted and obtained by help of aromatics, and in especial the bitter, or of volatile [alkaline] salts more tempered."[186]

The theory of coction, as accepted by the Empirical School, required disease to be understood as a process with several stages. Thus it was a historical approach to disease and health. Sylvius, like other Rationalist thinkers, converted disease and cure from a historical process into an analytical one and, by the same token, denied the value of medical history itself. Sprengel remarks that he "paid no attention to the progress of the *natura* in acute diseases nor to their periodization; he paid no attention to procatarctic causes or to pathognomic signs . . . thus the noblest of the arts become the plaything of the chemists' imagination, and they regarded all their predecessors with contempt."[187]

The physiology and therapeutics of Willis are also grounded in the concept of coction, which he interprets as fermentation.[h] Many other ideas, however, find a place in his doctrine: the salt, sulphur and mercury of Paracelsus, the acids and alkalis of Sylvius, animal spirits, etc., making an inconsistent and unwieldy mixture. He was entirely in error in claiming to follow the inductive method of Bacon.[188]

The two processes traditionally denoted by "coction"—the digestion of food vs. the "cooking" and neutralization of a morbific cause by the body's *physis*[i]—are combined in Willis' physiology of digestion. Food is converted into chyle in the stomach, passing from there to the bloodstream as *cruditas*. "Coction" is the second stage of digestion, performed by the heat[j] of the bloodstream and the animal spirits, which transforms this *cruditas* into blood and the other humors. These are both processes of fermentation: the food is fermented into chyle, and then, in the second stage, the blood boils up "and conceives a heat, almost after the same manner as new beer put into bottles."[189] This culminates in the "crisis" (and another simile from brewing): "the mass of liquor swells up, notably ferments, and by reason of the force of fermentation, oftentimes makes the bottle fly in pieces."[190] It is followed by the evacuation: "this matter [must] be gathered together in such a quantity that by its turgescency it may irritate the *natura* to a critical expulsion."[191]

The Galenic categories have been exploded by "our most famous Harvey [who] hath laid the circulation of the blood as a new foundation in medicine."[192] The four humors are now only products of fermentation, "recrements" of the

[h]"Yea, we also endeavor the cure of diseases by the help of fermentation: for to the preserving or recovering the health of man the business of a physician and a vintner is almost the same. The blood and humors, even as wine, ought to be kept in an equal temper and motion of fermentation . . . I could easily unfold the curatory intentions, as also the effects and operations of every medicine, according to the doctrine of fermentation." (*Dr. Willis's Practice of Physick,* Part I, 14).

[i]See *Divided Legacy,* I, 240-247.

[j]We have already noted that for Willis the body's vital force is reduced to the "flame" in the blood (see above, pp. 137-138).

blood "which ought continually to be separated from it. For in truth the blood is an only humor . . . and wheresoever it is carried through all the parts of the body, it is still the same and like itself."[193] "Tis almost the same thing to say an house consists of wood and stone as a body of four elements,"[194] and they are to be replaced by the Paracelsan "spirit, sulphur, salt, water, and earth" which are the components of the fermentation or combustion continually occurring in the blood.[195] Yellow bile consists of salt and sulphur with an admixture of spirit and water; black bile is the same with an admixture of earth.[196] The sulphur in the blood makes it red and furnishes material for combustion: "when by reason of too great crudity the sulphur is less dissolved, the blood becomes watery and pale."[197] The blood also contains salt: "If at any time the saline particles are not rightly exalted in the blood, by reason of ill digestion, but remain crude and for the most part fixed, from thence the blood becomes thick and unfit for circulation[k] . . . But when coction being rightly performed in the bowels and vessels, the salt is duly exalted, and being associated with the spirit, is volatilized, then by reason of its mixture the liquor of the blood more equally ferments."[198]

Willis saw his doctrine as superior to Descartes' in that fermentation is visible to the senses [*sic*] while Descartes' corpuscles are "only to be signified by conception." "Certainly [the corpuscular philosophy] deserves no light praise, but . . . it rather supposes than demonstrates its principles, and teaches of what figure those elements of bodies may be, not what they have been, and also induces notions extremely subtil and remote from the sense, and which do not sufficiently quadrate with the phenomena of nature when we descend to particulars."[199]

Actually, while hoping to render physiological processes visible by assimilating them to fermentation, Willis was only committing the common Rationalist error of assuming knowledge of invisibles.

In any case, "coction" is the point of departure for his

[k]Cf. the Cartesian "obstruction" (above, pp. 146-147).

physiology, pathology, and therapeutics. It occurs in the healthy, as well as in the sick, some hours after each meal.[200] It can proceed slowly or rapidly depending upon the degree of innate heat in the blood, yielding a different humor in each case and making the individual phlegmatic, choleric, etc.[201] If more raw juice is not introduced at regular intervals, the blood becomes overconcocted and sour—like wine which has turned to vinegar—but the coction can be perverted in other ways also, the blood becoming watery, cold, sharp, salt, acid, austere, etc.[202]

"Fever" is immoderate fermentation of the blood and humors leading to a loosening of the "frame of the liquor" which causes the "active particles" to "leap forth from the rest and strive to expand themselves on every side." They "rush with violence" through the vascular system and "by that means diffuse the effluvia of heat through the whole body."[203] When a person is underfed, too little *cruditas* is injected into the blood, and "by a too long coction [it] is burned and grows bilious . . . [the patient] becomes sad and melancholic." "Some diseases habitually induce such a disposition of the blood; such are the scurvy, the yellow jaundice [and others] in which the whole mass of blood passes from a spirituous into either a sour, sharp, or austere nature."[204] When improperly concocted chyle is passed along through the bloodstream, "whilst this juice, being little cocted or purged from dregs, is sent from the depraved blood to the nervous parts, 'tis wont variously to irritate them into cramps and convulsive motions; also no few symptoms in fevers arise by reason of the depravation and irregular motion of this juice."[205] In typhus, when the blood burns and gives off a "dusty" matter which shows up in the urine, the crisis will be successful only when the blood has been mostly consumed by fire: "because in the midst of its burning the *natura* is not at leisure for a crisis, nor is it ever prosperously endeavored, nor in truth procured by art with good success." The "spirit of the blood" must separate the "dusty" matter and render it liable to expulsion, for "otherways, tho' a copious evacuation happens, the *natura* will never be free from her burden."[206]

"Animal spirits" are introduced whenever the argument makes their presence necessary. While rejecting Van Helmont's *Archeus,* Willis notes "a very near relation and intimate sympathy between the spirits of the stomach and those of the brain."[207] A blow on the head causes vomiting "because the spirits within the brain, being disturbed, excite the others that inhabit the stomach into the same commotion, by the commerce or intercourse of the eighth pair of nerves."[208] These spirits become agents of disease when provoked by poisons, improper diet, or when "irritated or stirred up by some disturbance given to other spirits that are here and there dispersed at a distance, and do communicate their grievance to the stomach by the passages of the fibers or nerves."[209] An intermittent pulse is due to the "obstructed" movement of animal spirits out of the brain and into the nerves and tendons of the heart.[210] The *succus nutrivus* of the nerves can contract a taint from the blood and "be depraved in its disposition" or else "perverted from its equal motion." "From thence the rigor and pain, convulsions, delirium, frenzy, and many more symptoms of the nervous kind, usual in fevers, do arise."[211]

He divided medicines into those which act on the humors and those which affect the animal spirits (either directly or *via* the humors).[212]

Salt, sulphur, and iron medicines improve the temper or ferment of the blood.[213] Others have the opposite effect: fever, for example, is cured by an antipyretic which calms the fermentation process.[214] "When the blood grows too hot, even as wine, it is usual . . . to allay its fervor with temperate things."[215] Still other medicines thin out the thick and obstructed blood: cordials impregnated with a volatile salt "meet with either a fixed or acid salt, which they force into their embraces, and thereby open the mass of blood which is too much thickened and bound together by the feverish effervescence thereof, insomuch that they promote the separation and expulsion of the morbific matter."[216]

The traditional purgatives and vomitives were reinterpreted in terms of fermentation.[217] Sulphur and salt, the major ingredients of purgatives, "do not dissolve the blood like acids or other precipitating salts, that is to say, by embracing some parts of it more intimately and closely and so separating them from their associates to oblige them to become their own companions; but, on the contrary, the purging particles, being disagreeable to the whole mass of blood and all its particles, as also immiscible and untameable, put them all into confusion like themselves and excite them to an expurgative effervescence."[218]

All of these uses of remedies were thus justified by the doctrine of contraries, now presented as the acceleration or slackening of some process of fermentation.[1]

Willis' discussion of medicines which act on the animal spirits is reminiscent of Van Helmont: "[it] either provokes and moves them toward purgation, or . . . by assuaging of them appeases and removes all things that discompose or molest them, or lastly by overpowering of them lays their fury asleep."[219] Medicines against nausea "by their grateful allurements may entice the spirits thither in greater plenty and likewise refresh or recruit them when weak."[220] Purgatives sometimes provoke vomiting as well as evacuation "because the animal spirits being vehemently provoked, and exploded or discharged, fly differently sometimes into these, and sometimes into those ends of the fleshy fibers."[221] Vomitives cause an "explosion or a great expansion of the animal spirits that possess or inhabit [the fibers of the stomach wall]."[222] Or, as in the treatment of epilepsy, the medicine binds the spirits more firmly to the body's solids:

> When as we have already asserted the procatarctic cause of the epilepsy to consist in the heterogenous *copula* joining or cleaving to the spirits inhabiting the brain, and inciting them to preternatural explosions, it follows that

[1]The doctrine of contraries also appears in its pure Iatrochemical form: in phthisis the overacidity of the blood is neutralized by an alkaline medicine (*Dr. Willis's Practice of Physick,* Part IX, II, 41).

> those things which take away or resist such a cause must be of that nature that by strengthening the brain and binding up its pores, may exclude that *copula* and so fix, and as it were bind the spirits, flowing within the middle or marrow of the brain, from leaving their *copula,* that they shall not be any more apt or prone to irregular explosions.[223]

These medicines were also interpreted iatrochemically, in terms of contraries:

> I am of opinion that seeing the animal spirits are very subtle bodies, composed of a spirit and a volatile salt, both joined together and highly exalted, the opiates, on the contrary, are made of a stinking sulphur, that is, of sulphur united with fixed salt and earthy matter, raised to a violent degree; which kind of compositions, it is well known, are such great enemies to the subtle texture of the animal spirits, that sometimes at a distance, by mere emanations that flow out of them, though not perceivable to the smell, they overpower them.[224]

Some medicines act as "specifics." Such cure epilepsy "with a certain innate and secret virtue."[225] Or phthisis: "by a peculiar property, or a certain specific virtue, [they are] reported to heal the lungs."[226]

According to Cheyne the "body is nothing but a congeries of canals, the greatest . . . part of which is glands, properly so called, designed for the separation of some fluid."[227] Consequently, diseases are due to "a vitiation of the quantity, quality, or motion of the fluids, or to a bad disposition and texture, a distortion, distention, luxation, or dilaceration of their conduits, and the other solid parts of their bodies."[228] "The general and most effectual cause of all fevers is the obstruction or dilatation of (the complicated nerve and artery, the excretory duct, and conservatory one, or rather all these, which, as shall be afterwards shown, make up) the glands, and they receive their denomination as these or those glands are more or less obstructed or divided."[229]

"The most universal and comprehensive sources and causes of chronical distempers are a glewiness, sizyness, viscidity, or grossness in the fluids, either accidental or acquired."[230]

Hence physiology and pathology can be understood mathematically: "seeing all these are the modifications and qualities of material beings, which have the dimensions of bodies, and are therefore *quanta,* it necessarily follows that the only method of examining the effects and causes of these qualities is by applying to them the doctrine of quantity, i.e., geometry and numbers, and it is altogether unaccountable how the world has not been sufficiently aware of this till within these few years."[231] We have only to follow the path of "that stupendiously great man, Sir Isaac Newton."[232] "We want a *Principia Medicinae Theoreticae Mathematicae* [which] should contain the true nature of fluidity . . . the general laws of motion of all fluids . . . the nature and cause of electricity . . ."[233]

> When a person falls into a *Hectic* fever, we may suppose the Quantity of his Blood (because it is from the rest of the Fluids, which we are speaking of, generated) to be considerably abated: Let us suppose him from 20 pounds in his ordinary state, to have dwindled to 16; then, by *Lemma primum* and its *Scholium,*
>
> $\frac{aa}{a + 6}$ = 12 lbs., in case of a Subduple Dilatation;
>
> and
>
> $\frac{aa}{a + 6}$ = 12 4/5 pounds, in case of a Subtriple one,
>
> i.e., if there be (upon the aforesaid Account) supposed but 16 Pounds of Blood in a Hectic Person, as the *Media Quantitas,* and that to the Cylindrical Canals (equal to the whole Vessels of the Body, save the Intestines and Lacteals) there be added another, whose Orifice is equal to one half of the former (i.e. if the Vessels be dilated in their Orifices one half), then the Quantity of 16 Pounds of Blood in these so dilated

> Vessels, shall be but like 12 Pounds in these Vessels, if they had not been dilated, and produce but such effects, as such a Quantity would do in the Canals if they were in their ordinary State; and so in other Dilatations. From both these Considerations it is clear, we may suppose the Quantity in all Fluids of Hectic People abated at any required Rate of Minority.[234] [m]

As for therapy, "there is no surer or more general maxim in physick than that diseases are cured by the contrary or opposite method to that which produced them."[235]

Cheyne assimilates coction to cure through contraries (after a fashion) by interpreting it as a grinding or scouring process whereby the obstructed passages are cleared. The physician should follow the *natura* which "grinds and concocts" the morbid matter and the "material cause" of the disease, "and when this matter is sufficiently concocted by the distemper, then comes the *crise* to throw it out of the habit by some evacuation or other, as sweating, vomiting, purging, hemorrhage, urine, or coughing and spitting."[236] [n]

Cheyne had no patience with Iatrochemistry: "all is nonsense unless they first shew their systems and chemical effects to be necessary corollaries from the known laws of motion, i.e., unless all their philosophy, and chemistry too, be first mechanically explained."[237] Medicines act physically or mechanically: mercury by the heaviness, rotundity, and attractive power of its particles; salts by their sharp points, strong attractive power, and solidity; water by its moisture and thinness; sulphur by its fiery particles and heat; earth by conferring solidity and firmness; quinine by its vegetable stypticity; and steel by its astringency.[238] The two preeminent "specifics"—quinine and mercury—were thus thought by Cheyne to work on purely mechanical principles: Jesuit's Bark is the "only cool bitter astringent known to man." He denies that it has any specific effect on the salivary

[m]This mathematical fantasy went through *seven* editions.

[n]The Methodist School had interpreted coction as the mechanical grinding of food by the stomach walls (see *Divided Legacy,* I, 292).

glands.[239] Mercury breaks up obstructions in a purely mechanical way: it "digs out all the obstructions of the impassable canals like so many little bullets shot against a mud wall, every little bullet breaks down a part till the whole be levelled; and this it is the more able to perform both because it is exceeding weighty and makes therefore a greater and more forcible *ictus* and because its particles are exceeding small and are therefore to be considered as so many exceeding sharp wedges or *cunei.* Besides, by the smallness of its particles it is able to enter into these slender canals in which the blood cannot freely pass, and thereby to scour all the passages be they ever so small."[240] [o]

A good example of Cheyne's therapeutics is his treatment of the "English Disease," meaning "spleen, vapours, or lowness of spirits," which he calls a "nervous" disease due to "some gross concretions not sufficiently broken and divided by the digestive powers in the alimentary tube, retarding or stopping the circulation in the small vessels whereby the stagnant juices become sharp and corrosive and the salts have time, by their innate attractive quality, to crystallize or unite in greater clusters and exert their destructive force on the solids" or to "a too great laxity or want of due tone, elasticity, and force in the fibres in general, or the nerves in particular."[241]

The first therapeutic indication is to "thin, dilute, and sweeten the whole mass of the fluids" by bleeding, purging, and evacuations, or by mercury, antimony, and other metals "whose chief efficacy seems to lie in their weight after they have dropped their salts in the alimentary tube."[242] The second indication is to "divide, break, and dissolve the saline, acrid, and hard concretions generated in the small vessels and to destroy all sharpness and acrimony lodged in the habit." This is done by medicines which "blunt the acrimony of the salts and the sharpness of the juices" and "drive the ponderous medicines into the most remote capillaries."[243]

[o]In 1685 Robert Boyle published a work explaining the action of specific medicines in mechanical terms: *Of the Reconcilableness of Specifick Medicines to the Corpuscular Philosophy, to Which is Added a Discourse About the Advantages of the Use of Simple Medicines* (London, 1685).

Finally, certain medicines are used which are "more grateful to nature, strengthening the digestive powers, and making all the functions more full and strong, so that vigor and cheerfulness flow in daily." These are medicines of the "strengthening and astringent kind which contract, corrugate, wind up, and give firmness and force to the weak and relaxed solids, fibers, and nerves" such as bitters, aromatics, chalybeates, Jesuit's Bark, steel, gentian, zedoary, wormwood, oak bark, etc.—in short, everything that is subacid, whether mineral or vegetable.[244]

Hoffmann's pathology and therapeutics flow naturally from his physiology which defines "life" as: 1) the interaction of the fluids and solids, and 2) the animal spirits or *anima.*

The primary element here is the heartbeat and the circulation of the blood: "since the discovery of the circulation of the blood . . . will anyone deny that one can deduce from the movement of the blood and of the solids the causes of life, death, health, and sickness."[245] "The circulation is a vital movement which preserves the body from putrefying, to which it is extremely subject . . . To preserve the human body from disease, pain, sadness, is hence nothing other than to give it the necessary help and above all to prescribe for it a regimen which preserves the circulation and excretions in the state in which they should regularly be; and the treatment of all disease is nothing other than restoring the blood and the liquids to the state from which they had deviated."[246]

Diseases can arise in a variety of ways, and no real pattern can be discerned in Hoffmann's pathology. In one writing he attributes all diseases to irregularities in the systolic and diastolic motion of the heart: if the contraction of the heart (systole) is too long or too strong, it produces spasm in the solid parts of the body, causing fever, epilepsy, various kinds of pain, and derivation of the humors to inappropriate parts of the body.[247] If the dilatation of the heart (diastole) is excessive, it causes atony of the solid parts, stagnation of the blood and humors, engorgement of the viscera, obstructions, scirrhous concretions, corruptions, etc.[248] Systole is generally associated with acute diseases and diastole with chronic ones.[249]

Another group of diseases results from disproportion in the components of the blood: "either the mobile, volatile, saline, and sulphurous particles predominate in the blood and humors, and then a disproportion arises that is warm, saline, and sharp; or else the mucilaginous, acid, and fixed particles predominate, and then a disproportion results that is cold, acid, and melancholic."[250] "If viscid, fixed, and watery particles predominate in the humors, then both the internal and circulatory movements are diminished and slow; if, however, the volatile and spiritous particles predominate, then the motion is more rapid and depressed."[251]

A third set of diseases results from impaired motion of the animal spirits. "As the vital actions depend directly on the proper, laudable, and even motion of the fluid parts, especially the animal spirits, and the proper conformation of the solids, diminished and distorted vital actions arise from the impaired motions of the humors and the distorted conformation of the solids."[252] "Whatever injures or destroys the proportion and the laudable motion of the blood and nerve fluid, or the configuration of the solid parts (which consists in proper situation, number, and shape) deserves the title of morbific cause."[253] The passages in the nerves through which the animal spirits flow can be blocked, causing spasm, apoplexy, paralysis, stupor, lethargy, coma, catalepsy, vertigo, mania, delirium, headaches, etc. etc.[254]

Various "poisons" contribute their share to the production of diseases. Malignant diseases are those "caused by poison and those which arise from an extremely minute poisonous principle which, like a ferment, multiplies itself and thoroughly perverts and impairs the motion of the blood."[255] A major effect of atony is the accumulation of excrements in the intestines and colon; these then spread their poisons throughout the body and cause various diseases.[256]

"Fine, saline, acrid corpuscles, which irritate the membranes, can be a major cause of increased flow and of stasis."[257]

The effect of all of these morbific causes is usually some sort of blocked flow in the capillaries or other small passages in the body: the obstructed humors stagnate and corrupt, generating diseases of all varieties.[258]

Consequently, drugs and medicines must be understood to work primarily as removers of obstructions, acting on the humors directly or *via* the animal spirits. "The operation of drugs is wholly mechanical and can best be explained by size, shape, and the laws of motion."[259] "Whoever wants to know the nature and properties of drugs ought to know the states of matter and the laws of motion according to mechanics and be a good physicist."[260] "The nature of drugs and the manner in which they operate are best explained by the diverse *textura* of the particles, in respect to shape, size, and variety of motion."[261] "When the *textura* is changed, a different power and effectiveness arises in that object."[262] "Inasmuch as every disease is rooted in the fluid parts of the body which are defective in quantity, quality, or motion, drugs ought to regard the quantity, quality, or motion of those parts."[263] Mercurial and sulphurous remedies "operate directly on the nerves and their fluid, by stimulating and irritating them and communicating an impetus to the animal spirits."[264] "Cordials . . . provide elastic, finely ethereal, and favoring particles to the animal spirits and blood."[265] "Cephalics . . . re-open the obstructed pores of the brain and nerves [and] supply material to the animal spirits."[266]

Another group of drugs retards the movement of the humors when this is too rapid: "by their coarse particles, unsuitable for motion, they block up the very small passages; or they coagulate humors that are too fluid and thin, by means of particles that are angular and unsuitable for movement, and have a broad surface."[267] Of this type are all tinctures of iron having a vitriolic nature, all vitriols, alums, and harsh styptics.[268]

The traditional vomitives, purgatives, diuretics, sternutatories, diaphoretics, etc. were accepted by his doctrine, together with venesection.[269] "Diminished humors are restored by blood transfusion [*sic*], sound nourishment, use of highly nutritious foods that confer a plethora, and rest."[270]

A fourth group of drugs are the "alteratives" which alter the composition of the humors along chemical lines: "which correct the humors and harmful qualities and change them into their contraries."[271] Acids are corrected by alkalis; sharp and acrid saline humors by mucilaginous oily substances and various earthy materials; viscid tenacious humors by sharp oily volatile salts; gentle pituitous humors by bitters, balsams, and resins; bilious humors by the more bland acids; humors that are too dry and earthy by volatile, moistening, diluent, and nitrous substances, etc.[272]

A final group of drugs reflects Hoffmann's systole/diastole theory of disease origins: "spasm" is calmed or relaxed by sedatives and antispasmodics, while tone is restored to excessively flaccid parts by tonics.[273] Paralysis, for instance, due to a spasmodic stricture or compression of the membranes around the brain whereby the nervous fluid is impelled into the organs of motion and its passage into the sensorium interrupted, is cured by allaying the violent spasms of the dura mater with anodynes and sedatives.[274] Dropsy, on the other hand, being an atonic disease caused by laxity of the blood vessels and languidness of the circulation, is cured by such tonics as bitters, Peruvian Bark, and cascarilla.[275]

The two principal elements of the Empirical theory of therapeutics, the existence of "specific" remedies and cure through coction/evacuation, found a Rationalist interpretation in Hoffmann's doctrine.

The "specifics" are those remedies which, according to Galen, act "by the whole substance," are "appropriate to certain parts of the body and favorable to them," and "[oppose] a particular morbific cause, thus curing a particular disease."[276] The specific action of a drug can often be explained "through some mechanical configuration of particles."[277]

He interprets "coction" either mechanically or in terms of the "animal spirits." Urine with sediment foretells what the ancients called "coction," meaning "a morbid or febrile material that is not yet malignant or sharp and insurgent, but one that is covered by other fixed particles."[278] A "crisis," which is a "change in the *natura* for better or worse," "comes about by a laudable movement of the blood and spirits through the minute capillary vessels and excretory organs."[279] "The spirits are the healing agents of diseases; they are also the foundation of the crisis itself, and as their mixture or their movement are impaired either less or more, a better or worse crisis is to be expected."[280]

The beneficial effect of fever—a major point of Empirical doctrine—was attributed by Hoffmann to the more rapid movement of the blood in fever, cleansing the vessels and passages more thoroughly.[281]

Thus, while he accepts the existence of certain reflexes or reactions in the body, they are often immoderate and devoid of purpose, hence harmful.[282] And the reactive process itself he reduced to a simple mechanism, amenable to direction, regulation, and control through medicines which also act mechanically.

Boerhaave's pathology and therapeutics are no less complex than Hoffmann's. His humoral, mechanical, and chemical proximate causes are limited only by the power of his imagination.

Although he rejected Galen, Galenic humoral causes are a living part of his medicine. Yellow bile "produces many and malignant disorders, sickness and aversion to food, anxieties, hiccups, heartburns, vomiting, iliac passion, colics, gripes, flatus, rumbling noise in the bowels, etc."[283] Black bile "corrodes, burns, and dissolves the contiguous solid parts, excites inflammations, gangrenes, sphacelus, excruciating pains, and violent effervescences of the humors."[284] Any humor may be in excess or deficient.[285] A humor may be perverted and thus interfere with one of the functions performed by a solid.[286] "Internal causes for the most part injure first the humors and then the solid parts."[287]

But humoral diseases were also interpreted in terms of the corpuscles of Descartes, or "viscidities" and "acrimonies."[288] Humoral particles may be too large to pass through the walls of vessels; or they may be too small and pass through too easily; they can also be too elastic, causing other sorts of damage.[289] Saline acrimony causes "thirst, hoarseness, roughness, dryness, and stiffness of the solids, with acrimony in the humors, etc."[290] Spicy acrimony causes "thirst, dryness, heat, and inflammation, stimulates the solids, increases the velocity of the fluids, etc."[291] "Crude acid humors" cause a whole range of disorders.[292] And the blood also, "when charged with a predominant acid, alkaline, muriatic, saline, or oily acrimony, or with earth," produces the disorders associated with these substances.[293]

Another group of diseases was associated with "vital spirits": "when impelled into the muscular fibers of the heart," they cause a "violent and sensible contraction of it, accompanied with a great resistance to the blood expelled from the heart."[294] But this group is small in Boerhaave's pathology (compared to Willis or Hoffmann).

A large group of diseases was due to spasm or atony of the solids. The vessels can be stopped up, squeezed together, collapsed, or distended by "too great a distending force of the humors."[295] The solids can be deformed through injury.[296] Exposure to cold "shortens the solid fibers and renders them more dense and strong," causing a multitude of complaints.[297] Sometimes the solids are inactive and fail to expel the humors gathered there, allowing them to putrefy and become stagnant.[298] The cause of diabetes "is generally esteemed too great a relaxation of the fibers, accompanied with too thin a state of the humors, both which may proceed from the humors being too much diluted with water."[299] The pulsation of the heart can be a cause: "the alteration made in the blood by the heart is from its reception, stay, and expulsion, which motions being too quick, produce continual ardent and violent fevers; but if it stays longer than it ought in the heart, or if its expulsion from thence is too languid, the consequences are faintings, polypous concretions, cold, phlegm, chilliness . . . dropsy . . . and a long train of different disorders arising from these."[300]

If the humors are moving too rapidly through the vessels, "this will cause a compressure, attrition, attenuation, heat, and inflammatory disposition of the juices, with the ill consequences thereof already explained from too much exercise. But a too slow motion of the humors produces disorders like those before described from too much rest or inactivity of the body."[301]

Once these disease causes are known, the indication is to remove them.[302] Therapeutics means "to remove the cause of the disease . . . to take away the disease itself, and, lastly, to expel the present effects or symptoms of the disease."[303] Or an artificial change is to be produced in the body of the patient. "Therefore a physician ought first to know what alteration is necessary to be made in the patient, and by what means or remedies he is to bring it about."[304]

Here Boerhaave accepted all the traditional emetics, purgatives, issues, setons, diuretics, sudorifics, chylogogues, etc.[305] Phlebotomy is especially useful, as it

> lessens the quantity of humors both in the arteries and veins, and consequently it therefore lessens the resistance to be removed . . . thus it restores the over-distended vessels to their former contractions and elasticity, it rarefies or thins the humors, it occasions their parts to cohere less together, it dissolves those parts which are too gross or large, it removes obstructions, it promotes the circulation, secretion, and excretion of the humors, it makes a revulsion from other parts, and it cools the whole habit.[306]

Hence "bleeding removes a great many, and those very

different diseases, while at the same time it works very surprising changes."[307] [p]

If the humors are too thick, they can be thinned out by watery drinks, easily digestible foods, saline resolvants, etc.[308] If they are too thin, they can be thickened "by the use of jellies and gelatinous aliments taken from animals and vegetables, etc."[309] If the passages are blocked, they must be opened up, and if the humors are moving too rapidly through the solids, they must be slowed down with opiates or by bloodletting.[310]

Humors may be thickened or thinned chemically, using "those remedies which are diametrically opposite to the inspissating or coagulating cause in the humors, as of mild alkalis against a coagulating acid, and of saponaceous substances against an inspissating oily glue . . ."[311] Acid diarrhoea of children is treated by a gram of chalk dissolved in water.[312] Acid acrimony of the humors is treated by alkaline remedies, and alkaline acrimonies by acid remedies.[313] "The fumes of vinegar, spirit of salt, and the firing of gunpowder are serviceable in destroying caustic, alkaline, and putrid fumes; but acid poisonous exhalations are corrected by the odors of alkaline and oily spirits."[314]

Medicines also act by contrariety on the solid parts of the body. "Astringents . . . applied to the too flaccid fibers adhere with their particles so as to render them more firm or rigid"; "such things . . . by their austereness constringe and compact the fibers when relaxed or separated from each other, reducing them into one mass."[315] Similarly, too great rigidity of the parts requires relaxation.[316]

But, Boerhaave observes, the diseases of the solids generally depend upon a disorder of the fluids.[317]

Diseases arising from a state of putrefaction within the body "must be guarded against by those foods which by their acidity, saltness, or firmness are least disposed to this kind of corruption."[318] And the diet generally can be adjusted to

[p]But "Helmont exclaims that all bleeding is butchery" (*Dr. Boerhaave's Academical Lectures,* VI, 427).

treat particular diseased states. If an acid indisposition of the humors predominates, animal remedies are used: "the solid parts of animals, which by a long and gentle boiling dissolve in water and form thin broths, jellies, or soups."[319] "Especially birds or fowls which feed upon worms; nor is there any thing which more powerfully resists acidity than eggs, which putrefy sooner than any other thing."[320] "If a muriatic acrimony predominates, it will be convenient to use the aliments before-mentioned, free from salt or seasoning."[321] "But when an oily acrimony offends in the humors, the like aliments will be most convenient, after being plentifully diluted and perfectly freed from their fat or oily parts."[322]

A final class of medicines are the specifics. "The specific method . . . removes the cause of the disease barely by the application of such things as are known to be efficacious only from experience . . . This method, therefore, only requires the name of the disease and of the medicine; as in the case of an intermitting fever by the bark, of pains by the use of opium, and of every particular kind of poison by its proper and known corrector and antidote, to attract or expel the same."[323] [q] These are "hardly to be discovered but by accident and experience."[324] Van Helmont's "universal remedy" for quieting the *Archeus* was the specific, opium, in quince juice.[325] Paracelsus used the specifics, laudanum and mercury.[326]

Boerhaave devoted relatively little space to the specifics in his medical treatises, however, preferring a rational analysis of the powers of medicines. His rationalizing urge is seen, moreover, in his treatment of coction.

His eclecticism and respect for tradition compelled him to accept this concept: "Hippocrates considers the *natura* and the disease as two enemies betwixt whom the rencounter being severe, cannot remain long undecided, but one must overpower the other; and this state of combat he has termed

[q] But elsewhere he assimilates the action of poisons to the acid/alkali opposition (*Dr. Boerhaave's Academical Lectures,* VI, 341, 343, 346).

a crisis."[327] "The doctrine of crudity, concoction, crisis, and the changing of a disease into health . . . is a subject of the last importance to be considered in physick, and is that which properly distinguishes the rational physician from an Empiric."[328]

In the Empirical tradition, however, coction was an unknowable process which could be judged only by the external signs and the outcome, while Boerhaave subjects it to his mechanical mode of thinking and assumes that it can be understood.[r]

In the first place, "crudeness" (*cruditas*) only means any sort of morbific cause: "Hippocrates understands nothing mysterious in the term crudity, only he intends it for a general term to comprise every morbid cause in the body . . . as acrimonious, thick, or watery fluids; or, as Hippocrates speaks, a redundancy of sweet, bitter, salt, or acid . . . *even the most healthy blood itself will cause disease and be crude* [*sic*] if it abounds too much in the veins of a person weakened by disease."[329] "What has been said of the humors with respect to crudity is likewise true of the solids, so far as these last are disordered by the fluids."[330]

Thus, just as "crudeness" only means any one of the multifarious causes which can obstruct the circulation, "coction" only means restoration of the obstructed flow: "the cause changing the crude into concocted humors is the action of the remaining life or circulation, a spontaneous change of the morbific matter, with the assisting virtue of medicines."[331] "The matter of the disease being so far concocted or digested by the causes as to become like unto the healthy humors, the disease is then said to be resolved; and the action itself is termed resolution, which is always the most perfect way of curing the disease."[332] "If the morbific

[r]"Hippocrates . . . considered that we are altogether ignorant of what is performed within the body of the living patient, whether in health or diseased; and that we are only capable of knowing those changes which appear in diseases different from the appearances which we usually observe in health. These last changes, or appearances, are the effects of life remaining; but the cause exciting the morbid effects is that latent entity which we term the cause of the disease . . ." (*Dr. Boerhaave's Academical Lectures,* VI, 167).

matter first crude is so changed . . . and consequently disposed to abate the violence of the disease by the change thus wrought in the quantity, figure, cohesion, mobility, or inactivity in the matter of the disese, it is then said to be concocted."[333]

But how is the organism aroused to effect this coction? "The cause of this change in the morbific matter is the remaining *vis vitae* irritated by the said matter variously conditioned, so as to cause either a translation or a discharge of the matter, or kill the patient."[334]

The "remaining *vis vitae*" only means that part of the circulation still unaffected by the disease:

> This is what Hippocrates calls the *natura,* and what others term strength: namely, the powers of generating motion. Which powers being carefully examined, will be found to depend upon the remaining motion of the humors through the vessels, however conditioned that motion may be . . . the circulating motion of the humors through the heart, lungs, and cerebellum, in which therefore consists every the least force of life.[335]

And, in Boerhaave's view, the "crudeness" of the *disease* irritates this remaining *vis vitae* into a reaction: "the presence of those diseases in the body irritates it to exert a sort of mechanical impulse, or unconscious *automatic* motion, for their removal . . . By an automatic motion or impulse we therefore understand that motion which results from the mechanical structure of the human body, which we can neither produce nor destroy by the influence of the mind or will . . . even the smaller elastic solids, which are everywhere continued throughout the body, have a power by which they endeavor to resist and overcome everything injurious to the economy."[336]

The thrust of Boerhaave's argument is to deny any purposive capacity in the organism. The whole process is supposed to be one of mechanical reaction, so that the same solids which permit the disease to get a foothold in the organism at some subsequent stage react against it. But this mode of reasoning is illogical, since the material substrate cannot first accept the disease and then react against it unless permitted the attributes of autonomy and spontaneity. Galen had made the same attempt—deriving the attractive, retentive, and expulsive *dynameis* of each organ from the same substrate of the four qualities.[s]

Galen's and Boerhaave's reinterpretations of the body's vitality had an identical aim: to eliminate the purposiveness and spontaneity of the organism, its reactive capacity, and to subject it to the *a priori* rules and authority of the physician.[t]

Some form or other of this chemical-mechanical doctrine of obstructions was the dominant teaching in Paris and other centers of medical instruction up to the French Revolution.[u]

[s]See *Divided Legacy,* I, 307-310.

[t]See below, pp. 717-722.

[u]See below, pp. 433-434.

NOTES

[1] Charles Adam and Paul Tannery, *Oeuvres de Descartes* (Paris: Leopold Cerf, 1897-1913), VI, 9.

[2] *Ibid.*, VI, 10-11.

[3] *Ibid.*, VI, 28.

[4] J. R. Partington, *A History of Chemistry* (London: Macmillan, 1961-1964), II, 282.

[5] Kenneth Dewhurst, *Thomas Willis as a Physician* (Los Angeles: University of California Press, 1964), 3.

[6] *Ibid.*, 12.

[7] H. Isler, *Thomas Willis, 1621-1675* (New York and London: Hafner, 1968), 39 (citing a 1721 publication).

[8] *Ibid.*, 40

[9] Kenneth Dewhurst, *Dr. Thomas Sydenham (1624-1689)* (Berkeley and Los Angeles: University of California Press, 1966), 36.

[10] Alfred Meyer and Raymond Hierons, "On Thomas Willis's Concepts of Neurophysiology," *Medical History* IX (1965), 1-15, 142-155, at 147.

[11] Isler, *Thomas Willis*, 111.

[12] Meyer and Hierons, "On Thomas Willis's Concepts of Neurophysiology," 148.

[13] George Cheyne, *A New Theory of Acute and Slow Continued Fevers. To Which is Prefixed an Essay Concerning the Improvements of the Theory of Medicine.* Seventh Edition (London, 1753), 16 ff.

[14] *Ibid.*, 11.

[15] See his *De medicamentorum facultatibus cognoscendis et applicandis libri duo* (Jena, 1678), translated as *Introduction to the Whole Practice of Physick, Showing the Natures and Faculties of Medicines* (London, 1685).

[16] J. H. Baas, *History of Medicine* (New York: Vail, 1889), 604.

[17] F. Hoffmann, *Opera Omnia Physico-Medica* (Geneva: Fratres De Tournes, 1740). Six Volumes.

[18] *Oeuvres de Descartes*, VI, 64.

[19] *Ibid.*, VII, 40.

[20] *Ibid.*, VII, 165.

[21] *Ibid.*, VII, 22-23.

[22] *Ibid.*, VII, 20.

[23] *Ibid.*, VII, 438.

[24] *Ibid.*, VII, 18-20.

[25] *Ibid.*, X, 422-423.

[26] *Ibid.*, VI, 29.
[27] *Ibid.*, VI, 63-65.
[28] *Ibid.*, X, 427.
[29] *Ibid.*, VI, 63.
[30] *Ibid.*, VI, 67.
[31] Thomas Steele Hall, *Rene Descartes: Treatise of Man* (Cambridge: Harvard, 1972), 77.
[32] *Oeuvres de Descartes*, IX, 319.
[33] Hall, *Rene Descartes: Treatise of Man*, 4.
[34] *Ibid.*, 5.
[35] George Cheyne, *The Natural Method of Curing the Diseases of the Body and the Disorders of the Mind Depending on the Body* (London, 1742), 65.
[36] Cheyne, *A New Theory of Acute and Slow Continued Fevers*, 2.
[37] *Ibid.*, 4-5.
[38] *Ibid.*, 10-11.
[39] *Ibid.*, 26.
[40] F. Hoffmann, *Medicinae Rationalis Systematicae Tomus Prior* (Halle, 1718), 4.
[41] *Loc. cit.*
[42] *Ibid.*, c-3, 12.
[43] F. Hoffmann, *Fundamenta Medicinae* (London: Macdonald, New York: Elsevier, 1971), 6.
[44] *Ibid.*, 5.
[45] Hoffmann, *Medicinae Rationalis*, 40-41.
[46] *Ibid.*, 9. Sprengel, *Histoire de la Medecine*, V, 288.
[47] Hoffmann, *Fundamenta Medicinae*, 5.
[48] *Loc. cit.*
[49] Hoffmann, *Medicinae Rationalis*, a, 5-6, 9.
[50] *Ibid.*, 4, 5, 8, 9, 14, 40.
[51] *Ibid.*, 4, 9-12.
[52] *Ibid.*, c-3 ff.
[53] *Ibid.*, c-3 ff., 17.
[54] *Ibid.*, 30.
[55] *Ibid.*, 11.
[56] *Dr. Boerhaave's Academical Lectures on the Theory of Physic, Being a Genuine Translation of His Institutes and Explanatory Comment* (London, 1742-1746), VI, 352.
[57] *Ibid.*, I, 32.
[58] *Ibid.*, VI, 352.
[59] *Ibid.*, I, 10, 13, 20, 21, 58.
[60] *Ibid.*, I, 20-22.
[61] *Ibid.*, I, 42.
[62] *Ibid.*, I, 63, 74.
[63] *Ibid.*, I, 41.
[64] *Ibid.*, I, 64.
[65] *Ibid.*, I, 81.
[66] *Ibid.*, I, 58.
[67] *Loc. cit.*
[68] *Ibid.*, I, 57.
[69] *Ibid.*, I, 42.

[70] *Ibid.*, I, 60-61.
[71] *Loc. cit.*
[72] *Ibid.*, I, 63.
[73] *Ibid.*, I, 28.
[74] *Ibid.*, I, 27.
[75] *Loc. cit.*
[76] *Ibid.*, I, 43-44.
[77] *Ibid.*, I, 45.
[78] *Ibid.*, I, 44.
[79] *Ibid.*. I. 43.
[82] *Ibid.*, I, 1.
[83] *Ibid.*, I, 77.
[84] *Ibid.*, I, 78.
[85] *Ibid.*, I, 78-79.
[86] *Ibid.*, I, 55.
[87] *Loc. cit.*
[88] *Ibid.*, I, 57-58.
[89] Hall, *Rene Descartes: Treatise of Man,* 114.
[90] *Ibid.*, 10.
[91] *Ibid.*, 14.
[92] *Ibid.*, 11.
[93] *Ibid.*, 113.
[94] *Ibid.*, 114.
[95] *Oeuvres de Descartes,* VI, 46.
[96] Hall, *Rene Descartes: Treatise of Man,* 12, note 26.
[97] *Ibid.*, 10, note 21.
[98] *Ibid.*, 17, 19.
[99] See. O. Temkin, "Galen's Pneumatology," *Gesnerus* VIII (1951), 180-189.
[100] Hall, *Rene Descartes: Treatise of Man,* 35-36, 71-72.
[101] *Ibid.*, 21.
[102] *Ibid.*, 4.
[103] Sylvius, *Praxeos Medicae Idea Nova* (London, 1671), 359-360.
[104] *Francisci Deleboe, Sylvii, Opera Medica* (Amsterdam, 1679), 20-21.
[105] Sylvius, *Praxeos Medicae,* 732.
[106] *Ibid.*, 706.
[107] *Ibid.*, 636-637.
[108] *Ibid.*, 562.
[109] Thomas Willis, *Dr. Willis's Practice of Physick, Being the Whole Works of that Renowned and Famous Physician: Containing these Eleven Several Treatises, viz. I. Of Fermentation. II. Of Fevers. III. Of Urines. IV. Of the Accension of the Blood. V. Of Musculary Motion. VI. Of the Anatomy of the Brain. VII. Of the Description and Use of the Nerves. VIII. Of Convulsive Diseases. IX. Pharmaceutice Rationalis, the First and Second Part. X. Of the Scurvy. XI. Two Discourses concerning the Soul of Brutes* (London, 1684), Part IV, 20-27; Part VI, 87-91.
[110] *Ibid.*, Part IV, 21.
[111] *Ibid.*, Part IV, 22-23.
[112] *Ibid.*, Part IV. 26.

[113] *Ibid.*, Part IV, 27.

[114] *Ibid.*, Part VI, 87-91. Meyer and Hierons, "On Thomas Willis's Concepts of Neurophysiology," 2. Dewhurst, *Thomas Willis as a Physician*, 14.

[115] Meyer and Hierons, "On Thomas Willis's Concepts of Neurophysiology," 2.

[116] Cheyne, *A New Theory of Acute and Slow Continued Fevers*, 12-15. Cheyne, *The Natural Method of Curing*, 4.

[117] Cheyne, *The Natural Method of Curing*, 94.

[118] *Ibid.*, 4, 94.

[119] Hoffmann, *Fundamenta Medicinae*, 6.

[120] *Ibid.*, 2.

[121] *Ibid.*, 6.

[122] *Ibid.*, 13.

[123] *Ibid.*, 11.

[124] *Loc. cit.*

[125] *Loc. cit.*

[126] *Loc. cit.*

[127] Hoffmann, *Medicinae Rationalis*, b-2.

[128] Hoffmann, *Fundamenta Medicinae*, 17.

[129] Hoffmann, *Medicinae Rationalis*, 43.

[130] *Loc. cit.*

[131] *Ibid.*, 16.

[132] *Loc. cit.*

[133] *Ibid.*, 17.

[134] Hoffmann, *Fundamenta Medicinae*, 13.

[135] *Loc. cit.*

[136] *Loc. cit.*

[137] *Loc. cit.*

[138] *Loc. cit.*

[139] *Ibid.*, 24.

[140] *Ibid.*, 17.

[141] *Ibid.*, 2.

[142] *Dr. Boerhaave's Academical Lectures*, V, 273.

[143] *Ibid.*, V, 271.

[144] *Ibid.*, I, 90.

[145] *Ibid.*, VI, 290.

[146] *Ibid.*, V, 256-257.

[147] *Ibid.*, I, 92.

[148] *Ibid.*, VI, 292.

[149] *Ibid.*, V, 257.

[150] *Ibid.*, V, 259.

[151] *Ibid.*, V, 255.

[152] *Ibid.*, V, 258.

[153] *Ibid.*, I, 7, 71. Cheyne, *The Natural Method of Curing the Diseases of the Body*, 1. Hoffmann, *Medicinae Rationalis*, 20, 44.

[154] *Dr. Boerhaave's Academical Lectures*, I, 84.

[155] *Ibid.*, V, 288.

[156] *Oeuvres de Descartes*, VI, 62.

[157] Hall, *Rene Descartes: Treatise of Man*, 5-6.

[158] *Ibid.*, 7.

[159] *Ibid.*, 8.
[160] *Loc. cit.*
[161] *Ibid.*, 9.
[162] *Ibid.*, 15.
[163] *Ibid.*, 17.
[164] *Loc. cit.*
[165] Hoffmann, *Medicinae Rationalis*, 18-19.
[166] Sprengel, *Histoire de la Medecine*, V, 56 ff.
[167] Etienne Blankard, *Traite de la Verole, Gonorrhee, Chancres, Bubes Veneriens, & de leurs Accidens* (Amsterdam: Corneille Blankard, 1688), 23.
[168] *Ibid.*, 25.
[169] *Ibid.*, 31.
[170] Sprengel, *Histoire de la Medecine*, V, 63.
[171] Sylvius, *Praxeos Medicae Idea Nova*, 107-108.
[172] *Ibid.*, 109-112.
[173] Foster, *Lectures on the History of Physiology*, 156.
[174] Sylvius, *Praxeos Medicae Idea Nova*, 912-913.
[175] *Ibid.*, 66, 69.
[176] *Ibid.*, 914.
[177] *Ibid.*, 943.
[178] *Loc. cit.*
[179] *Ibid.*, 914.
[180] *Ibid.*, 921.
[181] *Ibid.*, 918, 922.
[182] *Ibid.*, 924 ff.
[183] *Ibid.*, 944.
[184] *Ibid.*, 946.
[185] *Ibid.*, 920.
[186] *Ibid.*, 923.
[187] Sprengel, *Histoire de la Medecine*, V, 68-69.
[188] *Dr. Willis's Practice of Physick*, Part II, 46.
[189] *Ibid.*, Part II, 57.
[190] *Loc. cit.*
[191] *Ibid.*, Part II, 79.
[192] *Ibid.*, Part II, 45.
[193] *Ibid.*, Part II, 48.
[194] *Ibid.*, Part I, 2.
[195] *Loc. cit.*
[196] *Ibid.*, Part II, 48.
[197] *Ibid.*, Part II, 49.
[198] *Loc. cit.*
[199] *Ibid.*, Part I, 2.
[200] *Ibid.*, Part II, 51.
[201] *Ibid.*, Part II, 48.
[202] *Ibid.*, Part II, 50-51.
[203] *Ibid.*, Part II, 54.
[204] *Ibid.*, Part II, 51.
[205] *Ibid.*, Part II, 52.
[206] *Ibid.*, Part II, 79.
[207] *Ibid.*, Part IX, I, 127.

[208] *Ibid.*, Part IX, I, 19.
[209] *Ibid.*, Part IX, I, 17.
[210] *Ibid.*, Part IX, I, 122.
[211] *Ibid.*, Part II, 47.
[212] *Ibid.*, Part IX, I, 2-3.
[213] *Ibid.*, Part IX, I, 117.
[214] *Ibid.*, Part II, 66.
[215] *Ibid.*, Part I, 14. Also Part IX, I, 2.
[216] *Ibid.*, Part IX, I, 107.
[217] *Ibid.*, Part IX, I, 41.
[218] *Ibid.*, Part IX, I, 43.
[219] *Ibid.*, Part IX, I, 2.
[220] *Ibid.*, Part IX, I, 34.
[221] *Ibid.*, Part IX, I, 35.
[222] *Ibid.*, Part IX, I, 16.
[223] *Ibid.*, Part VIII, 18.
[224] *Ibid.*, Part IX, I, 126.
[225] *Ibid.*, Part VIII, 20.
[226] *Ibid.*, Part IX, II, 51.
[227] Cheyne, *A New Theory of Acute and Slow Continued Fevers*, 33.
[228] *Ibid.*, 4.
[229] *Ibid.*, 40.
[230] Cheyne, *The English Malady: or, a Treatise of Nervous Diseases of All Kinds, as Spleen, Vapours, Lowness of Spirits* (London, 1733), 6.
[231] Cheyne, *A New Theory of Acute and Slow Continued Fevers*, 4.
[232] *Ibid.*, 19.
[233] *Ibid.*, 22.
[234] *Ibid.*, 122-123.
[235] Cheyne, *The English Malady*, 158.
[236] Cheyne, *The Natural Method of Curing the Diseases of the Body*, 75.
[237] Cheyne, *A New Theory of Acute and Slow Continued Fevers*, 8.
[238] Cheyne, *The Natural Method of Curing the Diseases of the Body*, 44.
[239] Cheyne, *The English Malady*, 145. *A New Theory of Acute and Slow Continued Fevers*, 107-108.
[240] Cheyne, *A New Theory of Acute and Slow Continued Fevers*, 103-104.
[241] Cheyne, *The English Malady*, 6-7.
[242] *Ibid.*, 112, 126.
[243] *Ibid.*, 113, 137.
[244] *Ibid.*, 143-144.
[245] Hoffmann, *Medicinae Rationalis*, c-3.
[246] *Ibid.*, a-3.
[247] *Ibid.*, b-3.
[248] *Loc. cit.*
[249] *Loc. cit.* Hoffmann, *Fundamenta Medicinae*, 41.
[250] Hoffmann, *Fundamenta Medicinae*, 16, 40.
[251] *Ibid.*, 40.
[252] *Ibid.*, 39.
[253] *Loc. cit.*
[254] *Ibid.*, 41, 67-68.
[255] *Ibid.*, 55.

[256] Hoffmann, *Medicinae Rationalis,* c.
[257] Hoffmann, *Fundamenta Medicinae,* 41.
[258] *Ibid.,* 41-42.
[259] *Ibid.,* 119.
[260] *Ibid.,* 118.
[261] *Ibid.,* 119.
[262] *Ibid.,* 120.
[263] *Loc. cit.*
[264] *Ibid.,* 136.
[265] *Ibid.,* 121.
[266] *Ibid.,* 122.
[267] *Ibid.,* 137.
[268] *Loc. cit.*
[269] *Ibid.,* 120.
[270] *Loc. cit.*
[271] *Ibid.,* 133.
[272] *Loc. cit.*
[273] Hoffmann, *Medicinae Rationalis,* b-3, c, 31.
[274] Hoffmann, *A System of the Practice of Medicine,* II, 3, 6.
[275] *Ibid.,* II, 380-383.
[276] Hoffmann, *Fundamenta Medicinae,* 121.
[277] *Ibid.,* 121.
[278] *Ibid.,* 86.
[279] *Ibid.,* 101.
[280] *Loc. cit.*
[281] *Ibid.,* 48. Hoffmann, *Medicinae Rationalis,* b-3.
[282] Sprengel, *Histoire de la Medecine,* V, 288.
[283] *Dr. Boerhaave's Academical Lectures,* V, 478.
[284] *Ibid.,* V, 479.
[285] *Ibid.,* V, 332-334.
[286] *Ibid.,* V, 335, 469 and VI, 359.
[287] *Ibid.,* V, 376.
[288] *Ibid.,* V, 417, 428.
[289] *Ibid.,* V, 336, 337, 348.
[290] *Ibid.,* V, 418.
[291] *Ibid.,* V, 422.
[292] *Ibid.,* V, 474.
[293] *Ibid.,* V, 481.
[294] *Ibid.,* VI, 41.
[295] *Ibid.,* V, 299, 301.
[296] *Ibid.,* V, 293.
[297] *Ibid.,* V, 390.
[298] *Ibid.,* V, 490.
[299] *Ibid.,* VI, 40.
[300] *Ibid.,* VI, 29.
[301] *Ibid.,* V, 469.
[302] *Ibid.,* VI, 313.
[303] *Ibid.,* VI, 277.
[304] *Ibid.,* VI, 278.
[305] *Ibid.,* VI, 382.

[306] *Ibid.*, VI, 420.
[307] *Ibid.*, VI, 421.
[308] *Ibid.*, VI, 361, 366.
[309] *Ibid.*, VI, 365.
[310] *Ibid.*, VI, 363, 368.
[311] *Ibid.*, VI, 361-362.
[312] *Ibid.*, VI, 368.
[313] *Ibid.*, VI, 370-373.
[314] *Ibid.*, VI, 316.
[315] *Ibid.*, VI, 303.
[316] *Ibid.*, VI, 358.
[317] *Ibid.*, VI, 359.
[318] Hermann Boerhaave, *Elements of Chemistry* (London: Pemberton, 1735), I, 55.
[319] *Dr. Boerhaave's Academical Lectures*, VI, 301.
[320] *Loc. cit.*
[321] *Ibid.*, VI, 302.
[322] *Loc. cit.*
[323] *Ibid.*, VI, 354.
[324] *Ibid.*, VI, 322.
[325] *Ibid.*, VI, 381.
[326] *Loc. cit.*
[327] *Ibid.*, VI, 175.
[328] *Ibid.*, VI, 167.
[329] *Ibid.*, VI, 169.
[330] *Loc. cit.*
[331] *Ibid.*, VI, 173.
[332] *Ibid.*, VI, 174.
[333] *Ibid.*, VI, 171.
[334] *Ibid.*, VI, 175.
[335] *Ibid.*, VI, 282.
[336] *Ibid.*, I, 7.

CHAPTER III

EMPIRICAL REACTIONS (1): THOMAS SYDENHAM AND GIORGIO BAGLIVI

These two thinkers initiate the Empirical response to Iatrochemistry and Iatromechanism. Relying on Bacon's critique of metaphysics and his call for a return to observation and experience, Thomas Sydenham (1624-1689) rejected Willis's chemical interpretation of physiology and therapeutics and proposed a revival of Hippocratic principles. Giorgio Baglivi (1668-1707), a younger colleague of the Italian Iatromechanists, Borelli and Bellini, took up Sydenham's argument and extended it with further references to Hippocrates, the ancient Empirical School, and Bacon.

Sydenham, furthermore, converted Bacon's neo-Platonic "form" into a wholly new concept—the "specific disease" (already suggested by Paracelsus' and Van Helmont's discussion of "specific" medicines).

Biographical

Thomas Sydenham was born to a middle-class Dorsetshire family and at age seventeen enrolled in Magdalen College, Oxford, to study classics. But when war erupted two months later between King and Parliament, he enlisted in the Puritan army together with his three older brothers. He remained a soldier for five years and returned to Wadham College in 1647; in 1648 he received the bachelor's degree in medicine through political influence (the accelerated graduation of

Puritan students was part of Parliament's technique for gaining control over royalist Oxford).

About his personal life thereafter little is known.[a] He was once thought to have studied with Charles Barbeyrac (1629-1699) in Montpellier, but this is now regarded as a legend. He was admitted to the College of Physicians in 1663, but his unorthodox medical opinions prevented his relations with other physicians from being more than lukewarm. He settled in Westminster and devoted himself strictly to the practical care of the sick:

> I have the happiness of curing my patients, at least of having it said concerning me that few miscarry under me; but I cannot brag of my correspondency with some others of my faculty who, notwithstanding my profoundness in palmistry and chemistry, impeach me of great insufficiency, as I shall likewise do my tailor when he makes my doublet like a hop-sack, and not before, let him adhere to what hypothesis he will.[1]

He was awarded the M.D. in 1676 by Puritan Cambridge and died of the gout in 1689.[b]

Sydenham wrote in English and with extreme reluctance. Most of his original manuscripts were lost after being translated and published in Latin, and only recently have some of them been recovered.[c] His *Art of Medicine* (1669), a criticism of the "faculty of medicine as it now stands in reference to diseases and their cure,"[2] was long thought to be from the pen of his intimate friend, John Locke (1632-1704).

Giorgio Baglivi, of Armenian parentage, was orphaned as a boy in a shipwreck off the coast of Ragusa (Dubrovnik) and consigned to the care of the Jesuits. He was adopted by an Italian family and studied medicine in Salerno, Naples,

[a]All available biographical detail on Sydenham is to be found in Kenneth Dewhurst, *Dr. Thomas Sydenham (1624-1689). His Life and Original Writings* (Berkeley and Los Angeles: University of California Press, 1966).

[b]In 1810 the College of Physicians made amends for its earlier hostility, erecting a statue of Sydenham in Westminster Abbey.

Bologna, and Rome (under Marcello Malpighi). He eventually became professor of theoretical medicine, surgery, and anatomy in the latter city.

Despite his professorial accomplishments, his heart was in practice. He took Sydenham as a model, calling him the "profoundest observer after Hippocrates,"[3] and his most important writing was on the reformation of practice.[d] He died of overwork at the young age of thirty-six.

The Critique of Rationalism

While Galenism was gradually disappearing in its pristine form, it had been replaced by its Iatrochemical and Iatromechanist revisions in which the doctrine of contraries was clothed in chemical or hydraulic garb. Hence, just as Bacon had cleared the ground by a sweeping condemnation of scholastic thought patterns in philosophy, Sydenham and Baglivi commence with a general condemnation of the philosophical bases of Rationalism.

These false doctrines are only "hypotheses" drawn from "speculation" which have "as much to do with treating sick men as the painting of pictures with the sailing of ships."[4] "A contrivance of the word-catchers, the art of talking rather than the art of healing."[5] "These empty impractical notions . . . are but the puppets of men's fancies and imaginations which, however dressed up, after forty years' dandling are but puppets still, void of strength, use, or activity."[6]

Infatuation with these hypotheses has stultified observation of the phenomena of disease and the powers of medicines.[7] "Subtle speculations are of higher value and give more pleasure than genuine practice."[8]

The pagan Arabs and Galenists used the Hippocratic writings merely as a source of theories and thus perverted the masculine medicine of the Greeks.[9] "No man can state the

[c]They have been published in Dewhurst, *Dr. Thomas Sydenham.*

[d]*De Praxi Medica ad Priscam Observandi Rationem Revocanda* (Rome, 1696), translated into French as *De l'Accroissement de la Medecine Pratique* (Paris: Labé, Librairie de la Faculté de Medecine, 1851).

errors that have been occasioned by these physiological hypotheses. Writers, whose minds have taken a false color under their influence, have saddled diseases with phenomena which existed in their own brains only, but which would have been clear and visible to the whole world had the assumed hypothesis been true."[10] No wise man will *jurare in verba magistri,* since there is no "certain experiment" by which these "speculative reasons" can be tested.[11]

These hypotheses are only "idols". Some stem from human weakness, i.e., are idols of the tribe: "the natural inclination to . . . have some basis to rest their thoughts upon and some grounds to guide them in the practice of their art."[12] Others are merely a means of acquiring glory, i.e., idols of the theater.[13] Like the idols worshipped by the Romans, these impart no movement or life, while the mechanical arts, nourished by experience, approach every day closer to perfection.[14] [e]

Physicians are bedazzled by these idols, which have "but confined and narrowed men's thoughts, amused their understanding with fine but useless speculations, and diverted their inquiries from the true and advantageous knowledge of things."[15] They inspect books and not the *physis.*[16] [f] Even the symptoms which they observe correctly are misinterpreted:

> If by chance some symptom really coincide accurately with their hypothesis, and occur in the disease whereof they would describe the character, they magnify it beyond all measure and moderation; they make it all in all; the molehill becomes a mountain; whilst, if it fail to tally with the said hypothesis, they pass it over either in perfect silence or with only an incidental mention, unless,

[e]Cf. *Novum Organum,* I, Aph. LXXIV.

[f]Baglivi recounts the story of Giovanni Argenterio (1513-1572): he had a tremendous grasp of medical theory, attributing all diseases to *ametria* (lack of proportion) in the solids, but patients were unwilling to come to him, fearing the consequences of his treatment. At length he retired to a monastery where he died (Baglivi, *De Praxi Medica,* 41).

> by means of some philosophical subtlety, they can enlist it in their service, or else, by fair means or foul, accommodate it in some way or other to their doctrines.[17]

While Galenism was one such idol, the new chemical doctrine of acids and alkalis is an even worse source of error in medicine:

> Supposing it were . . . sal, sulphur, and mercury, the volatile and the fixed of the chemists, that made disorders in the body, and we could come to know which of these in excess it was that produced this malady and where it was lodged; supposing, v.g., that too much acid in the blood or other juices caused the gout, a fever, or epilepsy, what indication would this give a practiced physician in the cure of either of these diseases? 'Tis truth, 'twill presently be suggested he must mortify this acidity, but will he be thence enabled to choose fit remedies and a due method of their application; will he conclude that pearl, coral, or egg shells, because they take away the acidity in vinegar, will be certain and effectual remedies in the removal of these maladies? He that shall proceed on such grounds as these may indeed constitute fine doctrines and lay plausible hypotheses, but will not have much to brag about of his cures.[18]

Their introduction of chemistry into medicine is equivalent to Plato's mixing of theology with science or Aristotle's reduction of the study of nature to logic and dialectic.[19] But mathematics, chemistry, rhetoric, and logic are misleading, since the causes they claim to disclose cannot actually be judged by the senses.[20]

Reliance on these hypotheses has unduly restricted the variety of diseases which physicians are willing to consider:

> It happens at present that many diseases, although included in the same genus, mentioned with a common nomenclature, and resembling one another in several symptoms, are, notwithstanding, different in their

> natures and require a different medical treatment . . . Although it may be true that all complaints are not liable to the same amount of variety, there are still many which authors treat alike, under the same heads, and without the shadow of a distinction, whilst they are in their natures as dissimilar as possible.[21]

> The evident diversity of [epidemic] diseases is palpably shown, both by the difference and the peculiarities of their symptoms, and by the variety of treatment that they require. From all which it is perfectly clear that, although the disorders in question may, to a certain degree, both in their external characters and in several symptoms common to many of them, appear to the careless observer to coincide, they are in reality, if we attend closely, of wholly different characters, as little like one another as coin and counters.[22]

The outcome is the deterioration of practice. The Galenists hold that every fever is from bile, and they evacuate bile, but when the bile in the system has been evacuated, the fever still remains.[23] The Iatrochemists focus only on acids and alkalis, but many diseases have nothing to do with acids and alkalis.[24] Man has a thousand ways of being sick, and medicine cannot be reduced to such a narrow compass.[25]

Physicians confuse diseases whose symptoms are similar, treating them with the same medicines and causing them to grow worse.[26] Misunderstanding the true development of disease they prescribe remedies too early, thus altering the symptom pattern, preventing the crisis from coming on, and transforming acute diseases into chronic ones.[27] "It often happens that the character of the complaint varies with the nature of the remedies and that symptoms may be referred less to the disease than to the doctor. Hence two patients with the same ailment, but under different treatment, may suffer from different symptoms."[28] [g]

[g]Baglivi followed Sydenham in prescribing no medicines at the outset, to avoid disturbing the natural course of the disease (Baglivi, *De Praxi Medica,* 200; *The Works of Thomas Sydenham* [London: Sydenham Society, 1848-1850], I, 33).

Observation and Experience

Sydenham and Baglivi accept the dichotomy between the world of nature and that part of it which can be comprehended by the human intellect. "It may be well conceived that the utmost that I can find out by adverting to the Great Theater bears but an inconsiderable share in the divine opifice, which is still more exquisite and more great than I (who lie grovelling upon the dirt of this Earth) have faculties to comprehend."[29] "For suppose an oyster has the faculty of reasoning, ought he then to conclude, because nature has endowed him with that one sense of tasting, and perhaps with that other of touching, therefore, there were no other objects in the world than those which answered to his two senses? So to think were to be more like an oyster than a man."[30]

The schools, however, are unaware of the distinction between these two worlds.[31] Whatever falls outside the circle of their speculation they regard as impossible.[32] But the laws of nature exist of themselves and are not assigned by man.[33] The products of the intellect are building-blocks, while nature is the plumb-line; the former must be accommodated to the latter, and not vice-versa.[34]

In medicine the division is between the world of the physician's intellect and that of the patient's *physis.*

The *physis* is the origin of all that transpires in the body and thus the basis of therapeutics: "by this ladder and by this scaffold did Hippocrates ascend his lofty sphere—the Romulus of medicine whose heaven was the empyrean of his art . . . He it was who then laid the solid and immoveable foundation for the whole superstructure of medicine when he taught that *our natures are the physicians of our diseases.*"[35] But the physician's intellect cannot penetrate inside the *physis* to cognize the sources of health and disease.[36] "That least and subtle texture of the solid and fluid parts of the living body is hidden from us and will ever remain hidden, not only from the senses but from the edge of the human mind."[37] "Curious speculators lose their labor, since the investigation and illustration of primary and ultimate causes is a neglect of our capabilities and a violation of the *physis.*"[38]

Physicians react to this situation in three equally incorrect ways. Either they deny the existence of the *physis* altogether, failing to comprehend its operations.[39] Or they try to understand it chemically: the Iatrochemists think they have discovered the composition of chyle when they can put two or three chemicals together in a retort and from them extract some kind of whitish liquid.[40] But the processes of the *physis* differ from those of chemistry.[41] Finally, they try to understand it through dissection of the body. But, "though we cut into their inside, we see but the outside of things, and make but a new *superficies* for ourselves to stare at."[42]

> That anatomy is like to afford any great improvement to the practice of physic, or to assist a man in the finding out and establishing a true method, I have reason to doubt. All that anatomy can do is only to show us the gross and sensible parts of the body, or the vapid and dead juices, all which, after the most diligent search, will be no more able to direct a physician how to cure a disease than how to make a man . . . For suppose any one shall have so sharp a knife and sight as to discover the secret and effective composure of any part, could he make an ocular demonstration that the pores of the parenchyma of the liver or kidneys were either round or square and that parts of urine and gall separated in these parts were in size and figure answerable to those pores? I ask how this would at all direct him in the cure either of the jaundice or stoppage of the urine? What would this advantage his method or guide him to fit medicines?[43]

Thus the Iatromechanists are in error: just as blacksmiths cannot comprehend the workings of a watch, so humans, "miserable wanderers from the bright path of knowledge, [are] incapable of comprehending the method of the supreme artificer in his wondrous and wise machinery."[44] [h]

[h]Baglivi's Iatromechanist views led him to differ with Sydenham on this point (*De Praxi Medica,* 31, 91). See below, pp. 195-196.

The physician must have a basic knowledge of the structure and functioning of the body, but, even so, acute diseases possess "some specific property which no speculations deduced from the contemplation of the human frame will ever be enabled to discover and exhibit."[45]

The effort to penetrate into the body only distracts man from what lies on the surface, available to his senses and experience: "and thus man, by desire to know more than was fit a second time, lost the little remainder of knowledge that was left him."[46] "So much is human genius limited by the limits of human nature that we just know what our five senses teach. Prudent a man may be. A philosopher in the most august sense of the term no man can be."[47] "All our knowledge is rough and gross, dealing only with the outer husk of the things that we would know, ascertaining only, at its highest level, *how* things are, but by no means guessing *why* they are so."[48]

Man achieves knowledge of the body's functions and processes only by observing them in sickness and health.[49] Medicine is created by a "diligent, wise, and accurate recording of the *physis.*"[50] Thus the histories of diseases and treatments are the basis of medical science.[51] "The history of diseases is a science *sui generis;* it does not draw its principles and increase from other sciences but from the purest and most salutary fountains of the *physis* . . . the histories of disease depend upon the sedulous and patient description of what the learned observer has noted of their invasion, progress, and disappearance."[52] Medicine turns away from what is hypothetical and searches for instruments consecrated by the experience of centuries.[53]

Sydenham wrote: "to some it may appear that the method which I adopt is based upon insecure foundations. I am, however, on my own part, fully convinced . . . that it is altogether proved by a manifold experience."[54] To a young physician recommended to him as a "ripe scholar, a good botanist, a skilful anatomist," he remarked: "This is all very well, but it won't do–anatomy, botany!! Nonsense, Sir! I know an old woman in Covent Garden who understands botany better, and as for anatomy, my butcher can dissect a joint full as well. No, young man, all this is stuff: you must go to the bedside, it is there alone you can learn disease."[55] [i]

This was the greatness of Hippocrates: scorning theoretical knowledge, he relied only on observation and experience.[56] His *Aphorisms* drew upon thousands of observations.[57] He spoke the language of the *physis,* not that of man.[58]

It would be a great service to mankind if an academy could be established to record and classify all observable data of sickness and disease.[59]

Just as we cannot acquire analytical knowledge of the organism, so we cannot obtain such knowledge of the working of medicines. Their mode of action is a thorny issue, indeed, and another academy would be needed to study it.[60] For the *physis* uses the remedy like a man in a deep hole to whom a plank is thrown; he turns it left and right, sticks it into the side of the hole, etc. until, one way or another, he extricates himself. The remedy sometimes arouses fermentation, somctimes eliminates harmful humors, sometimes extinguishes the fire in the solids, sometimes detaches viscosities. The *physis* uses it in a thousand ways, and they can only be learned empirically—by observation and experience.[61]

So-called "primary" and "secondary" qualities are all fictitious; neither are remedies "stronger" or "weaker", more powerful or less powerful.[62] Each is different from each other and acts in its own way on the organism; each is a specific.[63]

The physician cannot understand this mode of action: he cannot know that "rhubarb or pellitory have in them fit wedges to divide the blood into such parts as may be

[i]Hans Sloane (1660-1753) who later became president of both the College of Physicians and the Royal Society. A contemporary reported Sydenham's views on medical education: "Physick, says Sydenham, is not to be learned by going to Universities, but he is for taking apprentices; and says one had as good send a man to Oxford to learn shoemaking as practising physick" (Dewhurst, *Dr. Thomas Sydenham,* 17). Another great figure in British medicine, John Hunter, was of the same opinion (see below, p. 356*h*).

separable, urine in the one, or gall in the other, or any other particles in them fitted to open [passages in the liver or kidneys]."[64]

> For the alterations that both our food and physic receive in our mouths, stomachs, guts, glandules, etc. are so many and so unintelligible to us before they come to the places we design them, that they are quite another thing than we imagine, and work not as we fancy but as nature pleases . . . For it is not by any sensible qualities by which medicines work their effects on our bodies, and so cannot by these criteria be chosen and adapted to our hypothesis . . . The anatomist will hardly be enabled to tell us, therefore, what changes any particular medicine either makes or receives in the body till he can inform us by what artifice and in what shops nature makes in the bodies of animals volatile salts out of the juice of plants which appear not to have any such substance in them.[65]

The powers of specific medicines can be discovered only by accident or experience: "all our knowledge of their efficacy being to be acknowledged rather old women's experience than learned men's theories."[66] "I must limit the function of a physician to industrious investigation of the history of diseases and of the effects of remedies, as shown by the only true teacher—experience."[67]

> How regulate his dose, mix his simples, and prescribe all in a due method? All this is only from history and the advantage of a diligent observation of these diseases, of their beginning, progress, and ways of cure, which a physician may as well do without a scrupulous enquiry into the anatomy of the parts as a gardener may by his art and observation be able to ripen, meliorate, and preserve his fruit without examining what kinds of juices, fibers, pores, etc. are to be found in the roots, bark, or body of the tree.[68]

Theory and Practice

"Disease" is a "specific exaltation" or "specific alteration" of one of the body's humors.[69] [j] The *physis* struggles with the exalted humor, endeavoring to concoct it; the process comes to a climax on a given day, differing from one disease to another, and then (if the patient does not die) the concocted disease matter is expelled through the skin or through one of the body's orifices.[70]

Thus the ebullition or boiling of the humor is both the disease and the curative process.[71] An acute disease represents the body's reaction, "nothing more than an effort of the *natura* which strives with might and main to restore the health of the patient by the elimination of the morbific matter . . . Hence the *natura,* in the concatenation of symptoms, has provided a method for the elimination and exclusion of the peccant and foreign matter which otherwise would undo the whole fabric of our frame."[72] Plague is "a complication of symptoms which the *natura* puts in play in order that, through the natural eliminations, either in the way of abscesses or by the help of some other form of eruption, she may expel from the body those infectious particles that we have taken in along with the air that we breathe."[73]

The fevers, evacuations, skin eruptions, etc. which occur in disease represent part of this healing effort. Fever is used by the *physis* "for the isolation of the tainted particles from the remainder of the blood" and then "by diaphoresis or diarrhoea, by eruptions, or some other evacuation, she expels the particles thus isolated."[74] "Many different diseases are cured by their different appropriate evacuations . . . it is the evacuation that performs the cure."[75] Morbific matter in the intestines makes its escape *via* a severe dysentery.[76] In a quartan fever a skin eruption is extremely beneficial, and the fever and eruption will eventually disappear of themselves without any further treatment.[77] A petechial eruption in an advanced stage of any disease is a good sign, showing that

[j]See below, pp. 196 ff.

coction has commenced and that the disease is being resolved; at the outset of a disease, however, it marks a breakdown of the blood and is dangerous.[78] Gout is the *natura's* way of purifying the blood of old men and purging deep-lying parts of the body.[79] Long-lasting ulcers are another escape route for harmful matters.[80]

The *natura* thus possesses a method of combating disease. This method is both its theory and its practice, and the physician must model his own theory and practice upon it—observing the body's natural process of cure and striving by his treatment to imitate and reproduce it:

> As [the Hippocratic] theory was neither more nor less than an exquisite picture of the *natura*, it was natural that the practice should coincide with it. This aimed at one point only—it strove to help the *natura* in her struggles as it best could. With this view it limited the province of medical art to the support of the *natura* when she was enfeebled, and to the coercion of her when she was outrageous; the attempt on either side being determined by the rate and method whereby she herself attempted the removal and expulsion of disease.[81]

> That practice and that alone will do good which elicits the indications of cure out of the phenomena of the disease itself. This made Hippocrates divine . . . True practice consists in the observations of the *natura;* these are finer than any speculations. Hence the medicine of the *natura* is more refined than the medicine of philosophy.[82]

> I have often thought that provided with a thorough insight into the history of any disease whatsoever, I could invariably apply an equivalent remedy; a clear path being thus marked out for me by the different phenomena of the complaint. These phenomena, if carefully collated with each other, lead us, as it were, by the hand to those palpable indications of treatment which are drawn not from the hallucinations of our fancy, but from the innermost penetralia of the *natura.*[83]

This point is exemplified in the following quotation from Cicero (*De Oratore,* i, 6) found among Sydenham's papers: "But to my way of thinking the virtue in all rules is, not that orators by following them have won a reputation for eloquence, but that certain persons have noted and reduced to an art the doings of men who were naturally eloquent; eloquence is not the offspring of the art, but the art of eloquence."[84]

Hence, medical practice cannot be based on theories generated outside practice itself:

> He that thinks he came to be skilled in diseases by studying the doctrine of the humors, that the notions of obstructions and putrefaction assist him in the cure of fevers, or that by the acquaintance he has with sulphur and mercury he was led into this useful discovery that medicines and regimen as certainly kill in the latter end of some fevers as they cure in others, may as rationally believe that his cook owes his skill in roasting and boiling to his study of the elements and that his speculations about fire and water have taught him that the same seething liquors that boil the egg hard make the hen tender.[85]

Even anatomy must be interpreted in therapeutic terms: a contemporary wrote that Sydenham's books "will bring physicians about his ears, to decry the usefulness of natural philosophy and to maintain the necessity of knowledge in anatomy in subordination to physic."[86] Baglivi held that knowledge from autopsies is useful to the physician only if he is familiar with the disease history.[87]

Contemporary thinking about fermentation was given an original turn by Sydenham—being also subordinated to therapeutics (in contrast to its role for Willis). Mankind he divides into four physiological types: the sanguine, the melancholic, the bilious, and the phlegmatic—in function of the degree of heat possessed by the body and the time which the food takes to pass through the digestive tract and be excreted. The latter he calls the "vent," a term taken from beer-making: "from the proportion of the vent to the heat do arise all the internal diseases of the four constitutions."[88] If the vent is too small, the organism behaves like a keg of beer in which the bung is too tight: the gas cannot escape, and the typical diseases are those (like fevers) of superactive fermentation. If the vent is too large, the body behaves like a beer keg with an open bunghole: the fermentation process comes to a standstill, and the liquids putrefy—hence plague and also many chronic diseases.[89] "This inability of the *natura* to concoct the humors is the chief cause of most chronic diseases."[90]

Thus Sydenham was perfectly familiar with the corpuscular theory, contemporary speculation about chemistry and fermentation, etc., but refused to base therapeutics upon this knowledge.[91] Although admitting that the organism's functioning can be reduced ultimately to a "continuous flow of particles," he still ridicules the physician (as noted above) who thinks that "the notions of obstruction and putrefaction assist him in the cure of fevers."[92] Because the *physis* employs these chemical and other processes *in its own way:*

> Now it is certain and beyond controversy that nature performs all her operations on the body by parts so minute and insensible that I think nobody will ever hope or pretend, even by the assistance of glasses or any other invention, to come to a sight of them and to tell us what organical texture or what kind of ferment (for whether it be done by one or both of these ways is yet a question and like to be so always, notwithstanding all the endeavors of the most accurate dissections) separate any part of the juices in any of the viscera or tell us of what liquors the particles of these juices are.[93]

Speculation about corpuscles and fermentation is just "hypothesis" and useless to practice because not drawn from practice. "Hypotheses" are "stable and permanent" when "directly derived from the facts themselves and arising from those observations only which are suggested by practical and natural phenomena . . . the hypotheses themselves, so far as they are true and genuine, *themselves originated in practice.*"[94] The theory must arise out of the practice.

Baglivi's interpretation of the relationship between theory and practice is ambiguous, since he both follows Sydenham and—because of his own Iatromechanist proclivities—attempts a different approach.

Thus, certain passages in his writings support the classic Empirical view that theory emerges from observation of the phenomena. Astronomy is the best example: a mass of facts is collected by observation, and then a theory is formulated whose truth is seen in its predictive ability.[95] Medicine should follow the same course: after observing processes repeating themselves time after time, the physician formulates a hypothesis based upon the constant movements of the *physis* (*constantes motus naturae*).[96]

But then Baglivi goes on to hold that these "constant movements" follow Iatromechanist laws: the teeth are like scissors, the chest is a bellows, the viscera and glands are like sieves, the muscles behave like cords, and the cardiovascular system is a set of pumps and conduits.[97] The language of the *physis* is mechanical.[98] "It was doubtless the will of God who, in order that the structures of the body more readily obey the commands of the mind, is seen to have marked off the most highly ordered mathematical rules of proportion and movement in the human body as though with a ruler and chalk."[99] [k]

[k]He even cites ancient Methodism as authority for basing medicine on the "unshakeable foundations of mechanics." Caelius Aurelianus, a leading member of this School, "almost" surpassed Hippocrates in the accuracy of his disease descriptions, and Baglivi holds that Sydenham was greatly under his influence. Baglivi seems not to realize that Methodism rejected the *physis* entirely. Elsewhere, in any case, he criticizes this School for its "perverse" views. He also attacks "Descartes, the followers of Democritus [i.e., the school of Pierre Gassendi], the mechanists, and physico-mechanists who pronounced on medicine without knowing anything about it" (*De Praxi Medica,* 28, 91, 201, 235). His interpretation of Methodism is inaccurate, reflecting his own failure to overcome the conflict between his Hippocratic instincts and Iatromechanist training. On the ancient Methodist School see *Divided Legacy,* I, 291-301.

Baglivi's acceptance of these Iatromechanist assumptions of course violates his own principle that medicine is all based on observation, since such fancied mechanical processes within the body are not subject to observation. The conflict between these two sides of his mind ultimately vitiates much of his therapeutic philosophy and, in particular, confuses his discussion of theory and practice.

On this latter question he adopts a position different from that of either Empiricism or Rationalism, holding that theory and practice proceed from separate sources, lead separate lives, and do not interact with one another.[100]

In ancient times the two were not divided, and the split arose only with the Arabs.[101] Today the theory of medicine is taken from anatomical investigations and its practice from therapeutic observation.[102] The two should not be confused: vital phenomena cannot be explained in terms of suction, attraction, etc., and the moderns are mistaken in basing practice on such theories.[103] The physician's therapeutic efforts can be guided only by experience, since the *physis* is subtler than any mathematician.[104] The first book is the patient.[105]

As guides to anatomical theory Baglivi recommends Harvey and Sanctorius (1561-1636), to practice–Hippocrates and the sixteenth-century Hippocratic, Louis Duret.[106]

Disease Causes and Classification

Sydenham wrought a major change in the Hippocratic theory of coction, transforming it into a doctrine of "specific diseases" which was to have a long life in Western medicine.

Paracelsus had introduced the concept of the "specific medicine" which was further developed by Van Helmont. Sydenham merely shifted attention from "specificity" of the remedy to that of the disease:

> The . . . humors become exalted into a substantial form or species; and these substantial forms or species manifest themselves in disorders coincident with their respective

> essences . . . every specific disease is a disorder that originates from this or that specific exaltation or . . . from the specification of some juice in the living body. Under this head may be comprised the greatest part of those diseases which are reducible to some given form or type, in the production and maturation whereof the *natura* binds herself to a certain method as stringently as she does with plants and even animals.[107]

This shift, however small, was nonetheless decisive, representing the move from the Rationalist view that diseases consist of cognizable elements to the Empirical view that disease is a *divinum quid.*

Sydenham was aware of the logical difficulty of extracting a specific disease out of the Galenic humors: "it cannot be easily comprehended how the disease in question can arise from a combination of either principles or evident qualities."[108] He tries to draw a parallel with plants growing out of the earth:

> Now, putting all this carefully together, we find reasons for believing that this disease is a species equally cogent with those that we have for believing a plant to be a species. The plant springs from the earth; the plant blooms; the plant dies: the plant does all this with equal regularity. All its other affections are those of its essence . . . a plant is universally recognized as a substance and as a distinct species in nature.[109]

but concludes that whereas plants separate themselves from the earth when they become species, disease species remain attached to their humors in some mysterious way.[110]

Thus the proximate causes of diseases are "inscrutable and inexplicable."[111] In a pleurisy "a man may work much, and work in vain, before he will understand the vicious crasis and the incoherent texture of the blood which is the primary cause."[112]

But this knowledge is not needed for cure.[113] "If [the physician] rightly know the cause by which it is *immediately* produced, and if he can rightly discriminate between it and other diseases, he will be as certain to succeed in his attempts at a cure as if he had attended to idle and unprofitable searches into remote causes."[114]

Thus Sydenham urges attention to (1) the exciting causes of the "specific" changes in the humors and (2) the visible signs which distinguish one disease from another. This knowledge permits the physician to classify diseases correctly.

Theories which rely on assumed knowledge of disease "proximate causes" distract physicians' attention from their exciting causes, "those causes that ought to be, and which can be, understood; which lie before our feet; which require no rotten supports; which appeal to the understanding at once; which are revealed by either the testimony of our senses or by anatomical observations of long standing."[115]

For diseases all arise from the impact of some environmental or external factor on the organism: "since it is the will of God, the Supreme Arbiter and Regulator of all things, that the human frame be, by nature, adapted to the reception of impressions from without, it follows that it must also be liable to a variety of maladies."[116]

Of these external (exciting) causes the major ones are the six "non-naturals": the air, meat and drink, motion and rest, sleep and wakefulness, the emotions, the *secreta* and *retenta.*[117]

Some acute diseases "originate from the particular anomalies of particular bodies."[118] The humors "may act the part of poisons from the influence of some venomous contagion."[119] Changes in the weather are major exciting causes of disease:

> There exist different and peculiar temperaments or crases of the same year. Herein the fevers that occur are determined by the manifest qualities of the air . . . come on sooner or later, and take more or less the character of epidemics. Besides this, however, the fevers which I have

> called *intercurrent* and which occur in any or all years promiscuously, originate most especially in this or that manifest atmospheric temperament . . . pleurisies, quinsies, and other like ailments generally prevail when long and severe cold is rapidly succeeded by sudden heat . . . we must admit that even the *sensible* qualities of the atmosphere have a predisposing effect upon our bodies even in the development of epidemics.[120]

In addition to these perceptible weather and climatic changes, however, there is an additional environmental factor giving rise to disease. This is the "constitution"–Sydenham's great contribution to the theory of exciting causes and to Empirical medicine generally.

Early in life he noted that the incidence of morbidity followed a pattern different from that of the weather or climate.[121] To elucidate the underlying reasons for the changes in disease patterns he made observations for the fifteen years from 1661 to 1676 in London and concluded that longer cycles, which he called "constitutions," impressed their stamp on all diseases occurring within them:

> This is how it is. There are different constitutions in different years. They originate neither in their heat nor in their cold, their wet nor their drought; but they depend upon certain hidden and inexplicable changes within the bowels of the earth. By the effluvia from these the atmosphere becomes contaminate, and the bodies of men are predisposed and determined, as the case may be, to this or that complaint . . . Each and all of these general constitutions take the melancholy characteristic of some proper and peculiar form of fever.[122]

> Whether the inward bowels of the earth undergo various changes by the vapors which exhale therefrom, so that the air is tainted, or whether the atmosphere be changed by some alterations induced by some peculiar conjunction of any of the heavenly bodies, it is a truth that at particular times the air is stuffed full of particles which are hostile to the economy of the human body.[123]

The humors "contract a morbific disposition from the existing atmospheric constitution . . . [and] become exalted into a substantial form or species."[124]

The "constitution" thus owed something to astrology and something to the corpuscular theory. It had much in common with Van Helmont's "blas of the stars."[l]

The next important criterion of classification after the exciting cause is the visible symptom-pattern which characterizes each disease.

Here both thinkers look to the "substantial form," the neo-Platonic concept which had been generalized and popularized by Bacon.[125]

He had urged that "forms" be derived from a comparison of the "natures" in which the "forms" appear, and this was easily adapted to the elucidation of disease "forms" by comparing the "natures" of all the persons suffering from the same "disease."

Furthermore, in accepting the "form" as a basic article of doctrine Sydenham and Baglivi were only following in the footsteps of Paracelsus and Van Helmont who also looked for guidance to the "form" or the "formal cause."

Like the two latter thinkers, and like Bacon, Sydenham relied on the "form" because it was externalized—became visible—in the symptoms: "these substantial forms or species manifest themselves in disorders coincident with their respective essences. Of these disorders the symptoms . . . are the disorders that depend upon the essence of the said species recently exalted to the particular degree in question."[126] The "form" can be recognized from the symptoms, and the physician describes and classifies diseases by their symptoms just as the botanist classifies plants according to their external configuration.[127]

Baglivi also uses the term, "form" *(figura)*, which is an aspect of the "primary disease" but sometimes seems to be identical with it.[128] [m]

[l]Sydenham was familiar with Van Helmont and his *Archeus*, noting that it is identical with the *physis* of the ancients (Dewhurst, *Dr. Thomas Sydenham*, 92).

[m]On his "primary diseases" see below, p. 204.

Both thinkers stress the careful collection of symptomatic information. "The history of a disease consists in its symptoms alone."[129] A history must be both "graphic and natural . . . To draw a disease in gross is an easy matter. To describe it in its history so as to escape the censure of the great Bacon is far more difficult."[130] "In writing the history of a disease every philosophical hypothesis whatsoever that has previously occupied the mind of the author should lie in abeyance. This being done, the clear and natural phenomena of the disease should be noted, these and these only. They should be noted accurately, and in all their minuteness, in imitation of the exquisite industry of those painters who represent in their portraits the smallest moles and the faintest spots."[131]

> If one wants to give to the primary history of a disease all possible fidelity, the one who writes it down must include in his observations the exact indication of the slightest phenomena from day to day, their order of succession, their violence, their progress, and their outcome—good or bad. This is not all: he should, furthermore, note in the most minute detail the circumstances of time and place, the constitution of the year, the past or present causes, the therapeutic method, and the medicines employed. In a word, he should not leave out anything which has preceded, accompanied, or followed the disease whose history he is writing. However slight a circumstance may appear, the omission of any one will reduce the value of the observation as a whole or distort the consequences which one draws. It may be just this omission which constitutes a serious lacuna in the history of the disease.[132]

This means the observation of everything perceptible to the senses: "We require the evidence and confirmation of our senses. The speculations of reason . . . is what we do *not* require."[133] Existing disease descriptions are only vague pictures of the *physis,* taken as much from books as from the living patient.[134] A thoroughgoing reform is needed.[135]

Baglivi urges the physician to note critical days, metastases of disease from one part of the body to another, sympathies among regions of the body, disease periodicity, the onset of new symptoms, exacerbations, etc.[136] While the causes of these phenomena cannot be grasped, they are still not to be disdained; reason loses itself in the infinite variety of the symptoms, but true wisdom *(sapientia)* consists in noting the perceptible manifestations.[137] All efforts of the *physis* have a purpose, and the smallest is often the commencement of some major change.[138] The bad habits of physicians, who frequently scorn questioning patients about their symptoms, must be corrected.[139] He calls *medicina prima* the history of a disease taken from pure observation "at the very bedside of the patient, from the patient himself. Other sciences have nothing to do with this history, nor the reading of books; so that it should constitute a science of itself and depend on observation of the patient alone. Extrinsic factors here can only cause confusion and uncertainty."[140] "In *medicina prima* the physician is limited to the role of witness; he does not evaluate, and he does not behave like a poet–abandoning all connection with the phenomena in order to launch into a free flight of fancy. He must be the slave of things, vanquishing the *physis* by obeying her and discovering her language by his ability to learn it."[141] The physician "writes [the symptoms] down in their simplicity, adding nothing of his own, nothing from books, and nothing from the other sciences."[142]

The major problem here is that the data are virtually infinite: "so varying, manifold, and (if I may use the term) so delicate is the *natura,* and so much does she sport in the production of disease that it is not the work of one man's lifetime (long as it may be) to graphically depict their varied phenomena and their appropriate cures. Did I say one man's lifetime? Ten men, succeeding each other through ten lifetimes, would not do it."[143] But the Galenists are in error when they hold that disease is only a "blind and disorderly effort of the *natura,* without principles or rules."[144] The generality have considered that disease is but a confused and disordered effort of the *natura,* thrown down from her proper state and defending herself in vain; so that they have classed the attempts at a just description with the attempts to wash a blackamoor white."[145]

The disorder of the symptoms is only apparent: if allowed to follow their natural course, diseases will fall into a finite set of categories. The *natura* acts in a regular and methodical fashion.[146] "Each disease has its own peculiar nature, also its own certain and peculiar onset, increase, state, and decline."[147] "Etiology is a difficult and perhaps an inexplicable affair, and I choose to keep my hands clear of it. I am convinced, however, that the *natura* here, as elsewhere, moves in a regular and orderly manner."[148] "Where we lose sight of our best guide, the *natura,* and give ourselves up to the luxury of guesswork, we have as many species of ailments as we choose to devise."[149] "In the production and maturation [of diseases] the *natura* binds herself to a certain method as stringently as she does with plants and even animals."[150]

> The *natura,* in the production of disease, is uniform and consistent, so much so that, for the same disease in different persons the symptoms are, for the most part, the same; and the self-same phenomena that you would observe in the sickness of a Socrates, you would observe in the sickness of a simpleton. Just so the universal characteristics of a plant are extended to every individual of the species; and whoever (I speak in the way of illustration) should accurately describe the color, the taste, the smell, the figure, etc. of one single violet, would find that his description held good, there or thereabouts, for all violets of that particular species upon the face of the earth.[151]

In Baglivi's opinion the continuing validity of such Hippocratic writings as *Coan Prognosis, Aphorisms,* and *Prognosis* proves that the *natura* acts, and has always acted, in a regular manner.[152] While "secondary diseases" are extremely varied, the "primary diseases" which underlie them are limited in number.[153] [n]

In seeking the criteria for distinguishing one disease "form" from another on purely symptomatic grounds Sydenham and Baglivi revert to the classical doctrine of *propria* and *communia.*

Ancient theory had distinguished the symptoms common to many persons with more or less similar complaints *(communia, ta koina)* from those peculiar to the individual patient, which distinguish him from others with similar complaints *(propria, ta idia).*[o] Rationalism based its disease categories on the *communia,* while Empiricism relied on the patient's *propria* as the best guides to treatment.

Sydenham and Baglivi accept the Empirical position that the *propria* are of primary significance but now *attach them to the specific disease "form" rather than to the patient.*[p]

Sydenham writes: "it is not enough for a writer to merely note down the common phenomena of some multiform disease; for, although it may be true that all complaints are not liable to the same amount of variety, there are still many which authors treat alike, under the same heads, and without the shadows of a distinction, whilst they are in their nature as dissimilar as possible."[154] "It is necessary, in describing any disease, to enumerate the peculiar and constant phenomena apart from the accidental and adventitious ones: these last-named being those that arise from the age or temperament of the patient and from the different forms of medical

[n]Thus, while Sydenham was a consistent Empiric, accepting disease specificity and leaving unresolved the number of diseases in the world, Baglivi was led astray by his Iatromechanism and claimed inconsistently (1) that diseases are specific and (2) that the number of "primary diseases" is limited. The Rationalists limit the number of possible diseases by reducing them to a limited number of defined "proximate causes." Implied in the concept of disease "specificity" is rejection of the possibility of knowing the proximate cause. Thus Baglivi could not consistently adhere to both views. His "primary diseases" were probably the inspiration for Paul-Joseph Barthez' "disease elements" (see below, pp. 263-266).

[o]See *Divided Legacy,* I, 249-252.

[p]Laennec was to do the same two hundred years later. See below, p. 480.

treatment . . . Outlying forms of disease, and cases of exceeding rarity, I take no notice of. They do not properly belong to the histories of disease. No botanist takes the bites of the caterpillar as a characteristic of a leaf of sage."[155] "What short way, what way at all, is there towards either the detection of the morbific cause that we must fight against, or towards the indications of treatment which we must discover, except the sure and distinct perception of peculiar symptoms? Upon each of these points the slightest and most unimportant circumstances have their proper bearings."[156]

Baglivi adopts Sydenham's argument, urging the physician to pay attention to the "peculiar and constant" *(constantes et individuas)* symptoms and to ignore the "common" ones *(communes)*–meaning those common to other diseases *(communes aliis [morbis]).*[157] "I see nothing more harmful to medical progress than this perverse habit of discussing generally obvious phenomena, while the phenomena which are contemptible [*vilia*] or obscure are neglected."[158] But the physician must also distinguish the "peculiar and constant" symptoms from the "adventitious" ones *(adventitias).*[159] These latter "rather depend on the different therapeutic methods and the almost infinite concourse of causes than on the very nature of the illness."[160] The Hippocratic *Aphorisms* were based upon the "peculiar and constant" symptoms, while the "adventitious" symptoms were left up to the physician's prudence and wisdom.[161]

Thus the unusual and unexpected should not be suppressed, as is often done by physicians taking case histories: many phenomena appear useless only because they do not accord with the physician's preconceived idea of the disease; they may actually yield valuable curative indications.[162]

For both authors, therefore, the disease "form" is recognized from the "peculiar and constant" symptoms which are to be distinguished both from the "common" symptoms (found in many other disease "forms") and from the "adventitious" or "accidental" ones (peculiar to the given patient).

This was a neat resolution of an ancient argument and an attractive adaptation of traditional concepts to the new doctrine of specific diseases, but it was impossible to sustain in practice, since symptoms could not be characterized as "peculiar and constant," "common," and "adventitious" in the absence of some additional criterion.

This problem was to plague Empirical thinkers—especially Georg Ernst Stahl and the School of Montpellier—for more than a hundred years; it was solved only with Samuel Hahnemann's discovery of the "proving" as the needed external criterion for classifying symptoms into *propria* and *communia.*[q]

The Natural Therapeutic Method

The above considerations determine the physician's procedure in treatment. In acute diseases he reaches a conclusion about the disease "form" and then follows the method of treatment dictated by the *physis.* Chronic diseases are more complicated, since the *physis* is unable to cope with them, and here Sydenham and Baglivi look to the specific medicine.

Acute Diseases

Acute diseases are from "particles of the atmosphere . . . which are hostile to the economy of the human body." They "insinuate themselves amongst the juices of the body, disagree with them, mix themselves up with the blood, and finally taint the whole frame with the contagion of disease."[163] "Some are engendered through occult and inexplicable changes of the atmosphere. These taint the human frame, but they depend upon the peculiar crases of our blood and humors only so far as these occult atmospheric influences have made an impression on them."[164] They are cured by coction and crisis as first described by Hippocrates.[165]

The process of coction, however, differs from person to person and from disease to disease, and, in furthering it, the

[q]See below, pp. 351-371.

physician must possess a great deal of knowledge about various aspects of the disease.

It is extremely important to know the exciting cause.[166] Fevers caused by a chill are treated differently from those caused by a debauch, excessive sexual activity, or overexposure to the sun.[167] When confronted with a fever due to sunstroke the Iatrochemist will prescribe all sorts of diffusible alkalis to neutralize the acid, but this is an error, since such fevers should sometimes be calmed by softening remedies and sometimes heated further with alkaline ones.[168] Weather and climate, as well as the prevailing constitution, are important exciting causes. The warmer the climate, and the better the air, the more successful the crisis, as pure and elastic air promotes the insensible transpiration of the humors: this is why the crisis was always so successful in ancient Greece.[169]

Some preexisting disease can often be a disease cause, as "secondary diseases" are often caused by some underlying "primary disease."[170] A patient with sciatica could not be treated properly by Baglivi until he had discovered an underlying syphilis: when the syphilis had been cured, the sciatica disappeared of itself; phthisis, which the Galenists regard as a single specific disease, is not itself "primary" but "secondary" to syphilis, scurvy, asthma, chlorosis, or ulcers, and its treatment will vary in function of these antecedent causes.[171]

The proegumenal cause—the patient's temperament—must also be considered. Every man is not equally liable to become infected from a woman with venereal disease, and not everyone falls ill during an epidemic.[172] While we can only guess at the reasons for differences of temperament, this knowledge is still essential for treatment.[173]

Failure to elicit these causes properly leads to erroneous therapeutic procedures and worsens the disease; then the physician looks for some malignity upon which to cast the blame.[174]

Once he has settled on the exciting cause, the physician examines the patient's symptoms: "It is quite sufficient for him . . . to be able to distinguish with accuracy between the effects and symptoms of the complaint which he has at hand and those of some similar one."[175] This means very attentive observation of the tongue, eyes, face, morbid symptoms, excretions, pulse, respiration, mental state, etc., not omitting the unusual or unexpected which may often be the key to treatment.[176] "In respect to the histories of a disease, any one who looks at the case carefully will see at once that an author must direct his attention to many more points than are usually thought of."[177]

Particular attention must be paid to the patient at the outset of the disease. Sydenham writes: "Unless I use exceeding caution, and unless I exert the full energies of my mind, it is as much as (nay, it is more than) I can do to avoid risking the lives of one or two of the first who apply to me as patients. At length, however, I steadily investigate the disease, I comprehend its character, and I proceed straight ahead and in full confidence towards its annihilation."[178]

Information from anatomical investigations is of little value for therapeutic practice.[179]

The physician must understand correctly the meaning of the symptom—interpreting it as the sign of the organism's struggle against disease. "It becomes a matter of absolute necessity . . . that grave and terrible symptoms be associated with such an effort of the *natura;* for she is trying her strength and must either expel the mischief by a crisis or herself faint in the struggle."[180] "That practice, and that alone, will do good which elicits the indications of cure out of the phenomena of the disease itself."[181] "With the *natura* for my guide I should swerve not a nail's breadth from the true way."[182]

But most physicians do not recognize or accept this natural curative process, ridiculing the theory of coction and critical days.[183] Hence they prescribe at random, confusing the disease process, aborting acute diseases, and transforming them into chronic ones.[184]

In particular, they neglect the prognostic signs—the most important indicators of the disease course.[185] They despise such a mundane matter as farting. But if a dysentery patient has gas at a late stage of the disease, it is favorable for prognosis. In a serious enteritis, on the other hand, noisy and evil-smelling farts portend a rapid death.[186]

These and all other symptoms must be interpreted correctly to determine if the body's own vitality is capable of coping with the disease. Expectant treatment is often the best.[187] Hippocrates himself used no medicines in acute diseases, so as not to interrupt the crisis.[188] A good rule is "*multa scire et pauca agere.*"[189] We have to overcome the prejudice of patients in favor of many and expensive remedies.[190] The *natura* saves many whom science would kill.[191]

If the *physis* is not capable of handling the disease, however, the physician himself must be able to act decisively: "when once, by good fortune, I have hit upon the true and proper line of practice that this or that fever requires, I can (with the assistance of the Almighty) by taking my aim in the same direction, generally succeed in my results, respect being always had to the age and temperament of the patient."[192] As acute diseases have a regular course, the physician can observe this course and assist it using methods whose efficacy has been proven, not by theory or logic, but by experience.[193] Each species and sub-species of disease requires a slightly different mode of treatment.[194] Remedies must be varied according to the patient's temperament and age, the country, the exciting cause, and the prevailing constitution.[195]

Treatment on natural principles means assisting the organism to do what it is attempting to do itself. If the patient has vomited, or is nauseous, the physician administers an emetic.[196] Women with suppressed menses should be bled at the time the menses are due; otherwise their suppression will bring on a consumption.[197] In a woman whose fever and headache were caused by the artificial curtailment of a preceding dysentery, treatment was "substituting for the flux that had been checked some other evacuation. I cured her accordingly."[198]

Treatment is always governed by the progress of coction.[199] If it is languishing, spirits and diffusible stimulants are given; if it is too rapid, the physician moderates it with cooling medicines; this continues until the febrile humors have been brought to the degree of movement needed to concoct the *materies morbi* and evacuate it through sweat, *per anum, per urinas,* etc.[200] In autumnal intermittents Sydenham treated the patient by sweating him under a blanket.[201] He frequently resorted to "accubitus"—placing another person or a small dog into bed with the patient to provide additional heat.[202] Since fever is beneficial, Sydenham attacked his colleagues who prescribe cooling remedies in fevers:

> I cannot bring my brain to comprehend the meaning of those physicians that are continually talking about the administration of remedies that promote the concoction of the febrile matter . . . At the same time they have no hesitation in recommending medicines that are intended to control the fever. Why? The fever itself is the *natura's* instrument. By this she separates the pure parts from the tainted ones . . . To accelerate this we are not to meddle with temperants and I know not what; but we are to let the effervescence go on as long as the condition of the patient can bear with it; we are to watch for its crisis and declension; and when we discover that separation is taking place, we are to back it up with warm remedies . . . This is the true way of promoting febrile concoction. Your evacuants and refrigerants are but hindrances; they procrastinate recoveries; and, when health is coming of its own accord, they frighten it away.[203]

However, he introduced the "cooling treatment" in smallpox, opposing the diaphoretic treatment in vogue with his colleagues: "it is not reason but experience which teaches us what fevers are cured by diaphoresis and what by other evacuations."[204] Baglivi also used cooling remedies in some inflammations on the ground that excess heating of the blood caused its nutritive and chylous part to be separated off and coagulated.[205]

In everything timing is vital.[206] The physician should neither be ahead of nor behind the natural process itself: "We must be careful not to purge before the disease is wholly expelled. It is true, indeed, that by so doing the natural parts may appear to have been relieved of the foul humors that the fever has heaped upon them. Nevertheless, fresh matter is introduced, and they gradually increase. The fever supplies it; the action of the cathartics and the agitation of the humors having recalled the fever. Hence, all that we have done by our purging is to render the disease more obstinate. Daily examples tell us this."[207] He used purgatives on the same principle, administering them at the time the *physis* itself was preparing the evacuation: "I judge of this both from the signs in the urine of a laudable separation and from the palpable remission of the other symptoms. This purge draws off the miscellaneous sediment of the preceding fermentation. Miss the opportunity of this, and the chances are that they return to the blood and produce a relapse."[208] "In deference to the vulgar theory that a melancholy humor is the source and origin of the disease, and that in the removal of obstructions, and in the evacuation of this same humor, consists the chances of cure, patients are harassed during the decline of their complaint with repeated and punishing purges. Now, be the humors that are thus worked out and eliminated what they may, it is certain that their effect upon the fever is to make it root itself more deeply, and hold its ground more resolutely, than if it had never been meddled with."[209] However, Sydenham gave an emetic at the beginning of a fever: "By so doing we can ensure the patient against all those formidable symptoms which originate in the mass of impurities that lie lodged within the stomach and in the parts around it."[210]

Both Sydenham and Baglivi employed bloodletting. In a continued fever accompanied by "an inordinate commotion of the volume of the blood . . . excited by the *natura* in order that either some heterogenous matter incorporated with our humors and inimical to them may be eliminated, or else that the blood itself may be transmuted towards a better diathesis," the condition of the blood is the main indication: "we must keep it within its limits, so that it coincide with the intentions of the *natura.*" If it "rage too much, perilous symptoms will set in," and blood must be drawn; if the blood is weak, however, venesection is not used.[211] Baglivi used bloodletting as part of the cooling treatment in some inflammations as well as to resolve stasis of the humors.[212]

Treatment must ignore the internal (proximate) causes of diseases except where these are such palpable entities as kidney stones, pus (in empyema), water in the tissues (in dropsy), etc. where removal of the cause is indicated.[213] In a very few fevers, due to some sort of *aura* or poison in the atmosphere, to eating spoiled meat or the flesh of poisoned animals, etc., the peccant matter is evacuated right away.[214] In the great majority of cases, however, the physician waits for the onset of coction and crisis. The idea that the proximate cause of "fermentation" in the *secundae viae* is some kind of matter in the *primae viae,* and that the latter must be evacuated, is a "vision of the Arabs" and devoid of value.[215]

The harm done by supposedly causal treatment, which actually suppresses the symptoms, is seen from experience. Suppression of an ulcer of long standing can provoke a fatal disease of the chest.[216] Petechial eruptions should be encouraged with bezoar stone and diaphoretics, not suppressed by medicines which drive them into the interior of the body.[217] Suppression of scabies can cause spitting of blood, fevers, blindness, apoplexy, and dropsy.[218] In Book V of the *Epidemics* Hippocrates mentions a man in Athens who was treated for scabies with hot baths: the scabies disappeared, but after a time the man became dropsical and died.[219]

But Baglivi still applied certain treatments explicable more in terms of contraries than of coction. Malignant fevers are from two sources: excessive thickness of the body's fluids or their dissolution, and the treatment is to thicken or thin out these liquids, as the case may require.[220] The viscous, thick, and inert matter which produces an intermittent fever is cured by sharp and bitter remedies.[221] A slow fever is cured by a milk diet because the soft, sulphurous, and alkaline principles in the milk are the contrary of the morbid principles in the blood.[222]

Sydenham was not sure whether the best diet is contrary to the patient's temperament or similar to it: "I do affirm *contraria contrariis* are not always to be observed but *similia similibus.*"[223 r] Thus, milk is a phlegm-producing food, but phlegmatic children still benefit from it.[224] Likewise, old people (who are cold and dry) benefit more from cold dry foods than from hot wet foods.[225]

Finally, both authors were interested in the possibility of specific remedies for specific diseases. Sydenham wrote to Robert Boyle: "I have again taken breath and am pursuing my design of specifics which, if but a delusion, so closely haunts me that I could not but indulge the spending of a little money and time at it once more."[226] He distinguished between medicines "specific" to a particular evacuation and those "specific" to a disease: "in the first case we satisfy the curative indications and drive away the ailment; in the second, we take no cognizance of the indication or intention at all, while we destroy the disease directly and immediately."[227] While he hoped that specifics would one day be found for acute diseases, the existing ones, in his opinion, were no more specific to such diseases than is the lancet specific to pleurisy.[228]

Baglivi, writing some decades later, took a view more in line with Empirical tradition: all medicines are actually specifics, acting through humoral specialization.[229] Hot remedies cure hot diseases, and vice-versa, without provoking any evacuation.[230] The physician should search for more of the same, such as quinine and mercury, which are sure, constant, and specific against a given disease, extinguishing it *in ovo,* as it were, without coction, crisis, and evacuation.[231]

Chronic Diseases

Hippocratic doctrine held that an unsuccessful or aborted coction results in empyema—the formation of pus or a

[r]The ancients had also puzzled over this issue (*Divided Legacy,* I, 49).

concretion in the body which disappears, if at all, only after lengthy and inconclusive efforts by the *physis.* To this the Methodist, Caelius Aurelianus, in the fifth century, A.D. added the suggestion that such an unsuccessful coction gives rise to chronic disease which time and the *physis* alone cannot cure.[232] Caelius Aurelianus' theory was adopted by Sydenham: "the inability of the *natura* to concoct the humors is the chief cause of most chronic diseases."[233] They arise "either from the particular conformation of the part itself, as is the case with morbid matter impacted in the nerves of paralytics, and with the pus in the cavities of a thoracic empyema, or else from a deficiency of the natural heat and animal spirits, as is the case with the phlegm falling upon the lungs of old men worn with coughs."[234] Gout is caused by the "native heat not being strong enough to throw off the *materia morbifica* upon the joints."[235] Baglivi modified this doctrine considerably, holding that, while acute diseases mostly arise in the liquids, chronic ones arise in the solids (or, if in the fluids, because they are so viscous as to be impossible of coction): hence they are beyond the control of the *physis* and must be treated by medicines other than those which act on the *physis.*[236] [s] In general, while the phenomena of acute disease are relatively clear, those associated with chronic disease are less so.[237]

This impasse—the existence of chronic diseases which were incurable by any ordinary or known means—stimulated physicians to search for specifics.

The idea of the specific remedy, first suggested by Paracelsus, had been enormously strengthened by the introduction into European medicine of quinine (cinchona, Peruvian Bark, Jesuit's Bark, etc.) in 1665. The following year Sydenham was recommending it strongly in intermittent fevers.[238] In contrast to other "specifics," he maintained, quinine cured this disease without any visible evacuation, as it were, destroying the disease in its essence; this was the sign

[s]He states that, while the causes of acute disease cannot be known, those of chronic diseases can be known (*De Praxi Medica,* 98).

of the true specific–specific to the "disease" and not to some particular indication.[239] [t]

Both authors held that discovery of this specific, which did not substitute one "secondary quality" for another but actually uprooted the "disease" itself, finally proved the futility of Galenic reasoning in medicine.[240] Sydenham, however, was not convinced of the long-term effect of quinine and observed that it sometimes checks, but does not conquer, intermittent fever.[241]

For these same reasons, and also because they felt that some unpurged remnent must remain in the body of the patient when quinine was used, many of Sydenham's contemporaries objected to its employment.[242]

Baglivi urged physicians to find specifics for all chronic diseases, suggesting that they operate by heightening the tone of the solids, i.e., by counteracting atony.[243]

Sydenham, Baglivi, and the Empirical Tradition

The classic Empirical themes figure prominently in the thinking of Sydenham and Baglivi: physiological vitalism, the origin of practice in observation and experience, the emergence of theory from practice, the general orientation toward therapeutics, the concern with pharmacology, the rejection of logic and metaphysics as sources of medical knowledge.

Empiricism also emphasized the discovery of new knowledge and, especially, the significance of knowledge which was of direct therapeutic use, and this was followed by Sydenham and Baglivi:[u]

> I have always thought (and not without reason) that to have published for the benefit of afflicted mortals any certain method of subduing even the slightest disease was

[t]Thus Sydenham held mercury not to be specific to syphilis, only to salivation; the salivation, in his view, cured the syphilis and could as well have been provoked by any other sialogogue (*The Works of Thomas Sydenham,* I, 22; II, 44).

[u]Baglivi's openness to new knowledge led him to give a sympathetic reception to acupuncture, recently brought to the West in the writings of Willem G. Ten Rhyne (1647-1700) (*De Praxi Medica,* 237).

> a matter of greater felicity than the riches of a Tantalus or a Croesus.[244]

> I have ever held that any accession whatever to the art of healing, even if it went no further than the cutting of corns or the curing of toothaches, was of far higher value than all the knowledge of fine points and all the pomp of subtle speculations, matters which are as useful to physicians in driving away diseases as music is to masons in laying bricks.[245]

> Speaking here of the knowledge of natural bodies, the end and benefit whereof can be no other than the advantages and conveniences of human life, all speculations in this subject, however curious or refined or seeming profound and solid, if they teach not their followers to do something either better or in a shorter and easier way than otherwise they could, or else lead them to the discovery of some new and useful invention, deserve not the name of knowledge.[246]

> I always consider that in acute diseases it is not sufficient to do what is done by the rashest of old women—prove that the treatment is good from the event being favorable. More than this is required. The disease must be conquered easily, and, as far as its nature will allow, must go off of its own accord.[247]

Baglivi states that the physician, by following the *physis*, makes himself *useful.*[248] He praises Paracelsus and Van Helmont for their discovery of new remedies which improve practical medicine; the new observations and discoveries of their successors are making medicine a profound and liberal science.[249] He criticizes Galenism for its inability to make discoveries (*inventionis sterilitas*).[250]

Both physicians held that their method, based on observation and experience, conferred greater certainty upon medical practice:

> [Physicians] ought not to be satisfied with simply giving health to the sick, but they should strive to add greater

> certainty to the art that they administer; and they should so direct their experiments that the science of medicine may grow day by day more clear and more efficient. In this way the human race may reap the advantages thereof generally, and with safety, even after they themselves have been laid in their graves.[251]

Baglivi maintains that his method yields "knowledge, not opinion."[252]

And the pursuit of certainty is important because medicine is concerned with human lives and is thus a moral undertaking. The physician's responsibility has a religious basis. Sydenham writes:

> Whoever takes up medicine should seriously consider the following points: firstly, that he must one day render to the Supreme Judge an account of the lives of those sick men who have been entrusted to his care. Secondly, that such skill and science as, by the blessing of Almighty God, he has attained, are to be specially directed towards the honor of his Maker and the welfare of his fellow-creatures; since it is a base thing for the great gifts of Heaven to become the servants of avarice or ambition. Thirdly, he must remember that it is no mean or ignoble animal that he deals with. We may ascertain the worth of the human race, since for its sake God's only-begotten Son became man, and thereby ennobled the nature that he took upon him. Lastly, he must remember that he himself hath no exemption from the common lot, but that he is bound by the same laws of mortality, and liable to the same ailments and afflictions with his fellows. For these and like reasons let him strive to render aid to the distressed with the greater care, with the kindlier spirit, and with the stronger fellow-feeling.[253]

He wrote his works for "those of my fellow-creatures who unite the love of truth with the love of their kind."[254]

He attacks those physicians who:

> Will in no wise allow themselves to be regulated by these considerations, as is clearly manifest both from their practice and their way of life. Some are swollen up with pride and puffed out with the vain conceit of their knowledge; so that these matters seem small in their eyes. They can only come down to them negligently and contemptuously. They care nothing for the unfortunates committed to their charge. The Supreme Being they either disown or disregard. The others either gape and grow greedy for gain, or else are borne away by the hopes of some small celebrity; in either case looking to their purses or to their fame.[255]

Baglivi's medical views were not suffused with religious feeling, but he was equally critical of his colleagues' professional arrogance—their infatuation with hypotheses, their unwillingness to accept what disagreed with their preconceived opinions, their "martial airs" and "dialectics," and their habit of abandoning patients just before death to avoid the responsibility.[256]

These parallels with the Hippocratic and Empirical tradition raise the question of the attitude of Sydenham and Baglivi toward this tradition. With respect to the Hippocratic Corpus, both follow that group of works which accepts the process of coction and which we have characterized as the Empirical group.[v] Sydenham even makes reference to a major passage in *Ancient Medicine,* the keystone of this group of writings,[257] [w] and his seminal idea of the "specific

[v]See *Divided Legacy,* I, 10-33, 68-88.

[w]"Certain physicians and philosophers assert that nobody can know medicine who is ignorant what a man is; he who would treat patients properly must, they say, learn this. But the question they raise is one for philosophy; it is the province of those who, like Empedocles, have written on natural science, what man is from the beginning, how he came into being at the first, and from what elements he was originally constructed. But my view is, first, that all that philosophers or physicians have said or written on natural science no more pertains to medicine than to painting" (cap. XX). See *Divided Legacy,* I, 74.

exaltation" of a humor may well have been suggested by it.[x] But he did not know of the ancient Empirical School and, like Bacon, confused Empiricism with the practice of the uneducated "empirics" of his time.[258]

Baglivi also relied on the Empirical core of the Hippocratic Corpus: *Coan Prognosis, Aphorisms,* the books of the *Epidemics,* and *Prognosis*—which set forth the theory of coction—are most frequently cited by him, as well as *The Art.*[259] He refers with approval to Galen's *De Subfiguratione Empirica,* one of the ancient writings in which the Empirical principles are elaborated in detail.[260] [y] On the other hand, he was conscious of the disrepute of "empiricism" and wanted to avoid the accusation of having "gone over to the camp of the Empirics."[261] Hence his comments on this school were both positive and negative.

The Empirics were always talking about experience but rarely attained it, since they had no method.[262] They never sought the internal causes of disease but relied on the evident and palpable ones; Herophilos, however, was even worse, as he never took causes into account at all.[263] [z]

But since medicine is conjectural, according to Celsus, these visible causes should not be neglected.[264] Physicians scorn experience because of the old hatred of the Rationalists for the Empirics as a "vile commercial sect, unworthy of an educated person."[265] But the Empirics healed as well as the Rationalists with all their speculation about proximate causes.[266] They treated with specifics, and with success.[267]

Medical tradition is divided because some overstress experience and others reason.[268] The cure is to combine the

[x]"There is in man salt and bitter, sweet and acid, astringent and insipid, and a vast number of other things, possessing properties of all sorts, both in number and in strength. These, when mixed and compounded with one another, are neither apparent nor do they hurt a man; *but when one of them is separated off, and stands alone, then it is apparent and hurts a man"* (cap. XIV). See *Divided Legacy,* I, 74.

[y]See above, p. 89*y*.

[z]On Herophilos of Chalcedon see *Divided Legacy,* I, 194-199.

two, just as the bee (according to Bacon) occupies the middle ground between the spider and the ant.[269] We do not mean "stupid, erratic, oncc-only experience" but a scientific Empiricism: "a rational Empiricism, an Empiricism made literate, discovered by method and not by accident, fecundated in the intellect, based on daily exploration of the facts of disease."[270] Man has always exalted this Empiricism as a faithful reflection of the *natura.*[271] An Empiricism which is learned, impregnated by observation, and directed by the flame of intelligence.[272] As Galen wrote in *De Subfiguratione Empirica,* one man's life is too short to discover all the secrets of the science; all the observations of prior ages must be united into a single body, thus to make, of so many men separated by centuries, one single man and one infinite science.[273]

The debt of both physicians to Francis Bacon is enormous. Sydenham explicitly professes allegiance to his method, and Baglivi quotes him liberally throughout his *De Praxi Medica.* Bacon's critique of metaphysics, his distinction between the world of nature and that of the mind, gave them an instrument with which to attack Iatrochemical and Iatromechanist "idols" and "hypotheses." Bacon also urged reliance on observation and experience and provided them with the concept of the disease "form". All three saw the advancement of knowledge as consisting in the improvement of practice through experience or experiments.

Sydenham, like Bacon, drew inspiration for his scientific work from his strong religious feeling.

Reliance on the inductive method is implicit in their assumption that the disease "form" can be filtered out of the various "natures" in which it appears, but this side of Bacon's philosophy is not stressed. The inductive technique would see more extensive elaboration in the School of Montpellier.

Baglivi hoped to follow Bacon in unifying Empiricism and Rationalism into a single doctrine. As the discussion has shown, however, he was no more capable of this than the great Chancellor himself, and the outcome was only confusion and ambiguity in his medical philosophy.

The impact of Sydenham and Baglivi on medicine, however, was very beneficial. They were a necessary reaction and counterweight to the Rationalist exaggerations of Willis, Boerhaave, and Hoffmann. They remained a living example of Hippocratic and scientific thinking for many future generations of physicians.

NOTES

[1] Kenneth Dewhurst, *Dr. Thomas Sydenham (1624-1689). His Life and Original Writings* (Berkeley and Los Angeles: University of California Press, 1966), 34.

[2] A. G. Gibson, *The Physician's Art* (Oxford: University Press, 1933), 8.

[3] Georgii Baglivi, *De Praxi Medica ad Priscam Observandi Rationem Revocanda Libri Duo* (Rome, 1696), 238.

[4] Dewhurst, *Dr. Thomas Sydenham,* 40.

[5] *The Works of Thomas Sydenham.* (London: Sydenham Society, 1848-1850), I, 18.

[6] Dewhurst, *Dr. Thomas Sydenham,* 83.

[7] Baglivi, *De Praxi Medica,* 4.

[8] *The Works of Thomas Sydenham,* I, 10.

[9] Baglivi, *De Praxi Medica,* 3, 19, 43, 88.

[10] *The Works of Thomas Sydenham,* I, 14. See, also, Dewhurst, *Dr. Thomas Sydenham,* 80.

[11] *The Works of Thomas Sydenham,* II, 211.

[12] Dewhurst, *Dr. Thomas Sydenham,* 80.

[13] Baglivi, *De Praxi Medica,* 105.

[14] *Ibid.,* 93. Dewhurst, *Dr. Thomas Sydenham,* 82.

[15] Dewhurst, *Dr. Thomas Sydenham,* 80. Baglivi, *De Praxi Medica,* 4.

[16] Dewhurst, *Dr. Thomas Sydenham,* 93.

[17] *The Works of Thomas Sydenham,* I, 14. Cf. Baglivi, *De Praxi Medica,* 99, 163 (citing Bacon).

[18] Dewhurst, *Dr. Thomas Sydenham,* 93. Cf. Baglivi, *De Praxi Medica,* 213.

[19] Baglivi, *De Praxi Medica,* 159.

[20] *Ibid.,* 20, 212.

[21] *The Works of Thomas Sydenham,* I, 13.

[22] *Ibid.,* I, 32. Baglivi, *De Praxi Medica,* 206-207.

[23] Baglivi, *De Praxi Medica,* 233.

[24] *Ibid.,* 235.

[25] *Ibid.,* 237.

[26] *Ibid.,* 25, 214, 245, 247-248.

[27] *Ibid.,* 157, 200, 252.

[28] *The Works of Thomas Sydenham,* I, 14.

[29] Dewhurst, *Dr. Thomas Sydenham,* 145-146.

[30] *Ibid.,* 151.

[31] Baglivi, *De Praxi Medica,* 5, 7.

[32] *Ibid.,* 110.

[33] *Ibid.,* 5.

[34] *Ibid.,* 7.

[35] *The Works of Thomas Sydenham,* I, 16. Cf. Baglivi, *De Praxi Medica,* 236-237.

[36] Baglivi, *De Praxi Medica,* 237-238.

[37] *Ibid.,* 8. See, also, *ibid.,* 98, 214.

[38] *The Works of Thomas Sydenham,* I, 20.

[39] Baglivi, *De Praxi Medica,* 252.

[40] *Ibid.,* 104, 156-157.

[41] *Ibid.,* 104.

[42] Dewhurst, *Dr. Thomas Sydenham,* 88.

[43] *Ibid.,* 85-86.

[44] *The Works of Thomas Sydenham,* II, 84.

[45] *Ibid.,* II, 170. See Baglivi, *De Praxi Medica,* 109.

[46] Dewhurst, *Dr. Thomas Sydenham,* 82.

[47] *The Works of Thomas Sydenham,* II, 182.

[48] *Ibid.,* II, 171. See, also, *ibid.,* II, 60.

[49] Baglivi, *De Praxi Medica,* 6, 11, 155.

[50] *Ibid.,* 4.

[51] *Ibid.,* 21.

[52] *Loc. cit.*

[53] *Ibid.,* 3.

[54] *The Works of Thomas Sydenham,* I, 26.

[55] Dewhurst, *Dr. Thomas Sydenham,* 48.

[56] Baglivi, *De Praxi Medica,* 94, 211.

[57] *Ibid.,* 92.

[58] *Ibid.,* 2.

[59] *Ibid.,* 160-176. *The Works of Thomas Sydenham,* I, 39.

[60] Baglivi, *De Praxi Medica,* 251.

[61] *Loc. cit.*

[62] *Ibid.,* 245, 248.

[63] *Ibid.,* 245-246.

[64] Dewhurst, *Dr. Thomas Sydenham,* 86.

[65] *Ibid.,* 93.

[66] *Ibid.,* 93.

[67] *The Works of Thomas Sydenham,* II, 12.

[68] Dewhurst, *Dr. Thomas Sydenham,* 86.

[69] *The Works of Thomas Sydenham,* I, 19-20. Baglivi, *De Praxi Medica,* 235, 245.

[70] *The Works of Thomas Sydenham,* I, 21, 29. Baglivi, *De Praxi Medica,* 10, 14, 180, 239, 253.

[71] Baglivi, *De Praxi Medica,* 245, 247.

[72] *The Works of Thomas Sydenham,* I, 29-30.

[73] *Ibid.,* I, 30.

[74] *Ibid.,* I, 30. See, also, *ibid.,* I, 54.

[75] *Ibid.,* I, 22.

[76] *Ibid.,* I, 38.

[77] Baglivi, *De Praxi Medica,* 228.

[78] *Ibid.,* 114.

[79] *The Works of Thomas Sydenham,* I, 30.

[80] Baglivi, *De Praxi Medica,* 10.

[81] *The Works of Thomas Sydenham,* I, 16-17.

[82] *Ibid.*, II, 22.
[83] *Ibid.*, I, 16. See, also, Baglivi, *De Praxi Medica*, 7, 238.
[84] Dewhurst, *Dr. Thomas Sydenham*, 80, note 1.
[85] *Ibid.*, 81.
[86] *Ibid.*, 73.
[87] Baglivi, *De Praxi Medica*, 182.
[88] Dewhurst, *Dr. Thomas Sydenham*, 142.
[89] *Ibid.*, 140. See Baglivi, *De Praxi Medica*, 252-255.
[90] *The Works of Thomas Sydenham*, II, 139.
[91] *Ibid.*, I, 44.
[92] *Ibid.*, I, 11. Dewhurst, *Dr. Thomas Sydenham*, 81.
[93] Dewhurst, *Dr. Thomas Sydenham*, 85.
[94] *The Works of Thomas Sydenham*, II, 173.
[95] Baglivi, *De Praxi Medica*, 6, 106.
[96] *Ibid.*, 107.
[97] *Ibid.*, 97.
[98] *Ibid.*, 98.
[99] *Ibid.*, 28.
[100] *Ibid.*, 95, 109.
[101] *Ibid.*, 95.
[102] *Ibid.*, 92.
[103] *Ibid.*, 31, 95-96, 108-109.
[104] *Ibid.*, 92, 98-99, 109.
[105] *Ibid.*, 40.
[106] Haeser, *Geschichte der Medizin*, 606.
[107] *The Works of Thomas Sydenham*, I, 20. Baglivi, *De Praxi Medica*, 235.
[108] *The Works of Thomas Sydenham*, I, 20.
[109] *Loc. cit.*
[110] *Loc. cit.*
[111] *Loc. cit.*
[112] *Loc. cit.* Cf. Baglivi, *De Praxi Medica*, 235, 245.
[113] *Loc. cit.*
[114] *Loc. cit.*
[115] *Loc. cit.*
[116] *Ibid.*, I, 29.
[117] *Ibid.*, I, 18, 34. Baglivi follows Sydenham's doctrine of exciting causes (*De Praxi Medica*, 139, 211-218).
[118] *Ibid.*, I, 32.
[119] *Ibid.*, I, 19-20.
[120] *Ibid.*, I, 34.
[121] *Ibid.*, I, 33. See, also, *ibid.*, I, 40.
[122] *Ibid.*, I, 33.
[123] *Ibid.*, II, 138. See, also, Dewhurst, *Dr. Thomas Sydenham*, 66.
[124] *Ibid.*, I, 19. See, also, Baglivi, *De Praxi Medica*, 26, 163.
[125] *The Works of Thomas Sydenham*, I, 19.
[126] *Loc. cit.*
[127] *Ibid.*, I, 13, 40.
[128] Baglivi, *De Praxi Medica*, 108, 154, 205-207.
[129] *Ibid.*, 173.
[130] *The Works of Thomas Sydenham*, I, 12.

[131] *Ibid.*, I, 14.
[132] Baglivi, *De Praxi Medica*, 163.
[133] *The Works of Thomas Sydenham*, I, 40.
[134] Baglivi, *De Praxi Medica*, 93.
[135] *Ibid.*, 163.
[136] *Ibid.*, 174.
[137] *Ibid.*, 10-11.
[138] *Ibid.*, 169.
[139] *Ibid.*, 173.
[140] *Ibid.*, 152.
[141] *Loc. cit.*
[142] *Ibid.*, 21.
[143] *The Works of Thomas Sydenham*, II, 31. See, also, *ibid.*, I, 39 and Baglivi, *De Praxi Medica*, 162, 181, 237.
[144] Baglivi, *De Praxi Medica*, 152.
[145] *The Works of Thomas Sydenham*, I, 16.
[146] Baglivi, *De Praxi Medica*, 153.
[147] *Ibid.*, 7, 153.
[148] *The Works of Thomas Sydenham*, I, 72.
[149] *Ibid.*, I, 40.
[150] *Ibid.*, I, 19. See Baglivi, *De Praxi Medica*, 8, 153.
[151] *The Works of Thomas Sydenham*, I, 15.
[152] Baglivi, *De Praxi Medica*, 8, 153.
[153] *Ibid.*, 205.
[154] *Ibid.*, I, 13.
[155] *Ibid.*, I, 14.
[156] *Ibid.*, I, 15.
[157] Baglivi, *De Praxi Medica*, 9, 173.
[158] *Ibid.*, 169.
[159] *Ibid.*, 9, 173.
[160] *Loc. cit.*
[161] *Ibid.*, 9.
[162] *Ibid.*, 99, 163.
[163] *The Works of Thomas Sydenham*, I, 29; II, 138. Baglivi, *De Praxi Medica*, 245-247.
[164] *The Works of Thomas Sydenham*, I, 31.
[165] *Ibid.*, I, 19, 21, 30, 31. Baglivi, *De Praxi Medica*, 245-247.
[166] Baglivi, *De Praxi Medica*, 211-218.
[167] *Ibid.*, 213.
[168] *Loc. cit.*
[169] *Ibid.*, 256.
[170] *Ibid.*, 205.
[171] *Ibid.*, 206-207, 212, 215.
[172] *Ibid.*, 216, 218.
[173] *Ibid.*, 217-218, 249.
[174] *Ibid.*, 25.
[175] *The Works of Thomas Sydenham*, I, 20.
[176] Baglivi, *De Praxi Medica*, 111-129, 163, 221-222.
[177] *The Works of Thomas Sydenham*, I, 13.
[178] *Ibid.*, I, 33.

[179] Baglivi, *De Praxi Medica,* 215. Dewhurst, *Dr. Thomas Sydenham,* 85.
[180] *The Works of Thomas Sydenham,* I, 31.
[181] *Ibid.,* II, 22. Baglivi, *De Praxi Medica,* 180, 238-239, 247.
[182] *The Works of Thomas Sydenham,* I, 4.
[183] Baglivi, *De Praxi Medica,* 10-11, 14, 252-259.
[184] *Ibid.,* 247-248, 252-255. *The Works of Thomas Sydenham,* I, 89.
[185] Baglivi, *De Praxi Medica,* 14.
[186] *Ibid.,* 170.
[187] *Ibid.,* 247.
[188] *Ibid.,* 253.
[189] *Ibid.,* 249.
[190] *Loc. cit.* and 258.
[191] *Ibid.,* 250.
[192] *The Works of Thomas Sydenham,* I, 33.
[193] Baglivi, *De Praxi Medica,* 8, 23, 109, 153, 239, 245.
[194] *Ibid.,* 205.
[195] *Ibid.,* 238, 246, 249. *The Works of Thomas Sydenham,* I, 33, 39.
[196] *The Works of Thomas Sydenham,* I, 47.
[197] Dewhurst, *Dr. Thomas Sydenham,* 95.
[198] *The Works of Thomas Sydenham,* I, 181.
[199] Baglivi, *De Praxi Medica,* 109, 238.
[200] *Ibid.,* 239.
[201] *The Works of Thomas Sydenham,* I, 83.
[202] Dewhurst, *Dr. Thomas Sydenham,* 54-55.
[203] *The Works of Thomas Sydenham,* I, 54.
[204] *Ibid.,* II, 211.
[205] Baglivi, *De Praxi Medica,* 222.
[206] *Ibid.,* 233.
[207] *The Works of Thomas Sydenham,* I, 89.
[208] *Ibid.,* I, 57.
[209] *Ibid.,* I, 89.
[210] *Ibid.,* I, 49.
[211] *Ibid.,* I, 44-46.
[212] Baglivi, *De Praxi Medica,* 222, 227.
[213] *Ibid.,* 211, 220.
[214] *Ibid.,* 26, 255.
[215] *Ibid.,* 19.
[216] *Ibid.,* 10.
[217] *Ibid.,* 114.
[218] *Ibid.,* 228.
[219] *Loc. cit.* (see V, 209, Littre).
[220] *Ibid.,* 26.
[221] *Ibid.,* 226.
[222] *Loc. cit.*
[223] Dewhurst, *Dr. Thomas Sydenham,* 140.
[224] *Ibid.,* 141.
[225] *Loc. cit.*
[226] *Ibid.,* 164.
[227] *The Works of Thomas Sydenham,* I, 22.
[228] *Loc. cit.*

[229] Baglivi, *De Praxi Medica,* 236, 245.

[230] *Loc. cit.*

[231] *Ibid.,* 110, 236, 242, 245.

[232] Caelius Aurelianus, *On Acute Diseases and On Chronic Diseases.* Translated by I. E. Drabkin (Chicago, University of Chicago Press, 1950), 441 (*Chronic Diseases,* Bk. I, Preface).

[233] *The Works of Thomas Sydenham,* II, 139.

[234] *Ibid.,* I, 31.

[235] *Ibid.,* I, xxxviii.

[236] Baglivi, *De Praxi Medica,* 98, 153-154, 180.

[237] *Ibid.,* 180.

[238] *The Works of Thomas Sydenham,* II, 11. Dewhurst, *Dr. Thomas Sydenham,* 41.

[239] *The Works of Thomas Sydenham,* II, 11.

[240] *Ibid.,* I, 21; II, 161-162. Baglivi, *De Praxi Medica,* 234.

[241] *The Works of Thomas Sydenham,* I, 84; II, 11.

[242] *Ibid.,* II, 11.

[243] Baglivi, *De Praxi Medica,* 226, 236, 242, 245-246.

[244] *Ibid.,* II, 5.

[245] *Ibid.,* I, 119.

[246] Dewhurst, *Dr. Thomas Sydenham,* 83.

[247] *The Works of Thomas Sydenham,* I, 181.

[248] Baglivi, *De Praxi Medica,* 5.

[249] *Ibid.,* 6, 89.

[250] *Ibid.,* 93, 249.

[251] *The Works of Thomas Sydenham,* I, 26.

[252] Baglivi, *De Praxi Medica,* 110.

[253] *The Works of Thomas Sydenham,* I, 25.

[254] *Ibid.,* I, 26.

[255] *Ibid.,* I, 25.

[256] Baglivi, *De Praxi Medica,* 4, 110, 163, 249.

[257] *The Works of Thomas Sydenham,* II, 170.

[258] *Loc. cit.*

[259] Baglivi, *De Praxi Medica,* passim.

[260] *Ibid.,* 172-173.

[261] *Ibid.,* 5, 155, 215.

[262] *Ibid.,* 156.

[263] *Ibid.,* 215.

[264] *Loc. cit.*

[265] *Ibid.,* 155.

[266] *Ibid.,* 219.

[267] *Ibid.,* 242.

[268] *Ibid.,* 8.

[269] *Ibid.,* 104.

[270] *Ibid.,* 155.

[271] *Ibid.,* 156.

[272] *Ibid.,* 238.

[273] *Ibid.,* 172-173. Cf. with Karl Deichgraeber, *Die Griechische Empirikerschule* (Berlin/Zurich: Weidmann, 1930, 1965), 64.

CHAPTER IV

EMPIRICAL REACTIONS (2): GEORG ERNST STAHL AND THE SCHOOL OF MONTPELLIER

Another focus of Empirical thought in medicine at the dawn of the eighteenth century was the Halle professor, Georg Ernst Stahl (1660-1734), who influenced all his contemporaries–Hoffmann, Boerhaave, Baglivi,[1] and others –but was himself guided only by Hippocratic-Empirical principles and the doctrines of Pietism.

Stahl reworked the tenets of Empiricism into a new form which incorporated Harvey's discovery of the circulation and transformed the Hippocratic *physis* into the *Anima sensitiva.* In contrast to Boerhaave's mechanistic treatment of the circulation, Stahl's proved a fruitful source of new ideas, stimulating Theophile Bordeu (1722-1776), in particular, to pioneering investigations of the glandular system.

The *Anima sensitiva* remained influential in the School of Montpellier until the end of the nineteenth century.

Biographical

Stahl was born in Ansbach and (like Hoffmann) studied at Jena under Georg Wolfgang Wedel. In 1694 he was called to Halle by Hoffmann (from whom he was later estranged) as professor of pathology, dietetics, physiology, pharmacology, chemistry, and botany. He remained there until 1716 when he became physician-in-ordinary to the Emperor, residing in Berlin until his death.

Stahl was the leading chemist of his generation but (perhaps for this reason) postulated the inapplicability of this discipline to therapeutics.[2] He once wrote to a friend:

> Brought up in the principles of Sylvius and Willis, which referred all disease causes to particular acrimonies of the humors, I was amazed that the humors did not alter despite their continual and natural tendency to putrefaction, and that sphacelus (which is complete putrefaction) occurred only very rarely. I did not see the salts introduced every day into the body with the food causing the accidents generally attributed to saline acrimonies. I could not refer the diseases peculiar to certain ages and temperaments to any particular alteration of the humors. I then recognized the falsity of any application of the chemical sciences to the theory of diseases. Furthermore, I could not explain by mechanical laws the extraordinary and sudden changes due to the passions, which give rise to actions in the various parts of the body which are quite different from those resulting naturally from their mechanical conformation—these being so obviously caused by a disorder of the vital movements that it seemed absurd to accept the involvement of any material cause. Thus I felt the need to reconstruct medical theory on a firmer basis than chemistry and mechanics.[3]

This firmer basis was the Hippocratic *physis* to which Stahl added the attributes of Paracelsus' Alchemist and Van Helmont's *Archeus*, formulating a therapeutic doctrine which incorporated traditional Empirical assumptions about health and disease. He is a unique figure in having mastered both the chemical and the medical knowledge of his day while consistently maintaining a separation between the two disciplines.

The counterweight to the attraction of chemistry in Stahl's mind, and the force which strengthened his Empirical orientation, was Pietism.

We have maintained that the Empirical/Rationalist polarity exists in all of man's intellectual activities,[a] and this is preeminently true for religion. The Pietistic version of Lutheranism, which stood for the Empirical side of religious thinking in contrast to the increasing Rationalization of the established Lutheran church, gave comprehensive support to Stahl's doctrine of the *Anima* and to his Empirically structured therapeutics generally.[b]

With the establishment of Lutheranism as the state religion emphasis was laid increasingly on correct belief, rather than Christian conduct, as the key to salvation. Doctrine took precedence over behavior, theory over practice. The Pietist revival, led by Philipp Jakob Spener (1635-1705) and August Hermann Franke (1663-1727), drawing on Eckhart and other mystics, turned away from this intellectualized religion and appealed to the heart and will as manifested in Christian works and experience:

> Spener's basis was experience. Without attacking doctrine, he relegated it to a minor place, emphasizing the will rather than knowledge, and insisting that justification by faith must be by a faith supported by works, such as repentence, conversion, and a changed life . . . In the main, Pietism is justly to be called a movement of revaluation, which tried to attach to regeneration and sanctification as accomplished facts a higher value than to justification by faith as an approved theory . . . Pietism was the reaction of the spirit against the letter. It sprang

[a] See *Divided Legacy,* I, Introduction.

[b] J. H. Baas, in his incomparable way, draws attention to the tie between Stahl's religious and medical beliefs: "A thinker as profound as he was earnest . . . Stahl was a great Pietist and a man of stiff and rough manners, unchangeably true to his laboriously acquired convictions and bitter and reserved at their non-acceptance. For he held these convictions to be as important as a revelation from God (an expression of Pietistic pride) and in fact regarded them as such a revelation. The success of another thus seemed a personal injury to himself, and accordingly from a hypochondriacal croaker he became gradually a confirmed misanthrope, until finally his morbid reserve and gloomy moroseness ended in actual melancholy. Pecuniary profit, however, he never sought, and its pursuit he scorned" (*History of Medicine,* 608).

> up in protest against the formalism of its day . . . it represents a permanent spirit, for, just as tyranny provokes rebellion, so will formalism always call up some form of Pietism.[4]

Pietism incorporated the rigid Empirical distinction between the "inward" and the "outward." The believer's degree of piety, being "inward," was not knowable directly but became manifest in his conduct. Hence Pietism stressed active works of charity, founding a series of schools and orphan asylums as well as Halle University itself. The Moravian Church, an offshoot of Pietism, pioneered in Protestant missionary activity.[c]

The most important component of the "inward" life was the Holy Spirit, which acts on the will, strengthening it for charity and good works (in contrast to orthodox Lutheranism, which believed that the Holy Spirit enlightens the intellect). The religious image of an active agent within the body which guides it to salvation and preserves it from sin (Pietism even held that conversion is accompanied by a "crisis") fused in Stahl's mind with the Hippocratic *physis* and emerged as the *Anima* which directs and controls the organism in its struggle against harmful environmental influences.

Stahl exemplifies rigid adherence to principle combined with Christian devotion to the practical care of the sick. His

[c]John Wesley (1703 1791), the founder of Methodism, dated his own evangelical conversion to meetings with Moravians in Georgia (1736) and in England (1738). His medical handbook, *Primitive Physick, or an Easy and Natural Method of Curing Most Diseases* (Dublin, 1752), which passed through innumerable editions for many decades and was probably used by households even in the nineteenth century, is cast in a purely Empirical form: reliance on the innate healing power is best, remedies have all been discovered by chance, patients should avoid compound medicines which only "swell the apothecary's bill" and "possibly prolong the distemper, that the doctor and he may divide the spoil," all of medicine arises from experience, etc. "Thus ancient man, having a little experience, joined with common sense and common humanity, cured both themselves and their neighbors of most of the distempers to which every nation was subject" (Preface).

writings are permeated with charity for suffering humanity,[d] and he developed a complex series of arguments proving the existence of an *Anima* within the organism which protects it in health and cures it when diseased. In so doing the *Anima* follows a variety of different curative procedures, and the physician must understand them in order to provide assistance when needed.

But Stahl did not define or classify these procedures of the *Anima,* and did not create an elaborate doctrine of therapeutic intervention, leaving these two points to his followers for solution.

The first was attacked dramatically by Francois Boissier de la Croix de Sauvages (1706-1767) who introduced the Stahlian doctrine to Montpellier. An acute mathematician and Iatromechanist who felt that his mechanically conceived organism needed a motivating force, Sauvages followed the suggestions made by Sydenham and Baglivi and described in symptomatic terms all the illnesses and diseases known to medicine at the time—a total of about 2500. These patterns combined the impact of the morbific stimulus and the reaction of the *Anima.*[5] [e] Sauvages' therapeutics, however, remained conventional and eclectic.

He was followed by Theophile Bordeu, a more subtle and realistic thinker and one of the great figures of French medical history.

Bordeu demonstrated his Empirical love of practical healing at an early age, taking the degree of "physician-surgeon" upon completing his medical studies at Montpellier in 1744 (in 1743 the king had proclaimed the professional equality of the two branches of medicine).[6] Later in life he frequently took the side of the surgeons in their disputes with the physicians.[7]

[d]Stahl's charity was not extended to the Iatromechanists and other medical thinkers who disagreed with his "true medical theory" *(theoria medica vera).* "He could scarcely refrain from employing insulting epithets whenever he spoke of them" (Sprengel, *Histoire de la Medecine,* V, 200).

[e]See below, pp. 251-252.

His student years had coincided with the controversy between Sauvages and the pure Iatromechanists who rejected the *Anima* (his own dissertation on sensation and motion drew equally on Van Helmont and Stahl),[8] and Bordeu thus set himself the task of cleansing the Iatromechanist residuum from Sauvages' doctrine, carrying through to a finish what the latter had started: "Stahl spoke only of what is observed in the sick; he wanted to train physicians only to be practitioners, and his legitimate disciples have carried things so far as to doubt the very utility of medical schools; what would they have said at seeing medicine reduced only to physics, and Borelli and Bernouilli cited instead of Galen and Hippocrates?"[9] Iatromechanism, Bordeu held, was closer to the teachings of Cheyne and Pitcairn—the English Iatro-mathematicians—than to the "dream of Stahl . . . the dream of one of the greatest geniuses medicine has ever known."[10]

Bordeu aligned the *Anima* more closely with the Hippocratic *physis,* clothing it with the biological and physiological concepts developed by his contemporaries while retaining its purposiveness and spontaneity.[11] This led to an original and valuable interpretation of the glandular system (making him a pioneer of endocrinology) and an understanding of the voluntary and sympathetic nervous systems. But his pharmacology, like that of Stahl, was rudimentary.

The final apotheosis of Animism in Montpellier, lasting through the nineteenth century, was that of Paul-Joseph Barthez (1754-1806), a child prodigy and polyhistor born the year of Stahl's death who left a mark on three different fields.

He studied medicine at Montpellier and Paris and for several years taught it at Montpellier. Then he abandoned medicine for law and by 1780 had risen to *conseiller de justice.* He thereupon left law for philosophy and by 1785 was chancellor of Montpellier. During the Revolution he supported the aristocratic party, his official career went into eclipse, he returned to medicine, and in 1802 was personal physician to Napoleon. He died four years later.

During Barthez' years at Montpellier Iatromechanism was being taught in its pure form by Antoine Fizes (1689-1765),[f] Sauvages' modification of Iatromechanism was also popular, Haller's irritability and sensitivity were gaining support,[g] and Bordeu's neo-Hippocraticism was coming into vogue.[12] Barthez aimed to bring order into this situation by setting forth with precision all possible patterns of the *Anima's* reaction to morbific influences, thus continuing the work of Sauvages but assisted by Condorcet's analysis of the functions of the intellect. He also subscribed to Bacon's method of induction: while disease causes are unknowable (like all other "causes" in nature), precise observation will yield the patterns and laws of disease and health. Barthez hoped to develop therapeutics inductively: having classified the movements of the "vital principle" (his name for the *Anima*), the physician could experiment with various medicines for their effect on each pathological movement.

The development of therapeutic doctrine along these lines occupied Montpellier for a hundred years, generating what must be the most turgid and incomprehensible corpus of medical writing in the Western tradition. For these thinkers came late to the realization that the inductive method could not be applied in the absence of agreement on what was being observed.

At issue was the ranking of symptoms, the relative weight of the *propria* and *communia,* which had preoccupied Empirical thinkers since ancient times. The problem could not be resolved merely by gazing at the symptoms themselves, for however long a time, but required invocation of some external criterion. Montpellier, to its credit, rejected the proximate cause as the standard for evaluating symptoms but failed to come up with an alternative criterion for distinguishing important symptoms from unimportant.

[f] See his *Traite des Fievres* (Paris: Desaint and Saillant, 1757).

[g] One of the later leaders of Montpellier wrote: "the mediocrities of the town did experiments with Haller's irritability" (J. Lordat, *Essai d'une Caracteristique de l'Enseignement Medical de l'Ecole de Montpellier* [Montpellier: Castel, 1843], 32).

Medical theory hence turned in a vicious circle: the disease was defined by its significant symptoms, and the symptoms, in turn, took on significance from the disease in which they appeared.

Thus, while Montpellier advocated pure observation and experience, and felt itself thereby faithful to Hippocrates,[h] it committed the same error as the Rationalists—reading into observation a (changing) set of unconscious and *a priori* assumptions about the relative importance of symptoms.

When Samuel Hahnemann introduced a different criterion—that of the parallel sets of symptoms obtained from proving medicines on the healthy—he acquired some support in Montpellier but very little.[i]

Therapeutics in this school remained more stable than elsewhere but still fluctuated with doctrinal fashions. By the end of the nineteenth century Montpellier was only a country cousin of the dominant school of Paris.

The Source of Medical Knowledge. The Anima. Iatrochemistry and Iatromechanism

For Stahl the starting-point of a true understanding of the organism was the realization that, while composed of corruptible matter, it does not corrupt, being prevented by the presence of a force which he called the *Anima sensitiva, Anima rationalis,* or simply the *Anima,* and defined as a "habitual inclination to movement."[13] [j]

The *Anima* maintains health, and restores it when lost, by the circulation of the blood and the functioning of the organs

[h]Inscribed over the entrance of one of the main buildings was: *Hippocrates, olim Coensis, nunc Monspaliensis* ("Hippocrates, formerly of Cos, now of Montpellier").

[i]See below, pp. 559-560.

[j]Van Helmont had argued in favor of vitalism by invoking the difference between a live body and a corpse (*Oriatrike,* 471, 543). He also used the term, *anima sensitiva* (see above, p. 28).

which cleanse the body of impurities.[14] This process is identical with coction, the *Anima* is hence identical with the *physis,* and Harvey's discovery does not detract from Hippocratic doctrine.[15]

Stahl called the *Anima* "rational" to stress its independence of material constraints and determinants and to show that it must of itself learn how to cope with illness.[16] When the *Anima* makes an incorrect choice, the body succumbs to one of the morbific influences perpetually assailing it.[17] [k]

By thus assimilating man's rational faculty to his vegetative soul Stahl inverted the argument of Descartes and other Rationalists who had held that the vegetative functions could be interpreted in the *a priori* categories of *ratio.*

The physical body exists for the sake of the *Anima* and is its instrument.[18] The "life of man" (*vita hominis*) is the *Anima,* while the "life of the body" (*vita corporis*) reflects the impact of the *Anima* upon the organism.[19] The *vita corporis* can be understood only by reference to the *Anima,* not in isolation from it as the Iatrochemists and Iatromechanists attempt to do.[20] The presence of the *Anima* distinguishes the body not only from a mass of chemicals but also from a mere piece of machinery.[21]

The *Anima* is the formal and efficient cause of life, but it acts in response to the final cause which is God's will that man enjoy long life.[22] For this reason He placed the *Anima* in the body. Determined by this final cause, the *Anima* acts purposefully to select, among the variety of alternatives available at any time, the one which is most consonant with God's will that the organism be preserved from harm.[23]

Thus man *can possess causal knowledge of the organism* because he can observe the *visible* acts by which the *Anima*

[k] Because animals are closer to nature than man, with more highly developed sensory powers, the *Anima* of an animal is more skilful, and animals are hence less subject to disease (Stahl, *Theoria Medica Vera* [Leipzig: Choulant, 1831-1833], I, 102). Stahl has difficulty explaining death, since the *Anima* does not age, but it seems to be due to lack of resistance by the *Anima* (*ibid.,* II, 46).

preserves it from harm.[24] [1] This is necessary, since the human mind cannot perceive into the organism.[25] "It has not received from its Creator this privilege of intimate intuition."[26] It "can neither perceive, nor grasp by reasoning, any external object which does not appear in a sense-perceptible form."[27]

The Iatrochemists and Iatromechanists are mistaken in their doctrines for two reasons. They erroneously extrapolate into the organism from their chemical and mechanical experiments, and, in any case, the material causes which they are trying to elucidate are of secondary importance, being at all times subordinate to the formal and efficient causes (the *Anima*) and the final cause (the will of God) of the life of the organism.[28]

Iatrochemistry is a "lure for those of weak and credulous imagination," a pretended explanation of processes which chemists actually do not understand, leading them into frivolous experiments which harm and kill their patients.[29] They inject chemicals, hoping for the effect obtained in their retorts, but such reactions cannot take place without participation by the other substances in the body; furthermore, such experiments are done in the presence of air, while the chemistry of the body does not involve air.[30]

Anatomy also burdens medicine with incorrect ideas and is really useful only to surgery.[31] It reveals nothing about the body's functions: a corpse is like a run-down watch–mere inspection of the spring will not reveal that it is the source of the watch's movements, as this can be obtained only by observing the watch in motion.[32] Anatomy gives no guidance to therapy.[33]

Hence the Iatromechanists who rely on anatomy for conclusions about the body's functioning are in error. "Life" cannot be reduced to the mere circulation of the blood and other humors.[34] The body's movements are not determined

[1] **Stahl's "formal" and "efficient" causes serve the same function (of ensuring visibility) as the "formal causes" of Paracelsus, Sydenham, and Baglivi.**

by its material structure but reflect the presence of the *Anima* which does not act "generally" (like a piece of machinery) but "specifically."[35] It produces specific actions which are its response to a given set of circumstances, a given challenge or morbific influence, and are caused by the Divine Will that man enjoy long life.[36]

For all these reasons the source of medical knowledge is observation of the visible acts of the *Anima.*[37] "Everything in medicine is based on clinical practice and on precise observation of the facts furnished us by experience."[38]

Stahl ascribed all the movements of the body to the *Anima* which, among its other functions, reacts to external morbific influences. The number of such reactions was identical with the number of possible influences—i.e., infinite. Sauvages curtailed this freedom of the *Anima,* dividing the organism into an area subject to the *Anima* directly and a second area which, while ultimately dynamized by the *Anima,* functions as a hydraulic machine.[39] [m] The *Anima* possesses "animate forces," and the organism-as-hydraulic-machine functions through its "inanimate forces" which follow the ordinary laws of physics and chemistry.[40]

He thus attributed to the *vita corporis* what he had taken away from the *vita hominis.* The "inanimate forces" comprise the forces of gravity, cohesion, electricity, attraction, and elasticity as well as such processes as fermentation, condensation, etc.[41] All are intrinsic to the body's material structure.

Hence the physician obtains knowledge not only from sense-perception but also from mechanical and mathematical analogies, "syllogisms linked together geometrically," etc.[42]

Bordeu sought a middle road between the pure Stahlian *Anima* and Sauvages' neo-Iatromechanism. The *Anima* has

[m]This hydraulic machine is actuated by an "electrical" or "nervous" fluid—Sauvages' adaptation of the seventeenth-century "animal" and "vital" spirits (*Nosologie Methodique* [Paris: Herissant, 1770-1771], I, 341, 346, 348).

thrown Stahl's disciples into a "metaphysical labyrinth," but the Iatromechanists are also wrong in attempting to reduce the organism to a mere piece of machinery.[43] The laws of the living body are not physical, mechanical, or chemical, and medicine may not be dominated by these disciplines.[44] Knowledge of anatomical structure tells the physician nothing about function: anatomy must be "animated" and learned at the bedside. The chemists dissolve the body into its components and leave behind only the debris.[45] [n]

Nor is the reasoning power of any use, "a rule of lead and wax which can be lengthened, twisted, and accomodated to any bias and any measure" (quoting Montaigne).[46] In the words of Pierre Bayle, it is "a vague and spinning instrument which can be turned in any direction like a top."[47] [o] Reason can never prevail over observation.[48]

The science and art of medicine must not rely on these bodies of knowledge, but on the living human body itself.[49]

Bordeu resolved this problem by assimilating the *Anima* more closely to the coction/evacuation function of the Hippocratic *physis*. And he described this function more

[n]More about Bordeu's attitude toward his orthodox contemporaries may be ascertained from the book by his best friend, Louis de la Caze (1705-1765), who wrote that the assumption of an "obstruction" to the circulation as a primary cause of disease is purely arbitrary; these "obstructions" are supposed to be from diseased or putrescent matter, but rotten milk is thinner than healthy milk, and milk from diseased animals is thinner than that from healthy ones; the "chyle veins" from which chyle is supposed to be secreted have never yet been observed; chyle is supposed to make the blood thick, but blood is thicker than chyle already; if chyle mixed with blood causes the latter to stagnate, why does it not all stagnate at once instead of in just one place; why, in acute diseases, do the symptoms move around the body instead of being localized; the idea that chyle is loaded with acids or alkalis is disproved by persons with acid or alkaline indigestion who have no other ailment; one can only conclude that Boerhaave "substituted for the history and correct evaluation of the phenomena of the *natura* his own way of conceiving them" (*Idee de l'Homme, Physique et Moral, Pour Servir d'Introduction a un Traite de Medecine* [Paris: Guerin and Delatour, 1755], 28-36).

[o]Pierre Bayle (1647-1706) was a pioneer of the French Enlightenment who advocated religious scepticism and criticized rationalized religion (as well as all metaphysics generally), seeking to ground knowledge in sensory data.

comprehensively, expanding on Harvey's discussion of the circulation together with other increments of chemical and anatomical knowledge and continuing to interpret them in the light of Hippocratic principles.[50]

Each vital function is a mixture of sensation and motion, with "life" defined as the "alternation of evident motions and evident sensations with hidden motions and sensations."[51] "Motions," however, are of two different kinds, those in which the *Anima* plays a major role and those which are generated by the body's "innate principle of life and action."[52]

This "intermediate view" between Stahl and the Iatromechanists contains a residue of Sauvages' "inanimate forces" and, furthermore, was Bordeu's reaction to Haller's "sensitivity" and "irritability."[53] [p]

The heart, brain, and stomach are the locus of life and the centers of sensation and motion.[54] Physicians in the past have tended to underestimate the significance of the stomach—which is no less important than the other organs.[q]

> The latter's functions depend upon a reserve of sensitivity [*sensibilite*] which has been too ignored by all the practitioners of ordinary physiology; they have considered this viscera merely as an almost passive reservoir or, at the most, as one with only slight capacity for movement. In fact, it is endowed with a great deal of sensitivity whose various degrees (or various tastes) are manifested at every moment and thereby maintain or upset the progress and harmony of the whole animal economy.
>
> Thus the stomach or its appurtenances, which are a principal center of the body's movements, are equally a center of its various degrees of feeling. This is the long and short of the speculations of the most modern

[p]On Haller see below, pp. 279-282.

[q]Bordeu's first publication was on the digestive process, and he was intrigued by it throughout his career (*Oeuvres de Bordeu* [Paris: Caille et Ravier, 1818], I, iii, xvii).

> philosophers with respect to the principle of life and the organization of its functions.[55] [r]

Bordeu owes much here to Van Helmont but elaborates on his physiology, hypothesizing an intimate connection between the glands (connected by nerves to the brain) and the arterial system (driven by the heart), with the unity and equilibrium of the organism assured by the involvement of all parts in the circulation of the blood and other humors.[56] The parts of the body are continuously adapted and adjusted to each other through interaction between the glands and the circulating blood.

Bordeu was thus the first endocrinologist, and his interpretation of this area of physiology reflects his understanding of the *Anima* and the coction/evacuation process: for the "secretion" (whereby the glands extract what they need from the bloodstream) is controlled by the *Anima,* while "excretion" (by the glands into the bloodstream) is merely a new formulation of Hippocratic coction/evacuation!![s]

The blood both nourishes and cleanses the organs.[57] It is a sort of "circulating flesh" *(chair coulant)* which fills all the interstices of the body and contains extracts from all the glands.[58] Man can scarcely understand these processes which are solely within the purview of the *physis:* the chemist, in particular, can never understand them through experiments, since he starts by destroying that which he is to investigate. And the Iatromechanists, who consider the blood merely as a conglomeration of globules, are also far from the mark. These processes can be comprehended only by observing their visible effects:

> It must be agreed that this aim will never be reached—neither through anatomy or chemistry nor through

[r]On the function of "tastes" in the Empirical tradition see *Divided Legacy,* I, 74-77.

[s]Bordeu did not distinguish the ductless glands, whose product is absorbed by the lymph or the blood, from glands such as the lachrymals or mammaries which secrete from the blood for subsequent excretion from the body.

> physical or academical experiments. Only by following the course of diseases and meditating on them will we seize the true composition, the combinations, and the nature of the animal humors. This must be repeated time after time: a knowledge of the composition of the blood is inseparable from a calculation of the effects it produces unceasingly upon the sensitive organs. These effects are repeated at every instant of life—which is aimed specifically at preserving the individual and the mass of the humors. The *natura* has as its task the mixing, purification, destruction, and continuous reproduction of the materials of these humors. It thrives only in the resultant combinations of all of these seminal and living parts.[59]

While the heart, maintaining the blood and humors in circulation, is an important locus of life, the brain—together with the glands to which it is attached—is equally important. Bordeu observes that the glands are endowed with many more nerves than are needed merely to sustain life and concludes that these assure the processes of secretion and excretion.[60] Secretion is evidence of the *Anima's* capacity to perceive and select among alternatives: excretion, on the other hand, is a mechanical and involuntary effect of the body's "innate principle of life and action."[61]

Thus secretion is not a function of the circulation alone (as some Iatrochemists have held) but is initiated in the brain by the *Anima* and mediated through the nerves.[62]

Communication through the nervous system is not by "animal spirits," as claimed by Willis, Haller, and others. These were introduced arbitrarily to serve as a link between soul and body.[63] "By what fatality have the natural and vital spirits succumbed, while the animal spirits survived?"[64] Nor is such communication the function of some "nervous fluid."[65] Bordeu prefers to hold that the *Anima* communicates certain tensions and vibrations to the organs and glands through the nerves.[66]

Some have attributed secretion to attraction by an analogous humor outside the gland, but why, then, is natural secretion restored in a gland which has been (artificially) filled with some alien liquid?[67] Why do humors flow in greater quantity toward an actively secreting gland (e.g., the salivaries during meals)?[68] And why is glandular function reduced or curtailed altogether during sleep?[69] None of the accepted explanations are satisfactory.

Although secretion is not easy to understand, it seems to be due to the *Anima's* perception and selection at the glandular level. Each gland possesses its own "taste," its own sensation, by which it selects a part of the humors flowing by: the secretory duct of the gland possesses its own sphincter and its own nerves by which it opens or closes the gland and thus admits or excludes the appropriate humor.[70] Secretion is a "specific action whereby the organ, so to speak, prepares and disposes itself to separate a humor."[71] It is the "specific action" (*action propre*) of the organ; just as the function of the eye is vision, so each gland has its own specific function which is a sort of sensation.[72]

Just as the *Anima* possesses the capacity to select among alternatives at the level of the whole organism, so each gland possesses this same capacity at the glandular level.

Glandular excretion has been attributed by some to purely mechanical compression by the neighboring parts of the body.[73] [t] This, however, is unsatisfactory, and excretion must be interpreted in terms of Hippocratic coction and evacuation. All glands behave like the penis in the male which, when suitably excited, becomes hard and distended, "erect," and then during the "crisis" discharges its contents.[74] This excitement or stimulation is from the surrounding milieu: "each gland has, so to say, its own niche and can be shaken, agitated, or excited by the neighboring parts of the body without being compressed by them."[75]

While others have proposed some form of "irritation" as the basis of glandular function, they have omitted these important details.[76]

[t]Bordeu tested this theory by excising the parotid gland in the jaw of a dog, filling the cavity with a piece of sponge. Closing the dog's jaw did not compress the sponge, and Bordeu reasoned that the same must be true *a fortiori* for the internal glands (*Oeuvres de Bordeu,* I, 51, 57, 66-69, 100-106, 117).

But Bordeu guards against spurious precision in his "explanation" of glandular function. He is, in particular, imprecise about the division of roles between the *Anima* and the "animal being."[77] Thus the *Anima* plays a certain role in the excretory function also: "this should be added to all the other causes we have been discussing."[78] It is beyond man's grasp to give precise reasons for the behavior of the glands.[79] All of the body's movements and functions are continually being altered and adjusted through the pervasive presence of the *Anima.*[80]

> This is again one of those metaphors which should be pardoned us; persons who know these matters firsthand know how difficult it is to be clear in discussing the force which so precisely directs the thousand peculiar movements of the human body and its parts; one does not even know what language to employ to express, for example, certain movements of vegetables and even certain properties of minerals; there have been physicians who, struck by these movements, have resorted to particular causes . . . Stahl claimed that the *Anima* directs the whole animal organism. However that may be, we can say that all the living parts are directed by a conservative force which is unceasingly watchful; is this, in some respects, the essence of a portion of matter or a necessary attribute of its combinations? One more thing, we do not claim here to give more than a way of looking at things, metaphorical expressions, comparisons . . .[81]

He jokes that only a Descartes or a Leibnitz could give solid explanations of the harmony and laws of the human economy.[82]

Bordeu's indeterminacy is entirely Empirical, as he was far more concerned with the practical consequences of his glandular analysis than with pinpointing a series of "proximate causes": the essential is that the body functions as a unit pervaded by the *Anima.* While the nervous system and brain play major roles, as do the stomach and circulation, knowledge of these subsystems is not acquired through minute anatomical investigation. Bordeu amused himself with the observation that

> someone has discovered lymphatic veins in the testicles and attributes to them the function of returning semen to the blood: but we did not need any such discovery to know that such absorption must occur. This must be said for fear of some other anatomist coming along and telling us that these veins in the testicles do not exist. One must always beware of these petty anatomical assertions which in no way affect the absorption of the emanations from each organ.[83]

He reached his own conclusions by observing the temperamental differences between sterile women and women with children, between eunuchs and ordinary men, between women before and after puberty, etc.[84] Like all else of significance in medicine, these issues must be resolved by observing sick and healthy people, not on the basis of the "petty assertions" of the anatomists.

Barthez, in principle, accepted the Empirical vitalism of the organism and reliance on observation. "We only see the crust of things."[85] The "facts" making up the "science of man" are not taken from physics, chemistry, and mathematics, but are developed in the "science" itself.[86] [u] Proximate causes are unknowable and cannot be discovered by anatomical investigation.[87]

Medical knowledge is developed by observing the patient's symptoms, comparing them with one another, and through induction arriving at the laws which govern them. "The object of natural philosophy is to seek the causes of natural phenomena, but only insofar as they can be known through experience. Experience cannot tell us what is the essence of the action of any one of these causes . . . it can only manifest the order and rule which are followed, in their succession, by the phenomena which indicate these causes."[88] The many isolated facts of the "science of man"

[u]Barthez praises Hippocrates for separating medicines from the other sciences; he supports the latter's criticism of the Cnidians for presuming to classify diseases in terms of their seats and causes (J. Lordat, *Exposition de La Doctrine Medicale de P. J. Barthez* [Paris: Gabon, 1818], 369, 372).

must be collated to bring out the "general facts, or the results of experience."[89] "Causal" explanation of an event is only "showing that the phenomena of which it is composed occur in an order analogous to the order of succession of other facts which are more familiar and therefore seem better known."[90] [v]

But Barthez was at pains to distinguish his own vitalism from Stahl's and that of "my illustrious friend Bordeu."[91] Like Sauvages, he postulated two parallel sets of functions in the organism, the "voluntary," subject to the *Anima,* and the "involuntary," subject to the "vital principle."[92] Stahl erred in ascribing the latter to the *Anima* (which he defined metaphysically and even theologically), since digestion, menstruation, nutrition, and sensation all fall under the "vital principle."[93]

Barthez refused to define the distinction between the "vital principle" and the mere mechanics of the body: "one should maintain an invincible scepticism as to the nature of the vital principle in man."[94] He would not state whether or not it is a "modality of the living body" (*mode du corps humain vivant*).[95] "For the progress of the science of man, which is limited to combinations of correctly perceived facts, it suffices to conceive in an abstract and sceptical fashion this being with an unknown nature which is the vital principle in man."[96]

While Van Helmont (and Bordeu) ascribed a vital principle to each organ, undue multiplication of such fictive entities retards the progress of science.[97] For the "vital principle" represents the body's unity, the sympathy among its parts, ensuring that a stimulus applied at any point on the body will affect it as a whole.[98] This is why both pupils contract even though only one is touched by a beam of light.[99] Head wounds often cause liver abscesses, despite the absence of a direct connection between these two parts; a stomach wound can cause trembling of the hands; and

[v]He admired Hume's critique of causal thinking (P. J. Barthez, *Nouveaux Elements de la Science de l'Homme* [Paris: Goujon, 1806], I, notes: 12).

paralysis of the thumbs was found to be among the *sequelae* of a recent epidemic of colic.[100]

While the "vital principle" permeates all the solids and the blood, we do not know how it is associated with the body's movements and functions.[101] There is no reason to suppose that it acts through the nerve fibers or the "animal spirits"; more probably it acts directly on the molecules of the muscular fibers.[102]

Our ignorance of its mechanisms, however, does not prevent us from taking it as the only suitable foundation for medical practice.[103]

The School of Montpellier thus converted Stahl's Empirical *Anima* into Barthez' Rationalist "vital principle." The *Anima,* being unknowable *a priori,* was not acceptable in its pristine form, and Sauvages and Barthez succumbed to the impulse to single out areas of physiology and pathology in which the movements of the *Anima* could be determined and measured. By the end of the eighteenth century the greater part of diseases—especially the difficult and dangerous ones—had been classified in this area of pathology.

Symptoms. Diseases. Therapeutics

For Stahl there was no qualitative difference between sickness and health, since the *Anima* is at work in both states, and he denied that disease is a *res contra naturam.*[104] Just as the *Anima* organizes the harmony of the body's movements to preserve health, so it organizes similar movements to restore health and combat morbific influences.[105] A diseased state arises when the *Anima* is overcome (temporarily) by a morbific influence or when the crasis of the humors degenerates spontaneously.[106] Plethora is another cause of disease: the *Anima* becomes accustomed to producing blood in youth, when a large quantity is needed, and is unable to moderate the process later.[107] [w]

[w]That blood could be in excess, being relieved by hemorrhage, was a fundamental Hippocratic principle (*Divided Legacy,* I, 52).

Diseases can also arise from psychosomatic influences—the best evidence that physiological processes are vitalistic and not chemical or mechanical.[108]

Since "disease" symptoms in fact represent the *Anima's* reaction to the morbific cause, they point the way to health.[109] Fever, in particular, signifies that the *Anima* is accelerating the circulation of the blood and the action of the organs to cope with an increased burden of toxins.[110] Hemorrhages and hemorrhoids are particularly to be welcomed, showing that the *Anima* is ridding the body of the excess blood whose thickening—with consequent obstruction of vital functions—characterizes many diseases.[111] [x]

However, a small group of symptoms are actually morbific—i.e., the direct effects of the exciting cause. Stahl insisted that these are few in number, and his "special pathology" gives rules for distinguishing them from the far larger class of beneficial symptoms.[112]

The physician must grasp the harmony and periodicity of the *Anima's* movements, the regularities in the succession of the phenomena, the "customary facts."[113] The criterion of truth is the utility of these facts as interpreted in terms of their final cause—God's will that man enjoy long life.[114]

This raises the question of how the physician ranks the symptoms, which are more important and which less, and here Stahl went no further than Sydenham and Baglivi. While the physician must pay particular attention to "customary facts," "he will not consider it frivolous and useless to ascertain if movements outside the ordinary rule are really abnormal and defective, i.e., not only outside the ordinary law and type, but also contrary to all utility (as regards the integrity and needs of the body) and, what is more, entirely harmful and destructive."[115] Some movements, while deviating from "normality," are still natural and useful.[116] At the same time, one should not speculate and theorize from a few rare and exceptional cases.[117]

[x]A contemporary stated that Stahl gazed at his patients' bleeding hemorrhoids like a lover at the face of his mistress.

Stahl's therapeutics is fragmentary and disorganized, as the therapeutic section of the *Theoria Medica Vera* was never written.[118]

Treatment generally is designed to support the *Anima* when it is weak and calm it when it is too energetic.[119] The physician assists the *Anima* with the coction and evacuation of the morbific cause, being guided by the symptoms.[120] He pays particular attention to the various kinds of hemorrhage, in no circumstances interfering with them.[121] The suppression of hemorrhoids is particularly harmful.[122] Their excision can cause gout and other diseases which are benefited if the hemorrhoids are allowed to bleed freely.[123] The best treatment of any hemorrhage is further bloodletting, thus assisting the *Anima* to rid the organism of blood.[124] The physician should never lower a fever, as this would be working against the *Anima*.[125] Stahl particularly opposed the use of quinine for this purpose, and his influence led to a reduction in the prescribing of this remedy (at the same time, he stimulated an increase in bloodletting).[126]

He attacked the therapeutics of the Iatrochemists. When astringent medicines are given for blood in the urine (haematuria), the effect is ulceration of the legs and degeneration of the kidneys.[127] Persons stay healthy even though taking every day into their systems quantities of the acids, alkalis, and salts which the Iatrochemists view as disease causes and treat by contraries.[128] He opposed the concept of the "alterative" medicine, as no disease can be converted into another.[129]

He treated scorpion stings and rabid-dog bites by similars: some part of the animal (preferably the heart) was applied to the wound, neutralizing the poisonous effect.[130]

He accepted the existence of a few "specifics" whose action can be determined by experience.[131] In general, however, he had little confidence in these or other remedies.[132] He wrote extensively against the polypharmacy and large doses of his colleagues:

> Cleansing the pharmacy of our times is more than the labor of Hercules who undertook to cleanse the Augean

> stables. Here it is a stable, not of horses, but of asses. What honest practitioner who is skilful and serious does not realize that the modern pharmacopoeia abounds in superfluous, impotent, uncertain, absurdly compounded, and dangerous remedies bequeathed to us by the ancients as well as by the Greek and Arab pharmacologists. They have been further sullied by the audacious and imprudent lies of charlatans, hawkers at fairs, charcoal sellers, barbers, and stupid empirics and, accompanied by their **** comments resounding in superlatives, are so praised as to make those who sell them to the public at the fairs and markets—together with their **** eulogies—rightly ridiculous. Certainly these latter remedies are piles of ass **** which no river can ever wash away.[133]

His own practice was largely expectant—as the physician is needed not absolutely, but only accidentally, and, in general, art is no substitute for nature.[134] Frederick the Great's sister wrote that he always prescribed the same pills and "cooling powders," regardless of the disease.[135] [y] Bordeu states that he prescribed nothing but sea-salt, especially toward the end of his life.[136] Another authority, however, indicates that he employed salts of vitriol for suffocative catarrh, potassium-antimonium tartrate for asthma and intermittent fever, ipecac in dysentery, and aloes, rhubarb, and jalap as purgatives.[137]

Barthez thought him a rather ineffective practitioner.[138]

Stahl's expectancy laid him open to professional attack by colleagues who thought this detracted from the dignity of the profession. Gideon Harvey (*circa* 1640-1700) in 1689 had published his *Art of Curing Diseases by Expectation* which described expectancy as

> the applying of remedies that do little hurt and less good, from which the patient day by day frustraneously

[y] These were probably his "balsamic pills," composed of aloes, black hellebore, and bitters ("Stahlianisme, ou Mieux Stahlisme," *Dictionnaire des Sciences Medicales* [Paris, 1821]).

> expecting relief and benefit, is at last deferred so long that Nature and Time have partially or entirely cured the disease, which notwithstanding, the physician by subtlety, cunning, and officiousness, doth commonly with success insinuate that the patient is debitor for his life and recovery to the doctor's skill, judgment, method, and remedies.[139]

Stahl felt obliged to respond (even though Harvey's book was not directed against him), and his *Ars Sanandi cum Expectatione: Opposita Arti Curandi Nuda Expectatione* (1730) held that while many are cured without a physician, none are cured without medicine. This medicine, however, is methodical, not pharmacological.[140] The method is that of the *physis* which waits for maturation of the *materies morbi,* separates out the matured matter, and expels it from the body.[141] The *physis* is not a passive spectator but an active participant, and the physician must be the same.[142]

Sauvages' *Methodical Nosology* commenced with the observation that the physician must first recognize the disease species in the patient before him and then discover the true indications for treatment.[143] Existing writers (i.e., Stahl) have not provided assistance in this: instead of describing diseases in their variety, they announce a theory and leave its application to the individual physician.[144]

Hence there is no connection between theory and practice, and most fail to follow the theory they preach. The young graduate attempting to apply the theory he has learned in the schools meets only with failure: so he "assumes a grave and serious air, pronounces a few conventional phrases in a learned tone, and, after fooling others in this way for a long time, ends by fooling himself."[145]

Stahl had provided medicine with a nosology which was copious in its volume but indefinite in its details.[z] Sauvages resolved to reduce this disorder to a scientific classification. He quotes Sydenham: "There must be, in the

[z]He was not even certain that rabies is a specific disease (*Theoria Medica Vera,* III, 388).

first place, a history of the disease . . . There must be, in the second place, a Praxis or Methodus respecting the same, and this must be regular and exact."[146] And, despite Baglivi's complaint that this would require a whole academy, Sauvages decided to do it himself.[147]

Once a correct definition of the disease categories had been established, in Sauvages' opinion, the correct treatment for each category could be developed by trial and error, i.e., by experience.[148] He elaborated a systematic nosology of diseases, with ten major groups, 44 orders, about 315 genera, and 2400-2500 species.[a]

This precise and reliable classification of diseases *will take the place of lengthy experience.*[149] Once he has named the disease the physician has a clear idea of it—like the botanist with his plants.[150]

Sauvages' categories were based entirely upon symptoms, following Sydenham's warning against adopting a pathological hypothesis and then disregarding those symptoms which do not fit the hypothesis.[151] Galen's four humors and Paracelsus' three elements yield incorrect disease classes, since these internal causes will ever remain invisible and unknown.[152] Following such a causal criterion would be like classifying animals according to their "*ova,* or spermatic *animalculi,* or other mysteries of generation."[153]

The symptoms must be graded in the way suggested by Sydenham, following the "peculiar and constant phenomena, apart from the accidental and adventitious ones, these last-named being those that arise from the age or temperament of the patient and from the different forms of medical treatment."[154]

The physician need not fear lest the variety of diseases become too great when this method is followed, for "the

[a]Sauvages' first systematic attempt at disease classification was his *Nouvelles Classes de Maladies,* published in 1731, which inspired Carolus Linnaeus (1707-1778), originally a student of medicine, to undertake his life's work of botanical classification. Sauvages and Linnaeus never met but corresponded throughout their lives (see Knud Faber, "Nosography in Modern Internal Medicine," *Annals of Medical History* IV [1922], 1-63, at 7).

natura in the production of disease is uniform and consistent, so much so that, for the same disease in different persons the symptoms are, for the most part, the same."[155] Baglivi himself is authority for the proposition that the number of diseases is not infinite, and that they do not vary over time.[156]

Sydenham and Baglivi were right because the human body resembles a machine, reacting in the same way to the same stimuli: "unless this proposition is accepted, nothing could be certain either in medicine or in any other activity of life."[157 b]

Disease is a contest between the "inanimate forces" in the body and the "animate forces." The mechanically conceived "inanimate forces" give rise to the *materies morbi,* while the "animate forces" oppose and combat it. Disease can thus result from either an excess of "inanimate forces" or a dearth of "animate forces."[158] Some symptoms represent the curative effort of the *Anima,* but many others represent the disease, i.e., the "inanimate forces."[159 c]

Sauvages was attempting a fusion of Empirical and Rationalist principles (like Baglivi), but this led to conflict and ambiguity in his therapeutic philosophy. On one hand, he wanted the number of diseases to be finite, since they are a function of the "inanimate forces" which follow the ordinary laws of physics and chemistry and cannot be capable of purposeful adaptation to new morbific stresses. On the other hand, he ignored the "proximate cause," adhered to a purely symptomatic description of diseases and, in fact, preferred the *propria* to the *communia,* quoting Sydenham: "[the symptoms] should be noted accurately and in all their minuteness, in imitation of the exquisite industry of those painters who represent in their portraits the smallest moles and the faintest spots."[160]

[b]Claude Bernard said the same 200 years later (see below, p. 691).

[c]He also accepted Stahl's overproduction of blood as a major cause of disease (*Nosologie Methodique,* I, 346).

By seeking to base disease description on the *propria,* which by definition are infinite in number, Sauvages negated his own assumption that the "inanimate forces" in the body determine the classes of disease.

His philosophy is contradictory in other ways. He claimed that "proximate causes" cannot be known but assumed knowledge of the "inanimate forces."[d] He accepted Hippocratic coction but then went on to a therapeutic method based on contraries: the symptoms representing the curative efforts of the "animate forces" were to be stimulated along Hippocratic lines, but those representing the morbific efforts of the "inanimate forces" were to be treated with contraries.[161] This was equivalent to removing the disease cause.[162] He cited with approval Galen's injunction to correct the *physis* when it is doing wrong.[163]

Another mode of treatment was with specifics, especially quinine, which deprive the *materies morbi* of its power, make it fluid, and improve the elasticity of the blood vessels—correcting the *materies morbi* without any sensible evacuation.[164] In general, use of specifics is preferable to merely seconding the efforts of the *physis.*[165]

Sauvages is seen to have enlarged the role of Stahl's *vita corporis* at the expense of his *vita hominis.* By the same token, he expanded Stahl's small group of symptoms which do not represent the effect of the *Anima* but that of the disease.[166]

The *Methodical Nosology* created a sensation when it appeared and soon became extremely popular, in part, at least, because Sauvages' doctrinal contradictions permitted any kind of practice. While paying lip-service to Empirical principles, he was an influence for Rationalism, and his therapeutics was at best eclectic.[e] Sometimes the physician

[d]Thus fever can arise from heightened viscosity of the blood, greater velocity of the fluids, improper distribution of "nervous fluid" between the heart and the rest of the body, etc. (*Nosologie Methodique,* I, 341).

[e]Not surprisingly, he had been encouraged in his efforts by Boerhaave (*Nosologie Methodique,* I, 110).

assisted the *physis,* sometimes he opposed it, sometimes he used similars,[f] sometimes contraries.[167] Sometimes he treated the cause, sometimes the symptoms.[168] Sometimes Sauvages criticized polypharmacy, and sometimes he prescribed a different medicine for each symptom.[169] Although holding, in principle, that proximate causes are unknowable, he also states that they must be known if the physician is to prescribe correctly, etc. etc.[170]

Bordeu's therapeutics returned to the more rigid Empiricism of Stahl.

He accepted the Empirical assumption of a continuum between sickness and health: the glands perform the same functions of coction and evacuation in both states, and, in a sense, we are always sick, since we could always be in better health.[171] [g]

Each person's idiosyncrasy reflects a different relationship between the heart, brain, and stomach.[172] Disease is a derangement of the interaction among these three organs.[173] Disease of the stomach can cause a sympathetic disease at some other point in the body, and this can then take on independent life.[174] Even the *Anima* can become diseased.[175]

The physician does not base treatment on assumptions about proximate causes: the Galenic and Iatrochemical doctrines of viscous humors, "febrile and acrid matters in the *primae viae,*" etc. are entirely incorrect.[176] The physician need only know that disease is a process of coction, crisis, and evacuation, the crisis terminating with movement of the *materies morbi* to another part of the body or to the outside.[177]

This doctrine of crises is only for the superior physician: "those who are content with following their ideas and

[f]Scabies suppressed by incorrect treatment, thus assuming a more virulent form, was treated by clothing the patient in the garments of a person who had scabies: this returned the disease to the surface of the body (*Nosologie Methodique,* I, 33). For more on scabies (the itch) see below, pp. 397 ff., 468, 548*e*.

[g]See above, p. 247, and below, p. 670.

systems rather than the *physis* will only formulate romantic fictions, far removed from the proper goal."[178]

Bordeu's main diagnostic technique, other than direct observation of the patient, was by the pulse.

Two works on the pulse had been published when he was a young man, *Idioma de la Naturaleza* by the Spaniard, Solano de Luques, and *New and Extraordinary Observations Concerning the Prediction of Various Crises by the Pulse* by the Irishman, James Nihell, who had known Solano in Cadiz.[179] [h] Solano aimed to establish a therapeutic doctrine drawing equally on Hippocrates and the *Archeus:* the *physis (la naturaleza)* is the only source of true indications, showing by the pulse when it is opportune to give remedies.[180] By studying the *physis* and its dynamics the physician will realize that medicine is a certain, constant, and solid science.[181] Nihell was more purely Hippocratic and objected to the inclusion in Solano's book of "a thousand... impertinences from the Helmontian philosophy," but entirely accepted his pulse doctrine.[182] He attacked the "modern affected contempt of crises"; their judicious observation, on the contrary, is "consistent with a very vigorous method of practice."[183] [i] While some call pulse doctrine "delusive and imaginary, tending to revive in the practice of medicine the old exploded tenets of crisis established by Hippocrates," the reply is that it has been established by observation and must be refuted by observation.[184]

[h]Solano took his ideas, in turn, from John Floyer's *The Physician's Pulse-Watch. To Explain the Art of Feeling the Pulse and to Empire it by the Pulse-Watch* (London, 1707, 1710) which was itself derived from two books by former Jesuit missionaries in China: Michael Boym, *Clavis Medica ad Chinarum Doctrinam de Pulsibus* (Nuernburg, 1686) and Andreas Cleyer, *Specimen Medicinae Sinicae, sive Opuscula Medica ad Mentem Sinensium* (Frankfurt, 1692). These devote hundreds of pages to discussion of the Chinese pulse theory, and the modern European pulse doctrine is thus rooted directly in Chinese medicine. See Sprengel, *Histoire de la Medecine,* VI, 14. Bordeu notes that the Chinese are well-versed in pulse lore (*Oeuvres,* I, 257).

[i]Hippocratic medicine was always open to the criticism that it inhibited the physician's freedom of action.

His book gave many case histories where different pulse rhythms served to prognosticate crises three to four days ahead of time: a rebounding pulse at every thirtieth beat indicates a critical hemorrhage through the nose in four days; a rebounding pulse at every sixteenth beat indicates the same in three days; at every eighth heartbeat it indicates a hemorrhage in two or two and a half days. The shorter the interval between the rebounding pulses, the nearer the hemorrhage.[185]

Nihell insisted that a bloodletting or evacuation produced by the physician is not equivalent to the same operation done by the *physis:*

> Though the quantity thus evacuated may be equal or even superior to that which was to be naturally discharged, this is generally found an imperfect compensation, incapable of preventing a thousand disorders consequent to the suppression, because Nature is not relieved in that very way which the universal determination of the whole machine requires, nor this determination changed by the substituted artificial bleeding . . . on some occasions certain particular evacuations can alone discharge the body of noxious fluids or change the tone and tendency of the machine.[186]

Bordeu was very attracted by pulse doctrine and in 1754 published his 150-page *Recherches sur le Pouls par Rapport aux Crises* which added much material to that developed by Solano and Nihell.[187] He and his followers eventually distinguished more than 400 different pulses: critical, noncritical, simple pectoral, simple guttural, simple nasal followed by nosebleed, simple nasal followed by mucous secretion, the pulse presaging a copious sweat, the pulse presaging vomiting, evacuation *per anum,* evacuation *per urinas,* etc.[188]

He anticipated Rationalist criticism that life is too short to learn these subtle distinctions, that pulses resemble one another too closely, that such small differences cannot be important, etc.[189] [j] These very comments had been made to Solano, who had rightly disregarded them.[190] How can data of observation be refuted by mere theoretical objections? Pulse doctrine is based purely on practice; it is a history of observed facts; any theory must be rejected which casts doubt on such facts and thereby impedes the progress of observation.[191] The best answer to criticism of this kind (Bordeu observes) was his own experience teaching a young physician to diagnose and prognosticate from the pulse: after only four months' practice, he scarcely ever erred.[192]

There is no exact rule for pulse-taking; one learns to judge from experience.[193] Every physician has his own style, like every painter: the differences among pulses are clear and striking to physicians who have had practical experience with them.[194]

Knowledge of the different pulses is indispensable for correct practice, since they indicate both the organ where coction is taking place and the one through which the concocted *materies morbi* will be evacuated. Pulse knowledge is thus a combination of diagnosis and prognosis; it is diagnosis through prognosis.[195]

Early in the disease the pulse is not yet critical; the critical pulse comes on as the organism prepares for the crisis, and it shows where the coction will occur.[196] If coction and evacuation occur without a critical pulse, the patient will suffer a relapse, and the disease will be prolonged.[197]

Bordeu assumed that the pulse depends on the nerves of the heart and arteries.[198] All functions are a mixture of sensation and motion: the pulse is one in which motion is more evident and sensation less so. Each organ makes its contribution to the pulse, one quite imperceptible in normal

[j]A hostile obituary of Bordeu stated that his book on the pulse made his reputation even though he was only 34 years old and had scarcely had the opportunity to experience each variety of pulse two or three times: "Soon one saw young men practicing pulse-taking following Bordeu's method; the subject was interesting, enthusiasm was generated, but enthusiasm in some cases resembles a rocket in flight which starts off rapidly and, after blowing up, leaves behind nothing but a little smoke which is soon dissipated by the wind" (*Journal de Medecine, Chirurgie, Pharmacie* XLVII [1777], 184).

health but which becomes increasingly apparent as the organ prepares for a critical effort.[199] [k]

The physician assists the efforts of the *physis*.[200] Fever is the latter's principal technique, and the physician must at times augment the fever.[201] When the secretions or excretions are suspended, the physician must bring them on again, inducing vomiting, purging, sweating, etc. at the very time when the *physis* is doing the same.[202]

Bordeu attributed chronic disease to suppression of the crisis in acute diseases by wrongful use of medicines.[203] Chronic diseases have the same periods as acute but spaced at longer intervals.[204] Treatment should convert them back into acute diseases, particularly by inducing a fever.[205]

He agreed with Stahl's therapeutics but regarded it as too expectant.[206] Medicines and bloodletting are perfectly allowable if they restore a natural function or bring on a salutary hemorrhage.[207] Complex diseases should be converted into simple ones.[208] He used many of the same remedies as his colleagues: purgatives and vomitives to rid the system of acid humors, absorbants, quinine to aid the digestion, antiscorbutics, etc.[209] He held timing to be as important as the actual medicine employed.

He criticized his colleagues for their abuse of drugs and phlebotomy: "This profusion of medicines makes the disease unrecognizable and forms a major obstacle to cure . . . I seem to hear the *physis* crying out to be left alone to perform the cure."[210]

His pharmacology centered on remedies which affect the coction process. Mineral springs, for instance, can convert chronic diseases into acute ones and thus make them curable.[211] [l] Theriac he called the "masterpiece of Empiri-

[k]Modern Chinese pulse theory, of course, also associates different pulses with different internal organs. See Reuben B. Amber and Anna Babey-Brooke, *The Pulse in East and West* (New York: Santa Barbara Press, 1966).

[l]Bordeu's fondness for mineral waters is also to be explained by his inherited position as superintendant of the springs of Aquitaine. He wrote several works on the virtues of these springs (see his *Lettres Contenant des Essais sur l'Histoire des Eaux Minerales du Bearn et de Quelques Cures* [Amsterdam, 1746]).

cism"—a universal remedy with the virtues needed to cure every disease.[212] [m] It awakens the *physis* and drives away its sadness, languor, and weakness; it arouses coction and digestion and excites the body to a tumult of drunkenness; theriac succeeds in a thousand different diseases because it possesses a thousand aspects favorable to health: "it combines, so to speak, all possible tastes of all stomachs."[213] He thought a mixture of unfermented fruit pulps would be a similar universal remedy in acute diseases (presumably because their subsequent fermentation would stimulate coction): "with this and the ancient theriac one could go far in medicine."[214]

Thus Bordeu's feeling that medicines should affect the whole organism led him to mineral springs and theriac. He did not approve of specifics which were said to cure directly, bypassing the stages of coction: "Why worry about the ancients if specifics will do the trick?"[215] He doubted the existence of "alteratives": Stahl has observed that an alterative medicine is a *rara avis in terris*, and "who will oppose the voice of this reformer in medicine?"[216] Boerhaave thinks that an alterative thins the crude humor down to its natural consistency, but how can he bypass the critical days? In any case, according to Hippocrates, coction *thickens* the crude humor and prepares it for evacuation.[217] If the alterative can thin the crude humor, why wait for the *physis*.[218]

Bordeu's relations with his colleagues were hostile and unsettled, reproducing the typical conflict between Empiricism and Rationalism.

He attacked Albert von Haller at the height of the latter's reputation.[219] He criticized Boerhaave's theory of coction as entirely un-Hippocratic, and, through the pen of his close associate, Louis de la Caze, carried the attack even further: Boerhaave presents too many facts and classifies

[m]Theriac was composed of the remnents of all the prescriptions made up in a day's work by the apothecary. Claude Bernard found it still in use in early nineteenth-century France (see below, p. 643*h*).

them in a way which is useless for practice. He published his *Institutes of Medicine* and his *Aphorisms* after only seven or eight years' experience, *"et encore, d'une pratique peu heureuse."*[220] His reputation was thus due less to his own successes than to the systematic ideas he presented in his *Institutes:* "Boerhaave's very methodical mind had mastered a number of fields of knowledge: there was no more certain way of attracting the admiration of his listeners, since it is known that students–most of whom are young and avid for knowledge–are very disposed to accept as truth whatever is presented to them in a facile way. All his students thus became his passionate admirers who took home with them the ideas he had dispensed and subsequently called on him for consultation at every important occasion."[221]

This sort of assault on heroes of Rationalism was resented, and Bordeu's colleagues reciprocated in kind, ridiculing his theory of pulses as lacking theoretical justification and calling his ideas vague and contradictory.[222] "One feels that the pen was carried away by a rapid imagination which brooked no hindrance, took no time for reflection, and still less could retreat from any opinion once formulated. The author has a talent for writing, his style is often picturesque, animated, and bold, but is it always sufficiently accurate? Is it not jerky and uneven? The inexperienced reader will take sophisms for proofs, paradoxes for truths, adroitly presented inductions for axioms, isolated observations for incontestable facts."[223] Fortunately, "the paradoxes too thickly scattered through his works prevented people from being seduced."[224]

The Paris Faculté's hostility to Bordeu (who, in addition to all else, was considered an ally of the surgeons) went so far as to provoke the accusation that he had stolen the watch and snuffbox of a noble patient on a trip south to the springs of Aquitaine; the charges, countercharges, and hearings lasted three years before Bordeu was cleared.[225]

The therapeutics of P. J. Barthez carried the Iatromechanism of Sauvages to its culmination. Where the latter had interpreted disease and cure as a struggle between the "animate" and "inanimate" forces, the former left the "animate" forces out of consideration entirely, *even with respect to the curative process.*

Thus disease is not a conflict between "animate" and "inanimate" forces but represents the impact of some morbific influence on the "vital principle." "Diseases are essentially the consequence of affections of the vital principle in man . . . in general determined automatically by the action of external or internal morbific causes–in conformity with the laws (neither mechanical nor arbitrary) established by the vital principle."[226]

Of these diseases a small number, "especially the simpler ones," are amenable to cure by the "natural method."[227] Here the "vital principle" cures by producing coction and evacuation, and the physician aids either actively or by expectancy.[228] But this effort of the "vital principle" is not autonomous or spontaneous; *it is the consequence of the morbific influence itself:* "by a wonderful work of God there are several diseases . . . in which the very affections which constitute the disease can produce effects which change the behavior [*la maniere d'etre*] of the vital principle, introducing other affections which restore it to health."[229] And the power of this principle should not be exaggerated: Barthez reproached Hippocrates and Stahl for overestimating its efficacy.[230]

Thus Barthez greatly restricted the scope of the *physis* and, what is more, rejected its autonomy and spontaneity in favor of a reductionist interpretation which made it a mere reflex of the morbific influence. Thereby he enlarged the potential role of the physician. In his other two classes of disease, those responding to "empirical" and "analytical" treatment, even this reflex action of the "vital principle" disappeared completely, and treatment was by the physician alone.

"Empirical treatment" was divided into perturbative, imitative, and specific.[231]

"Perturbative" is the same as "alterative" treatment and means "substituting" for the existing disorder of the "vital principle" some other disorder which is more easily cured.[232] Barthez prescribed "perturbative" treatment for iliac colic, which cannot be treated "naturally" (since the "vital principle" is ineffectual there) or "analytically" (since the disease is one and unitary, and cannot be divided into its "elements").[233]

Here the physician does not know how his remedies operate but uses ones which experience has shown to be effective.[234] They act on the disease as a whole, not on its component "elements."[235]

"Imitative" treatment resembles "natural" treatment in imitating the action of the "vital principle": if the disease is usually cured by a hemorrhage, the physician stimulates the organism to a hemorrhage.[236]

"Specific" treatment consists in using quinine for intermittent fever, mercury for syphilis, and a few other specifics (sulphur, iodine, arsenic, etc.) which cure by incompatibility between the diseased modification of the "vital principle" and the modification introduced by the remedy.[237]

"Analytical treatment," which was Barthez' major contribution to the School of Montpellier, was used in all the complex and difficult diseases which the "vital principle" is unable to cure and which can be broken down into their "elements," i.e., the great majority of diseases to which man is subject.[238] This method shows the influence of Lavoisier's table of the chemical elements (published in 1789) and of Condillac's analysis of intellectual operations into their simplest components[239]; it was also an extension of Sauvages' attempt to define and classify all the reactions of the *Anima.*[n] Barthez thought to reduce all diseased states to their component "elements," develop a rational or empirical treatment for each "element," and in this way prescribe an individualized course of treatment for each sick person. As typical "elements" he proposed: alterations of the sensitivity, unusual acts or functions, aberrations in the chemical constitution of the humors, excess or insufficient intensity of

[n]See below, p. 459.

the vital action, lesions of the solids and fluids inhibiting the exercise of a function, etc.[240]

While he assumed some "elements" to be beneficial, the greater part were harmful and required correction. The physician sets himself *against* the "vital principle," and Barthez criticized Baglivi for teaching that the "vital principle" should never be opposed by the physician.[241]

The treatment adopted for each "element" was usually based on contraries, hence "analytical," but could also be developed empirically—by experience.[242] An unchanging and independent disease component was isolated for which treatment could be worked out by induction, following Baconian principles, and the School of Montpellier made frequent references to Bacon throughout the nineteenth century.[243] Barthez called this doctrine "reasoned empiricism," thinking (like Bacon) to have combined Empiricism and Rationalism.[244]

"Morbid elements" were the basis of Montpellier medicine for many decades after the death of Barthez. In 1815 they were given as: pain, spasm, plethora, fluxion, phlogosis, nervous erethism, erethism of the vascular system, bilious state, phlegmatic state, cachexia, putrid state, weakness, malignity, lesion of the understanding, lesion of the will or feelings, rheumatic or catarrhal state, gouty state, herpetic state, scrophulous state, rachitic state, cancerous state, periodicity, virulent infection or poisoning, foreign body, change in the composition of the tissues, tension of the tissues, relaxation of the tissues, unnatural union of organs, solution of continuity (with or without loss of substance), loss of an organ—making 32 in all.[245] During the following decades different lists of "elements" were proposed by others, with a greater or lesser number of categories. One physician had 35, another 20.[246] At mid-century J. Quissac devoted two volumes to demonstrating that there were only eleven in all.[247] Twenty years later F. A. Jaumes expanded their number to virtual infinity.[248] Some of the tables included all the phenomena of health and disease, others only those useful to therapeutics.[249]

Characteristic of all these tables of "elements" was a devotion to the sense-perceptible, as Montpellier prided itself on abjuring pathological speculation where *"le terrain est glissant."*[250] But this plunged it straightaway into the problem of the relative significance of symptoms, and Montpellier oscillated back and forth between an instinctive preference for the unusual phenomena and the necessity—inherent in its method—of focussing on the common ones.

Barthez had observed that the "rare and peculiar" facts, "provided they are credible," are of special value in formulating medical doctrine.[251] "The aberrations of the *physis* outside its customary course sometimes cast more light on obscure matters than the ordinary and regular course of the *physis.*"[252] J. Lordat, Montpellier's leading nineteenth-century philosopher, devoted the first lecture of his course in physiology to "The Necessity of Studying Rare Cases," denying the Rationalist dictum that *rara non sunt artis* and claiming with Bacon that a true induction must cover all cases—rare as well as common.[253] The physician ascertains not only the common symptoms but also those which are scarcely perceptible, which are "disdained as accidental, the anterior and fugitive circumstances, heredity, procatarctic [exciting] causes, etc., like a jury which, seeking the perpetrator of a crime, pays little attention to the depositions of certain witnesses which are seemingly weighty and legally irreproachable but draws conviction from the statements of persons which a defective legislation had formerly barred from testifying, and from accessory circumstances which had formerly been neglected and qualified as simple presumptions."[254]

This was all well and good, and quite in line with the Empirical tradition which Montpellier claimed to follow, but it was incompatible with the doctrine of "elements"—a reductionist technique designed to elucidate what differing phenomena had in common.

Thus, even though rejecting internal pathology and pathological anatomy as the foundations of disease description and treatment, Montpellier fell into the same reductionist trap as Paris.[o] A writer in 1886 observed that the "elements" are those facts and symptoms which have the most pronounced and striking character.[255] F. A. Jaumes wrote that the discipline is developed by comparing similar phenomena for what they possess in common: on this basis one elucidates the general laws governing them.[256]

> Let us then accept as certain that, however diverse, pathological species grow from a common source and are reducible to certain elementary actions; then the pathological circle becomes much smaller, and we recognize that a restricted number of modalities, associated in different ways, gives rise to a multiplicity of diseases. The possibility and utility of simplifying in this way is the *raison d'etre* of general pathology and reveals its function. All the sciences are of this same character.[257]

Stahl suffered the same fate in Montpellier as Hippocrates in the writings of Galen or Paracelsus in the Iatrochemical school: an Empirical doctrine relying on observation and experience was devitalized and restructured along Rationalist lines. Where Stahl had held that one vital force in the body is enough, Sauvages and Barthez subdivided it into "animate" and "inanimate" forces and shifted medical practice to the latter. Where Stahl had held disease to be unitary, Barthez accepted the coexistence of several different diseases in the body.[258] Where Stahl had viewed the symptoms as positive phenomena, Barthez interpreted many or most of them as negative—representing the impact of the morbific cause on the mechanical "vital principle."

While Montpellier was a valuable corrective to the pathological-anatomical excesses of nineteenth-century Paris medicine and always claimed to represent an independent Hippocratic tradition, after Barthez it veered increasingly toward Rationalism. Although rejecting the "proximate

[o]See below, Chapter VII.

cause," it established its disease classes reductively, and its treatment was largely based on "contraries."

Methodologically unstable, it could not maintain and develop an independent medical tradition, and in the late nineteenth century Montpellier fell into line behind Paris, fully accepting the dominant Rationalist assumptions in therapeutics.

NOTES

[1] "Giorgio Baglivi," in *Biographie Universelle, Ancienne et Moderne* (Paris, 1811).

[2] Partington, *History of Chemistry,* II, 653 ff.

[3] Albert Lemoine, *Le Vitalisme et l'Animisme de Stahl* (Paris: Bailliere, 1864), 33.

[4] E. S. Waterhouse, "Pietism," in *Encyclopedia of Religion and Ethics* (New York: Scribners, 1928).

[5] See *The Works of Thomas Sydenham,* I, 12, 39. Baglivi, *De Praxi Medica,* 170-176. Francois Boissier de Sauvages, *Nosologie Methodique dans Laquelle les Maladies sont Rangees par Classe suivant le Systeme de Sydenham et l'Ordre des Botanistes* (Paris: Herissant, 1770-1771), I, 110.

[6] *Oeuvres de Bordeu* (Paris: Caille et Ravier, 1818), I, iv.

[7] *Journal de Medecine, Chirurgie, Pharmacie* XLVII (1777), 182.

[8] T. Bordeu, *Dissertatio Physiologica de Sensu Generice Considerato* (Montpellier: Rochard, 1742). *Oeuvres de Bordeu,* I, iii.

[9] *Oeuvres de Bordeu,* I, 205.

[10] *Ibid.,* I, 206, 224.

[11] *Ibid.,* I, 209-252.

[12] J. Lordat, *Exposition de la Doctrine Medicale de P. J. Barthez et Memoires de la Vie de ce Medecin* (Paris: Gabon, 1818), 31 ff.

[13] Georg Ernst Stahl, *Theoria Medica Vera, Physiologiam et Pathologiam tanquam doctrinae medicae partes vere contemplativas e naturae et artis veris fundamentis intaminata ratione et inconcussa experientia sistens* (Leipzig: Choulant, 1831-1833), I, 106-109, 141, 224, 233; II, 25.

[14] *Ibid.,* I, 78, 136, 242, 252, 476, 485-486.

[15] *Ibid.,* I, 45, 75-80, 117-118, 223-224, 249-252, 474-476, 481-487.

[16] *Ibid.,* I, 27, 32, 36-37, 76, 102, 141, 224, 238, 240, 476, 481.

[17] *Ibid.,* I, 102.

[18] *Ibid.,* I, 41-43.

[19] *Ibid.,* I, 75, 107.

[20] *Ibid.,* I, 107-109, 229.

[21] *Ibid.,* I, 63-66, 74.

[22] *Ibid.,* I, 7-10, 484, 488-489.

[23] *Ibid.,* I, 17-18, 34.

[24] *Loc. cit.*

[25] *Ibid.,* I, 238-240.

[26] *Ibid.,* I, 10.

[27] *Ibid.,* I, 240.

[28] T. Blondin, ed. *Oeuvres Medico-Philosophiques et Pratiques de G. E. Stahl* (Paris: Bailliere, 1859-1864), II, 648, 660, 667.
[29] Stahl, *Theoria Medica Vera,* I, 70, 73, 110.
[30] *Ibid.,* I, 128.
[31] *Ibid.,* I, 69; II, 4.
[32] *Ibid.,* I, 481. Blondin, *Oeuvres de Stahl,* VI, 79, 255-256.
[33] Stahl, *Theoria Medica Vera,* I, 63, 68, 225.
[34] *Ibid.,* I, 75, 113, 226.
[35] *Ibid.,* I, 17-18, 22, 25, 34, 156.
[36] *Loc. cit.*
[37] *Ibid.,* I, 10, 238-240; II, 3, 77.
[38] Blondin, *Oeuvres de Stahl,* II, 711.
[39] Sauvages, *Nosologie Methodique,* I, 45, 65-78.
[40] *Ibid.,* I, 78.
[41] *Loc. cit.*
[42] *Ibid.,* I, 5-7, 14, 25, 45, 59, 63, 89.
[43] *Oeuvres de Bordeu,* I, 204-205, 224.
[44] *Ibid.,* II, 804, 831, 930.
[45] *Ibid.,* I, 45-48; II, 933-946.
[46] *Ibid.,* I, 254.
[47] *Loc. cit.*
[48] *Ibid.,* I, 254.
[49] *Ibid.,* I, 421; II, 831, 942.
[50] *Ibid.,* I, 209-253; II, 800.
[51] *Ibid.,* II, 667-669.
[52] *Loc. cit.*
[53] *Ibid.,* II, 667 668.
[54] *Ibid.,* I, 174; II, 831.
[55] *Ibid.,* II, 669.
[56] *Ibid.,* II, 839-840.
[57] *Ibid.,* II, 946.
[58] *Ibid.,* II, 946, 1006-1007.
[59] *Ibid.,* II, 1007.
[60] *Ibid.,* I, 156-157; II, 938.
[61] *Ibid.,* I, 50 ff.
[62] *Ibid.,* I, 160-162, 202-203.
[63] *Ibid.,* I, 85.
[64] *Ibid.,* I, 85, 87.
[65] *Ibid.,* I, 154.
[66] *Ibid.,* I, 1, 202-203.
[67] *Ibid.,* I, 153.
[68] *Ibid.,* I, 155, 161.
[69] *Ibid.,* I, 155.
[70] *Ibid.,* I, 162-163; II, 942.
[71] *Ibid.,* I, 156.
[72] *Ibid.,* I, 144, 157, 163.
[73] *Ibid.,* I, 144.
[74] *Ibid.,* I, 144-148.
[75] *Ibid.,* I, 144.
[76] *Ibid.,* I, 51, 144.

[77] *Ibid.*, II, 667.
[78] *Ibid.*, I, 203.
[79] *Ibid.*, I, 202.
[80] *Ibid.*, I, 203.
[81] *Ibid.*, I, 163.
[82] *Ibid.*, I, 208.
[83] *Ibid.*, II, 945.
[84] *Ibid.*, II, 951.
[85] P. J. Barthez, *Nouveaux Elements de la Science de l'Homme* (Paris: Goujon, 1806), I, 96.
[86] *Ibid.*, I, 18, 19, 33-37, 55, 85; II, 11.
[87] *Ibid.*, I, 37.
[88] *Ibid.*, I, 5.
[89] *Ibid.*, I, 40.
[90] *Ibid.*, I, 7-8.
[91] P. J. Barthez, *Nouveaux Elements de la Science de l'Homme*, I, 26, 73-74, notes: 24.
[92] *Ibid.*, I, 20.
[93] *Ibid.*, I, 19-20, 90.
[94] *Ibid.*, I, 27.
[95] *Ibid.*, I, 83.
[96] *Ibid.*, I, 84.
[97] *Ibid.*, I, 21.
[98] *Ibid.*, II, 1, 12.
[99] *Ibid.*, II, 27.
[100] *Ibid.*, II, 18, 20.
[101] *Ibid.*, I, 221, 224, 236.
[102] *Ibid.*, I, 119.
[103] *Ibid.*, I, 42, 110, notes: 96.
[104] Blondin, *Oeuvres de Stahl*, II, 651.
[105] Stahl, *Theoria Medica Vera*, I, 230, 474.
[106] *Ibid.*, I, 480.
[107] *Ibid.*, II, 73, 78; III, 4. Blondin, *Oeuvres de Stahl*, II, 681.
[108] Blondin, *Oeuvres de Stahl*, VI, 683. Stahl, *Theoria Medica Vera*, I, 119-122.
[109] Blondin, *Oeuvres de Stahl*, II, 651, 655, 671, 713. Stahl, *Theoria Medica Vera*, I, 47; II, 29, 35, 40, 41, 54.
[110] Stahl, *Theoria Medica Vera*, I, 242; II, 306.
[111] *Ibid.*, II, 86 ff.; III, 1-228.
[112] *Ibid.*, II, 35, 40, 54, 79.
[113] *Ibid.*, I, 72-73, 476-477; II, 4. Blondin, *Oeuvres de Stahl*, II, 694.
[114] Stahl, *Theoria Medica Vera*, I, 73, 151, 487; II, 41.
[115] *Ibid.*, I, 478.
[116] *Loc. cit.*
[117] Blondin, *Oeuvres de Stahl*, II, 694.
[118] "Stahlianisme, ou Mieux Stahlisme," in *Dictionnaire des Sciences Medicales* (Paris, 1821).
[119] Stahl, *Theoria Medica Vera*, I, 132, 490.
[120] *Ibid.*, I, 76, 131-132, 139-140, 150, 489; II, 31.
[121] *Ibid.*, II, 86 ff.; III, 1-128.

[122] *Ibid.*, III, 67-88.
[123] *Ibid.*, II, 195.
[124] *Ibid.*, II, 73.
[125] *Ibid.*, II, 306. Blondin, *Oeuvres de Stahl*, II, 699.
[126] Lemoine, *Le Vitalisme et l'Animisme de Stahl*, 82. E. Ackerknecht, "Aspects of the History of Therapeutics," *Bulletin of the History of Medicine* XXXVI (1962), 389-419, at 414.
[127] Stahl, *Theoria Medica Vera*, II, 150.
[128] *Ibid.*, II, 15.
[129] *Ibid.*, I, 130. Blondin, *Oeuvres de Stahl*, VI, 181.
[130] Stahl, *Theoria Medica Vera*, III, 390.
[131] *Ibid.*, II, 289. Blondin, *Oeuvres de Stahl*, VI, 181.
[132] Stahl, *Theoria Medica Vera*, II, 289.
[133] Lemoine, *Le Vitalisme et l'Animisme de Stahl*, 103.
[134] *Ibid.*, 100. Stahl, *Theoria Medica Vera*, I, 76, 156.
[135] J. Lordat, *Exposition de la Doctrine Medicale de P. J. Barthez*, 51.
[136] *Oeuvres de Bordeu*, II, 598.
[137] "Stahlianisme, ou Mieux Stahlisme," 440.
[138] P. J. Barthez, *Memoires sur le Traitement Methodique des Fluxions et sur les Coliques Iliaques qui sont Essentiellement Nerveuses* (Montpellier: Sevalle, 1816), 94.
[139] G. Harvey, *The Art of Curing Diseases by Expectation: with Remarks on a Supposed Great Case of Apoplectick Fits* (London: Partridge, 1689), 2.
[140] G. E. Stahl, *Ars Curandi cum Expectatione, Opposita Arti Curandi Nuda Expectatione. Satyra Harveana Castigata* (Paris: Horth-hemels, 1730), 16.
[141] *Loc. cit.*
[142] *Ibid.*, 136-137.
[143] Sauvages, *Nosologie Methodique*, I, 1.
[144] *Ibid.*, I, 1-2.
[145] *Ibid.*, I, 2.
[146] *Ibid.*, I, 11 (see *The Works of Thomas Sydenham*, I, 12).
[147] *Ibid.*, I, 110.
[148] *Ibid.*, I, 11.
[149] *Loc. cit.*
[150] *Ibid.*, I, 42.
[151] *Ibid.*, I, 12-13, 26.
[152] *Ibid.*, I, 12, 24.
[153] *Ibid.*, I, 25.
[154] *Ibid.*, I, 13 (Sauvages quotes from Sydenham: see *The Works of Thomas Sydenham*, I, 14).
[155] *Ibid.*, I, 26 (Sauvages quotes from Sydenham: see *The Works of Thomas Sydenham*, I, 15).
[156] *Ibid.*, I, 33 (Sauvages quotes from Baglivi, *De Praxi Medica*, 207).
[157] *Ibid.*, I, 27.
[158] *Ibid.*, I, 92-104.
[159] *Ibid.*, II, 29, 35, 40, 55.
[160] *Ibid.*, I, 12 (see *The Works of Thomas Sydenham*, I, 14).
[161] *Ibid.*, I, 112, 341-347, 351.
[162] *Ibid.*, I, 347.

[163] *Ibid.*, I, 350.
[164] *Ibid.*, I, 344.
[165] *Loc. cit.*
[166] *Ibid.*, I, 350.
[167] *Ibid.*, I, 33, 347, 350.
[168] *Ibid.*, I, 354.
[169] *Ibid.*, I, 348, 350.
[170] *Ibid.*, I, 341, 353.
[171] *Oeuvres de Bordeu*, II, 832.
[172] *Ibid.*, II, 831.
[173] *Ibid.*, II, 832.
[174] *Ibid.*, II, 839, 841.
[175] *Ibid.*, II, 856.
[176] *Ibid.*, II, 840.
[177] *Ibid.*, I, 209-252; II, 845-846.
[178] *Ibid.*, I, 251.
[179] Solano de Luques, *Idioma de la Naturaleza* (Cadiz: Geronymo de Peralta, 1737). James Nihell, *New and Extraordinary Observations Concerning the Prediction of Various Crises by the Pulse* (London: Society of Booksellers for Promoting Learning, 1741).
[180] Solano de Luques, *Idioma de la Naturaleza*, 519.
[181] *Loc. cit.*
[182] Nihell, *New and Extraordinary Observations*, xxii.
[183] *Ibid.*, 102-104.
[184] *Ibid.*, 74-79.
[185] *Ibid.*, 2.
[186] *Ibid.*, 96, 100.
[187] *Oeuvres de Bordeu*, I, 253-421.
[188] *Ibid.*, I, 256, 259, 269, 277, 281, 284, 287, 301.
[189] *Ibid.*, I, 254, 256.
[190] *Ibid.*, I, 256.
[191] *Ibid.*, I, 254, 421.
[192] *Ibid.*, I, 254.
[193] *Ibid.*, I, 261.
[194] *Ibid.*, I, 254.
[195] *Ibid.*, I, 255.
[196] *Ibid.*, I, 258-267.
[197] *Ibid.*, I, 267.
[198] *Ibid.*, I, 421.
[199] *Ibid.*, I, 420-421.
[200] *Ibid.*, II, 844-846.
[201] *Ibid.*, II, 846.
[202] *Ibid.*, I, 45; II, 794, 844-846.
[203] *Ibid.*, II, 847.
[204] *Loc. cit.*
[205] *Loc. cit.*
[206] *Ibid.*, I, 224.
[207] *Ibid.*, II, 795.
[208] *Ibid.*, II, 845.
[209] *Ibid.*, I, 443-444; II, 931.

[210] *Ibid.*, II, 794, 795.

[211] *Ibid.*, II, 806, 844, 914-929.

[212] *Ibid.*, II, 564.

[213] *Loc. cit.*

[214] *Ibid.*, II, 565-566.

[215] *Ibid.*, I, 173, 228.

[216] *Ibid.*, I, 173.

[217] *Ibid.*, I, 228.

[218] *Loc. cit.*

[219] Lordat, *Exposition de la Doctrine Medicale de P. J. Barthez,* 54.

[220] *Loc. cit.* Louis de la Caze, *Idee de l'Homme Physique et Morale, Pour Servir d'Introduction a un Traite de Medecine* (Paris: Guerin et Delatour, 1755), 47, 51.

[221] *Ibid.*, 54.

[222] *Journal de Medecine, Chirurgie, Pharmacie* XLII (1774), 314.

[223] *Ibid.*, XLVII (1777), 184, 186.

[224] *Ibid.*, XLVII (1777), 180.

[225] Gaston Castaigna, *Etude sur Bordeu* (Montpellier Thesis, 1878), 114-120.

[226] Barthez, *Nouveaux Elements,* I, 43-44.

[227] *Loc. cit.* P. J. Barthez, *Memoire sur le Traitement Methodique des Fluxions,* 89, 92. Lordat, *Exposition de la Doctrine Medicale de P. J. Barthez,* 294-295.

[228] Lordat, *Exposition de la Doctrine Medicale de P. J. Barthez,* 295. P. J. Barthez, *Traite des Maladies Goutteuses* (Paris: Deterville, 1802), I, xi. Barthez, *Nouveaux Elements,* I, notes: 26-27.

[229] Barthez, *Nouveaux Elements,* I, 44.

[230] *Ibid.*, I, notes: 26-27. Barthez, *Memoire sur le Traitement Methodique des Fluxions,* 91-92.

[231] Barthez, *Traite des Maladies Goutteuses,* I, xv.

[232] *Loc. cit.*

[233] Barthez, *Memoire sur le Traitement Methodique des Fluxions,* 89-90.

[234] Lordat, *Exposition de la Doctrine Medicale de P. J. Barthez,* 302-303.

[235] *Loc. cit.*

[236] Barthez, *Traite des Maladies Goutteuses,* I, xvi.

[237] *Ibid.*, I, xvii. Lordat, *Exposition de la Doctrine Medicale de P. J. Barthez,* 306-307.

[238] Lordat, *Exposition de la Doctrine Medicale de P. J. Barthez,* 296. Barthez, *Memoire sur le Traitement Methodique des Fluxions,* 94-99.

[239] Lordat, *Exposition de la Doctrine Medicale de P. J. Barthez,* 289-290. Barthez, *Nouveaux Elements,* I, notes: 19-21.

[240] Lordat, *Exposition de la Doctrine Medicale de P. J. Barthez,* 125-127, 289-290.

[241] *Ibid.*, 71, 290-292.

[242] Francois de la Mure, *Nouveaux Elements de Matiere Medicale* (Montpellier: Tournel, 1784), 239-241, 386-393 *et passim.* J. Quissac, *De la Doctrine des Elements et de son Application a la Medecine-Pratique* (Montpellier: Sevalle, 1850), I, 193 ff.

[243]Barthez, *Nouveaux Elements,* I, 3. J. Lordat, *Essai d'une Caracteristique de l'Enseignement Medicale de Montpellier* (Montpellier: Castel, 1843), 7, 32. J. Lordat, *Premiere Lecon du Cours de Physiologie* (Montpellier: Martel, 1840), 26. J. Lordat, *De la Necessite de Creer dans Chaque Faculte de Medecine une Chaire de Philosophie Naturelle Inductive* (Montpellier: Castel, 1846), *passim.*

[244]J. Lordat, *Exposition de la Doctrine Medicale de P. J. Barthez,* 72.

[245]"Elements," *Dictionnaire des Sciences Medicales* XI (Paris, 1813), 58 ff.

[246]"Elements," *Dictionnaire Encyclopedique des Sciences Medicales, Premiere Serie,* 33 (1886), 380-404, at 394.

[247]J. Quissac, *De la Doctrine des Elements,* I, 8.

[248]F. A. Jaumes, *Traite de Pathologie et de Therapeutique Generales* (Paris: Masson, 1869).

[249]"Elements," *Dictionnaire Encyclopedique des Sciences Medicales,* 33 (1886), 397.

[250]*Ibid.,* 402.

[251]Barthez, *Nouveaux Elements,* I, 29.

[252]*Ibid.,* II, 6.

[253]J. Lordat, *Premiere Lecon du Cours de Physiologie,* 12, 15, 24, 26, *et passim.*

[254]J. Lordat, *Exposition de la Doctrine Medicale,* 66-67.

[255]"Elements," *Dictionnaire Encyclopedique des Sciences Medicales,* 33 (1886), 403.

[256]F. A. Jaumes, *Traite de Pathologie et de Therapeutique Generales,* 1-2.

[257]*Ibid.,* 2.

[258]J. Lordat, *Exposition de la Doctrine Medicale,* 297.

CHAPTER V

FROM RATIONALISM TO METHODISM: WILLIAM CULLEN AND JOHN BROWN

While the Stahlian tradition was undergoing Rationalization in Montpellier, the Boerhaavian legacy was being transformed into Methodism.

Medical Rationalism aims to reduce the data of experience to a limited number of hypothesized "causes" at work in the organism and its environment. Methodism is the final stage in this process, with the variety of proximate causes accepted by medicine limited to a mere two or three.

Methodism first appeared in history just prior to the Christian era, out of the wreckage of pre-Galenic Rationalism.[a] It reemerged in the physiology of Descartes and the therapeutics of his followers. And it came to the fore a third time in the systems of William Cullen (1710-1790) and his disciple, John Brown (1735-1788).

Ancient Methodism was based on the atomic or corpuscular theory of Democritus, Epicurus, and Lucretius. Descartes also adopted a corpuscular theory. But physiological processes could be simplified in other ways as well, and the Scottish Methodists looked rather to the ebb and flow of nervous energy for the ultimate determinants of disease and health. Their hypotheses about nervous energy yielded therapeutic doctrines identical in structure to those of the ancient Methodist School.[b]

[a]See *Divided Legacy,* I, 291-301.

[b]For more discussion of Methodism see below, pp. 653, 675, 690 ff.

Biographical

The son of the estate agent of a Scottish nobleman, Cullen studied surgery and practiced several years as a surgeon before graduating as a physician in 1740 at Glasgow. In 1751 he became professor of medicine at this university, in 1757 he began to give clinical lectures at the hospital, and in 1766 he became professor of the theory and practice of medicine at Edinburgh where he remained. His *Lectures on the Materia Medica* (1772), *Treatise of the Materia Medica* (1789), *Synopsis of Methodical Nosology* (1772), and *First Lines of the Practice of Physic* (1778) shaped the thinking of generations of students and were considered the acme of late eighteenth-century medical progress.

Cullen's most famous pupil was John Brown, the son of a farm worker. His father died early, and Brown's stepfather, a weaver, at first apprenticed him to this trade, but the lad's great intellectual promise at length induced family and friends to allow him an education. He acquired great proficiency in Latin and in his early twenties earned a living tutoring the Edinburgh medical students in this language, translating their theses into Latin, and, if need be, writing the theses himself.[c] He frequented medical lectures for more than ten years where he was befriended by Cullen and eventually taken into the latter's home as tutor and instructor of his children.

[c]He was "at all times ready to furnish an original dissertation according to the system his employer preferred" (the fee for a translation was only five guineas, for an original composition—ten). Opinions as to Brown's Latinity differ according to the political standpoint of the commentator. The *Dictionary of National Biography* remarks on "the purity of his Latin style," while the posthumous editor of Brown's *Elements of Medicine* (translated by Brown himself from his own Latin original) writes: "In his translation Dr. Brown seems to have exceeded his usual negligence. His English, it is true, when he is unfettered by the Latin idiom, shows that he was poorly qualified to do his own work justice, had he exerted his utmost care—These two causes conspired with the laboured perplexity of his Latin style to render the translation disgustingly uncouth throughout . . . nor do I doubt but that the author considered his Latin text as sacred, both on account of the purity of the style and the excellence of the doctrine . . . few readers, I conceive, will regard it with the same reverence" (John Brown, *Elements of Medicine* [Portsmouth, New Hampshire: Treadwell, 1804], iv, xxii).

For a while the two were intimate friends, Brown repeating in the evening the lecture which Cullen gave in the morning, but they fell out over Brown's application for the post of professor of theoretical medicine.[d] Thereupon Brown developed his own system, which he preached and propagated with some success among the medical students—even though his suspected sympathizers were rigorously failed on examination.

Brown's years as a perpetual student came to an end in 1779: since the Edinburgh degree was barred to him, he obtained one from St. Andrew's and set up as a private instructor in medicine.[e] Although popular with the younger men, his irregular habits and spendthrift nature landed him for a time in debtor's prison (where he continued to lecture), and he finally removed to London where he died in 1788 of a stroke.

His only important work was the *Elementa Medicinae* (1780) which sets forth his doctrines in wearisome and repetitive detail. Of all medical systems known to history this most peculiarly bore the personal imprint of its inventor: Brown suffered from gout and, finding that whiskey and opium relieved his pain—most effectively when consumed at the same time, he spun a whole theory of health and disease from this single observation. He lectured with a glass of whiskey and opium on the lectern; red meat and "diffusible stimulants" had a prominent role in his therapeutics; and the drug-addiction and drunkenness which his system promoted contributed greatly to its roaring popularity.

Some have thought that Brownism (also called Brunonianism) was conceived purely to spite Cullen, or perhaps as a hoax, but Brown was sincere and honest despite his marked

[d]Brown did not have Cullen's support for this application, and when the magistrates entrusted with the appointment asked who this unknown candidate was, Cullen "after some real or affected hesitation, is said to have exclaimed in the vulgar dialect of the country: 'Why, sure, this can never be our Jock!" (Brown, *Elements of Medicine,* xxvi).

[e]Brown's attitude toward therapeutics becomes easier to comprehend when it is realized that he practiced little or no medicine himself but made a living first as a translator and then as a teacher.

failings, "a legitimate physician and in no sense a quack or charlatan."[1] He was endlessly charitable to his friends and followers, which helps explain his perpetual poverty. And his teachings, while bizarre to modern eyes, make some sense when seen as a reaction against the sadistic modes of treatment of the times—especially in public hospitals.

The system's fantastic simplification of diagnosis and therapeutics brought it many adherents after Brown's death, and it was an important component of medical practice in the early nineteenth century.

The Definition of Life. Physiology

The thinking of Cullen and Brown was the final stage of Rationalism's effort to come to terms with Stahl's *Anima.*

By postulating the existence of this vegetative soul which governs and controls the movements of the body the Halle philosopher had deflected attention from Boerhaave's chemical and hydraulic humoralism and placed on the agenda the idea that the body is a system of solids moved by forces. Stahl's personality and the power of his arguments led to a certain acceptance of his ideas. As has been noted, Frederick Hoffmann recognized the *Anima* and made provision for it in his system. But Rationalism instinctively rejects the concept of an autonomous or indeterminate force in the organism, and it was more natural for Hoffmann (and others) to materialize or hypostatize the *Anima* as immanent energy bound to, and determined by, the body's solids. His "spasm" and "atony," reflexes of the heart's systole and diastole and determining each a whole class of diseases, were an effort to narrow down the *Anima's* autonomy and purposiveness in the same way that Sauvages' "inanimate" forces encroached on the "animate."

> Only spasm and simple atony, by disturbing and perverting the equal, free, and proportionate movement of the blood and all similar fluids (by which the succession of excretions and integrity of the *Anima* and the body are caused to flourish) undermine and destroy the whole vital

> economy; from this it appears that a universal pathology can more correctly and easily be deduced and explained from vitiated microcosmic motions in the solids than from the various affections of vitiated humors. Thus all internal diseases are to be referred to preternatural affections of a nervous type . . . Attentive observation teaches that all kinds of morbific movements principally have their seat and exercise their tyranny in the nervous parts of the body whose channels derive their strength from systolic and diastolic motion . . . All causes of disease have their most powerful effect on the parts endowed with motion and sense.[2]

Hoffmann saw this as an improvement on Boerhaavian orthodoxy ("on all of these matters the accepted doctrine of medicine preserves a lofty silence"), reflecting the great volume of research on the nervous system in the early eighteenth century.[3]

The next advance in neurological research came fifteen years later with Albert von Haller's *Dissertation on the Sensible and Irritable Parts of Animals* (1753).[4] Where Boerhaave had ascribed to all parts of the body both "sensitivity" (the capacity to feel pain) and "irritability" (the capacity to contract when stimulated), Haller refined the analysis, showing that certain parts (the nerves and the solids endowed with nerves) possess sensitivity, others (the muscles) irritability, and still others (the heart, stomach, intestines, etc.) both sensitivity and irritability.[5]

Like Hoffmann, Haller was arguing against Stahl and his followers: they hold that the "tone" and "natural contraction" of the fibers (i.e., their irritability) are due to the *Anima,* but, "as they have always had an aversion to anatomy, they have made no experiments to illustrate this."[6] The solids are not moved by the *Anima* but by an immanent quality of the solids themselves: "neither irritability depends upon the *Anima,* nor is the *Anima* what we call irritability in the body."[7] Irritability "does not depend upon the nerves but on the original fabric of the parts which are susceptible of it."[8]

> What therefore should hinder us from granting irritability to be a property of the animal *gluten,* the same as we acknowledge attraction and gravity to be properties of matter in general, without being able to determine the cause of them. Experiments have taught us the existence of this property, and doubtless it is owing to a physical cause which depends upon the arrangement of the ultimate particles, though the experiments that we can make are too gross to investigate them.[9]

Thus, in Haller's view, the body possesses an immortal soul whose "indestructibility by death is proved by a very common phenomenon, for many people, when their bodily powers are wasted and spent, give evident proofs of a highly serene, vigorous, and even cheerful mind."[10] [f] But Stahl's *Anima* has disappeared, reduced by Haller's 190 vivisectionist experiments[g] to (1) the "irritability" and (2) Sauvages' "nervous fluid . . . thin and invisible and destitute of all taste and smell"[11] which coordinates the movements of the organism and provides it with sensitivity.

The Stahlians, who viewed the nerves as vibrating cords connecting the *Anima* in the brain to all parts of the organism, were triumphantly refuted, and the Galenic "animal" and "vital" spirits—under the name of "nervous fluid"—were restored to their traditional role of filling the cracks and chinks in a reductionist theory of physiology.[12] [h]

To prove that irritability is independent of the *Anima* Haller demonstrated that the irritable parts of the body are least subject to the will or the mind.[13] To prove it a

[f] *L'Homme Machine* (1748) by De la Mettrie (1709-1751) had sought to explain even the immortal soul in terms of irritability. This was indignantly rejected by Haller (*Dissertation,* 3, 45).

[g] "A species of cruelty for which I felt such a reluctance as could only be overcome by the desire of contributing to the benefit of mankind" (*Dissertation,* 7).

[h] Haller was instinctively hostile to Bordeu's neo-Hippocratism in which the glands, as the agents of the *physis,* performed functions of coction and evacuation. He declared, in opposition to the latter, that the glands possess very *few* nerves rather than very many (*Dissertation,* 23).

property of matter he removed the heart and other muscles from animals and found that for days and even weeks they retained the capacity to contract.[14]

Naturally, the heart as the most vital organ is also the most irritable.[15] The cause of its motion, and of the motion of other irritable muscles, lies "in the muscles themselves."[16] "Wherefore the heart is moved by some unknown cause, which neither depends upon the brain nor the arteries but lays concealed in the very structure of the heart itself."[17] "Perpetual irritation alone [is] the cause of the continuation of motion in the vital organs."[18]

> When the auricle is relaxed, it is filled by the muscular force of the contiguous veins, and so the heart in like manner contracts itself, when it is irritated by the blood conveyed through the auricle. Therefore, the heart, when it has received the blood, in consequence of that irritability and stimulus by which its fibers are excited to action, contracts, empties itself of the blood, and, being freed from the stimulus, rests and becomes relaxed . . . Nor do I believe any thing more required than a continual stimulus applied to a part irritable in the highest degree.[19]

"Life" (just as with Hoffmann) was identified with the heart considered as a *perpetuum mobile.* And aging and dying were interpreted in the same terms. As it grows older the heart becomes less irritable: "the nerves become more and more callous and insensible to the impressions of the senses, and the muscles to irritation; thus the contractile force of the heart, and the frequency of its pulsations, is diminished, and therefore every force which impels the blood into the ultimate vessels."[20] "The heart becomes unable to propel the blood to the extremities, the pulse and heat desert the feet and hands . . . now the heart itself, being totally deprived of its powers, and not irritable by the blood to any effectual motion, cannot propel the blood through the lungs, that the aorta may receive its due quantity."[21] "I shall call that death when the heart has become totally deprived of irritability."[22]

The physician need not look behind the sensitivity and irritability:

> The theory why some parts of the human body are endowed with these properties, while others are not, I shall not at all meddle with. For I am persuaded that the source of both lies concealed beyond the reach of the knife and microscope, beyond which I do not choose to hazard many conjectures.[23]

In other words, the physician need give no thought to an autonomous vital principle. The living body has become an "irritable" solid whose motions can be defined, determined, and classified *a priori.*[i]

Cullen was trained in the system of Boerhaave, "and even when I came to take a professor's chair in [Edinburgh] University, I found that system here in its entire and full force."[24] His own research aimed to replace this dominant humoralism by a greater concern for the solids and their motions:

> Although it cannot be denied that the fluids of the human body suffer various morbid changes; and that upon these diseases may primarily depend; yet I must beg leave to maintain that the nature of these changes is seldom understood, and more seldom still is it known when they have taken place: that our reasonings concerning them have been, for the most part, purely hypothetical; have therefore contributed nothing to improve, and have often misled, the practice of physic. In this particularly they have been hurtful, that they have

[i]The word, "irritability," with which Haller hypostatized Stahl's *Anima,* had been popularized in the medical vocabulary seventy-five years earlier by Francis Glisson (1597-1677) in an attempt to subject the Helmontian *Archeus* to the same reduction. Glisson defined "irritability" as a "natural perception" dependent upon the *Archeus.* See Owsei Temkin, "The Classical Roots of Glisson's Doctrine of Irritation," *Bulletin of the History of Medicine* XXXVIII (1964), 297-328, at 325; Walter Pagel, "Harvey and Glisson on Irritability With a Note on Van Helmont," *Bulletin of the History of Medicine* XLI (1967), 497-514, at 500; Stephan D'Irsay, *Albrecht von Haller: Eine Studie zur Geistesgeschichte der Aufklaerung* (Leipzig: Georg Thieme, 1930), 46-56.

> withdrawn our attention from, and prevented our study of, the motions of the animal system, upon the state of which the phenomena of diseases do more certainly and generally depend.[25]

Here the pioneering breakthrough was Hoffmann's discovery that the fluids are governed by the "microcosmic motions" of the solids, and ultimately by the spasm and atony of the heart.[26] However, Hoffmann was still too infected with Stahl's *Anima* and the associated (humoral) "plethora."[27] Hence Cullen (who translated Haller's *Primae Lineae Physiologiae* into English) modified Hoffmann by incorporating into his physiology the concepts of sensitivity and irritability.[28]

He divides the body's solids into "simple" and "vital," the former identical with inanimate matter and the latter endowed with both *vis insita* and "nervous power" from the brain.[29] Thus the "vital" solids possess both sensitivity and irritability, and Cullen—whose thinking generally effaces distinctions among concepts—assimilated the *vis insita* (irritability) and "nervous power" (sensitivity) to each other: "it is probable that the nervous and inherent powers are somewhat of the same nature; and it is also probable that, in entire and living bodies, both the nervous and inherent powers have a constant dependence upon the animal."[30]

"Life," then, "so far as it is corporeal, we suppose to consist in the excitement of the nervous system, and especially of the brain, which unites the different parts and forms them into a whole."[31]

As Cullen debased Haller's physiology, so Brown debased Cullen's, building on his definition of "life" as "excitement of the nervous system" to develop a whole doctrine. To Brown "life" is "excitability," an unknown quantity which fills the organism and follows its own laws.[32] Each person is fueled at birth with sufficient "excitability" to last him until old age if burned at a normal rate. The flames of this combustive process are called by Brown "excitement," and excitability is enkindled into "excitement" by various external and internal "exciting powers"—just as a fire is made to burn more brightly by adding air. If the "exciting powers" are too strong, the "excitability" is used up too rapidly (the body is in a state of excess "excitement"), and if the "exciting powers" are too weak, there is too little "excitement" (like a fire which is smothered through lack of air). Health consists in a balance between the inherent "excitability" and the internal or external "exciting powers."[33]

Pathology and Therapeutics. The Classification of Diseases

Both Cullen and Brown defined "disease" as a deviation from normal physiology, and therapeutics as restoring the physiology to normality.

Cullen divided most existing diseases into four classes in function of the flux of nervous energy through the organism: a) those in which the nervous energy is weak or debilitated, b) those in which the flow of energy is blocked or intermittent, c) those in which the body is diseased without any apparent disturbance in the flow of energy, and d) local diseases involving weakness or impairment of energy flow.[34] [j]

His first class, the "fevers," includes the greatest number of diseases, and Cullen gives a precise analysis of the causal relationships which bring on a "fever." Finding that all "fevers" can be divided into a stage of "debility," a "hot" stage, and a "cold" stage, Cullen connects the three stages as follows:

> Our doctrine of fever is explicitly this: the remote causes are certain sedative powers applied to the nervous system, which, diminishing the energy of the brain, thereby produce a debility in the whole of the functions, and particularly in the action of the extreme vessels. Such, however, is, at the same time, the nature of the animal economy that this debility proves an indirect

[j] He admits that some diseases may have been overlooked, about some others too little is known, and a third group do not fit his nosology (William Cullen, *A Synopsis of Methodical Nosology* [Philadelphia: Parry Hall, 1793], xi).

> stimulus to the sanguiniferous system; whence, by the intervention of the cold stage, and spasm connected with it, the action of the heart and larger arteries is increased and continues so till it has had the effect of restoring the energy of the brain, of extending this energy to the extreme vessels, of restoring therefore their action, and thereby especially overcoming the spasm affecting them; upon the removing of which the excretion of sweat, and other marks of the relaxation of excretories, takes place.[35]

He introduces the *vis medicatrix naturae* (the *physis*) at various points in his reasoning to assure the necessary connections among the stages:

> How the state of debility produces some of the symptoms of the cold stage may perhaps be readily explained, but how it produces all of them I cannot explain otherwise than by referring the matter to a general law of the animal economy whereby it happens that powers which have a tendency to hurt and destroy the system often excite such motions as are suited to obviate the effects of the noxious power. This is the *vis medicatrix naturae,* so famous in the schools of physic, and it seems probable that many of the motions excited in fever are the effects of this power.[36]
>
> The idea of fever, then, may be that a spasm of the extreme vessels, however induced, proves an irritation to the heart and arteries, and that this continues until the spasm is relaxed or overcome . . . It will still, however, remain a question what is the cause of this spasm; whether it be directly produced by the remote causes of fever, or if it be only a part of the operation of the *vis medicatrix naturae.*[37]

Hoffmann's "spasm" is, clearly, well provided for in Cullen's etiology of fever. His "atony" has been transformed into "debility" of the nervous functions. But the word, "atony," itself is also employed: "the symptoms of anorexia, nausea, and vomiting . . . depend upon a state of debility or loss of tone in the muscular fibers of the stomach [and] it may be presumed that these symptoms in the beginning of fever depend upon an atony communicated to the muscular fibers of the stomach from the muscular fibers of the extreme vessels on the surface of the body."[38]

Hence "atony," resulting from a "diminution of the energy of the brain," is a principal component of the proximate cause of fever.[39]

Treatment is with contraries, applied to the various stages of fever. The reaction of the sanguiniferous system is moderated by bloodletting, acids, neutral salts, purges, sedatives, and exercise. "Spasm" in the peripheral vessels is reduced or eliminated by diluents, neutral salts, sudorifics, emetics, antispasmodics such as opium and camphor, blistering, and warm baths. Underlying debility or "atony" is remedied by tonics and stimulants which increase the power of the heart. And the tendency of the body's fluids to putrefaction is obviated or corrected by fresh air, changing the bed-clothes, avoidance of meat, frequent evacuation of the intestines, diuretics, sudorifics, diluents, and antiseptic medicines administered internally.[40]

Cullen provided equally complex etiologies for the various *sequelae* of "fever," and they also were treated by contraries. Hemorrhage, for instance, is due to "some inequality in the distribution of the blood [which] occasions a congestion in particular parts of the sanguiniferous system; that is, a greater quantity of blood is poured into certain vessels than their natural capacity is suited to receive. These vessels become, thereby, preternaturally distended; and this distension proving a stimulus to them, excites their action to a greater degree than usual, which, pushing the blood with unusual force into the extremities of those vessels, opens them by anastomosis or rupture."[41] It is treated with cold air, cold drinks, astringent remedies such as alum, lead, or iron, and, finally, by quinine and bloodletting.[42]

Inflammation ("some causes of inequality in the distribution of the blood may throw an unusual quantity of it upon particular vessels, to which it must necessarily prove a stimulus") is treated: 1) with alkaline remedies if caused by an acid, and with acid remedies if caused by an alkali; 2) otherwise with demulcent (saponaceous) medicines; and 3) the underlying "spasm" is removed with blisters, sinapisms, and warm baths.[43]

Cullen's second class, called "neuroses" or "nervous diseases," are "all those preternatural affections of sense or motion which are without pyrexia as part of the primary disease; and all those which do not depend upon a topical affection of the organs, but upon a more general affection of the nervous system . . . they consist either in the interruption and debility of the powers of sense and motion or in the irregularity with which these powers are exercised."[44] [k]

A typical member of this class is apoplexy: "occasioned either by some compression of the origin of the nerves or by something destroying the mobility of the nervous power."[45] Most commonly it is due to an accumulation of blood in the brain which presses on the nerve, and it is treated by bloodletting, purging, and blistering.[46]

His third class, the "cachexies," are defined as "a depraved state of the whole, or of a considerable part, of the habit of the body, without any primary pyrexia or neurosis combined with that state."[47] To these diseases (including scrophula, rickets, syphilis, scurvy, jaundice, elephantiasis, and others) Cullen cannot assign a proximate cause and occasionally falls back on the concept of inheritance or constitutional predisposition.[l] He resorts to traditional therapies without (usually) providing any explanation. Rickets, for instance, arises from "some weakness, and pretty frequently from a scrophulous habit, in the mother . . . a predisposition . . . from the parents."[48] "The nature of [scrophula] is not easily to be ascertained. It seems to be a peculiar affection of

[k]He observed that this is to some extent a misnomer, since every disease affects the nervous system: "neuroses" proper are those "which attack that system almost alone or at least primarily and do not affect the circulation at the same time, nor the disposition or state of the fluids unless secondarily" (*A Synopsis of Methodical Nosology,* 86).

[l]On "predisposing causes" see below pp. 466-468.

the lymphatic system . . . probably, however, there is a peculiar acrimony of the fluids that is the proximate cause of the disease; although of what nature this is, has not yet been discovered."[49] Syphilis is "most commonly contracted in consequence of coition with an infected person, but in what manner the infection is communicated is not clearly explained."[50] It is treated with mercurials.[51]

Cullen's "local diseases"—his fourth class—are also (distantly) associated with spasm and atony and include: blindness, deafness, satyriasis, nymphomania, hemorrhages, enuresis, gonorrhoea ("preternatural flux of a humor from the urethra in males, with or without lust"), constipation, amenorrhoea, tumors, aneurism, herpes, *tinea capitis,* psora ("pustules and itching, little ulcers, contagious, afflicting the hand"), fractures, caries of the bones, and many others.[52] Gonorrhoea (regarded as a variety of syphilis) is treated by diet, bloodletting, injections of lead and other astringents into the urethra, and mercury in obstinate cases.[53] "As most of the symptoms arise from the irritation of a stimulus applied, the effects of this irritation may often be lessened by diminishing the irritability of the system; and it is well known that the most certain means of accomplishing this is by employing opium."[54]

In discussing his nosological method Cullen employed the traditional concepts of *propria* and *communia,* analyzing their relationship to the proximate cause.

Previous nosologists, such as Sauvages, have "overdone the thing" by failing to distinguish the "common and inseparable" symptoms from the "uncommon symptoms and those not necessarily connected." "Whilst they were endeavoring to render the history of disorders very full, which might assist to distinguish one from another, they have missed it; nay, they have made it more difficult."[55] In particular, they have considered certain diseases as primary when actually they were only symptomatic variants of others.[56]

Cullen prided himself on having reduced the number of disease genera: "many that are accounted for and set down as different by others, are no ways different, and therefore placed by us under one head."[57] He did this by choosing, as his criteria of classification, the *communia* and the proximate cause.

His classification started with the symptoms, "the external marks that are easily to be observed, having let alone, or rather rejected, any conjectures about the internal state of the body. Moreover, I have always rather preferred those perceptible symptoms such as were obvious to the physician than those perceived by the patient."[58] Diseases are to be distinguished into genera on the basis of "the general as well as the more particular symptoms."[59]

In other words, he preferred the *communia,* which are "easily to be observed," to the *propria* which required attentive examination of the patient or were elicited only by questioning him.

If the patient lacked some of the essential symptoms of the given species, his disease was regarded as a "variety" or sub-species. When he manifested additional symptoms, "if the added ones can rather be looked upon as symptoms of symptoms than symptoms of the cause of the disorder, they only constitute a variety." "Again, when the added symptoms are altogether unusual to the given species, and at the same time the chief circumstances of the disorder appear little or not at all altered, this also is to be looked upon as a variety . . . Likewise, the genus may be of a different species from the diversity of its seat; but as often as neither the structure of the part nor the mode of function differs, although the seat be different, this is nevertheless to be looked upon only as a variety."[60] [m]

In any case, it is clearly necessary to distinguish symptoms into degrees of significance, and Cullen criticized Joseph Lieutaud's *Synopsis of the Universal Practice of Medicine*

[m]He holds that "species are formed by nature," suggesting that the genera are artificial constructions, but he then states that a nosology is essential ("for if anyone denies this, he might as well have said that there is nothing in the medical art") and that treatment must be accommodated to the genus as well as to the species and the sub-species (*A Synopsis of Methodical Nosology,* vii, ix, xiv).

(1765), written on Hippocratic and Empirical principles, as merely a mass of symptoms, manifesting a "total want of method, arrangement, system, or decision."[61] [n] "The distinction of the genera of diseases, the distinction of the species of each, and often even that of the varieties, I hold to be a necessary foundation of every plan of physic, whether Dogmatical or Empirical. But very little of this distinction is to be found in the work of Mr. Lieutaud . . . his method of managing his subject must certainly interrupt and retard all methodical nosology."[62]

He further criticized Lieutaud for neglecting the study of proximate causes and for failing to associate his symptoms with anatomical changes.[63] In view of the work done by Morgagni on the causes and seats of diseases "it may well seem surprising that Lieutaud should find the whole of proximate causes *atra caligine mersas*[o] and that he should never have thought of applying his dissections toward the ascertaining of at least some of these."[64] [p]

Thus, while symptoms are important, the character of a disease is mainly determined by its cause.[65] Diseases with the same symptoms can differ in their "nature" or "proximate cause" and thus demand different modes of treatment.[66] "Some similarity of the cause argues a similarity of the disorder produced by it," especially in the case of contagious diseases.[67] [q] Cullen decided that this is true also for most "epidemic fevers," disputing Sydenham who had regarded

[n]Lieutaud (1703-1780) studied medicine at Aix-en-Provence and then at Montpellier. He eventually became physician to Louis XV. His writings emphasized the importance of the *physis*, the relative lack of efficacy of medicines, the impossibility of discovering proximate causes, and the ignorance of physicians (see Joseph Lieutaud, *Synopsis of the Universal Practice of Medicine. Exhibiting a Concise View of all Diseases, Both Internal and External: Illustrated with Complete Commentaries.* [Philadelphia: Richard Parker, 1816], 2-9).

[o]"immersed in darkness"

[p]The *De sedibus et causis morborum per anatomen indagatis libri quinque* (Venice, 1761) of Giovanni Baptista Morgagni (1682-1772) was a major effort to associate disease symptoms with internal pathological alterations.

[q]But, on the other hand, he argues that *contagia* have only one effect on the organism—that of increasing debility (see below, p. 295).

these later as differing one from the other according to the prevailing constitution.[68]

Brown carried nosological simplification to ridiculous lengths, arranging all diseases along a spectrum representing the balance between the body's "excitability" and the external or internal "exciting powers." When the latter are weak, the "excitability" is not sufficiently aroused, "excitement" is low, and the patient suffers from one of the "asthenic" diseases marked by "direct debility." If the "exciting powers" are somewhat too strong, the "excitement" rises, and the patient has a "sthenic" disease. If these powers are much too strong, the "excitement" is at a peak: this leads to collapse, with an ensuing train of diseases of "indirect debility."

Brown urged the physician to ignore most symptoms in assigning diseases to one class or another: "Though excitement regulates all the phenomena of life, yet the symptoms of diseases which either its excess or deficiency produces, *do not of themselves lead to any proper judgment respecting it;* on the contrary, their fallacious appearance has proved the source of infinite error."[69] [r]

> The mistake of symptoms in consequence of judging of their interior nature from the similarity or dissimilarity of their appearance is [a] false idea . . . it is to be observed that symptoms the most similar to each other in their appearance are, in reality, the most different, and those that have the least resemblance in their appearance have the nearest affinity in their interior nature, and indeed are one and the same, with no other difference but a difference of degree, and even that often very slight, sometimes next to none at all. The great variety of symptoms that distinguish the whole form of asthenic diseases affords . . . many proofs of the truth of this proposition.[70]

[r]How did he square this with his boast to be "a sure and cautious observer of the phenomena of nature . . . to view every object of observation by nature's clearest light"? (*Elements of Medicine,* 215). See below, pp. 692 ff.

He had a low opinion of the efforts of nosologists, who cannot see the forest for the trees: "The truth is that systematics, who were otherwise no nosologists, have made too much work about eruptive and contagious diseases, and have never dived into the interior nature either of them or almost of any other. They have all followed each other from their first leader, and never once deigned to turn a glance of their eye upon the phenomena of nature as these arose before them. Hippocrates misled his followers, they misled theirs from age to age, and they all misled the poor nosologists."[71]

But the physician should also ignore all proximate and other causes: their discussion "must cease in the medical language, and attention will be turned away from the endless pursuit of distinctions without a difference to the study of the solid and useful facts that nature holds up to contemplation in great abundance."[72]

These "solid and useful facts" are precisely the most common of the *communia*. "The onset of every sthenic disease is announced by shivering . . . the pulse is stronger, harder, fuller, and somewhat more frequent than in the healthy state . . . redness of the surface of the body which is often preceded by paleness . . . delirium . . . thirst and heat . . . etc."[73] And the asthenic diseases? "Shivering is not unusual at the commencement of asthenic diseases of any considerable severity . . . the pulse is weak, small, soft, and very quick . . . paleness and dryness of the skin . . . checked perspiration . . . headache . . . delirium . . . thirst and heat . . . want of appetite and loathing of food . . . etc."[74]

The truth is that to Brown all sick persons looked more or less alike: "Instead of the infinite differences of habits and temperament, I have found every individual precisely the same as every other. Whatever produces the gout in one will produce it in another prepared to receive its influence. And whatever cures it in any one, cures it also in every other; and so forth with respect to every other disease. The deeper we explore the works of nature, the more shall we be convinced of this wonderful simplicity, so that, to a philosopher, all nature would appear the effect of one single instrument in the hand of the all-wise, all-powerful Creator."[75]

Among the "asthenic" diseases of "direct debility" were ranged: intermittent fever, mild colic, dyspepsia, hypochondria, rheumatalgia, cholera, epilepsy, St. Vitus' Dance, rickets, scrophula, typhus, lead colic, gout, tetanus, scurvy, diabetes, dropsy, jaundice, and others. These were all to be treated with remedies which supported the "excitement"—application of heat, roast beef, opium, exercise, whiskey, wines, spirits, and other "diffusible stimuli."[76]

The "sthenic" diseases, requiring a "lowering treatment" (bleeding, application of cold, vomiting, sweating, a starvation diet), were: phrenitis, inflammatory sore throat, continued fever, mild smallpox, measles, peripneumonia, dysentery, mania, miliary fever, chicken pox, ophthalmia, rheumatism, catarrh, and scarlet fever.[77]

And, finally, the highly sthenic diseases resulting in "indirect debility" were apoplexy, palsy, plague, malignant fever, gangrenous sore throat, confluent smallpox, hydrothorax, phthisis, and contagious dysentery.[78] These all required the same treatment as the "asthenic" diseases of "direct debility."

In Brunonian practice, therefore, nearly all diseases were ascribed to "debility," whether "direct" or "indirect," and very few required remedies which reduced "excitement." Brown's leading French disciple estimated 95% of all urban diseases, and 98% of all diseases in the countryside, to be asthenic.[79] [s]

[s]To do Brown justice, it must be borne in mind that his therapeutics aimed, *inter alia,* at getting food into hospital and other patients who were being bled, purged, and starved literally to death. At the Edinburgh Royal Infirmary in 1782 the piece of "steak" which the patients received from time to time was not more than 1 5/16" long and 7/8" wide. Brown's followers wrote to the director asking if he would choose to be fed in this fashion if sick: "Your victuals are not only scanty but bad. Your porridge is sometimes boiled almost into water-gruel; your broth is commonly much better qualified to operate as an emetic than to nourish the system . . . your beer is not always tolerable even to the palate of an alehouse scullion" (Brown, *Elements of Medicine,* xxxvii). Whiskey and the other "diffusible stimulants" did not seem harmful, nor did opium—the medicine which Brown prescribed virtually to the exclusion of any other (although his followers

The Triumph of Brownism

The simplification of disease categories meant a simplification of therapy. Cullen's "spasm," "atony," and "debility" were universal solvents of medical facts and observations, as were Brown's "excitability," "excitement," and "exciting powers."

Cullen's principal medicines were those which affected the "nervous power" or "nervous fluid": astringents, tonics, stimulants, sedatives, antispasmodics, etc.[80] Their action was on the vital solids "in consequence of which a motion is propagated from the place of impulse along the course of the nerves to their origin in the brain or *medulla spinalis.*"[81] Antispasmodics were especially valuable, since, in addition to their power over the "nervous fluid," they give "a tone and steadiness to the energy of the brain so as to prevent those sudden alternations of excitement and collapse in which so many convulsive disorders consist."[82] [t]

With Brown, of course, simplification reached the absurd: "The same debilitating remedies which remove any one sthenic disease remove that whole set of diseases; and the same stimulant means which cure any one asthenic disease remove all the rest. Are not palsy, insofar as it is curable, and dropsy, insofar as it is a general affection, as well as the gout and fevers, both relieved and removed by the same remedies? And are not peripneumony, the smallpox, the measles, rheumatism, and catarrh removed by the same remedies, to wit, evacuants, cold, and starving?"[83]

All individual differences disappeared in the flux of nervous forces and excitabilities. Brown denied the existence of differences in temperament. Cullen reduced them to (*inter alia)* variations in the nervous system, "different states of its

enlarged the Brunonian pharmacopoeia). Furthermore, he held that therapy should effect change gradually and by degrees (citing the case of the Highland chieftain who cured himself of drunkenness by pouring, every day, a little more wax into his *queich* [Brown, *Elements of Medicine,* lxvi]). To some extent, therefore, professional opposition to Brownism reflected dislike for his more humane treatment of patients.

[t]He also had a class of medicines with a mechanical effect on the "simple solids": emollients, astringents, corrosives, etc. (William Cullen, *Treatise of the Materia Medica* [Edinburgh: Charles Elliot, 1789], II, 3, 4, 116, 128).

sensibility, its irritability, and its strength."[84] "Idiosyncrasy" is a "preternatural degree of the sensibility or irritability of certain parts of the system, or a peculiar sensibility or irritability of the whole body, or particular parts of it, with respect to certain applications."[85] Specific contagia, a problem already exercising some medical minds and which would shortly emerge as a major theme of speculation,[u] were reduced by Cullen to "debilitants" and by Brown to "stimulants."[86]

> It appears that the [bubonic] plague is especially distinguished by a specific contagion, often suddenly producing the most considerable symptoms of debility in the nervous system or moving powers . . . and it is from a consideration of these circumstances as the proximate cause that I think both the prevention and cure of the plague must be directed.[87]

> The smallpox and measles are cured by the same means as peripneumonia or any other sthenic disease; and, excepting the contagious matter, arise from the same stimulant hurtful powers; they must, therefore, with the same exception, be the same. The only difference is that they are accompanied with a contagious matter, and the other sthenic diseases are not.[88]

Both philosophers denied the existence of "specifics." Cullen observed that "many, dissatisfied with the reasonings of dogmatic physicians, have been led into pursuits of specifics. If this could be done with success, it would certainly be very desirable; but at this day I know no medicine whose action I do not think I can explain by its answering a particular indication, which entirely destroys the notions of a specific."[89] He urged his contemporaries to reduce their indications to "more simple operations"; this "would almost entirely destroy the doctrine of specifics which must otherwise continue upon the most mysterious and uncertain foundation."[90] "Many, perhaps, we may be

[u]See below, pp. 463-464 and 514-518.

still obliged to leave among that number, but surely we ought to endeavor to leave as few as possible."[91] Brown carried the argument against specifics to an even further degree of simplification:

> The notion of some powerful remedies, as opium, mercury, and Jesuit's Bark [quinine], etc., acting by an operation peculiar to each and different from every other power in nature, was long prevalent in the schools of medicine. Those they called *specifics,* altogether contrary to sound philosophy, since the more careful our inquiries into nature's operations are, the more and more reason have we to be convinced that simplicity and uniformity everywhere pervade the whole phenomena of the universe. Accordingly, in the exciting powers that act upon the excitability of our bodies, we find only one action, that of stimulating, varying only in its degree, to take place in all animal as well as vegetable bodies, nay, in every thing that we know to possess life in the universe. We also find to the same extent only one property in living systems upon which it acts, that is, the excitability; and one effect produced by the mutual relations betwixt them in that respect, to wit, the excitement. Instead of the distracted notion of vortices, or atmospheres in rapid motion, governing the motion of the planets, Sir Isaac Newton found the whole planetary systems of the universe governed in their motions by one single principle.[92] [v]

The two specifics *par excellence* at this time were quinine and mercury.

According to Cullen, however, quinine should not be considered a specific.[93] "I consider the Peruvian bark . . . to be a substance in which the qualities of bitter and astringent are conjoined . . . As a bitter and astringent conjoined, I

[v]A similar argument is presented by Iago Galdston, "I have a conviction . . . that the concept of the specific in medicine, whenever it dominates in medical theory, deleteriously affects its practice and retards its further development" ("The Concept of the Specific in Medicine," *Transactions of the College of Physicians of Philadelphia,* IX [1941-1942], 25-34, at 26).

consider the bark as a powerful tonic. As we have before shown that these qualities in their separate state give tonic medicines, so it will be readily allowed that, conjoined together, they may give one still more powerful."[94] "No body doubts of its being a tonic with regard to the stomach; and it is equally well known that the state of the stomach is readily communicated to the rest of the system. It is in no instance, however, more remarkable than in the cure of intermittent feyers . . . the bark in this instance operates by a tonic power exerted in the stomach."[95]

According to Brown, quinine is merely another tonic among tonics and not very effective in the treatment of intermittent fever, which is better handled by exposure to the sun and administration of spirituous liquors.[96]

Cullen (like Sydenham) regarded mercury as merely another sialogogue (i.e., causing salivation), curing syphilis by an evacuation through the salivary glands.[97]

> This leads to consider the question, if the disease is to be cured by evacuation, why other evacuations, however diligently employed, do not cure the disease as well as those by mercury? The answer to this may be that all other evacuations are partial only; they may largely diminish the quantity of the fluids, but they draw them off by one way only, and without being attended with any general increase of excretion. They for the most part diminish all the excretions except that which is on the occasion, by special means, increased; and it is mercury only that, under proper management, can be employed to increase the whole excretions at the same time. It seems to be by this peculiar mode of operation that it is peculiarly fitted to cure the venereal disease.[98]

Brown did not discuss syphilis or mercury in his *Elements of Medicine,* but the pharmacopoeia of his French disciple, J. F. Chortet, devoted twenty-five pages to mercury as a leading "negative stimulant" used in treating the "sthenic disease," syphilis.[99]

Cullen's, and especially Brown's, simplifications of therapeutics swept the medical world in the late eighteenth and early nineteenth centuries. The philosophical and scientific problems of differences among patients, diseases and medicines over which physicians had toiled for centuries were abolished by *fiat* of the Scottish Methodists, and the practitioner needed to bear in mind only a few basic indications:

> Such is the simplicity to which medicine is thus reduced that when a physician comes to the bedside of a patient, he has only three things to settle in his mind. First, whether the disease be general or local; secondly, if general, whether it is sthenic or asthenic; thirdly, what is its degree? When once he has satisfied himself in these points, all that remains for him to do is to form his indications or general view of the plan of cure and carry that into execution by the administration of proper remedies.[100]

Philippe Pinel (1755-1826) wrote disapprovingly that Brownism admitted of no obstacles to conquer, recognized no difficulties in acquiring a precise idea of the disease, called for no preliminary study of physics, anatomy, or physiology, and required no skill in observation.[101] A German professor, Johann Andreas Roeschlaub (1768-1835) reduced the whole system to thirty propositions which could be mastered in a few weeks.[102]

In these very respects Brownism resembled the Methodist doctrine of antiquity, as was noted at the time by perceptive observers.[103]

Brown's *Elementa Medicinae* was reprinted in Milan in 1792 and 1794. The English translation was published in London in 1795 and 1804 and in the United States (Philadelphia and elsewhere) in 1790, 1791, 1793, 1795, 1797, 1804, and 1806. German translations appeared in Frankfurt (1795, 1806), Vienna (1796), and Copenhagen (1798, 1804). Italian translations came out in Naples (1796) and Venice (1800), and there were three French editions, the last in 1805. An edition in Spanish was published in Madrid in 1800. A large volume of secondary literature appeared in all of these languages plus Portuguese (in Lisbon and also Brazil).

"As late as 1802 the University of Goettingen was so convulsed by controversy on the merits of the Brunonian system that contending factions of students in enormous numbers, not unaided by professors, met in combat in the streets on two successive days and had to be dispersed by a troop of Hanoverian horse."[104] In Great Britain it "wrought a memorable change in medical opinions and practice."[105] Giovanni Rasori (1766-1837) in Italy based on it a whole system of "contrastimulism" which survived well into the nineteenth century. Brownism was for a while official doctrine in the Austrian Army, "although the rescript was recalled owing to professional opposition."[106] Napoleon was interested in it as a system of treatment for his troops, and, although it never acquired extreme popularity in France, the system was defended in debates at the Institut National des Sciences by the country's two leading chemists, Claude-Louis Berthollet (1748-1822) and Antoine-Francois Fourcroy (1755-1809).[107] In the United States it became orthodoxy in the version of Benjamin Rush (1745-1813) who had known Cullen and Brown during his medical studies in Great Britain and admired both extravagantly; he copied most of the worst features of the two systems and promulgated them for decades as professor of medicine at the University of Pennsylvania.[w]

An American physician wrote retrospectively in 1860:

> The Brunonian system . . . exercised an extensive sway, for nearly twenty-five years, over the minds of many otherwise enlightened practitioners whose enthusiasm seemed to have been carried away by it to the utmost stretch of the imagination. Many of them, indeed,

[w]See *Divided Legacy,* III, 5-73.

supposed that they had actually discovered the philosopher's stone in regard to the treatment of disease . . . John Brown, the author of this practice, was almost deified . . . The opinions of Brown exerted so wide a sway in Great Britain as to affect, for a time, the whole practice of medicine. In Italy his works were translated by the celebrated Rasori, with notes and annotations; and so great was their influence in that country that there was hardly an intelligent pupil who did not openly avow himself a Brunonian. The "doctrine" also speedily found its way into Germany and France, in both of which, but especially in the former, it made numerous converts, and long maintained its hold upon the profession. In a number of the continental universities its principles were formally expounded by the professors. In Germany, writes an anonymous author, Brown was hailed as a medical Luther, and so great were the dissensions among the pupils of some of the leading schools in regard to the claims of the Northern Light that it was not uncommon for them to come to blows. At Goettingen the Brunonians were so rebellious as to require the authority of the military to keep them in subjection. Of the extent to which the new doctrine had enslaved some of the German practitioners a correct idea may be formed when it is stated that at the hospital in Bamberg the attending physician, Dr. Marcus, a man of eminence, considered himself justified in distributing, as an average allowance, among nearly five hundred patients affected with various kinds of diseases, a drachm of opium, with three times that quantity of camphor, and a pound of alcohol, together with numerous other stimulants. This was at the close of the last century.[108]

NOTES

[1] L.S. King, *The Medical World of the Eighteenth Century* (Chicago: University of Chicago Press, 1958), 147.

[2] Frederici Hoffmanni consiliarii medici, *Medicinae rationalis systematicae tomus primus - quartus* (Venetiis: Ex typographia Balleoniana, 1737), III, 45-46.

[3] See J. N. Langley, "Sketch of the Progress of Discovery in the Eighteenth Century as Regards the Autonomic Nervous System," *Journal of Physiology* L (1916), 225-258.

[4] London, 1755 (reprinted Baltimore: Johns Hopkins University Press, 1936, with an Introduction by Owsei Temkin). See, also, *Albertus de Haller de Partibus Corporis Humani Sensibilibus et Irritabilibus. Die 22 April. 1752.* in *Commentarii Societatis Regiae Scientiarum Gottingensis. Tomus II. Ad annum MDCCLII.*

[5] *Ibid.*, 8-9, 26.

[6] *Ibid.*, 43.

[7] *Ibid.*, 46.

[8] *Ibid.*, 25.

[9] *Ibid.*, 42.

[10] Albert von Haller, *First Lines of Physiology* (Troy, New York: Obadiah Penniman, 1803), 470.

[11] *Ibid.*, 182.

[12] *Ibid.*, 181. Haller, *Dissertation,* 20. Sprengel, *Histoire de la Medecine,* V. 328.

[13] Haller, *Dissertation,* 41.

[14] *Ibid.*, 27, 28, 34, 41.

[15] *Ibid.*, 37, 40.

[16] *Ibid.*, 43.

[17] *Ibid.*, 44.

[18] *Loc. cit.*

[19] Haller, *First Lines of Physiology,* 52-53.

[20] *Ibid.*, 466.

[21] *Ibid.*, 469.

[22] *Ibid.*, 470.

[23] Haller, *Dissertation,* 8.

[24] William Cullen, *First Lines of the Practice of Physic* (Edinburgh: Bell and Bradfute, 1796), I, 29.

[25] *Ibid.*, I, 33.

[26] *Ibid.*, I, 20-21.

[27] *Ibid.*, I, 24.

[28] *Ibid.*, 23-24, 47.

[29] William Cullen, *Institutions of Medicine: Part I. Physiology* (Edinburgh and Boston: Reprinted by John Norman, 1788), 8.

[30] *Ibid.*, 39.

[31] *Ibid.*, 55. See also, Cullen's definition of the "vital principle" in *Treatise of the Materia Medica* (Edinburgh: Charles Elliot, 1789), I, 59.

[32] John Brown, *The Elements of Medicine* (Portsmouth, New Hampshire: Treadwell, 1804), lxii-lxvii.

[33] *Ibid.*, lxiv-lxv.

[34] William Cullen, *A Synopsis of Methodical Nosology, in Which the Genera of Disorders are Particularly Defined and the Species Added, with the Synonimous of Those from Sauvages* (Philadelphia: Parry Hall, 1793).

[35] Cullen, *First Lines of the Practice of Physic*, I, 92.

[36] *Ibid.*, I, 81.

[37] *Ibid.*, I, 83-84.

[38] *Ibid.*, I, 87.

[39] *Ibid.*, I, 89-90.

[40] *Ibid.*, I, 244-247.

[41] *Ibid.*, II, 305-306.

[42] *Ibid.*, II, 355, 359, 397.

[43] *Ibid.*, I, 272, 295-297.

[44] *Ibid.*, III, 142-143.

[45] *Ibid.*, III, 153.

[46] *Ibid.*, III, 167, 182, 184, 186.

[47] *Ibid.*, IV, 199-200.

[48] *Ibid.*, IV, 354-355.

[49] *Ibid.*, IV, 392.

[50] *Ibid.*, IV, 406.

[51] *Ibid.*, IV, 432.

[52] Cullen, *Synopsis of Methodical Nosology*, 142ff.

[53] Cullen, *First Lines of the Practice of Physic*, IV, 415, 421, 423.

[54] *Ibid.*, IV, 428.

[55] Cullen, *Synopsis of Methodical Nosology*, v.

[56] *Ibid.*, x.

[57] *Loc. cit.*

[58] *Ibid.*, xv.

[59] *Ibid.*, viii.

[60] *Ibid.*, xiii.

[61] Cullen, *First Lines of the Practice of Physic*, I, 36.

[62] *Loc. cit.*

[63] *Ibid.*, I, 39.

[64] *Ibid.*, I, 40.

[65] Cullen, *Synopsis of Methodical Nosology*, xvi.

[66] *Ibid.*, iii.

[67] *Ibid.*, xiii-xiv.

[68] *Ibid.*, xiv.

[69] Brown, *Elements of Medicine*, 116 (stress added).

[70] *Ibid.*, 228.

[71] *Ibid.*, 307.

[72] *Ibid.*, 119.

[73] *Ibid.*, 163-164.

[74] *Ibid.*, 178-179.

[75] *Ibid.*, 243.

[76] *Ibid.*, Table of Diseases.

[77] *Loc. cit.*

[78] *Loc. cit.*

[79] J. F. Chortet, *Traite de Pharmacologie (Matiere Medicale) Base sur la Theorie de Brown Suivi d'un Nouvel Essai sur l'Art de Formuler* (Luxembourg: Lamort, 1806), 48.

[80] William Cullen, *Treatise of the Materia Medica* (Edinburgh: Charles Elliot, 1789), II, 4, 53-54, 131-132, 348, *et passim.*

[81] *Ibid.*, I, 57.

[82] *Ibid.*, II, 359.

[83] Brown, *Elements of Medicine,* 125.

[84] Cullen, *Treatise of the Materia Medica,* I, 89.

[85] *Ibid.*, I, 119.

[86] Cullen, *First Lines of the Practice of Physic,* I, 79. Brown, *Elements of Medicine,* 91, 117.

[87] Cullen, *First Lines of the Practice of Physic,* II, 238-239.

[88] Brown, *Elements of Medicine,* 117.

[89] William Cullen, *Lectures on the Materia Medica* (Philadelphia: Robert Bell, 1775), 43-44.

[90] Cullen, *Treatise of the Materia Medica,* I, 30.

[91] Cullen, *Lectures on the Materia Medica,* 288.

[92] Brown, *Elements of Medicine,* 242-243.

[93] Cullen, *Lectures on the Materia Medica,* 288.

[94] Cullen, *Treatise of the Materia Medica,* II, 90.

[95] *Ibid.*, II, 91.

[96] Brown, *Elements of Medicine,* 429-430.

[97] Cullen, *Treatise of the Materia Medica,* II, 440-454.

[98] *Ibid.*, II, 151.

[99] Chortet, *Traite de Pharmacologie (Matiere Medicale) Base sur la Theorie de Brown,* 252-276.

[100] Brown, *Elements of Medicine,* 119.

[101] Philippe Pinel, "Brownisme," *Dictionnaire des Sciences Medicales* (Paris, 1812).

[102] *Loc. cit.* K. Sudhoff, *Kurzes Handbuch der Geschichte der Medizin* (Berlin: Karger, 1922), 340.

[103] For example, Pomme, *Refutation de la Doctrine Medicale du Docteur Brown* (Paris: Cussac, 1808), 10.

[104] "John Brown," *Dictionary of National Biography.*

[105] Brown, *Elements of Medicine,* Editor's Introduction, xi.

[106] "John Brown," *Dictionary of National Biography.*

[107] Bernhard Hirschel, *Geschichte des Brown'schen Systems und der Erregungstheorie* (Leipzig: Arnold, 1850), 129. Pomme, *Refutation de la Doctrine Medicale du Docteur Brown,* iv.

[108] S. D. Gross, "Brunonianism, Toddism, and other Isms," *North American Medico-Chirurgical Review* V (1861), 66-83, at 69, 72 (Paper read before the Philadelphia County Medical Society, November 11, 1860).

CHAPTER VI

EMPIRICAL REACTIONS (1): HAHNEMANN AND HOMOEOPATHY

The history of Cullen and Brown shows that medical Rationalism becomes increasingly alienated from therapeutic reality, reaching a culmination in Methodism. The biography of Samuel Hahnemann (1755-1843) exemplifies the next stage in the movement of medical thought: the abstract nature of Methodism and the ensuing failures in practice provoke a reaction; there is a proliferation of mutually inconsistent eclectic systems and, at length, a return to the principles of Empiricism.

A German medical professor in 1810 called his age one of "uncertainty, contention, and contradiction."[1] Another wrote in 1819:

> We are now in a time when the most varied systems are blended and amalgamated. The mechanical and chemical views of the organism have joined and subordinated—or at least taken a position beside—the dynamico-vitalistic view. The humoral and solidist theories have joined together and been reduced to the idea of the reciprocity of the solid and liquid parts of the organism. The individual organs and functions are recognized both as integral parts of the organism and as manifestations of its life, and the seat and essence of the various diseases are sought in them. But no individual function, regardless of how widespread it may be in the organism (for example, irritability, sensitivity, excitability, nutrition), no individ-

> ual organ system, regardless of how completely it may permeate all the organs (such as the vascular and the nervous systems) is taken as the sole source of diseases . . . The evacuating and irritating, the depleting and strengthening, as well as many other opposite methods of treatment stand peacefully side by side in general therapy and reciprocally restrict one another; our learned contemporaries make use of all these systems in the various diseases, although each one may have his own preference.[2]

To this intellectual disarray was added the upheaval occasioned by the French Revolution and the ensuing decades of war—civil, national, and international. These political and social hurricanes, which reached into the home of every citizen, cost every state thousands of lives, reconstituted the political boundaries of many countries and reordered the internal polity of most, shook the foundations of thought as well. They cleared away the debris of centuries and permitted the emergence of two new Empirical departures in therapeutics—Hahnemann's doctrine, which he called "homoeopathy," and the series of new systems and concepts (from 1790 to about 1860) known as the "Paris School."

Both were reactions to the domination of theory by Rationalism and Methodism. Both were attempts to return to first principles, renouncing a therapeutics based upon hypothetical proximate causes and seeking a method relying on observation and experience. Thus both accepted the traditional Empirical principles as guides to therapeutics.

They diverged, however, in one major point. The Paris School was late in coming to terms with contemporary pharmacological and chemical learning, while homoeopathy, as Hahnemann suggested, was the Hippocratic method combined with knowledge of pharmacology.[3] In a new and original interpretation of pharmacology Hahnemann found the key which Empirical thinkers had been seeking for centuries; one which brought all elements of Empirical doctrine together in a new crystallization and gave them a new focus. It was this which has enabled the homoeopathic system to outlive all its competitors and, in fact, to survive and flourish to the present day.[a] The Paris School, on the contrary, despite its profusion of eminent intellectuals and personalities, many of them motivated by the sincerest desire to benefit the sick, could not elaborate a doctrine to withstand the test of time. The thinking of these physicians slowly ran into the sand while the valid part of their pharmacology was borrowed from homoeopathy.[b]

The present chapter traces the history of Hahnemannism in medicine, and the two following are devoted to the Paris School.

Biographical

Hahnemann's medical outlook, like that of Paracelsus, was shaped by his early life. The moral fervor which permeates the thinking of both was instilled by their upbringing and early professional experience. The parallels between their careers, as between their medical doctrines, are striking.

Hahnemann was born in 1755 in Meissen, a town in the Electorate of Saxony famous for its porcelain. His father, uncles, and grandfathers were all painters and designers of porcelain (Hahnemann's father published a small book on watercoloring techniques), and there was a strong artistic streak in the family.[4]

Although socially and economically superior to the peasants and lowest class of townspeople, Hahnemann's family was still poor, and their only son passed a childhood without amenities. The sole luxury they could afford was his education. Hahnemann was an excellent student and, in view

[a] Since the homeopathic system is still practiced in most countries of the world, it deserves more extended treatment than we have given to doctrines of purely historical interest. Furthermore, Hahnemann's life and thought have not yet been analyzed competently by any historian outside the ranks of the homoeopathic school, even though, as an influence on medical thought, he ranks with Paracelsus and the Hippocratic authors.

[b] See below, pp. 569 ff.

of his poverty and promise, both elementary and secondary schools absolved him of the obligation to pay fees.

The family lived at all times on the edge of poverty, as is seen in the occasional attempts by Hahnemann's father to terminate his education and put him to work. He was for a while apprenticed to a green-grocer, and when he ran away and returned home, his mother had to hide him for several days until the father's wrath had abated. Even so, Hahnemann was removed from school for varying periods of time—months and perhaps even years, which explains why he remained so long at the secondary level.

The stubbornness which is so prominent a trait of his character was tempered by this long struggle for an education. He wrote later that he knew no childhood and that his whole formative period was consumed by the effort to become educated: "Mental exertion and study are unnatural occupations for young people whose bodily development is not yet complete, especially for those who are endowed with sensitive feelings. This nearly cost me my life during the period from 15 to 20 years of age."[5]

In spite of his father's reluctance to see Hahnemann's education through to the end, he seems to have affected the boy beneficially. An associate later recalled that "before going to the factory [he] used frequently to lock his son in a room, close the shutters, and give him a difficult sentence to ponder over, of which he had to give an account on his father's return. This contributed to making the son into an original thinker."[6] Later in life, Hahnemann remembered his father with great respect, writing in an autobiographical fragment (1791):

> To act and live without pretence or show was his most noteworthy precept, which impressed me more by his example than by words. He was frequently present, though unobserved, where something good was to be accomplished. Should I not follow him? In his deeds he differentiated between noble and ignoble to so fine a degree of correctness and practical delicacy of feeling as

to be highly creditable to him; in this also he was my teacher. His ideas on the first principles of creation, the dignity of mankind, and its lofty destiny, seemed consistent in every way with his mode of life. This was the foundation of my moral training.[7]

Hahnemann's biographer surmises that the future physician was raised on Rousseauian principles as developed into a pedagogical system by J. B. Basedow (1723-1790)–about whom Windelband comments: "the complete development of the individuality was the main thing, from which the turning away from learned one-sidedness, the direction of attention to the real and practical, the appeal to perception, and the use of individual instead of general truths in instruction and education, followed as a matter of course . . . the school of German philanthropy . . . under the lead of Basedow, combined the principle of natural development with that of utility."[8]

Whether or not the legacy of Basedow and the elder Hahnemann, all of these themes emerge repeatedly in homoeopathy and in Hahnemann's later life.

His career was distinguished by rigid determination to be true to his own self.[c] An early medical writing (1784) describes the true physician as the one who: "sworn to no system, rejects nothing not investigated by himself, nor takes the word of another, and has the courage to think for himself and to treat accordingly."[9] At age 74 he wrote to a friend: "Let me go down to posterity only as the image of my inner self, which can easily be discerned in my writings. My vanity goes no further than this."[10]

In homoeopathy the theme of individualization is embodied in the insistent demand that each patient receive the remedy precisely suiting his own individual needs.

Basedow's concern for utility, the "real and practical", is central to homoeopathy which sets itself the goal of making all pharmacological knowledge useful to the practitioner immediately and without the intervention of theory. Hahne-

[c]Like Paracelsus' *Alterius non sit qui suus esse potest* (*Divided Legacy,* I, 352)

mann asked to have the words, *Non inutilis vixi,* inscribed on his coffin.[11]

Basedow's "appeal to perception", of course, figures in Hahnemann's exclusive stress on symptoms as the source of medical knowledge.

In 1775 Hahnemann left Meissen to study medicine at Leipzig. He supported himself by tutoring other students in languages and making translations from English, but his studies seem to have been a disappointment (the medical curriculum included no clinical training), and after two years he left for Vienna to study with the Royal physician, Dr. Joseph von Quarin (1734-1814), who had access to a hospital. Although von Quarin singled him out as a student of promise, and even helped him financially, Hahnemann's resources were at an end after nine months, and he had to go as librarian to the governor of Transylvania at Hermannstadt (Sibiu).

He spent almost two years there, cataloguing the governor's library and pursuing the study of languages. When he had accumulated the funds to continue his medical education, he enrolled at Erlangen (where fees were lower) and there, after a single term, obtained the degree in 1779. He was twenty-four years old.

He set up practice in a small copper-mining town north of Dessau but, unlike Paracelsus, derived no inspiration from this environment. In 1781 he removed to Dessau, but practice was slow, and he passed his time studying chemistry and translating chemical works from French and English. In 1782 he married the daughter of the local apothecary.

The next twenty years were a time of great hardship, even by Hahnemann's unpretentious standards. He was gradually becoming disillusioned with the doctrines he had learned, and this made practice difficult. He rarely stayed longer than a year or two in a single location, changing residence seventeen times between 1782 and 1805 when he settled in Torgau. In these years he underwent a crisis brought on by conflict between the need to support a growing family and his inability to find his way in the thicket of late eighteenth-century systems:

> It was painful for me to grope in the dark, guided only by our books in the treatment of the sick—to prescribe, according to this or that (fanciful) view of the nature of diseases, substances that only owed to mere opinion their place in the materia medica; I had conscientious scruples about treating unknown morbid states in my suffering fellow-creatures with these unknown medicines which, being powerful substances, may, if they were not *exactly* suitable (and how could the physician know whether they were suitable or not, seeing that their peculiar special actions were not yet elucidated) easily change life into death, or produce new affections and chronic ailments, which are often much more difficult to remove than the original disease. To become in this way a murderer or aggravator of the sufferings of my brethren of mankind was to me a fearful thought—so fearful and distressing was it that shortly after my marriage I completely abandoned practice and scarcely treated any one for fear of doing him harm, and—as you know—occupied myself solely with chemistry and literary labors.[12]

Thus, like Paracelsus and Van Helmont, he was disillusioned with the prevailing ideas and retired from practice to think out a new approach. From 1782 to 1796 he earned a living largely through chemical research, translations, and writings.[d]

[d]Here is not the place to discuss Hahnemann's qualifications as a chemist. A detailed account of the development of his chemical views and activities can be found in Wilhelm Ameke, *History of Homoeopathy* (London: Gould, 1885). On Hahnemann's place in the history of chemistry Von Lippmann wrote: "he does not possess absolute significance for this science but, relatively, significance without question, far outstripping any of his numerous, even chemical, contemporaries." (Edmund O. Von Lippmann, *Beitraege zur Geschichte der Naturwissenschaften und der Technik.* Zweiter Band [Verlag Chemie, GMBH. Weinheim, 1953], 298). In addition to his original contributions to chemistry Hahnemann translated works from English, French, Italian, and Latin. Furthermore, he wrote a number of works on medicine, hygiene, and pharmacology before his homoeopathic period. Of these the most substantial are: *Directions for*

But he could not easily abandon the profession to which access had been won at such cost. Furthermore, he had an increasing family which needed medical assistance: "children were born to me, several children, and in course of time serious diseases occurred, which, because they afflicted and endangered the lives of my children—my flesh and blood—caused my conscience to reproach me still more loudly, that I had no means on which I could rely for affording them relief."[13] Thus, during these years of professional stagnation he was searching for some reliable basis upon which to resume practice. The fruit of these investigations appeared in his 1796 "Essay on a New Principle for Ascertaining the Curative Powers of Drugs, with a Few Glances at Those Hitherto Employed"[14] where he advocated the use of "provings"[e] to determine the curative powers of remedies. Medicines were to be administered to healthy individuals and a record made of the symptoms which they produced: a given substance was then to be used to treat the patient whose symptoms were identical with the symptom-pattern developed in the "proving" of this substance. This interpretation of the traditional Empirical principle of "cure through similars" was called by Hahnemann the "law of similars" and was thenceforth the basis of homoeopathic practice.

After this time Hahnemann rejoined his profession, following exclusively the principles of his developing

Curing Old Sores and Ulcers (1784, 192 pages), *On Poisoning by Arsenic: its Treatment and Forensic Detection* (1786, 276 pages), *Instructions for Surgeons in Venereal Diseases* (1789, 292 pages), *The Friend of Health* (1792 and 1795, 196 pages), and *Pharmaceutical Lexicon* (in four parts: 1793 [280 pages], 1795 [244 pages], 1798 [259 pages], 1799 [498 pages]). This last was a general guide to the preparation of medicines and a handbook for pharmacists; in it Hahnemann collected, compiled, revised, and edited all existing pharmacological knowledge. It was very well received by the medical profession at the time of its appearance (see the review in *Journal der Pharmacie* [1794], II, St. 1, 185). In fact, Hahnemann was one of the most learned men of his generation in matters medical, chemical, and pharmacological, and his later attacks on physicians and pharmacists were based upon firsthand knowledge. A complete bibliography of his original writings and translations is given in Richard Haehl, *Samuel Hahnemann, His Life and Work* (London: Homoeopathic Publishing Co., 1922), II, 511-515.

[e]In German, *"Pruefung"*—a "test" or "trial."

homoeopathic system. On it he wrote over forty essays (collected in his *Lesser Writings)* and three major works: the *Fragmenta de Viribus Medicamentorum Positivis Sive in Sano Corpore Observatis* (1805),[15] the *Organon of Rational Healing* (1810),[16] and the *Chronic Diseases, Their Nature and Homoeopathic Treatment* (1828).[17]

The rest of his life was spent in the effort to convert other physicians to his views, but the irreconcilability of the homoeopathic doctrines and the existing Rationalist and Methodist systems made this a hopeless undertaking from the start. Its difficulty was compounded by Hahnemann's rigid intolerance toward his opponents[f] as well as toward those of his followers who refused to follow him precisely and absolutely.[g] The appearance in 1810 of the *Organon,* which contained a systematic exposition of all elements of the homoeopathic doctrine, aroused his colleagues' opposition to a high pitch and led eventually to a split in the medical profession.

For a time there even existed a special journal devoted solely to attacks on Hahnemann—the *Anti-Homoeopathisches Archiv,* published in Hamburg.

Hahnemann at length wearied of his own generation and decided to appeal to youth by teaching at the University of Leipzig. In 1812 he submitted the dissertation required for those intending to lecture—an analysis of the use of hellebore *(Veratrum)* in the Hippocratic Corpus—which demonstrated a knowledge of the sources not only in Greek and Latin but also Hebrew and Arabic as well as the modern languages.[18] It

[f]Whom he called "allopaths" (see below, p. 365 and note).

[g]"There are but two principal methods of cure . . . the homoeopathic . . . and the heteropathic or allopathic. Each opposes the other, and only he who does not know either can hold the delusion that they can ever approach each other or even become united, or to make himself so ridiculous as to practice at one time homoeopathically, at another allopathically, according to the pleasure of the patient; a practice which may be called criminal treason against divine homoeopathy." (S. Hahnemann, *Organon of Medicine.* Translated from the German of the Sixth Edition by William Boericke [Calcutta: Roysingh, 1962], Section 52).

was accepted without demur despite the author's already controversial reputation.[19]

His course of lectures, however, was quite unsuccessful. By this time he was fifty-seven years old, accustomed to a solitary life with his family and patients, and could not adjust his manner of presentation, tempered by a decade of polemics with his profession, to the needs of young students. An eyewitness account of his style gives an impression of Hahnemann's personality:

> Think of the tension of the audience before his arrival, who as yet did not know the enthusiastic reformer, or perhaps were rubbing their hands in joyous anticipation of the volcanic eruptions—and you will tender forgiveness for the smile when you hear the outer door open and hear his step in the adjoining room, where he remains standing at the door, clears his throat, and then turns the key round twice in the lock; the door which is usually locked is seen to open, and a man enters of middle height and strong build; the few hairs of the thoughtful head are carefully curled and powdered, inspiring respect for his advanced age, which would have been apparent even if the bald crown and white hair had not been powdered; add to that the beautiful white linen round the neck and on the chest. The black waistcoat and the short black trousers; on the button of the latter was fastened the strap of his shining black top boots, above which appeared the finest white stockings. Think of this figure as, after three measured steps, he gives an almost imperceptible nod of the head, as a sign of greeting, then takes three more steps and having arrived at his chair, in front of which is a little table, he sits down with pathos after removing carefully the shining tails of the coat, opens the book, takes out his watch and puts it on the table before him, then clears his throat, reads the respective paragraph with ordinary voice, but becomes more ecstatic during his explanations, with shining and sparkling eyes, and great redness of the forehead and

> face—I ask how could it be possible to keep a serious face in front of such a Spanish grandezza which appears in the same way every time; in young years when one is inclined to ridicule everything and not even spare old age. . . . Unfortunately the lectures were not fitted to win friends and followers for his theories or himself. For, whenever possible, he poured forth such a flood of abuse against the older medicine and its followers, with the result that his audience lessened every hour and finally consisted of only a few of his students. . . . Any others were present not for the subject matter but to hear the unfortunate method of presentation, so that their sense of humor might be freely tickled.[20]

Hahnemann continued his lectures for several years, but the audience was small, and he eventually decided upon a different pedagogical technique, gathering a limited group of students and collaborators to observe his practice and help with the "provings."

The hostility of the profession was extended to these helpers as well:

> Perpetual raillery from the students, poisonous looks from most of the professors, anxious desire of everybody to avoid more intimate intercourse with us—as if we were infected with some pestilential eruption—all this made my stay in Leipzig really painful, and consequently a visit to another university, at any rate for a short time, highly desirable.
>
> Even under the best circumstances [we] had to tolerate much mockery and irony and in malicious cases, hatred and persecution, not only during the student years but far beyond them. I can always remember how Hornburg [one of the collaborators] was worried in his final examination by the old pates and only just managed to escape being failed, whilst miserable thick-heads, not fit to wipe Hornburg's boots, passed *cum laude* and are now flourishing aloft here—narrow-minded but successful physicians.[21]

This was a foretaste of the reaction of other medical schools, later in the century, to the suspicion of homoeopathic sympathizers in their midst.[h]

But homoeopathy itself was spreading. An impetus was given by its apparent efficacy against the typhus epidemic of 1813, the endemic scarlet fever which could assume epidemic proportions at any time, and, finally, the Asiatic Cholera which swept west from Russia and the Orient in 1831 and 1832.[22]

This success was over the bitter opposition of Hahnemann's allopathic colleagues, for he was by now attacking most of their techniques of treatment—in particular, blood-letting:

> Although there probably never was a drop of blood too much in the living human body, yet the Old School practitioners consider an imaginary excess of blood as the main material cause of all hemorrhages and inflammations, which they must remove and drain off by venesections, cupping, and leeches.[23] [i]

> Anyone who has felt the tranquil pulse of a man an hour before the occurrence of the rigor that always precedes an attack of acute pleurisy, will not be able to restrain his amazement if told two hours later, after the hot stage has commenced, that the enormous plethora present urgently requires repeated venesections, and will naturally inquire by what magic power could the pounds of blood that must now be drawn off have been conjured into the blood-vessels of this man within these two hours, which but two hours previously he had felt beating in such a tranquil manner. Not a single drachm more of blood can now be circulating in those vessels than existed when he was in good health, not yet two hours ago.[24]

[h]See *Divided Legacy,* III, 207-213.

[i]Homoeopaths called themselves the "New School" and their orthodox ("allopathic") colleagues the "Old School."

> How did they pretend to let out the impure blood only? What magician's wand could separate, as through a sieve, the depraved from the good blood within the blood-vessels, so that only the bad would be drawn off and the good remain? What head is so rudely organized as to believe that they could effect this? Sufficient for them that streams of blood were spilt, of that vital fluid for which even Moses showed so much respect, and that justly.[25]

As early as 1792 he had vented his indignation at the death of Leopold II of Austria, due largely to the excessive letting of blood by his physicians. He commented as follows on the physicians' bulletins which appeared at the time:

> The bulletins state: "On the morning of February 28th, his doctor, Lagusius, found a severe fever and a distended abdomen"—he tried to fight the condition by venesection, and as this failed to give relief, he repeated the process three times more, without any better result. We ask, from a scientific point of view, according to what principles has anyone the right to order a second venesection when the first has failed to bring relief? As for a third, Heaven help us! but to draw blood a fourth time when the three previous attempts failed to alleviate! To abstract the fluid of life four times in twenty-four hours from a man who has lost flesh from mental overwork combined with a long continued diarrhoea, without procuring any relief for him! Science pales before this.[26]

This attack, by an unknown physician, upon the most illustrious *medici* of the Austrian Empire "produced a sensation no less vivid among the public than among the practitioners" (to quote a contemporary).[27]

A prominent patient entered Hahnemann's life in 1820 when Prince Schwarzenberg, commander of the allied armies against Napoleon, came to Leipzig for treatment of a stroke which had paralyzed his left side.[j] For several weeks

Hahnemann paid him regular visits but eventually quarreled with the Prince's personal physicians, who were bleeding him between the homoeopathic remedies, and relinquished the case. Schwarzenberg died five weeks later of a second stroke, and his physicians blamed homoeopathy for "delaying the application of more powerful measures" (i.e., more blood-letting).[28]

Schwarzenberg's death aroused public opinion against Hahnemann. At this time he was also troubled by political maneuvers of the pharmacists to bar him from dispensing his own medicines. These were administered in extremely small doses and prepared according to a method which the pharmacists did not know and could not, in Hahnemann's view, be trusted to follow diligently.[k] He therefore insisted that homoeopathic physicians prepare their own medicines and dispense them. The pharmacists felt this as an economic hardship and accused Hahnemann of "entrenching upon their privileges by the dispensing of medicines."[29] At a trial the judge found in their favor, and Hahnemann was compelled to change residence once again.

The Duke of Anhalt-Koethen invited him to live in his principality where he was allowed to prepare and dispense his own drugs, and Hahnemann remained there from 1821 until 1835. His wife died in 1830, and for several years Hahnemann, now over seventy-five years old, lived in virtual isolation. In 1835, however, he married a thirty-five year old Frenchwoman who was well-born, beautiful, and capable, and had apparently journeyed to Koethen (dressed as a young man) with the express purpose of marrying him. Since she was younger than nine of Hahnemann's eleven children,

[j]Hahnemann's refusal to come to Vienna to treat Schwarzenberg caused another sensation. Goethe, in this connection, wrote to a friend: "Now Prince Schwarzenberg, very ill and probably incurable, has confidence in this new Theophrastus Paracelsus and begs for leave of absence from the Emperor to seek a cure across the border"(Haehl, *Hahnemann,* I, 113).

[k]See "On the Preparation and Dispensing of Medicines by the Homoeopathic Physicians" (S. Hahnemann, *Lesser Writings* [New York: Radde, 1852], 696-712).

this marriage provoked discord within the family and astonishment outside. Moreover, the new Mme. Hahnemann insisted on removing her husband to Paris, and his last years were passed in this cultural center of the world where he was (at first) warmly welcomed by the French homoeopaths.[1] He was idyllically happy with his new wife, who plunged him into the thick of society, and rapidly acquired a fashionable and flourishing practice.

The political significance for homoeopathy of this move to Paris cannot be overestimated: it placed Hahnemann and his system at the center of world attention and gave him a platform of which he made full use. He died there in 1843 at the age of eighty-eight. He was buried in the Montmartre Cemetery, and his wife never remarried.

The early history of homoeopathy was shaped by Hahnemann's character and background.

He was from the borderline between the petty bourgeoisie and the laboring class, was the first in his family to achieve physician's status, and had to work long and hard for it. He had idealized the physician's calling during his many years of gazing at this unattainable goal. When he did attain it, and found the comportment of his colleagues to fall below the standards he had imagined existed, his disappointment was all the greater.

Although, with two wives and eleven children, he had more personal contacts than Paracelsus, Hahnemann was still a solitary person in whom the dearth of human relationships was replaced by an abstract love for humanity.

His lower-class origin, the isolation of his life, and his idealization of the physician's calling alienated him from his more aristocratic and well-connected colleagues. Although for years he endeavored to maintain good relations with them, he was willing to strike an independent course when the need arose.

[1]See below, p. 544.

Hahnemann's refusal to succumb to professional pressure enabled homoeopathy, the newest avatar of medical Empiricism, to assume an independent position in the world.

Hahnemann's Criticism of the Medical Profession

Much of Hahnemann's literary output was criticism of the theoretical errors and practical shortcomings of his colleagues, most of whom he felt unworthy of the name of physician.[m] His suggestions for reform follow the already familiar lines of the Empirical critique of medical Rationalism and Methodism, and he resembles Van Helmont in elucidating the tie between Rationalist-Methodist medical science and the socio-economic needs of the practitioner.

The brunt of his ideological critique is directed at the time-honored Rationalist claim to know the proximate causes of diseases:[n]

> Two thousand years were wasted by physicians in endeavoring to discover the invisible internal changes that take place in the organism in diseases and in searching for their proximate causes and *a priori* nature, because they imagined that they could not cure before they had attained to this *impossible* knowledge . . .[30]
>
> All that inflated bombast, passing for demonstration, abounding in words but void of sense—all the antics and curvets of the sophists about undiscoverable things, are ever vain and to the modest spirit of the true philosopher perfectly insufferable.
>
> We cannot even conceive a path that should lead us to such knowledge.

[m]"A number of causes . . . have for several centuries reduced the dignity of that God-like science, practical medicine, to a wretched breadwinning, a glossing over of symptoms, a degrading commerce in prescriptions—God help us!—to a trade that mixes the disciples of Hippocrates with the riffraff and medical rogues in such a way that one is indistinguishable from the other!" (*On Poisoning by Arsenic, the Remedies for It, and Its Medico-Legal Investigation,* quoted in Haehl, *Hahnemann,* I, 33).

[n]By this Hahnemann did not mean that exciting (procatarctic) causes should be neglected (see below, p. 392 and note).

> No, not a glimpse shall frail mortality ever obtain of that which lies deep hidden in the sacred recesses of the Divine Creating Mind, far, immeasurably far, beyond the grasp of human comprehension![31]

Four sciences are mistakenly invoked by physicians as auxiliaries in the search for causes: physiology, anatomy, pathology, and chemistry:

> *Anatomy* shows us the outside of every part which can be separated with the knife, the saw, or by maceration; but the deep internal changes it does not enable us to see . . . We see only the outside of organs, we see only their grosser substance; but into the innermost depths of their being and into the connection of their secret operations no mortal eye can ever pierce.[32]

> *Physiology,* until Haller's time, looked only through the spectacles of hypothetical conceits, gross mechanical explanations, and pretensions to systems, until this great man undertook the task of founding the knowledge of the phenomena of the human body upon sensible observation and truthful experiment alone . . . [but] little has been incontrovertibly established.[33]

> *Pathology,* a science in which that same love of system which has crazed the brains of the metaphysical physiologists, has caused a like misapplication of intellect in the attempt to search into the essential nature of diseases, that whereby affections of the system become manifest diseases. This they term the doctrine of *proximate, internal causes.* No mortal man can form a clear conception of what is here aimed at, to say nothing of the impossibility of any created intelligence, even in imagination, finding a road to an intimate view of what constitutes the essence of disease.[34] [o]

[o]About the application of Haller's sensivity and irritability to therapeutics Hahnemann writes: "what imaginable expedient have they for ascertaining *the exact degree* to which the sensibility, irritability, or reproduction they themselves (arbitrarily) dealt out to each of the organs are, in individual cases, increased,

But "none of the preliminary sciences has assumed so arrogant a place as chemistry."

> It is indeed a fact that chemistry explains certain appearances of the healthy as well as the diseased body, and is a guide to the preparation of various medicines; but it is incredible how often it has usurped the right of explaining all physiological and pathological phenomena, and how much it has distinguished itself by authorizing this or that medicine.[35]

The information obtained from investigations in these sciences is systematized in accordance with the rules of logic: "conjectures, opinions, definitions, postulates, and predicates, linked together by scholastic syllogisms."[36] This leads to arbitrary and incorrect classification of diseases and obstructs all practical efforts at healing.[37]

The theoretical problem engendered by the search for the "proximate cause" is that of distinguishing the "disease" itself from the "disease cause," the patient's organism, and the prominent symptoms:

> [The internal pathological process is] a dim picture of the imagination which theoretical medicine regarded as its *prima causa morbi,* and thus it was at one and the same time the *proximate cause of the disease* and the internal essence of the disease, the *disease itself*—although, as sound human reason teaches us, the cause of a thing or event can never be at the same time the thing or the event itself.[38]

> The physician of the Old School erroneously alleged the various, often purely imaginary, characters and phenomena of chronic diseases to be their *cause* (whereas they

diminished, or changed in quality . . . what is the part played by each organ with reference to these three great divisions in any given case of disease, and what intimate and absolute condition of the whole system thence arises, whence it may be clearly seen what is the appropriate, and in every respect suitable, remedy? What an insoluble problem! And yet its solution is indispensable to the practitioner, if he is to make any use of the system!" (*Lesser Writings,* 495).

> are but the products and expressions of that cause) . . . They imagined these conditions to be the cause *(causa)* of the chronic diseases which had to be removed, and the diminution or suppression of these by means of the treatment hitherto prevalent to be cures of the cause. . . . . Whence did these actually and *originally* come, since they are nothing more than single . . . expressions (symptoms) of the indwelling malady . . .?[39]

Because of this incorrect understanding of the nature of disease, therapeutics takes one of three equally incorrect forms: (1) treatment of the disease name:

> "If the patient has the gout, give him sulphuric acid; the remedy for rheumatism is mercury; cinchona is good for ague, simaruba for dysentery, squills for dropsy." Here the mere name of the supposed disease is sufficient to determine the parempiric for a remedy which crude undiscriminating experience has sometimes found useful in diseases that have been superficially termed gout, rheumatism, ague, dysentery, dropsy, but have neither been accurately described nor carefully distinguished from similar affections.[40] [p]

(2) treatment of the prominent symptom or symptoms:

> In all times the Old School physicians, not knowing how else to give relief, have sought to combat, and if possible to suppress by medicines, here and there, a *single* symptom from among a number in diseases—a *one-sided* procedure which, under the name of *symptomatic treatment,* has justly excited universal contempt because by it not only was nothing gained, but much harm was inflicted. A single one of the symptoms present is no more the disease itself than a single foot is the man himself.[41]

> The combatting of a single [symptom] (under the false title of *cause*) with medicines is truly nothing else than

[p]On "empiricism" and "parempiricism" see below, p. 687 and note.

> (blameworthy) *symptomatic treatment* which these gentlemen with unwarrantable pretension allege to be rational *treatment of the cause.*[42]

or (3) treatment of the assumed proximate cause:

> [Some] thought to persuade us that a predominance of acid was the proximate cause of all diseases, and they prescribed nothing but alkalis. An attempt to ally itself with them was made by the old sect which referred all kinds of acute diseases, especially the epidemic maladies, to a common poison which they contended often developed itself in the interior of the body, and sought for the antidote of this poison, which they believed to be the general excitant of most diseases, in absorbent alkaline earths . . . C. L. Hoffmann imagined that he had an equal right to set forth as a universal truth his own particular notion that almost all diseases arose from a kind of putridity, and were to be cured with remedies which his school denominates antiseptics . . . The more refined humoralists, in addition to the impurities in the blood, alleged besides, the existence of a pretended, almost universal plethora, as an excuse for their frightful merciless bloodlettings; they also gave out that these acted derivatively, depressed the tone, and ascribed many other subtle scientific effects to them. They acted, as we see, like other sects, quite arbitrarily, but obviously with an endeavor (not, indeed, to cure, that would be vulgar, no!) to give to their arbitrary procedures the highest possible coloring of rationality.[43] [q]

Here what the physician usually regards as a disease "cause" is actually the disease product: "the Old School regarded all those matters which were altered by the disease, those abnormal matters that occurred in congestions, as well

[q]The "old sect" to which Hahnemann refers is Iatrochemistry. Christian Ludwig Hoffmann (1721-1807) derived his pathology from Glisson, Haller, Sylvius, and Boerhaave and concluded that diseases are from a septic substance within the organism.

as those that were excreted, as disease-producers or at least, on account of their supposed reacting power, as disease maintainers, and this latter notion prevails to this day."[44]

> A favorite idea of the ordinary school of medicine until recent (would that I could not say the most recent!) times was that of morbific matters (and acridities) in diseases, excessively subtle though they might be thought to be, which must be expelled from the blood vessels and lymphatics, through the exhalants, skin, urinary apparatus, or salivary glands, through the tracheal and bronchial glands in the form of expectoration, from the stomach and bowels by vomiting and purging, in order that the body might be freed from the material cause that produced the disease, and a radical causal treatment be thus carried out.[45]

Hahnemann's comment on this was: if "the foul, often disgusting excretions which occur in diseases [were] the actual matter that produces and keeps them up . . . the most inveterate coryza should be certainly and rapidly cured by merely blowing and wiping the nose carefully."[46] Actually, of course, the mucus and coryza in the common cold, like all other material manifestations of disease, are the product of a non-material disease cause.[r]

The other major line of Hahnemann's criticism was directed against the medical profession's claim to understand *a priori* the mechanism of action of medicines: to a theoretically defined disease cause they oppose a medicine whose mode of action is also theoretical.

A number of such theories of the operation of remedies were current. Galen's doctrine that the secondary quality of a medicine (its action on the organism) can be determined

[r]He extends this line of reasoning even to worms in the intestines: "Are you sure that your worm-symptoms, a distended abdomen, bulimia alternating with anorexia, itching of the nose, blue rings surrounding the eyes, dilated pupils, etc., and even the discharge of *lumbrici*, are incontestable symptoms of vermicular disease? May they not rather be symptoms of a state of ill-health coexisting along with an accumulation of *lumbrici*, which may be the cause and not the effect of the collection of worms?" (*Lesser Writings*, 542).

from its primary quality (its taste or smell) was still alive. Cullen's ascription of the medicinal effect of quinine to its bitterness and astringency encouraged German physicians, barred from access to Peruvian quinine by the British blockade of Napoleon's Europe, to propose various mixtures of vegetable substances as substitutes for this sovereign "tonic."[47]

Others hoped to attain to this knowledge by chemical analysis, and they ranked medicines according to their content of carbon, hydrogen, or nitrogen.[48] [s]

A third group experimented by adding drugs to human blood in a glass jar, deducing the effect on the body from the observed reaction.[49]

Some experimenters administered medicines to sick animals in the hope of ascertaining their therapeutic qualities.[50]

Plants of the same botanical family were assumed to have identical medicinal powers, and some physicians invoked the doctrine of signatures—attempting to deduce the medicinal properties of a substance from its external form.[51]

Hahnemann rejected all of these procedures.

No substance has the same medicinal power as another merely because of similarity of taste: "a mixture of calmus, gentian, and gall-nuts may indeed be much more aromatic, more bitter, and more astringent than cinchona bark, but it can never be cinchona bark."[52]

Of the chemical investigation of remedies he observes: "but cabbage, roast beef, and wheaten cakes contain also plenty of nitrogen, carbon, or hydrogen—where then do we discover in them those properties which were so liberally allotted to these elementary substances?"[53] Test-tube experiments with human blood are pointless: "as if the medicine

[s]Cullen attributed the therapeutic action of mercury to its "particular disposition to unite with ammoniacal salts" (*Treatise of the Materia Medica,* II, 446). The French Brunonian, J. F. Chortet, explained it by the oxygen in mercurous oxide (*Traite de Pharmacologie,* 253). A pharmacological treatise of the time stated." "The knowledge of the principles contained in medicines which chemistry gives us can along determine the efficacy of remedies" (quoted in *Lesser Writings,* 675).

must not first undergo an infinity of changes in the digestive canal before it can get (and that only by a most circuitous method) into the blood."[54] Saltpeter, which is antiseptic and prevents dried meat from putrefying, has the opposite effect when given in "putrid fevers" (typhus) with tendency to gangrene—accelerating the morbific process by weakening the vitality of the organism. He concludes that chemistry can as little explain the powers of drugs as it can explain magnetism.[55] [t]

About experiments in animals he observes that medicines have a different effect on animals than on humans. Pigs can safely eat *Nux vomica* in quantities which would kill a human many times over; dogs can swallow *Aconitum napellus* without injury, although it is a deadly poison to man; yew leaves are poisonous to man but can be eaten by some animals, etc.[56]

Botanical affinity is a deceptive guide: "there are many examples of opposite, or at least very different powers, in one and the same family of plants, and that in most of them."[57] And the doctrine of signatures is one of the "suppositions of our superstitious forefathers" whose efficacy rests only "on the authority of old women's tales."[58]

Hahnemann rejected efforts to ascertain the curative properties of drugs *ab usu in morbis*—by administering them to the sick and observing the effect. His reason was that, except for a very few diseases of relatively constant character caused by a specific miasm,[u] diseases are infinitely varied, and a clearcut classification is impossible; furthermore, they have been described so carelessly by physicians that the information is of no value. In addition, medicines are almost never prescribed singly, but usually in a mixture with others, thus depriving such investigations of value.[59]

[t]On Francois Magendie's experiments with human blood, see below, pp. 628 ff. Hahnemann recognized that chemistry was occasionally useful to medicine—particularly in the discovery of antidotes to poisons (*Lesser Writings*, 252, 506 note).

[u]See below, pp. 392-397.

> Am I told, "The properties of medicines are not unknown"? I ask: "Are the half-dozen words which the Materia Medica contains regarding each to be called information?"... Often it is nothing more than a list of names of diseases, in all of which the substance in question is said to have been useful... Names of diseases, did I say? Heaven knows to what states of body these names were given, and what wisdom presided over the assigning of them![60]

What, then, explains the persistence of medical Rationalism? If the whole effort to elucidate the causes of diseases and the mechanism of action of remedies is valueless, where is the source of the vitality of this doctrine which, throughout history, has been espoused by a majority of the medical profession?

Here Hahnemann abandons scientific criticism for sociological analysis, pointing out the psychological and economic roots of medical Rationalism.

In the first place, this system panders to the physician's sense of self-importance by providing him with *explanations* of all phenomena. This is their principal error: "the *vain fancy that the business of the medical profession is to explain everything.*"[61] [v]

[v]Hahnemann is especially critical of the so-called *"Naturphilosophie"* of his contemporaries, Johann Gottlieb Fichte (1762-1814) and Friedrich Schelling (1775-1854) which was an attempt to "explain" all natural phenomena in neo Platonic, mystical, vitalist terms: "Now we were fooled by the natural philosophers. For of such seers there was no lack; each fell on a new aspect of things—each wove a different system, having nothing in common but the morbid propensity, by inward self-contemplation, not only to give an exact *a priori* account of the nature and universal constitution of things, but, moreover, to look on themselves as the authors of the whole, and, according to their own fashion, to construct it for and out of themselves. Every hint they deemed themselves to have gathered on life in the abstract and the essential nature of man was—like their whole conception—so unintelligible, so hollow and unmeaning, that no clear sense could be drawn from it. Human speech, which is only fitted to convey the impressions of sense and the ideas immediately flowing from them—generalizations, each one of which is easily insulated into concrete examples and thus brought home and typified to the sense—refused to embody their conceits, their extravagant fantastic visions; and, therefore, they had to babble them forth in

> *They placed the essence of the medical art, and their own chief pride, in explaining even much of the inexplicable.* They imagined it impossible to treat scientifically the abnormal states of the human body (diseases) without possessing a *tangible* idea of the fundamental laws of the normal and abnormal conditions of the human frame.
>
> This was the first and great delusion they practiced on themselves and on the world. This was the unhappy conceit which, from Galen's day down to our own, made the medical art a stage for the display of the most fantastic, often most self-contradictory, hypotheses, explanations, demonstrations, conjectures, dogmas, and systems, whose evil consequences are not to be overlooked. Even the student was taught to think he was master of the art of discovering and removing disease when he had stuffed his head with these baseless hypotheses, which seemed made for the express purpose of distracting his brains and leading him as far as possible away from a true conception of disease and its cure.[62]

> Our system-builders delighted in these metaphysical heights where it was so easy to win territory; for in the boundless reaches of speculation every one becomes a ruler who can effectually elevate himself beyond the

new-fangled, highsounding words, superlunary collocations, eccentric rhapsodies, and unheard-of phrases without any sense, and got involved in such gossamer subtleties that one felt at a loss to know which was the most appropriate—a satire on such a misdirection of mental energy or an elegy on its ill success. We have to thank the natural philosophers for the disorder and dislocation of many a young doctor's understanding. Moreover, their self-conceit was yet too inflated for them to bring forward many views on diseases or their cure, except what they now and then put forward on their dualism, their polarization and representation, their reflex, their differentizing and indifferentizing, their potentizing and depotentizing. This natural philosophy still lives and flourishes in a forced animation of matter and in ecstatic hallucinations concerning the modelling and ordering of the world and its epitome—man. Incorporeal and ethereal, it still soars aloft beyond our solar system, beyond the bounds of the actual; and does not seem likely yet a while to descend from its super-sublime elevation to the lowly sphere of practice (the cure of man's diseases), nor, indeed—so far has it overstrained its power—to be able to do so" (*Lesser Writings,* 494-495). As a practical physician Hahnemann could have only contempt for such extremes of abstraction, totally divorced from any observable reality and devoid of any empirical foundation.

> domain of the senses. The superhuman aspect they derived from the erection of these stupendous castles in the air concealed their poverty in the art of healing.[63] [w]
>
> Innumerable and dissimilar ideas respecting the nature of diseases and their remedies sprang from so many dissimilar brains, and these theoretical views gave rise to the so-called *systems*, each of which was at variance with the rest and self-contradictory. Each of these subtle expositions at first threw the readers into stupefied amazement at the incomprehensible wisdom contained in it, and attracted to the system-monger a number of followers, who re-echoed his unnatural sophistry; to none of whom, however, was it of the slightest use in enabling them to cure better, until a new system, often diametrically opposed to the first, thrust that aside, and in its turn gained a short-lived renown. None of them, however, was in consonance with nature and experience; they were mere theoretical webs, woven by cunning intellects out of pretended consequences, which could not be made use of in practice, in treatment at the sick-bed, on account of their excessive subtlety and repugnance to nature, and only served for empty disputations.[64]

He concludes: "they have never yet taught us how to cure our fellow men in a manner that shall satisfy our conscience, but only how we may present to the people an appearance of learned wisdom and deep penetration."[65] The claim to understand proximate causes is "flattering, indeed, to the vanity of the learned theorist but usually leading astray when used as a guide to practice . . . wherein there was evidenced more of ostentation than of an earnest search for the curative indication."[66]

[w]Hahnemann may perhaps have been thinking of Locke's comment: "I see it is easier and more natural for men to build castles in the air of their own than to survey well those that are to be found standing"—*a propos* Sydenham's criticism of his own Rationalist contemporaries (Dewhurst, *Dr. Thomas Sydenham,* 59). Such a remark was preeminently applicable to "*Naturphilosophie.*"

He describes as follows the physician who has succumbed to the temptation to believe that he has plumbed the pent secrets of nature:

> Look how A. walks into the assemblage that reverentially expects him, with carefully measured steps, with expanded chest and elevated head; how he announces the dignity of his great person by a gracious slow inclination of his body, and how he decides the most important questions with a few short words and a disdainful air. He only honors the great people in the company with his notice, he flatters them in high-sounding phrases, in order to be entertained by them in return, and he talks about the highest personages in the land and the greatest savants as he would about the most ordinary trifles which may be estimated with the fifth part of a glance. Merit rewarded or neglected, heart-breaking domestic occurrences, danger and delivery, life and death, are all the same to him; nothing produces any change in his frigid manner, or at the most they elicit from him a witty remark, which the crowd of his admirers do not omit to acknowledge with their plaudits. He talks the modern languages with the most refined accent; his house is the model of fashion and the furniture in the best taste. . . . Who can be surprised that the details of a case of disease are tiresome to him, and that he defers till tomorrow doing anything for the urgent support of some poor man, the sole support of a wretched family, because he must go and leave his card on some lord who is passing through the town. His medical wisdom must, in the face of all these fashionable accessories, be but a thin coating which he has enough to do to keep well polished, so that all uninvited inquiring glances may be arrested by its mirror-like gloss, and be repelled without having penetrated its shallow depth.[67]

In the second place, Rationalism is a structure of thought "cunningly devised for the convenience of therapeutics,"[68] a procrustean bed which fits the needs of the physician at the expense of the patient. It "attribute[s] a false character to the acute diseases it [has] to cure in order that they might conform to the plan of treatment once adopted for them."[69] "Our dear ordinary system of medicine, whose maxim seems to be to leave everything in the old way, to take everything quite easily, and to spare ourselves as much reflection as possible."[70]

To be more specific, the reductionist urge of Rationalism is designed: 1) to curtail the variety of diseases in the world by eliminating many of the symptoms, and 2) to curtail the variety of remedies by assuming a limited number of medicinal "powers" of significance for therapeutics. Instead of accepting the full variety of diseases and remedies which exists in nature, and incorporating this variety in the therapeutic system, Rationalism finds least common denominators in each and bases its thought on these.

The linking of each diseased state to a hypothesized internal (proximate) cause means neglect of many of the patient's symptoms and thus an unjustified simplification of disease patterns:

> The Old School physician gave himself very little trouble in this matter in his mode of treatment. He would not listen to any minute detail of all the circumstance of his case by the patient; indeed, he frequently cut him short in his relation of his sufferings, in order that he might not be delayed in the rapid writing of his prescription. . . . At subsequent visits he only asked a few general questions, went through the ceremony of feeling the pulse at the wrist, looked at the tongue, and at the same moment wrote another prescription on equally irrational principles, or ordered the first one to be continued . . . and with a graceful bow, he hurried off to the fiftieth or sixtieth patient he had to visit, in this thoughtless way, in the course of that forenoon.[71]

> The physician who was called in to a case, to determine, as the rules of his art enjoined, the nosological name of the disease his patient labored under, must take for

granted, in reference to some symptoms that the pathological works describe as belonging to this form of disease, that they are merely accidentally absent in his patient, that they *might* very well be there, *although they are not*—the remaining often very numerous and serious sufferings and symptoms which the patient was really affected with, but which do not occur in the definition of the nosological name in the pathological work, he must, so the rules of his art required, regard as unessential, as accidental, as unimportant, as wild, exuberant offshoots so to speak—symptoms of symptoms—which he need not pay attention to.[72] [x]

"What do we care," say the medical teachers and their books, "what do we care about the presence of many other diverse symptoms that are observable in the case of disease before us, or the absence of those that are wanting? The physician should pay no attention to such empirical trifles; his practical tact, the penetrating glance of his mental eye into the hidden nature of the malady, enables him to determine at the very first sight of the patient what is the matter with him, what pathological form of disease he has to do with, and what name he has to give it, and his therapeutic knowledge teaches him what prescription he must order for it."[73]

Instead of taking a careful description of the patient's symptoms, the physician "delights to invent a fixed name, by preference a Greek one, for the malady, in order to make the patient believe that he has long known this disease as an old acquaintance and hence is the fittest person to cure it."[74] This permits him to diagnose rapidly and thus to treat 60 or 80 patients in a single day:[75]

See: by half-past four in the morning he is in his carriage, for this morning he has thirty visits to pay to patients.

[x]Cullen was only the most recent (after Galen, Boerhaave, and other Rationalists and Methodists) to employ the expression, "symptom of a symptom" (*Synopsis of Methodical Nosology,* xiii).

His horses foam with the rapidity of the pace, and have to be changed for fresh ones in a few hours. Whilst he drives along he is seen to bend in deep meditation over a long clearly-written list, wherein the names and abodes of the patients who are sighing for him, and the minute at which he believes he will be at each of them, are carefully marked. He looks at his watch which indicates the seconds, he calls to the coachman who instantly draws up. Out he jumps, says a few words to his servant and runs up the stairs. Doors fly open at his approach, three steps bring him to his patient's side. He feels his pulse, asks him a couple of questions, and without waiting a reply he calls for pen, ink, and paper: and after deep reflection for two seconds in his chair he suddenly dashes off the complex prescription, politely hands it to the patient for his uninterrupted use with a few solemn words, rubs his hands together, makes his bow, and disappears, in order to be with another patient six seconds afterwards, on whom also he bestows his two minutes of advice; for his presence is in such great request that he is perfectly unable to devote a longer period to each patient. He wipes the perspiration from his brow, complains of having too much to do, makes his servant call him half a dozen times out from a party where he stays altogether only half an hour; beckons to him every surgeon he meets, in order to whisper a few important words in his ear, pointing at the same time to some houses or streets. At his consultation hour, his anteroom teems with the friends of patients, sick-nurses, mid-wives, surgeons, and patients. There he dispenses in profusion prescriptions, recommendations, advice—like tickets for the theatre.[76]

The extreme of over-simplification was reached in Brunonian Methodism:

> In dialectic sophistries, in bold assertions, (in shameless self-praise), and in disregard of the infinite multiplicity of nature, manifested in the varieties presented by diseases and by their remedies, all known founders of medical

> sects were far surpassed by that deceiving parempiric, Brown, who, though not himself engaged in the treatment of diseases, limited all possible curative indications to exciting and diminishing excitement, and presented to the eyes of the world the greatest of all medical absurdities: "that there can be only two or three diseases which are distinguished from each other by no other difference besides a plus and minus of excitement and a corresponding accumulation of excitability."[77]

"God help us, what a mass of nonsense a single impractical book-maker can rake together and inflict on weak, lamb-like mortality, in defiance of all common sense!"[78] [y]

Just as the quest for proximate causes suits the convenience of physicians, so does the Rationalist analysis of drugs. Although each medicinal substance in the world differs from each other, these physicians group them into classes which are periodically reorganized to reflect prevailing pathological and therapeutic fashions:

> The remedies employed by the ancients as *alexipharmaca, cephalica, splenica, uterina* had afterwards to undertake the office of antispasmodic and antinervous remedies. When the prevailing system assumed tension and laxity of the fibers as the foundation of disease, the very same medicines which had hitherto performed a different part were forced to be twisted into one of these two directions . . . Then, when Brown needed for his system only *stimulating* and *debilitating remedies,* those very remedies which formerly had been marshalled under many other titles are immediately enlisted in the two new regiments . . . just as if one had but to utter the fiat, and the substances could not choose but obey the commands of the exalted man, at his pleasure to enter on one or the other function.[79]

[y] See, also, "Fragmentary Observations on Brown's *Elements of Medicine,*" in *Lesser Writings,* 350-361: "Heaven help us! throughout the whole transparent work he has dazzled as with a flaring straw fire, here it sinks down into ashes, and he leaves us, with a smile, surrounded by a howling wilderness in the darkness of night."

Then several drugs are prescribed at a time, to combat the presumed proximate causes:

> In a mixed prescription . . . the prescribing doctor determines for each ingredient the part it is to play in the human body. This one shall be the *basis*, this other the *adjuvans*, a third the *corrigens*, that one the *dirigens*, and the other the *excipiens*. Imperiously I command that none of these ingredients shall dare to leave its appointed post in the human body! I command that the *corrigens* shall not fail to cloak over the vices of the *basis*, and shall gloss over and turn to advantage all the wickedness of the main remedy and the *adjuvans*. That this same *corrigens* should leave its place and take up on its own authority some post—it may be in opposition to the *basis*—I must herewith strongly forbid . . . Do you seriously believe that the mixture will perform what you expect of all the ingredients, as if they were things which do not act reciprocally on one another, influence one another or not, regardless of your desire. Does it not occur to you that two dynamic agencies together can never effect that which each individually might, administered at different times? Do you not see that a middle effect must take place, which is not to be foreseen *a priori* . . . The heights of parempiricism are reached by prescribing multiconstituted prescriptions—perhaps many times a day . . . It is as though one should throw blindfold a handful of balls of various kinds upon an unknown billiard table with cushions of various angles, and should pretend to decide beforehand what effect they would all conjointly produce . . . And yet the results of all mechanical forces are much more easily determined than those of dynamic forces.[80]

Hahnemann was the first to raise his voice against the compounding of prescriptions, holding that the effects of compounds in disease could never be known precisely:[z]

[z]Equally important was his conviction that medicines are by nature harmful to the organism, and consequently should not be administered in greater quantities than necessary (see below, pp. 362 and 369).

> What shall we say to the alleged powers of drugs in this or that disease, when we know that the materia medica has obtained its information thereupon . . . generally with a mixture of drugs . . . *to ascribe any powers to a medicinal substance which has never been tested purely, that is, unless along with others, consequently might as well have been never tested at all, is to be guilty of deception and falsehood.*[81]

Another reason for the prevailing polypharmacy was the ignorance of physicians about any one medicine—their failure to acquire even such information as was available in the schools:

> This motley mixing system is nothing but a convenient shift for one who, having but a slender acquaintance with the properties of a single substance, flatters himself, though he cannot find any one simple suitable remedy to remove the complaint, that by heaping a great many together there may be one amongst them that by a happy chance shall hit the mark.[82]

Most physicians do not even compound a prescription for each patient but use the ready-made formulas in stock at the apothecary. The economic benefit is obvious, as the physician "gets four pence for every prescription. So the same for a prescription which he copies out of printed recipe book as for one that takes him an hour to compose! . . . Of course he prefers making use of borrowed, ready-written (i.e. unsuitable) prescriptions; he can write a number of such ones in the course of a forenoon—but he must write a *great many, more than are good for the patient,* because he is paid by the number of his prescriptions, and because he requires many four-pences in order to live, to live well, to live in style!"[83]

Hahnemann appreciates the strong psychological drives supporting Rationalist and Methodist medicine:

> It is the natural tendency of the human mind to seek for the exciting causes of the phenomena he sees about him, and hence we see that no sooner does a disease show

> itself than everyone occupies himself with attributing it to some source, that which seems to him to be the most likely one. But we should be greatly mistaken if, from this irresistible propensity to seek a cause for an effect, we should infer a necessity for such knowledge in order to effect a cure.[84]

> I admit it was more convenient for the weakness of humanity to assume that, in the diseases they were called on to cure, there existed some morbific material of which the mind might form a conception (more particularly as the patients readily lent themselves to such a notion), because in that case the practitioner had nothing further to care about than to procure a good supply of remedies for purifying the blood and humors, exciting diuresis and diaphoresis, promoting expectoration, and scouring out the stomach and bowels.[85]

But the physician must not yield to such impulses: "the essential nature of diseases and their cure will not adapt themselves to such fantasies, nor to the convenience of medical men."[86]

Actually, the physician often abandons his theories when faced with a difficult case:

> His learned theoretical apparatus leaves him in the lurch; he then runs over, in a purely empirical manner, just like the most unreflecting routine practitioner, a number of names of medicines—"there, make what you can of that! you may put all the names together into a bag and according to your fancy draw out one or several, it is quite immaterial, you may use this one or that one!" Here, where the question is to afford relief, we find the most stupid syncretism and empiricism . . . [87]

Therapeutic techniques which make a visible impact on the patient appeal to the physician's pride in himself as scientist and engineer:

> It is undoubtedly very agreeable for the physician to feel himself so powerful, or at all events to appear to be able

to promote perspiration here, urine there, to lull pain here, to excite there, to bind here, to loosen there, to incise here, to expel there, to strengthen here, to cool there, to check spasms here, and putridity there, to accomplish all that he commands his cohorts of medicines to do. . . . But admitting there were such general remedies that would here and there certainly promote perspiration, assuredly cause a flow of urine, strikingly soothe pain, infallibly strengthen, undeniably resolve, loosen, purge, and cause vomiting, powerfully act upon the secretion of mucus, in every case cool, allay every spasm, and check every inordinate discharge, unhesitatingly transfer congestions from a more to a less important seat, will all this, supposing it went on ever so beautifully, cure the disease? Oh no, in most cases not. Something striking has been performed, *but health has not been restored,* and that was what had to be done.[88]

The physician who is consulted diagnoses [a] malady to be gastric; he purges and re-purges. But behold the fever increases, the taste becomes more disagreeable, the breath and the excrements more fetid, the sclerotic yellower, the tongue more furred and browner, the ideas get confused, the lips tremble, stupifying slumber takes the place of sleep, etc. He is sorry to see his patient hurrying on toward his grave, but he is happy that he possesses the power of energetically purging away the impurities. What is the matter with you? "I put myself in a violent passion, my head is like to burst, I have spasms in my stomach, the bile rises incessantly into my mouth." You will, perhaps, take a bilious fever, take this emetic immediately. Look! he throws up bile, he vomits again and again, he will vomit up his very insides—the night of death obscures his sight, whilst he is bathed in cold perspiration. "I have done my duty," says the doctor to himself, "I have done all I could to clear away the bad bile."

And thus it is with the whole array of general remedies. The respectable doctor does much, only not

> what he ought—he produces remarkable effects, but very seldom health.[89]

Hahnemann's comment: "What a calumniation of the nature, what a dangerous insinuation for the ordinary half-instructed practitioner, already too officious! What a ministration to his pride to be deemed the lord and master of the nature!"[90]

This system permits them to blame their failures on "the incurableness of the disease . . . the disobedience of the patient, and . . . other insignificant circumstances."[91]

But there is another, rather unattractive, side to this activism of the physician. His feelings of mastery are reinforced even further when he inflicts paid and suffering:

> By treatment the ordinary physician often understands nothing more than a powerful violent attack upon the body with things that are to be found in the chemist's shop, with an alteration of the diet, *secundum artem,* to one of a very extraordinary, very meagre character. "The patient must first be powerfully affected before I can do him any good; I wish I could but once get him regularly laid up in bed." But that the transition from bed to the straw and the coffin is so very easy, infinitely easier than to health, he says nothing about that.
>
> The physician of the stimulating [Brunonian] school is in the habit of prescribing in almost every case an exactly opposite diet (such is the custom of his sect): ham, strong meat soups, brandy, etc. often in cases where the very smell of meat makes the patient sick, and he can bear nothing but cold water; but he too is by no means sparing in his use of violent remedies in enormous doses.
>
> The schools of both the former and the latter class authorize a revolutionary procedure of this sort: "No child's play with your doses," they say, "go boldly and energetically to work, giving them strong, as strong as possible!" And they are right if treating means the same thing as knocking down.[92]

> When physicians of the Old School do not know what to do in a chronic disease, they treat it blindly with their

> so-called *alterative* remedies *(alterantia);* among which the horrible *mercurialia* (calomel, corrosive sublimate, and mercurial ointment) occupy the foremost place—which they allow to act in such large quantities and for so long a time on the diseased body . . . that at last the health is by their destructive effects completely undermined. They thus certainly produce great alterations, but invariably such as are not beneficial, and they always, utterly ruin the health by their improper administration of this excessively dangerous metal.[93]
>
> In every acute or chronic disease that comes under their notice, they earnestly insist on a very complicated *artificial system of diet,* withholding many things and ordering a host of others.
>
> Do we physicians, however, know with such extreme precision the effects of all kinds of food, as to be able with certainty to say, in this case such and such an article of diet is to be taken, and this and that other to be avoided? How does experience refute our fancied omniscience![94]

The violent treatment of mental patients current in Hahnemann's time was another abuse against which he raised his voice:[a]

> I never allow any insane person to be punished by blows or other painful corporeal inflictions, since there can be no punishment where there is no sense of responsibility, and since such patients only deserve our pity and cannot be improved, but must be rendered worse, by such rough treatment. [A patient] often showed me with tears in his eyes the marks of the blows and stripes his former keepers had employed to keep him in order.[95]
>
> It is impossible not to marvel at the hard-heartedness and indiscretion of the medical men in many establishments

[a]In a 1796 article describing his own treatment of a mental patient in 1792—thus at least a year prior to Philippe Pinel's introduction of mild treatment of the insane at the Bicetre Hospital in Paris (see below, p. 448).

> for [the insane], who . . . content themselves with torturing these most pitiable of all human beings with the most violent blows and other painful torments. By this unconscientious and revolting procedure they debase themselves beneath the level of the turnkeys in a house of correction, for the latter inflict such chastisements as the duty devolving on their office, and on criminals only.[96]

Hahnemann concluded that existing forms of therapy cater to the ignorance and indolence of the average physician as well as to a certain sadistic streak: "the most important of all human vocations, I mean *the observation of the sick and of the infinite varieties of their disordered state of health,* can only be pursued in such a superficial and careless manner *by those who despise mankind.*"[97]

If their routine practice effects a cure, it is accidental—like a number in roulette which, if played time after time, will finally win.[98] "Not a single founder or follower of any of the many medical systems could or . . . would dare to carry out his system faithfully and vigorously into practice, without doing the greatest injury to his patients; so that they would have been far better off wanting medical aid altogether."[99] Many of them abandon active medicine entirely and practice pure expectancy.[100]

At any event the existing systems are mutually incompatible: "all these modes of treatment, many directly opposite to one another, have each their authorities and illustrious supporters; but nowhere do we find a universally applicable standard of treatment accredited in all ages."[101] Hahnemann concludes that "*the medical art stands in need of a thorough reform from head to foot* . . . The evil has become so crying that the well-meaning mildness of a Jan Hus no longer avails, but the fiery zeal of a rock-firm Martin Luther is needed to sweep away the monstrous leaven."[102]

His Reversion to Empirical Assumptions

He felt that reform would come from three sources: enhancement of the moral qualities of the practitioner, greater willingness to devote hard thought to medicine, and, finally, adoption of a correct method of analyzing and solving therapeutic problems.

In his 1792 domestic guide, *The Friend of Health,* Hahnemann gave the following description of the good family physician:

> Search for some plain man of sound common sense, who takes great pains to ascertain the truth of all he hears and says, and does not merely look to its passing muster, who knows how to give clear and condensed information respecting everything that belongs to his art, and never obtrudes his opinion unasked or at an improper time, and who is no stranger to everything else important for man as a citizen of the world to know. More especially let the man you choose be one who does not show temper nor get angry, except when he beholds injustice, who never turns away unmoved from any except flatterers, who has but few friends but these men of sterling principle, who listens attentively to the complaints of those who seek his aid, and does not pronounce an opinion without mature reflection.[103]

In the same work he places in the mouth of Socrates a eulogy to the benevolence of the true physician:

> Knowest thou the man that has just passed us clad in a coarse woollen garment? In his venerable aged form beams universal philanthropy. That is Eumenes the physician. The many thousands that he yearly makes by the practice of his art, he does not spend on fine country houses and on the other vain trifles of the luxurious. His happiness consists in doing good! About the tenth part of his large income he uses for his limited wants, the rest he puts out to interest in the state. And how? thou askest me. To the poor he gives his aid, his medical skill. With his stores he supports the convalescent families until they can again help themselves, and with the costliest of his wines he revives the dying. He seeks out the miserable in

> their dirty hovels and appears to them as a beneficent divinity . . . even at midnight he appears in the huts of the miserable to assist them, and lavishes on them consolation, advice, and aid . . .[104]

These qualities alone, however, were not enough. Medicine demands hard thought as well, "the most laborious of all work under the sun."[105] He urged his colleagues to improve their intellectual and other skills: "Let us become better, and all will soon go better."[106]

But "becoming better" presupposed knowledge of the direction in which to improve, and here Hahnemann urged a reconstruction of therapeutic thinking along Empirical lines. His proposals for change are the mirror-image of his criticism of Methodism and Rationalism.

In opposition to their materialization of the proximate cause, he holds that this internal cause is "spiritual" *(geistlich)* or dynamic and "can never be ascertained by mortal reason."[107]

> The causes of our maladies cannot be material, since the least foreign material substance, however mild it may appear to us, if introduced into our blood-vessels, is promptly ejected by the vital force, as though it were a poison; or when this does not happen, death ensues . . . . can it be supposed that in the case of a cutaneous disease of twenty years' standing, for instance, this indefatigably active vital principle will quietly endure the presence of such an injurious foreign, material, exanthematous substance, such as a herpetic, a scrofulous, a gouty acridity, etc. in the fluids of the body? Did any nosologist ever see with corporeal eyes such a morbific matter, to warrant him in speaking so confidently about it, and in founding a system of medical treatment upon it? Has anyone ever succeeded in displaying to view the matter of gout or the poison of scrofula?[108]

> As regards most diseases [the proximate cause] will remain forever concealed from human weakness.[109]

Hahnemann (like Stahl) cites psychosomatic diseases and physical diseases provoked by emotional upset as evidence for the dynamic or spiritual nature of the "proximate cause":

> How often has it happened that an irritating word has brought on a dangerous bilious fever; a superstitious prediction of death has caused the fatal catastrophe at the very time announced; the abrupt communication of sad or excessively joyful news has occasioned sudden death? In these cases where is the material morbific principle that entered in substance into the body, there to produce and keep up the disease, and without the material expulsion and ejection of which a radical cure were impossible. The champions of this clumsy doctrine of morbific matters ought to be ashamed that they have so inconsiderately overlooked and failed to appreciate the spiritual nature of life, and the spiritual dynamic power of the exciting causes of diseases.[110]

Finally, the proximate cause must be spiritual because it is a derangement of the vital force of the body, i.e., the *physis* of Hippocrates which acts purposively to maintain the organism in health and cure it when sick.[111]

The curative reaction of the *physis* (*die Natur*) to morbific stimuli is manifested in many ways. "For instance, the vital force of our organism that is always exercising a preservative function protects the sensitive parts of the palm of the hand of the pavier (as also of the worker among fire, the glassblower, and the like) against the scratching and lacerating sharp angles and points of the paving stones, with a hard, horny covering, to protect the skin with its nerves, blood-vessels, and muscles, from being wounded or destroyed."[112] [b] When the stomach is overloaded with food, it responds by vomiting.[113] "If even the minutest splinter penetrates a sensitive part of our organism, the vital principle everywhere present in our body never rests until it is removed by pain, fever, suppuration, or gangrene."[114] "A so-called

[b]He criticized Brown for ignoring this factor in cure (*Lesser Writings,* 547).

critical perspiration or diarrhoea produced by the ever-active vital force after a sudden indisposition . . . will be much more successful, at least for the time, in relieving the acute disease, than all the sudorific or purgative drugs in the pharmacopoeia."[115]

This protective force sometimes takes the form of an instinct in the patient to do what is needful for health. In animals this instinct is strong enough to constitute actual knowledge of many remedies.[116 c] In man the instinct is weaker, but the equivalent in him is the urge to eat the right foods and follow the correct regimen in disease. In *The Friend of Health* Hahnemann advises his readers to eat the foods which a "sound and unperverted instinct" recommends:

> What mutilator of the rights of man could have told you that our beneficent mother Nature has not endowed us with just as much instinct as we require? Who teaches the infant to prefer its mother's milk to pastry? Who instructs him that is sunk in grief and distress to take a glass of wine? Who tells the patient ill of a bilious fever to avoid meat, the dysenteric patient to pant for grapes? Who tells us when we are hungry, when thirsty?[117 d]

This instinct is also active in disease: "in acute disease the awakened instinct of the patient is often considerably wiser than the physician who does not consult the nature in his prescriptions." "The patient's own feelings are a much surer guide than all the maxims of the schools."[118] "An individual affected with an acute fever smells from afar the approach of an animal soup, to which the new wakeful, still unknown, life-preserving faculty evinces the greatest repugnance. He

[c]Note Paracelsus: "Now as the snake knows her help and knows the herb, there is also such an understanding in you. Therefore do not be astonished that the snake knows medicine" (*Divided Legacy,* I, 373). Hahnemann recounts the case of a man poisoned with *Arnica montana* who instinctively drank its antidote—vinegar (*Lesser Writings,* 325).

[d]Of course, the idea of the beneficence of the natural instincts is fundamental to Rousseau's *Emile* (on this see Haehl, *Hahnemann,* I, 53, 55).

would vomit violently were we to bring it too near to him. If lemon-juice is good for him—see, at the very mention of it his countenance expresses pleasure and desire, and yet when he was well, how indifferent were they both to him."[119]

For this reason he criticizes the self-assertive physician who prescribes a rigid diet for his patient and, in effect, denies the patient's instinctive capacity to eat what he needs:[e]

> In numerous instances many a prostrate patient has effected a miraculous cure upon himself not only by refusing the physician's medicine, but by secretly transgressing his artificial and often mischievous system of diet, in obedience to his own caprice, which is in this instance an imperious instinct impelling him to commit all sorts of dietetic paradoxes.[120]

When confronted with a disease cause, this dynamic force within the body attempts to overcome it through coction, crisis, and evacuation:

> In order to relieve the primarily affected organ by a crisis, an increased—often violent—activity is excited in the excretory organs to draw away the disease from the former to the latter; there ensue vomitings, purgings, diuresis, diaphoresis, abscesses, etc., in order by this irritation of distant parts to effect a sort of derivation from the primarily diseased part, and the dynamically affected nervous power seems to unload itself in the material product.[121]

Since this force acts purposively to protect the organism in health and cure it in disease, the physician must understand its operations if he is to do the same. But this does not mean a material knowledge of the body and its elements. It does not mean (as the Rationalist and Methodist physicians claim) assimilating the functioning of the human

[e]Yet Hahnemann himself was famous for the rigid regimen he prescribed for his patients.

body to processes described in the language of some other scientific discipline:

> It is impossible that either physician or teacher, when caring for mind or body, should require such foreknowledge of his subject-matter as shall lead him by the hand, as it were, to the completion of his work, as, perhaps, a knowledge of the physical and chemical properties of the materials helps and conducts the metallurgist, the tanner, and other such craftsmen, to the perfection of theirs. The vocation of these others demands quite another kind of knowledge, just as their object, a living individual, is quite different.[122] [f]

The living organism is *sui generis* and must be understood in its own terms, in the light of its own laws:

> To the explanation of human life, as also its twofold conditions, health and disease, the principles by which we explain other phenomena are quite inapplicable. With nought in the world can we compare it save with itself alone: neither with a piece of clockwork nor with a hydraulic machine, nor with chemical processes, nor with decompositions and recompositions of gases, nor yet with a galvanic battery, in short with nothing destitute of life. Human life is *in no respect* regulated by purely physical laws, which only obtain among inorganic substances.[123]

> Though all the component parts of the human frame are to be found in other parts of nature, they act together in their organic union to the full development of life and the discharge of the other functions of man in so *peculiar* and anomalous a manner (which can only be defined by the term *vitality*) that this peculiar *(vital)* relation of the parts to one another and the external world cannot be judged of or explained by any other rule than that which itself supplies; therefore, by none of the known laws of mechanics, statics, or chemistry. All those

[f]Thus Hahnemann rejects Aristotle's parallel between healing and building a house (*Parts of Animals* 639b 16-640a 8. See *Divided Legacy,* I, 148). His assimilation of healing to teaching shows Rousseauian influence.

> theories, to which age after age has given birth, when brought in contact with simple experience, and tried by an impartial test, have ever been found to be farfetched and unfounded.[124]

How, then, is the physician to go about comprehending the operations of this *sui generis* organism?

During his years in the wilderness, after abandoning his profession and while seeking a more reliable basis of thought and practice, Hahnemann was bolstered by his religious faith. He wrote later to his friend, C. W. Hufeland (1762-1836), in a letter "Upon the Necessity of a Regeneration of Medicine":

> But perhaps it is in the very nature of this art, as great men have asserted, that it is incapable of attaining any greater certainty.
>
> "Shameful, blasphemous thought," I exclaimed, —What, shall it be said that the infinite wisdom of the eternal Spirit that animates the universe could not produce remedies to allay the sufferings of the diseases it allows to arise? . . . Shall He, the Father of all, behold with indifference the martyrdom of His best-loved creatures by disease, and yet have rendered it impossible to the genius of man, to which all else is possible, to find any method, any *easy, sure, trustworthy* method, whereby they may see diseases in their proper point of view and whereby they may interrogate medicines as to their special uses, as to what they are *really, surely,* and *positively* serviceable for?
>
> Sooner than admit this blasphemous thought, I would have abjured all the medical systems in the world . . .
>
> Well, thought I, as there *must* be a sure and trustworthy method of treatment, as certainly as God is the wisest and most beneficent of beings, I shall seek it no longer in the thorny thicket of ontological explanations, in arbitrary opinions, though these might be capable of being arranged into a splendid system, nor in the authoritative declarations of celebrated men—no, let me seek it where it lies nearest at hand.[125]

In his pamphlet, *The Medicine of Experience* (1805), he wrote:

> As the wise and beneficent Creator has permitted those innumerable states of the human body differing from health, which we term diseases, He must at the same time have revealed to us a *distinct* mode whereby we may obtain a knowledge of diseases that shall suffice to enable us to employ the remedies capable of subduing them. He must have shown us an equally distinct mode whereby we may discover in medicines those properties that render them suitable for the cure of diseases–if He did not mean to leave His children helpless or to require of them what was beyond their power.
>
> This art, so indispensable to suffering humanity, cannot therefore remain concealed in the unfathomable depths of obscure speculation, or be diffused throughout the boundless void of conjecture; it must be accessible, *readily accessible* to us, within the sphere of vision of our external and internal perceptive faculties.[126]

Thus the source of medical knowledge must be man's perceptive faculties, his ability to observe the phenomena before him:

> Now, as in a disease . . . we can perceive nothing but the morbid symptoms, it must . . . be the symptoms alone by which the disease demands and points to the remedy suited to relieve it–and, moreover, the totality of these its symptoms, *of this outwardly reflected picture of the internal essence of the disease, that is, of the affection of the vital force,* must be the principal, or the sole means, whereby the disease can make known what remedy it requires–the only thing that can determine the choice of the most appropriate remedy–and thus, in a word, the totality of the symptoms must be the principal, indeed the only thing the physician has to take note of in every case of disease and to *remove* by means of his art, in order that the disease shall be cured and transformed into health.[127]

It was this capacity for observation that made Hippocrates great:

> This attentive unsophisticated observer sought nature in nature. He saw and described the diseases before him accurately, without addition, without coloring, without speculation. In the faculty of pure observation he has been surpassed by no physician that has followed him.[128]

And this observation can only be of the patient's symptoms: "We have no way of reaching with our senses, or of gaining essential knowledge as to the process of life in the interior of man."[129] "Besides a historical acquaintance with the constitution of the human frame in a healthy state, the physician needs but in the same way to know the symptoms of the particular malady (further, indeed, he cannot explore, as it would serve him nothing) in order to remove it."[130] What the physician cannot discover from the symptoms is not needed by him to treat the patient: "it is one of the regulations that most clearly mark the wisdom of the all-consistent, all-merciful Creator that what would be useless to man has been rendered impossible to him."[131]

This, of course, does not mean that the physician is barred from using his mind. Where God endowed animals with sufficient instinct to cope with the challenges they encounter in life, "man alone painfully escapes from his mother's womb, soft, tender, naked, defenceless, helpless, and destitute of all that can render his existence supportable." But, "Behold, the Eternal Source of all love only disinherited man of the animal nature in order to endow him all the more richly with that spark of divinity—a mind—which enables man to elicit from himself the satisfaction of all his requirements."[132]

By manipulating the data of observation in his mind, therefore, the physician acquires *experience:* "the knowledge of disease can be neither a metaphysical problem nor the product of fantastic speculation, but is an affair of pure experience by the senses, because disease as a manifestation can only be apprehended by observation."[133] "Medicine is a science of experience; its object is to eradicate diseases by means of remedies."[134] "Pure experience, the sole and infallible oracle of the healing art . . ."[135] "Experience, the teacher of truth . . ."[136]

The only way to acquire medical knowledge is thus through medical practice—by healing people. Here the epistemological side of Hahnemann's doctrine fuses with its moral side—for the physician's duty, in any case, is to cure people of their diseases. The first sentence of the *Organon* reads:

> The physician's high and *only* mission is to restore the sick to health, to cure, as it is termed.[137]

And the Introduction states:

> Without disparaging the services which many physicians have rendered to the sciences auxiliary to medicine, to natural philosophy and chemistry, to natural history in its various branches, and to that of man in particular, to anthropology, physiology, and anatomy, etc., I shall occupy myself here with the practical part of medicine only, with the healing art itself . . .[138]

Like all other Empirics before him, therefore, Hahnemann insists that therapeutic theory arises out of therapeutic practice. Practice is always prior to theory. The physician comes to know man only by curing him.

The Discovery of the Proving. The Law of Similars. Iatrogenic Disease

By dissolving the Rationalist/Methodist metaphysic of disease causes in the acid of Empirical analysis, Hahnemann abolished the existing doctrinal basis for prescribing remedies:

> It is impossible to divine the internal essential nature of diseases and the changes they effect in the hidden parts

> of the body, and it is absurd to frame a system of treatment on such hypothetical surmises and assumptions; it is impossible to divine the medicinal properties of remedies from any chemical theories or from their smell, color, or taste, and it is absurd to attempt, from such hypothetical surmises and assumptions, to apply to the treatment of diseases these substances which are so hurtful when wrongly administered. And even were such practice ever so customary and ever so generally in use, were it even the only one in vogue for thousands of years, it would nevertheless continue to be a senseless and pernicious practice to found on empty surmises an idea of the morbid condition of the interior, and to attempt to combat this with equally imaginary properties of medicines.[139]

Ancient Empiricism had matched sick persons and their remedies only through a process of trial-and-error guided by accurate historical records. Paracelsus had postulated the doctrine of similars as a therapeutic guide but had left unclear its precise content—not indicating how the medicine was "similar" to the sick person except within the framework of a system of cosmological concordances whose all-important details were not provided.

Hahnemann wrestled with this key problem of medical Empiricism: the criterion for finding the precise remedy needed by each sick person.

Not that he objected in principle to trial-and-error. To date, he observes, the countless trials conducted over the ages in domestic practice have provided us with virtually all existing valid therapeutic knowledge. "Who knows how many centuries the inhabitants of deep valleys were forced to suffer from their goiters before accident, after thousands of drugs and domestic nostrums had been tried in vain, put it into the head of an individual that *roasted sponge* was the best thing for it; at all events it was not until the thirteenth century that Arnold of Villanova notices its *power of curing goiter.*"[140] The same is true for syphilis: it was treated with purgatives and other useless techniques for years after its appearance "until, at last, after many attempts and repeated trials of an innumerable multitude of things by empirical physicians on many thousands of patients who sought their aid, *mercury* was hit upon, and proved itself specific in this dreadful scourge, in spite of all the violent theoretical opposition of the pedantic physicians of the Arabian School."[141] Quinine was discovered in the same way by the Peruvian indians as the specific for intermittent fever, "probably after innumerable trials of other drugs."[142] The consequences of bruises and contusions were long endured by humanity "ere chance revealed to the laboring classes who principally suffered from such accidents the specific virtues of *Arnica* in such cases."[143]

> *These few specifics in these few diseases constitute all the truth which is contained in the voluminous materia medica in common use;* and these are, for the most part, I may say, almost entirely derived from domestic practice.[144]

But Hahnemann objects to this method of discovery for several reasons.

In the first place, it is slow, painful, wasteful, and laborious.

In the second place, it is effective only in diseases which are well-defined and relatively unchanging. These are especially what he calls "miasmatic," meaning "produced by a miasm which continues the same through all generations," of which the chief example is syphilis:[145] [g]

> By an infinite number of trials of all imaginable simple substances used in domestic practice, in a *well-defined disease, which shall constantly present the same characters,* a true, certainly efficacious specific remedy for the greater number of individuals and their friends suffering from the *same* disease *might* certainly be discovered, though only *casu fortuito.*[146]

[g]On "miasmatic diseases" see below, pp. 392-397.

Other unchanging conditions are those—such as intermittent fever, goiter, and bruises—which always arise from the same exciting cause.

Except for these, however, the trial-and-error method does more harm than good: "these very chance cases of accidental cures, when they have occurred to physicians, have done most to fill the materia medica with false seductive declarations respecting the curative actions of particular medicines *ab usu in morbis.*"[147] Physicians stumble by accident upon the cure and then (usually after conferring a Latin or Greek name upon the condition cured) vaunt their remedy as the specific for this condition. Since the description of the condition is always imperfect, quite different cases are grouped together under this particular name, and

> he who, thereafter, is inclined to regard a case occurring to himself as the same pathological species of disease (and why should he not? the schools teach him to do so) has nothing to do but resort immediately to this magnificent recipe, this splended specific, at the bidding of the first recommender, or by the advice of the materia medica. But he certainly has, under the same illusory pathological name, a case before him vastly different in the detail of its symptoms, and hence happens what was inevitable, the medicine does no good; it does harm, as might have been anticipated.[148]

But the most important reason for rejecting trial-and-error is that it slights the dignity of man—that is, the intellect with which God has endowed him. "The Father of Mankind has chiefly reckoned on this faculty of the human mind to discover remedial agents, for his protection from the maladies and accidents to which the delicate organism of man is exposed."[149] "What crude nature presents to us should not form the limit for the relief of our necessities; no, our mind should be able to enlarge her resources to an unlimited degree for our perfect well-being."[150] Furthermore, the forms of disease are always changing, and the laborious trial-and-error process would have to be started anew continually:

> Sad is the thought, that the noblest, the most indispensable of arts, is built upon accident, which always presupposes the endangering of many human lives. Will the chance of such discoveries suffice to perfect the healing art, to supply its numerous desiderata? From year to year we become acquainted with new diseases, with new phases and new complications of diseases, with new morbid conditions. . . . Sadly we look forward into future ages, when a peculiar remedy for *this* particular form of disease, for this particular circumstance, may, *perhaps,* be discovered by chance, as was bark for pure intermittent fever, or mercury for syphilitic disorders.
>
> Such a precarious construction of the most important science—resembling the concourse of Epicurean atoms to make a world—could never be the will of the wise and most bountiful Preserver of mankind. How humiliating for proud humanity, did his very preservation depend on chance alone. No! it is exhilarating to believe that for each particular disease, for each peculiar morbid variety, there are peculiar directly-acting remedies, and that there is also a way in which these may be *methodically* discovered.[151]

Hahnemann has in mind a *method* for discovering the curative powers of medicinal substances, one which will fill the gap in the existing Empirical therapeutic method. This method must be quite different from trials *ab usu in morbis:*

> When I talk of the *methodical discovery of medicinal powers still required by us,* I do not refer to those empirical trials usually made in hospitals, where in a difficult, often not accurately noted case, in which those already known do no good, recourse is had to some drug, hitherto either untried altogether, or untried in this particular affection, which drug is fixed upon either from caprice and blind fancy, or from some obscure notion, for which the experimenter can give no plausible reason, either to himself or to others. Such empirical chance trials are, to call them by the mildest appellation, but foolish risks, if not something worse.[152]

He has also rejected *a priori* methods relying on chemistry, botany, signatures, astrology, or physics. The problem was to develop a new approach.

This new approach—the technique of drug provings first announced in Hahnemann's 1796 "Essay on a New Principle for Ascertaining the Curative Power of Drugs"—was inspired by the writings of the profoundly original and pathbreaking Scottish physician, John Hunter (1728-1793).

In 1789, when Hahnemann was thirty-five years old, he published a long treatise on syphilis and gonorrhoea which contained several of the key ideas he was later to incorporate in the concept of the drug proving. This *Instruction for Surgeons Respecting Venereal Diseases,*[153] makes over twenty references to Hunter's *Treatise on the Venereal Disease* (1786),[154] and the parallels between the two works are striking. To Hunter is thus due a share of the credit for Hahnemann's discovery of the drug proving.

John Hunter was the tenth child of a middle-class Scottish family.[155] As a boy he preferred sports to books and was allowed to neglect his education. He studied cabinet-making instead and became extremely proficient at it. In 1748 he went to London to help his elder brother, William Hunter (1718-1783), at the time a prominent surgeon, obstetrician, and anatomist, and his manual dexterity soon made him an excellent dissector. "He was very popular with the 'resurrection men' who were then essential to the anatomist, was fond of lively company and of the theater, and was familiarly known as 'Jack Hunter.' " In 1755 "Jack Hunter" was sent to St. Mary's Hall, Oxford, but stayed only a month.[h]

He returned and started assisting his brother in lecturing. From 1760 to 1763 he was a staff surgeon on various military expeditions. In 1773 he began to lecture on his own

[h]"In later years Hunter told Sir Anthony Carlisle, 'They wanted to make an old woman of me, or that I should stuff Latin and Greek at the university, but,' he added, significantly pressing his thumbnail on the table, 'these schemes I cracked like so many vermin as they came before me.' "

and was the first to devise "principles of surgery," establishing it as an independent discipline. In 1790 he became inspector-general of hospitals and also surgeon-general.

Hunter's great luck was never to have received formal training in medicine, but to have learned it from observation and practice. "He read comparatively little and could never adequately expound the information already accessible on any subject. Most of what he knew he had acquired himself, and he attached perhaps undue importance to personal investigation. Few men have ever done so much with so little book-learning . . . He felt that, although he was really a mere pigmy in knowledge, he was a giant compared with his contemporaries."

In physiology he was a vitalist, holding (with Harvey) that the blood is alive and that this vital force exists prior to the physical structures and parts of the body which it generates. He had advanced ideas in many areas, claiming that the embryo in the womb passes through a series of stages in each of which it resembles the adult form of some lower creature—thus anticipating Darwin's theory by many decades—and advancing extremely accurate and modern views on the nature of geological change.[i]

Venereal disease was one of his major medical concerns, and he actually inoculated himself with syphilitic matter to study the development of the disease at first hand. The subject from whom the matter was taken, however, had gonorrhoea as well, leading Hunter to the conclusion that both diseases are from the same cause.[156] [j] His *Treatise on the Venereal Disease,* setting forth the result of his thought and experimentation, contained a theory of the disease "peculiar to myself."[157]

[i]His papers on geology were only published posthumously due to the objections of a friend who pointed out that they made the earth look much older than 6000 years.

[j]When it affected the mucous membranes, it was gonorrhoea; when it affected the skin, it was syphilis (Hunter, *Works* [London: Longman, 1837], II, 316).

Hunter came to the idea that neither the whole organism nor any part of it can be diseased in two ways simultaneously: "no two actions can take place in the same constitution, nor in the same part, at one and the same time . . . it naturally results from this principle that no two different fevers can exist in the same constitution, nor two local diseases in the same part, at the same time."[158] While he accepted the existence of local venereal disease, the "irritation" by the "venereal poison" causing "inflammation," the whole constitution eventually becomes diseased through infection with pus from the original sore or else through the "sympathy" of the whole organism with each part.[159]

The venereal disease is a specific disease.[k] The first sign is a generalized inflammation "beside which inflammation the parts so contaminated have a peculiar mode of action superadded, different from all other actions attending inflammation; and it is this specific mode of action which produces the specific quality in the matter."[160]

The subject's predisposition is important, since not everyone is equally susceptible.[161] "The effects produced by the venereal poison appear to me to arise from its peculiar or specific irritation, joined with the aptness of the living principle to be irritated by such a cause."[162][l]

Hunter's ideas on the operation of medicines were also original. Mercurial medicines (the cure for syphilis) introduce an artificial irritation into the economy which overcomes and extinguishes the "irritation" from the venereal poison. Mercury induces a "mercurial fever" in the organism, a new

[k]This conclusion, obviously owing much to Sydenham, was one of the sources of the doctrine of "specific diseases" which emerged 25 years later in the Paris School (see below, pp. 502 ff.).

[l]The concepts of "diathesis" and "predisposition" were widely employed by Brown, but he reduced them to nothing more than varying degrees of "excitability." "Predisposition" is a mild state of the disease: "it arises from the same exciting powers acting upon the same excitability from which both health and disease arise and is an intermediate state between both" (*Elements of Medicine,* 116-117). See below, pp. 466-468.

disease—and since two fevers or "actions" cannot coexist in the body, the mercurial fever annihilates the venereal one.[163]

Of importance is Hunter's claim that mercury acts on the constitution of the patient, not on the "disease" or its "poison."[164] He specifically denies that mercury acts through chemical neutralization of the venereal "poison."[165] Nor does it act, as Cullen had claimed,[m] by the evacuation it produces—only by its "stimulating power" on the organism.[166]

Hunter's ideas affected Hahnemann profoundly, but he went beyond the Scotsman in several respects, even in this early work.

He accepts Hunter's identification of syphilis and gonorrhoea as well as his belief that the venereal disease is first local—systemic absorption of matter from this local infection producing the constitutional form.[167 n] The syphilis is a "peculiar irritation of a specific character distributed throughout the whole organism" or "perhaps only in the lymphatic system."[168]

It is cured by mercurial medicines administered internally (and Hahnemann proposed a new form of soluble mercury for this disease). No topical application of mercury to the bubo or chancre is needed.[169]

The mercury does not act through salivation, diarrhoea, diuresis, diaphoresis, or any other evacuation.[170] Nor does it act by its irritant, antiseptic, corrosive, or dessicant power on the organism.[171] But Hahnemann was unable to decide if cure comes about through chemical action of the mercury on the venereal "virus" or through the "specific irritation which it excites in our body . . . that specific alteration of the body

[m]See above, p. 297.

[n]He agreed with Hunter that perhaps once in 10,000 cases syphilis assumes its constitutional form without first producing the local lesion (*Lesser Writings,* 88). Later he reversed himself and held that in syphilis, as in all other diseases, the initial affection is constitutional, the local disease appearing only as the result of the constitutional one (*ibid.,* 647-650). See below, p. 417.

which may not inaptly be termed *mercurial fever.*"[172] In any case, it is by virtue of mercury's "specific powers."[173]

One grain of soluble mercury is often sufficient for cure, although Hahnemann occasionally raised the dose to as much as sixty grains.[174] [o] Treatment should be discontinued once the "mercurial fever" has appeared.[175]

In this early work Hahnemann had thus already advanced to the idea that cure is through incompatibility between two "fevers" or "irritations" in the body. He does not yet feel that incompatibility is greater in the case of two "similar" irritations, remarking, in fact, that mercury cures by the "gradual or sudden *antipathic* irritation of the fibres of a specific nature."[176] [p]

Probably within a few months of publishing this work Hahnemann experimented upon himself to discover more about the fever-producing potential of substances used as drugs. He selected quinine—the specific against intermittent fever (malaria)—and reported on it the following year in his translation of Cullen's *Treatise of the Materia Medica.* Where the Scotsman observes that Peruvian Bark cures "by a tonic power exerted in the stomach . . . a substance in which the qualities of bitter and astringent are conjoined," Hahnemann appended the following note:

> By combining the strongest bitters and the strongest astringents we can obtain a compound which, in small doses, possesses much more of both these properties than the bark, and yet in all Eternity no fever specific can be

[o] Hahnemann clearly underestimated the difficulty of curing syphilis.

[p] However, there is a hint of his future doctrine in his warning against overdosing with mercury through confusion between the symptoms of mercurial medicines and the symptoms of syphilis which they closely resemble (*Lesser Writings,* 140). Hunter had stated the same: the effects of the mercurial drug were often confused with the symptoms of venereal rheumatism, leading to the administration of more mercury than was necessary (*Works,* II, 470).

> made from such a compound. The author should have accounted for this. This discovered principle of the effect of the bark is probably not very easy to find. Let us consider the following: substances which produce some kind of fever (very strong coffee, pepper, arnica, ignatia-bean, arsenic) counteract these types of intermittent fever. I took, for several days, as an experiment, four drams of good china [quinine] twice daily. My feet and finger tips, etc. at first became cold; I became languid and drowsy; then my heart began to palpitate; my pulse became hard and quick; and intolerable anxiety and trembling (but without a rigor); prostration in all the limbs; then pulsation in the head, redness of the cheeks, thirst; briefly, all the symptoms usually associated with intermittent fever appeared in succession, yet without the actual rigor. To sum up: all those symptoms which to me are typical of intermittent fever, as the stupefaction of the senses, a kind of rigidity of all joints, but above all the numb disagreeable sensation which seems to have its seat in the periosteum over all the bones of the body—all made their appearance. This paroxysm lasted from two to three hours every time and recurred when I repeated the dose and not otherwise. I discontinued the medicine, and I was once more in good health.[177]

This was his description of the symptoms of quinine poisoning—called (in its chronic form) "cinchonism" after it had become generally recognized by the medical profession fifty years later.[q] Significant above all else in Hahnemann's

[q]See *Divided Legacy,* III, 246-249. In 1899 Louis Lewin, the Berlin pharmacologist, wrote: "The much discussed and contested quinine fever occurs fairly frequently alone or in connection with other side-effects of quinine. . . . There is no doubt that, for its manifestation, only a certain individual susceptibility is required. With such a special susceptibility even very small amounts of cinchona, such as 0.06 gram, produce this condition every time. . . . On the other hand, cases have been observed in which quinine fever occurred in the absence of this susceptibility. Therefore, the observations of Hahnemann on himself, who, after taking a substantial dose of cinchona bark, was attacked by a cold fever similar to malaria, must be considered reliable" (L. Lewin, *Die Nebenwirkungen der Arzneimittel. Pharmacologisch-Klinisches Handbuch.* Dritte, neu bearbeitete Auflage [Berlin: August Hirschwald, 1899], pp. 421-422).

observations was that the symptoms obtained from quinine were "typical of intermittent fever." This experiment made him certain that one "fever" cures another by the *similarity* between them, and he presented these insights in his 1796 "Essay":

> *Every powerful medicinal substance produces in the human body a kind of peculiar disease; the more powerful the medicine, the more peculiar, marked, and violent the disease.*
>
> *We should imitate the nature* which sometimes cures a chronic disease by superadding another, *and employ in the* (especially chronic) *disease we wish to cure, that medicine which is able to produce another very similar artificial disease,* and the former will be cured: *similia similibus.*[178]

This principle, which he called the "law of similars," was thenceforth the foundation of homoeopathic practice. Every medicinal substance acts through the "artificial fever" it arouses when given to a healthy person; this "artificial fever" is curative when the substance is administered to a sick person whose symptoms are similar to those of the "artificial fever"; hence, a reliable guide to the administration of any drug can be found in the symptoms it arouses in the healthy.[r]

Hahnemann called the "law of similars" a "law of nature" discovered "by the observation of nature and my own experience."[179] This path to the discovery of the curative action of drugs satisfied the requirements of the Empirical tradition:

> This spirit-like power to alter man's state of health which lies hidden in the inner nature of medicines can in itself never be discovered by us by a mere effort of reason; it is

[r]Hahnemann coined the word, *Arzneikrankheit* (drug disease, medicinal disease), for this "artificial fever" in his 1813 article, "The Spirit of the Homoeopathic Doctrine of Medicine" (reprinted in *Reine Arzneimittellehre,* II [1816], 16; see *Lesser Writings,* 617-631, at 629). It then appeared in the second edition of the *Organon* (Dresden: Arnold, 1819), 179.

> only by experience of the phenomena it displays when acting on the state of health of man that we can become clearly cognizant of it.[180]

Since almost no knowledge was available of the effects of medicines on the healthy,[s] Hahnemann set afoot an extensive program of provings:

> There is . . . no other possible way in which the peculiar effects of medicines on the health of individuals can be accurately ascertained—there is no sure, no more natural way of accomplishing this object, than to administer the several medicines experimentally, in moderate doses, to *healthy* persons, in order to ascertain what changes, symptoms, and signs of their influence each individually produces on the health of the body and of the mind.[181]

Only "the great and immortal Albert von Haller" had ever advocated this procedure (in the preface to his *Pharmacopoeia Helvetica*) "but no one, not a single physician, attended to or followed up this invaluable hint."[182]

The results of Hahnemann's initial provings, on himself and his family, were presented in his *Fragmenta de Viribus Medicamentorum Positivis* (1805) which gave the symptoms of 27 medicines with references from the literature on poisonings and occasional clinical observations. The *Reine Arzneimittellehre* (1811-1821) enlarged on the *Fragmenta,* presenting the symptomatology of 62 substances. By the end of his life Hahnemann had conducted or supervised the provings of over 200 substances, and more than 600 others had been added to the homoeopathic pharmacopoeia by the end of the century.[183]

This close inspection of the action of medicinal substances on the healthy led to a major discovery—the biphasic action of drugs. In his 1796 "Essay" Hahnemann wrote:

[s]Something was known of the effects of drugs when given to the *sick,* but "the reaction of the diseased organism . . . to an untested or imperfectly tested remedy gives such intricate results that their appreciation is impossible for the most acute physician" (*Lesser Writings,* 263).

"most medicines have more than one action: the first a *direct* action which gradually changes into the second (which I call the indirect secondary action). The latter is generally a state exactly the opposite of the former . . . It may be almost considered an axiom that the symptoms of the secondary action are the exact opposite of those of the direct action."[184] [t]

This observation was merely a generalization of the Empirical postulate that the organism at all times reacts to external morbific (or other) influences:

> According to a wonderful provision of the nature, organized living beings are not regulated by the laws of unorganized (dead) physical matter; they do not receive the influence of external agents, like the latter, in a passive manner, but strive to oppose a contrary action to them. The living body does indeed allow itself to be in the first instance changed by the action of physical agents; but this change is not in it, as in inorganic substances, permanent . . . on the contrary, the living human organism strives to develop, by antagonism, the exact opposite of the affection first produced in it from without.[185]

That *disease* symptoms reflect in part the impact of the morbific cause and in part the organism's reaction is a theme which reappears periodically in medical thought, but it had never been dealt with methodically and never extended to cover the action of drugs.[186]

Discovery of the biphasic action of drugs immediately raised the question: does the "similarity" necessary for cure lie between the primary or the secondary drug symptoms and those of the patient? For Hahnemann this could not be answered *a priori,* but experience showed similarity to lie between the patient's symptoms and the primary symptoms

[t] Relying on this discovery and that of the small dose (see below, p. 401) allopathic medicine later in the century formulated the Arndt-Schulz Rule: "small doses kindle vital activities, moderate increase them, large depress them, and largest remove them" (Linn J. Boyd, *A Study of the Simile in Medicine* [Philadelphia: Boericke and Tafel, 1936], 303).

of the drug; then the secondary symptoms of the drug (i.e., the symptoms of the patient's reaction) remove the disease.[187] He named his emerging system "homoeopathy" from the Greek words, *homoios* ("like") and *pathos* ("feeling," "suffering"), to indicate that cure results from similarity between the symptoms of the patient and the primary symptoms of the drug:

> If in the treatment of a disease we administer those medicines whose primary symptoms, or those of its positive action, present the greatest similarity to the phenomena of the disease, this is a *positive* or *curative* mode of treatment, that is to say, there occurs . . . rapid permanent amelioration.[188]

Proof that the prescription is correct is the slight aggravation of his symptoms which the patient feels immediately after taking the similar remedy—from reinforcement of the disease symptoms by the primary symptoms of the medicine.[189]

The other possibility was similarity between the secondary drug symptoms and those of the patient, i.e., contrariety between the primary drug symptoms and those of the patient. This Hahnemann called "enantiopathic" treatment (from Greek *enantios*—"opposite"—and *pathos*), also "antipathic" and "palliative," and held that it served only to render the disease more serious. "All pure experience . . . and all accurate research convince us that persistent symptoms of disease are far from being removed and annihilated by *opposite* symptoms of medicines (as in the *antipathic, enantiopathic,* or *palliative* method), that, on the contrary, after transient apparent alleviation, they break forth again, only with increased intensity, and become manifestly aggravated."[190]

Hahnemann charged that nearly all current practice embodied enantiopathic or allopathic[u] modes of prescribing in

[u]He coined the word, "allopathy," from Greek *allos* ("other," "different") to designate the existing orthodox system of practice in which the relationship

which the effect of the drug was only palliative, leading to an eventual exacerbation of the disease:

> If (according to the ordinary mode of procedure, *contraria contrariis curantur*) the primary action of the medicine we employ be just the *opposite* of the symptoms of the disease (for instance, if we give opium for habitual sleeplessness or chronic diarrhoea, wine for debility, or purgatives for chronic constipation), only a *palliative* relief, only an amelioration for a few hours will be the result, for, after these few hours have passed, the period for the second stage of the medicinal action comes on, which is the contrary of the first action and the analogue of the morbid state it is sought to cure—consequently, it causes an addition to the disease and an aggravation of it.[191]

When drugs are selected whose primary symptoms are the "opposite" of the disease symptoms, the secondary symptoms only reinforce the existing symptom-pattern:

> For a persistent tendency to sleepiness during the day the physician prescribed coffee, whose primary action is to enliven; and when it had exhausted its action, the day-somnolence increased; for frequent waking at night he gave in the evening, without heeding the other symptoms of the disease, opium, which by virtue of its primary action produced the same night (stupefied, dull) sleep, but the subsequent nights were still more sleepless than before; to chronic diarrhoeas he opposed, without regarding the other morbid signs, the same opium, whose primary action is to constipate the bowels, and after a transient stoppage of the diarrhoea it subsequently became all the worse . . . weakness of the bladder, with consequent retention of urine, was sought to be conquered by the antipathic work of cantharides to stimulate the urinary passages, whereby evacuation of the urine was

between remedies and diseases was neither homoeopathic nor enantiopathic but vague, indefinite, and indeterminate (*Organon,* Sec. 22, Note 12).

> certainly at first effected, but thereafter the bladder becomes less capable of stimulation and less able to contract, and paralysis of the bladder is imminent; with large doses of purgative drugs and laxative salts, which excite the bowels to frequent evacuation, it was sought to remove a chronic tendency to constipation, but in the secondary action the bowels became still more confined . . . The Old School physician rejoices that he is able to reduce for several hours the velocity of the small rapid pulse in cachetic patients with the very first dose of uncombined purple foxglove [*Digitalis purpurea*] (which in its *primary* action makes the pulse slower); its rapidity, however, soon returns; repeated, and now increased doses, effect an ever smaller diminution of its rapidity, and at length none at all—indeed—in the *secondary* action the pulse becomes uncountable! sleep, appetite and strength depart, and a speedy death is *invariably* the result, or else insanity ensues. How often, in one word, the disease is aggravated, or something even worse is effected by the secondary action of such antagonistic (antipathic) remedies, the Old School with its false theories does not perceive, but experience teaches it in a terrible manner.[192]

Thus he was not only accusing his colleagues of ignorance and carelessness in their prescribing of remedies, he was undermining the very doctrinal basis of orthodox medical practice.

He frequently criticized his fellow-physicians for their antipathic or palliative prescribing which only engrafted new and incurable chronic drug-diseases upon the patient's existing natural disease:

> By such large doses of the . . . medicine . . . he creates new morbid states which are often more difficult to cure than the original malady, and which often enough terminate in death.[193]
>
> The individual, naturally so irritable in disease, is readily aggravated by so many blindly instituted experiments,

> and may even fall a victim to them, especially since the recent fashion of prescribing large doses of powerful medicines has been adopted.[194]
>
> [The physician] is proud of his power of palliating, and of being able to allay pains for a few hours: but the after-effects—they do not trouble him. *Nil nisi quod ante pedes est.*[195]
>
> These insidious medicinal diseases produced *secundum artem* by such admirable modes of treatment become, on account of this pitiless robbery of the vital force, so *incurable* that recovery is not to be thought of, and a miserable death can alone release the patient from the maltreatment of his physicians and from his nameless torments.[196]
>
> Do not the poor, who use no medicine at all, often recover much sooner from the same kind of disease than the well-to-do patient who has his shelves filled with large bottles of medicine? The latter often remains much longer poorly after his treatment is finished, and must often go from one watering-place to another in order to get free from the after-sufferings left in him by the monstrous quantity of powerful drugs he took, which were usually totally inappropriate and consequently hurtful in their character.[197]

He urged his followers "not to receive at any price those patients who have been injured to the verge of incurability by the allopathic exterminating art, nor, by undertaking such impossibilities, to expose themselves to the scornful laughter of the renowned physicians of the Old School, who have already taken the greatest pains to make them utterly incurable for hard cash."[198] [v]

[v]The presence of these drug-induced diseases was an additional reason to reject the validity of data from internal pathology: "there is displayed *not what was present before your treatment,* as you would fain persuade the relatives, *but what was produced by your treatment—the incurability of the deceased was not before but after your treatment*" (*Lesser Writings,* 749).

Thus the other side of the homoeopathic coin was the iatrogenic disease. Since every substance is capable of arousing a "medicinal disease" *(Arzneikrankheit)* or "drug fever" in the organism, the repeated incorrect use of such substances will ultimately engraft an incurable medicinal disease upon the unfortunate patient. Hahnemann warned: *"all things that can be termed medicinal are per se hurtful substances, injurious in general to the health of man, which can only become wholesome where each exactly corresponds in its injurious power to the case of disease specially adapted for it."*[199]

This congeries of ideas was unwelcome to the medical profession which preferred to believe (in Hahnemann's words) *"that drugs, even in large, oft-repeated, and increased doses, are one and all per se and absolutely in all cases wholesome things."*[200]

Actually, the opinion of the profession was more complex, since physicians could not and did not imagine that such poisons as arsenic, *Aconitum napellus,* and *Strychnos nux vomica,* which Hahnemann was proving on himself, his children, and his followers, were "in all cases wholesome things." Thus the profession held *both* that the proving of remedies on healthy persons was dangerous (and useless) *and* that drugs could not have an adverse effect on the sick person's health.[w]

A few years after the appearance of the *Fragmenta* the royal physician of Brunswick wrote: "Should Mr. Hahnemann continue to conduct many more such experiments on his own person, I should be afraid of an undermining of his whole system and particularly of his brain. Really these experiments should be conducted on criminals who have merited death. If all physicians were obliged or were willing to make such experiments on themselves, I fear they would all be mutilated in soul and body."[201] An 1810 review of the *Organon* states the same in less jocular language.[202] At

[w]Such contradictions are not at all uncommon in medical Rationalism. Physicians are rarely aware of them. See below, p. 724.

the same time physicians wanted to believe that the "disease" was an entity separate and apart from the organism and that the (even poisonous) remedies they used in treatment affected only this entity. Typical here was the attitude of Johann Christian August Heinroth (1773-1843), professor of mental diseases at Leipzig, who wrote in his 1825 *Anti-Organon:*

> The idea of testing medicines on healthy persons is repugnant to reason and repellent to common sense . . . Only sick persons, and not healthy ones, have made us familiar with the curative properties of medicines; and it is just as impossible to discover these properties when in health as it is only possible to gain this experience in a diseased condition. Diseases and their remedies are correlatives in the same way as health and food. It would be just as senseless to try to ascertain the effects of medicines on healthy persons as it would be to seek to discover the effects of food on patients. Medicines show their power only in the diseased condition, as food does only in the healthy condition.[203]

This self-contradictory attitude toward the proving is understandable only as a visceral reaction to its corollary—that orthodox prescribing, even though in strict accord with the principles set forth in the books, *could actually make the patient worse.* Some of Hahnemann's critics accepted his assault on the abuse of drugs, but none would admit that physicians who followed the principles of the schools could have a destructive effect on their patients.[x] This was cutting too close to the bone by far and raised in a radical form the question of the relationship between the medical profession and the public:

[x]Thus A. F. Hecker, professor of medicine at Berlin, welcomed Hahnemann's advocacy of the single remedy as perhaps leading to a reduction in the overprescribing of most physicians but was indignant at Hahnemann's charge that allopathic treatment is mainly palliative and especially resented his rejection of bloodletting "which occupies one of the leading places among all the techniques which we employ on a rational basis" (*Annalen der gesammten Medicine* II [1810], 70, 254, 256).

> What will the reflecting public say when it learns that the physicians of the Old School of medicine . . . still go on to this day, giving their drugs to patients day after day in several doses a day, each dose of which is disturbed in its action by the one that speedily follows it, so that from their ignorance no dose is allowed one hundredth part of the time required for the completion of its action—an overloading of the body outside and in with the same medicinal mixture, wherefrom only injury to the health can be effected, but never anything good, appropriate, beneficial!![204]

Thus, while many of the elements of homoeopathy contributed to its unpopularity with the medical profession, the stage for the forthcoming clash between the New School and the Old was set by Hahnemann's advocacy of the proving to elucidate the curative powers of drugs.[y]

Historical Evidence for the Law of Similars

Hahnemann did not claim to have discovered the law of similars, only to be the first to teach it and apply it consistently.[205] To make this law more palatable to his

[y]Today, when the morbific potential of drugs is a commonplace of medical doctrine (although often enough lost sight of in practice) the effort is made to deprive Hahnemann of credit for this discovery. W. L. Von Brunn, for instance, cites works from 1816 (J. C. Reil), 1835 (F. G. Gmelin), 1838 (F. A. Schill), and 1840 (F. A. Schill)—i.e., from 20 to 45 years after the appearance of Hahnemann's 1796 "Essay"—as evidence that his ideas about the "drug disease" were "in tune with the thought of the times", meaning not original with him ("Homoeopathie als medizingeschichtliches Problem," *Sudhoffs Arkhiv* 48 [1964], 137-156, at 137).

Contemporaries, however, attributed the idea strictly to Hahnemann. A. F. Hecker, writing in 1810, states that fourteen years earlier Hahnemann offered this new principle for ascertaining the curative virtues of medicines and quotes the 1796 "Essay" (*Annalen der gesammten Medicin* II [1810], 34). Hahnemann himself invented the word, *Arzneikrankheit,* in 1813, and the earliest work cited by Von Brunn, J. C. Reil's *Entwurf einer allgemeinen Pathologie* (Halle: Curt, 1816) gives what is almost a direct quote from Hahnemann's 1796 "Essay" (III, 190).

The errors and carelessness, not to mention prejudice, of scholars who write about homoeopathy are the real *"medizingeschichtliches Problem."* The article by Von Brunn is not the most egregious—dozens of others could be cited.

colleagues he adduced evidence in support of it from medical history and practice:

> I do not bring forth the following passages from authors who had a presentiment of homoeopathy as proofs in support of this doctrine, which is firmly established by its own intrinsic merits, but in order to avoid the imputation of having suppressed these foreshadowings with the view of claiming for myself the priority of the idea.[206]

This evidence was of two kinds: cures by "similar" medicines and cures of diseases by other, "similar," diseases.

In respect of the former Hahnemann mentions the Hippocratic writing, *Places in Man,* [z] which calls for heating drinks in fevers; a Danish physician of the early eighteenth century who cured "a tendency to acidity of the stomach by a very small dose of sulphuric acid with the most successful result"; Anton von Stoerck (1731-1803) who, in the 1760's, published a series of works on the treatment of diseases with poisons according to the principle of similars, and others.[207] [a]

He also calls attention to certain medicines used professionally and in domestic practice whose beneficial effect in diseases is due to their homoeopathicity. Of these the two most striking were precisely the specifics, mercury and quinine, in syphilis and malaria, but Hahnemann mentions several others as well: parsley juice for ineffectual urge to urinate, juniper berries for uterine bleeding, opium for certain kinds of constipation, rhubarb in certain diarrhoeas, belladonna in hydrophobia, etc.[208]

He mentions favorably the use, in domestic practice, of heat as a treatment for burns and cold applications on frozen

[z]See *Divided Legacy,* I, 205-207.

[a]Information about other predecessors of Hahnemann who experimented with poisons or advocated such experiments (Gesner, Mattioli, Sydenham, Hoffmann, Quarin, De Haen, Sennert, Baglivi, etc.) is given in Boyd, *A Study of the Simile in Medicine,* 104. Even Galen mentions persons of his time who experimented with medicines on healthy persons (*Opera Omnia,* ed. Kuehn, XIV, 215).

limbs: "in recent cases of frost-bitten limbs frozen sauerkraut is applied or frictions of snow are used. The experienced cook holds his hand, which he has scalded, at a certain distance from the fire, and does not heed the increase of pain that takes place at first, as he knows from experience that he can thereby, in a very short time—often in a few minutes, convert the burnt part into healthy painless skin."[209] He notes that John Hunter had suggested the same[b] and that Sydenham had treated burns with alcohol.[210 c] The British physician, Edward Kentish, was applying heated turpentine or alcohol to the skin of miners injured in firedamp explosions.[211 d] In such cases cold water or cold applications only cause blistering and prolong the time of recovery: "Thus Benjamin Bell, in the case of a lady who had scalded both arms, caused one to be covered with *oil of turpentine* and made her plunge the other into *cold water.* In half an hour the first arm was *well,* but the other continued to be painful for six hours longer; when it was withdrawn one instant from the water, she experienced much greater pain in it, *and it required a much longer time than the first for its cure.*"[212 e]

Evidence in favor of the law of similars is also drawn by Hahnemann from the interaction of diseases.

[b]Hunter writes that application of cold to a burn takes away the pain, but the pain is more intense when the cold is removed. Hence, "it is recommended that when a part is burnt to hold it to the fire as close and as long as it can be held, which undoubtedly lessens the succeeding inflammation and soon gives ease" (*Works,* III, 265).

[c]"Foment the parts with linen rags dipped in spirits of wine until the pain departs. Dip the rag afresh, and apply it two or three times a day to the part affected" (Sydenham, *Works,* II, 290).

[d]See Edward Kentish, *A Second Essay on Burns, in Which an Attempt is Made to Refute the Opinions of Mr. Earle and Sir W. Farquhar, Lately Advanced on the Supposed Benefit of the Application of Ice in Such Accidents* (Newcastle on Tyne: Walker, 1800) which details a series of cases of burns from fire, boiling water, gunpowder, etc. in which application of oil of turpentine relieved the pain and promoted healing.

[e]*Physisch-Medicinisches Journal* (Leipzig) II (1801), 428.

If a sick person is exposed to another disease, several different outcomes are possible.

When the diseases are dissimilar, and the older one is stronger, the newer one cannot get a hold on the organism: thus a person with a severe chronic disease will not be affected by a moderate acute one. Edward Jenner (1749-1823) states that vaccination will not take effect in a person with rickets.[213]

If the new dissimilar disease is stronger, it will temporarily efface the older one, and when the new disease has run its course, the older one will return: if a child with measles catches smallpox, the smallpox must run its course, and then the measles returns to run *its* course (but the comparatively weak smallpox inoculation is temporarily suspended by an outbreak of measles).[214]

Sometimes the two dissimilar diseases coexist in the body: Jenner reports a case of cow-pox which ran its course during mercurial treatment for syphilis. "The stronger suspends the weaker (when they do not complicate one another, which is seldom the case with acute diseases), but they never cure one another."[215]

However, if the diseases are similar, the stronger cures the weaker. Smallpox gives rise to ophthalmia, and physicians have cured ophthalmia by inoculating the patient with smallpox.[216] Smallpox has also cured chronic conditions such as amaurosis, deafness, swelling of the testicle, and chronic dysentery, which resemble the *sequelae* of smallpox.[217] "The cow-pox, a peculiar symptom of which is to cause tumefaction of the arm, cured, after it broke out, a *swollen*, half-paralyzed arm."[218] In general, cow-pox homoeopathically lessens the severity of supervening smallpox and makes it much milder: "this seems to be the reason for this beneficial remarkable fact, namely, that since the general distribution of Jenner's Cow Pox vaccination, human smallpox never again appeared as epidemically or virulently as 40-50 years before when one city visited lost at least one-half, and often three-quarters of its children, by death of this miserable pestilence."[219] [f]

Doctrinal Corollaries of the Law of Similars

The Empirical tradition had always looked favorably on cure through similars, but the definition of "similarity" had remained unclear. By interpreting it in terms of drug provings Hahnemann defined the concept unambiguously, and all elements of traditional Empiricism were now restructured in function of Hahnemann's new definition of "similarity."

Symptoms and Pathology. Disease Classification. Propria and Communia. Local Disease and General Disease. Mental Disease

Since the only useful knowledge of remedies was that obtained from provings, and the provings yielded only symptoms, it followed that the only useful way to describe diseases was in terms of their symptoms.

> The disease, being but a peculiar condition, cannot speak, cannot tell its own story; the patient suffering from it can alone render an account of his disease by the various signs of his disordered health, the ailments he feels, the symptoms he can complain of, and by the alterations in him that are perceptible to the senses. But the pseudo-wisdom of ordinary physicians thinks all this scarcely worth listening to; and even if they listen to it, they allege that it is of no importance, that it is empirical and expressed in a very unlearned manner by the nature, that it does not coincide with what their pathological books teach them and is, therefore, not available for their purpose, but in place thereof they put forward a figment of their learned reveries as the picture of the internal (never ascertainable) state of the disease, in their folly

[f] In 1927 Julius Wagner-Jauregg (1857-1940) was awarded the Nobel Prize in medicine for work indicating the possibility of curing persons with advanced syphilis by inoculating them with tertian malaria.

> substitute this delusive pathological picture for the individual state of each case of disease as the nature faithfully delineates it, and direct their medical weapons against this trumped-up phantom of their imagination, the production of what they call their "practical tact."[220]

The Empirical position that knowledge of internal pathology is valueless and even misleading was thus reinforced by the proving. Since the prover could not be autopsied to determine changes in his heart, lungs, or liver, this information had to be excluded—on purely methodological grounds—from the diagnosis and treatment of diseases.

By symptomatic description of disease, however, Hahnemann did not mean the cursory procedures of his colleagues: "The ordinary physician seldom or never describes the case of disease correctly, and, indeed, considers the circumstantial description of a case of disease in all its symptoms as useless, if he cannot bestow on it a pathological name."[221]

> The sensations that differ so vastly among each other, and the innumerable varieties of the sufferings of the many different kinds of patients, were so far from being described according to their divergences and varieties, according to their peculiarities, the complexity of the pains composed of various kinds of sensations, their degrees and shades, so far was the description from being accurate or complete, that we find all these infinite varieties of sufferings huddled together under a few bare, unmeaning, general terms such as *perspiration, heat, fever, headache, sore throat, croup, asthma, cough, chest-complaints, stitch in the side, belly ache, want of appetite, dyspepsia, back ache, coxalgia, hemorrhoidal sufferings, urinary disorders, pains in the limbs* (called according to fancy, *gouty* or *rheumatic*), *skin diseases, spasms, convulsions,* etc. With such superficial expressions the innumerable varieties of sufferings of patients were knocked off in the so-called observations, so that—with the exception of some one or other severe,

> striking symptom in this or that case of disease—almost every disease pretended to be described is as like another as the spots on a die.[222]

Hahnemann describes as follows how the interview between physician and patient should proceed:

> The patient details the history of his sufferings; those about him tell what they have heard him complain of, how he has behaved, and what they have noticed in him; the physician sees, hears, and remarks by his other senses what there is of an altered or unusual character about him. He writes down accurately all that the patient and his friends have told him *in the very expressions used by them.* Keeping silence himself, he allows them to say all they have to say, and refrains from interrupting them unless they wander off to other matters. The physician advises them at the beginning of the examination to speak slowly, in order that he may take down in writing the important parts of what the speakers say.[223] [g]

and how it usually did proceed:

> The Old School physician gave himself very little trouble in this matter . . . He would not listen to any minute detail of all the circumstances of his case by the patient; indeed, he frequently cut him short in his relation of his sufferings, in order that he might not be delayed in the rapid writing of his prescription . . . No allopathic physician, as has been said, sought to learn all the minute circumstances of the patient's case, *and still less did he make a note in writing of them.* On seeing the patient again several days afterwards, he recollected nothing

[g]Stahl had also urged the physician to take an accurate symptomatic record, and he also refines the existing symptom categories—distinguishing, for example, among ten different kinds of pain: two burning pains (*dolor urens* and *dolor ardens*), erosive pain, lancinating pain, biting pain, tensive pain, heavy pain, cold pain, sharp pain, acute pain, boring pain, etc. What is particularly interesting is that he describes these pains *in German* in the midst of his Latin text, prefacing each such instance with the words: "Germans usually express these sorts of sensations in the following way . . ." (*Theoria Medica Vera,* II, 223ff.).

> concerning the few details he had heard at the first visit (having in the meantime seen so many other patients laboring under different affections); he had allowed everything to go in at one ear and out at the other. At subsequent visits he only asked a few general questions, went through the ceremony of feeling the pulse at the wrist, looked at the tongue, and at the same moment wrote another prescription, on equally irrational principles, or ordered the first one to be continued . . . and, with a graceful bow, he hurried off to the fiftieth or sixtieth patient he had to visit, in this thoughtless way, in the course of that forenoon. The profession which of all others requires the most reflection, a conscientious, careful examination of the state of each individual patient, and a special treatment founded thereon, was conducted in this manner by persons who called themselves physicians, *rational practitioners.* The result, as might naturally be expected, was almost invariably bad; and yet patients had to go to them for advice, partly because there were none better to be had, partly for fashion's sake.[224]

Hahnemann thus subscribed fully to the Empirical principle that proper observation of the patient is the primary prerequisite for treatment. In a short article, "The Medical Observer," he discussed the bad habits of his colleagues in this respect: "the medical practitioner must possess . . . the capacity and habit of noticing carefully and correctly the phenomena that take place in natural diseases as well as those that occur in the morbid states artificially excited by medicines when they are tested upon the healthy body . . . [which] is not met with among ordinary physicians even in a moderate degree . . ."[225] "Poetic fancy, fantastic wit and speculation, must for a while be suspended, and all overstrained reasoning, forced interpretation, and tendency to explain away things, must be suppressed."[226] "This capability of observing accurately is never quite an innate faculty;

it must be chiefly acquired by practice, by refining and regulating the perceptions of the senses."[227]

And the best practice in observing is acquired from provings: "the experimenter, after he has taken the medicine, has all his attention strained towards all the alterations of health that take place on and within him, in order to observe and correctly to record them . . . the experimenter attains the capability of observing all the sensations, be they ever so complex, that he experiences from the medicines he is testing, and all, even the finest shades of alteration of his health, and of recording in suitable and adequate expressions his distinct conception of them . . . He will thus acquire practice to enable him to make equally accurate observations on others also."[228]

Hahnemann's reasoning yields a solution to the perennial problem of the *communia* and *propria*.

In diagnosis the physician's main difficulty is to distinguish his patient from all others with a similar disease or disorder, a problem similar to that of the portraitist trying to capture a "likeness":

> No portrait painter was ever so careless as to pay no attention to the marked peculiarity in the features of the person he wished to make a likeness of, or to consider it sufficient to make any sort of a pair of round holes below the forehead by way of eyes, between them to draw a long-shaped thing directed downwards, always of the same shape, by way of a nose, and beneath this to put a slit going across the face which should stand for the mouth of this or of any other person; no painter, I say, ever went about delineating human faces in such a rude and slovenly manner; no naturalist ever went to work in this fashion in describing any natural production; such was never the way in which any zoologist, botanist, or mineralogist acted. It was only the semeiology of ordinary medicine that went to work in such a manner when describing morbid phenomena.[229]

Thus the key to the individuality of each patient is not found in the symptoms he has in common with others but in those which distinguish him from others. It is not the possession of a nose which renders a person distinctive, but the particular shape of this organ. Possessing a nose makes him like everyone else, while his own individual shape of nose makes him a unique individual.

The same is true in disease. The peculiar and unique features which distinguish one morbid process from another are those most valuable to the physician: "the most singular, most uncommon signs furnish the characteristic, the distinctive, the peculiar features."[230]

Thus, like other Empirical thinkers, Hahnemann urges reliance on the *propria* rather than the *communia.* But he went beyond them in pointing out a technique for distinguishing between the two.

Where Sydenham and others had defined the *propria* as the "peculiar but constant" symptoms, i.e., a contradiction in terms, leaving the decision to the judgment of each physician, Hahnemann solved the problem: the "common" symptoms of the medicine were manifested when it was taken in larger doses, its "peculiar" effects (*propria*) when taken "in high dilutions potentized by proper trituration and succussion." The latter were to be matched with the same "peculiar" symptoms of the patient.

> In this search for a homoeopathic specific remedy, that is to say, in this comparison of the collective symptoms of the natural disease with the list of symptoms of known medicines, in order to find among these an artificial morbific agent corresponding by similarity to the disease to be cured, the *more striking, singular, uncommon, and peculiar* (characteristic) signs and symptoms of the case of disease are chiefly and most solely to be kept in view; for it is *more particularly these that very similar ones in the list of symptoms of the selected medicine must correspond to,* in order to constitute it the most suitable for effecting the cure. The more general and undefined

> symptoms; loss of appetite, headache, debility, restless sleep, discomfort, and so forth, demand but little attention when of that vague and indefinite character, if they cannot be more accurately described, as symptoms of such a general nature are observed in almost every disease and from almost every drug.[231]
>
> If the . . . list of symptoms of the most suitable medicine contain those peculiar, uncommon, singular, and distinguishing (characteristic) symptoms, which are to be met with in the disease to be cured in the greatest number and in the greatest similarity, *this* medicine is the most appropriate homoeopathic specific remedy for *this* morbid state . . .[232]

The more common symptoms of the patient and the drug should also, generally speaking, be matched, but the medicine will not be effective if similarity lies *only* between the *communia* of the drug and the patient and not between their *propria:*

> If . . . among the symptoms of the remedy selected there be none that accurately resemble the distinctive (characteristic), peculiar, uncommon symptoms of the case of disease, and if the remedy correspond to the disease only in the general, vaguely described, indefinite states (nausea, debility, headache, and so forth) . . . in that case the physician cannot promise himself any immediate favorable result from the employment of this unhomoeopathic medicine.[233]

Thus, in the treatment of malaria (intermittent fever) Hahnemann notes that the paroxysms of fever (*communia*) are of little use in the selection of the remedy, since they are experienced by everyone. Instead, the physician should look to the patient's symptoms between the seizures of fever (*propria*), since these differ greatly from one patient to the next.[234]

He provides the following case from his own practice, showing the relative importance of the *communia* and *propria:*

Sch–, a washerwoman, somewhat above 40 years old, had been more than three weeks unable to pursue her avocation when she consulted me on September 1, 1815.

1. On any movement, especially at every step, and worst on making a false step, she has a shooting pain in the *scrobiculus cordis* that comes, as she avers, every time from the left side.[h]

2. When she lies, she feels quite well, then she has no pain anywhere, neither in the side nor in the *scrobiculus.*

3. She cannot sleep after three o'clock in the morning.

4. She relishes her food, but when she has eaten a little she feels sick.

5. Then the water collects in her mouth and runs out of it, like the water-brash.

6. She has frequent empty eructations after every meal.

7. Her temper is passionate, disposed to anger. —Whenever the pain is severe, she is covered with perspiration. —The catamenia were quite regular a fortnight since.

In other respects her health is good.

Now, as regards symptom 1, *Belladonna, China,* and *Rhus toxicodendron* cause shootings in the *scrobiculus,* but none of them *only on motion,* as is the case here. *Pulsatilla* certainly causes shootings in the *scrobiculus* on making a false step, but only as a rare alternating motion, and has neither the same digestive derangements as occur here at 4, compared with 5 and 6, nor the same state of the disposition.[i]

Bryonia alone has among its chief alternating actions, as the whole list of its symptoms demonstrates, pains

[h] *Scrobiculus*—the pit of the stomach.

[i] "The state of the disposition of the patient often chiefly determines the selection of the homoeopathic remedy, as being a decidedly characteristic symptom which can least of all remain concealed from the accurately observing physician" (*Organon,* Sec. 211).

> *from movement* and especially shooting pains, as also stitches beneath the sternum (in the *scrobiculus*) on raising the arm, and on making a false step it occasions shooting in other parts.
>
> The negative symptom 2 met with here answers especially to *Bryonia* . . .
>
> Symptom 3 is met with in several medicines, and also in *Bryonia*.
>
> Symptom 4 is certainly, as far as regards "sickness after eating," met with in several other medicines . . . but neither so constantly and usually, nor with relish for food, as in *Bryonia*.
>
> As regards symptom 5 several medicines certainly cause a flow of saliva like water-brash, just as well as *Bryonia;* the others, however, do not produce the remaining symptoms in a very similar manner. Hence *Bryonia* is to be preferred to them in this point.
>
> Empty eructation (of wind only) after eating (symptom 6) is found in a few medicines, and in none so constantly, so usually, and to such a great degree, as in *Bryonia*.
>
> To 7—one of the chief symptoms in diseases . . . is the "state of the disposition," and as *Bryonia* causes this symptom also in an exactly similar manner—*Bryonia* is for all these reasons to be preferred in this case to all other medicines as the homoeopathic remedy.[235]

Whereas the washerwoman complained of a pain in the pit of her stomach, Hahnemann was guided, in selecting the remedy, by: pain only on motion, a feeling of nausea after eating, empty eructations after eating, and the patient's choleric disposition.

By shifting the physician's focus from the *communia* to the *propria* Hahnemann destroyed all existing nosological classifications based on the common symptoms, the attempt to localize diseases in the body, the distinction between somatic and "mental" diseases, etc. The allopaths "imagined that their business was to select, from the apparently infinite variety of different morbid phenomena which the nature displays, a number of diseased states, all resembling each other in having some particular prominent symptom in common, as fundamental forms, and, having assigned to them general symptoms that were of not unfrequent occurrence in diseases and bestowed on them special names, to give them out for constant distinct diseases that always remained the same."[236] "The similarities of many [diseases] were investigated, and those that were considered to be connected were united in classes, orders, and species, etc. according to the similarity of their exciting causes, the functions that were deranged, the identity of their seat in the body, the peculiar tone of the fibers, and some common symptoms."[237]

> How were it possible to arrange such *inconjugabilia* into classes, orders, genera, species, varieties, and sub-varieties, like organic beings, and to give *names* to such states of the extremely composite psychico-corporeal microcosm, subject as it is to an infinity of modifications and shades of difference! The millions of morbid cases that occur perhaps but once in the world require no names—we only require to cure them.[238]

Thus he at a stroke reverted to the Empirical doctrine that diseases are infinite in number, "as diverse as the clouds in the sky."[239] "The nature presents an infinite variety of diseases that are often confounded with one another; it is excessively rare that exactly the same disease is met with twice."[240] "The morbific agencies that act on the human body are so numerous, their intensity and duration of action so various, that the diseases they give rise to must present a great variety of character."[241] "Each case of disease that presents itself must be regarded (and treated) as an individual malady that never before occurred in the same manner and under the same circumstances as in the case before us, and will never again happen precisely in the same way!"[242]

Physicians hitherto have "collected the infinite variety of diseases into a few arbitrarily formed classes of diseases."[243] Take the well-known class of intermittent fever (malaria):

"My friend, do you never suspect that all these were different kinds of agues, or rather intermittent diseases, differing completely from one another? . . . Do you not suspect that there may be perhaps twenty different kinds of intermittent fever, which parempiric imbecility has included under one head, has asserted all to belong to a single species (intermittent fever), and has sought to combat all with a single remedy, whereas each requires its peculiar remedy, without thereby deserving to be called capricious or obstinate."[244]

Nosological classifications do not reflect the true course of the nature but are designed rather for the comfort and convenience of the physician: "the collection of these forms of disease manufactured by themselves they asserted to constitute the whole range of the world of disease, in other words, *pathology, in order that they might be able to lay down special modes of treatment for these their imaginary morbid pictures,* and this constituted the science of *therapeutics.* Thus they made a virtue of necessity, but they did not consider the evil that must arise from this perversion of the nature, they did not reflect that this arbitrary procedure . . . did violence to the nature."[245]

The only true and natural disease class is that defined by the symptoms of a remedy, as developed in a proving, and Hahnemann urged physicians to stop using conventional disease names.[246]

The Rationalist nosological urge has created whole classes of supposedly "local" diseases: "by which term is signified those changes and ailments that appear on the external parts of the body. Until now the idea prevalent in the schools was that these parts were alone morbidly affected, and that the rest of the body did not participate in the disease—a theoretical, absurd doctrine, which has led to the most disastrous medical treatment."[247]

All diseases are, in fact, diseases of the whole organism:

> No external malady . . . can arise, persist, or even grow worse without . . . the cooperation of the whole organism, which must consequently be in a diseased state. It

> could not make its appearance at all without the consent of the whole of the rest of the health, and without the participation of the rest of the living whole (of the vital force that pervades all the other sensitive and irritable parts of the organism); indeed, it is impossible to conceive its production without the instrumentality of the whole (deranged) life, so intimately are all parts of the organism connected together to form an indivisible whole in sensations and functions.[248]

> The local affection depend[s] solely on a disease of the rest of the body and should only be regarded as an inseparable part of the whole, as one of the most considerable and striking symptoms of the whole disease.[249]

All diseases have both a physical and a mental aspect, both somatic and mental symptoms. The latter are as diverse as the former, and Hahnemann's provings yielded a copious variety.[250] The "mental diseases" are thus nothing more than diseases of the whole organism which have developed on their mental side, becoming localized in the body's intellectual and emotional centers.[j] They "do not constitute a class of disease sharply separated from all others, since in all other so-called corporeal diseases the condition of the disposition and mind is *always* altered, and, in all cases of disease we are called on to cure, the state of the patient's disposition is to be particularly noted, along with the totality of the symptoms, if we would trace an accurate picture of the disease."[251] [k]

The key to Hahnemann's solution of the problem of disease classes lies in his statement: "the millions of morbid cases that occur perhaps but once in the world require no

[j]Hence the physical symptoms decline as the mental ones are exacerbated (*Organon,* Sec. 215).

[k]Hahnemann treated mental and emotional diseases homoeopathically, i.e., with similars (*Organon,* Sec. 230). Note the importance he attached to the washerwoman's "choleric disposition" as a curative indication.

names—we only require to cure them." Rejecting the Rationalist technique of defining the cause and then proceeding to treatment, Hahnemann accepted the Empirical principle that treatment points to cause, that theory arises out of practice, that by healing his patients the physician comes to know them.[1]

The physician can understand his patient's needs *only through his own knowledge of remedies,* that is, from the provings. When he knows how to treat, he will then understand the nature of the patient's ailment and its relationship to other diseases.

The Single Remedy. Specificity. Chronic and Miasmatic Diseases

The classes of diseases are given by the classes of remedies:

> Of a truth it is only by a very considerable store of medicines accurately known in respect of these their pure modes of action in altering the health of man that we can be placed in a position to discover a homoeopathic remedy, a suitable artificial (curative) morbific analog for *each* of the infinitely numerous morbid states in nature, for *every* malady in the world.[252]

> Whichever of these medicines that have been investigated as to their power of altering man's health we find to contain in the symptoms observed from its use the greatest similarity to the totality of the symptoms of a given natural disease, this medicine will and must be the most suitable, the most certain homoeopathic remedy for the disease . . .[253]

The medicine which is homoeopathic to the illness of a given patient cures that illness and thereby identifies it, classifies it. This is the true meaning of "specificity"—the "specific" remedy is the one which is homoeopathic to a given "case of disease."[254]

[1]See *Divided Legacy,* I, 262-274.

> I do not expect, and do not believe, there can be a thoroughly specific remedy for any "disease," of such and such a name, burdened with all the ramifications, concomitant affections and variations, which, in pathological works, are so often inconsiderately detailed as essential to its character, as invariably pertaining to it . . . I am, on the other hand, convinced that there are as many specifics as there are different states of individual diseases . . .[255]

Thus God has provided a remedy for each "case of disease," each sick person, *and it is the physician's duty to find this remedy.* "Take comfort, sick humanity! What are still required for your relief are free sagacious men who have the strength to emancipate themselves from the strong slave-chains of ancient prejudice and theories."[256] Even chronic diseases have their medicines: "The Creator of these sufferers [has] provided remedies for them also . . . [this] source of boundless goodness . . . compared to which the tenderest mother's love is as thick clouds beside the glory of the noonday sun."[257]

The corollary of this principle is that each medicinal substance must be different from each other one:

> Each one of the many thousand genera of plants must possess a different medicinal action; in truth, even the several species must differ from each other in this respect, for their permanent differences of appearance announce them as things differing in kind. Here, then, we have fulness and abundance, here we have a divinely rich store of curative powers![258]

> As every species of plant differs in its external form, in its peculiar mode of existence, in its taste, smell, etc., from every other species and genus of plant—as every mineral substance, every salt differs from all others both in its external and internal physical qualities, so do they all differ among themselves in their medicinal properties, that is to say, in their morbific powers; each of the substances effects an alteration in our state of health in a peculiar, determinate manner.[259]

> Every plant has its own peculiar medicinal mode of action that is not to be found in any other plant in the world.[260]

> No substance in nature possesses the same qualities as any other, nor is it possible that it can, for they are characteristically different in externals, and as veal cannot turn into mutton or pork, neither can quitch-grass be transformed into sarsaparilla.[261]

Just as the disease is an alteration of the dynamic power which fills the whole organism, so is the remedy also a dynamic power which acts as a whole upon the whole human organism in disease or in health:

> This *dynamic* action of medicines, like the vitality itself by means of which it is reflected upon the organism, is almost purely *spiritual* in its nature . . . This dynamic property is so pervading that it is quite immaterial what sensitive part of the body is touched by the medicine in order to develop its whole action . . . immaterial whether the dissolved medicine enter the stomach or merely remain in the mouth, or be applied to a wound or other part deprived of skin.[262]

The particular case of disease is cured when the physician administers the single remedy whose symptomatology most closely matches that of the patient.[263] This was not, Hahnemann claimed, "symptomatic treatment": "in the cure effected by the removal of the whole of the perceptible signs and symptoms of the disease the internal alteration of the vital principle to which the disease is due—consequently the whole of the disease—is at the same time removed."[264] "It is not conceivable, nor can it be proved by any experience in the world, that, after removal of all the symptoms of the disease, and of the entire collection of the perceptible phenomena, there should or could remain anything else besides health, or that the morbid alteration in the interior could remain uneradicated."[265] [m]

[m]C. W. Hufeland wrote, in a critique: "Homoeopathy can remove the symptoms, but the disease remains." Hahnemann commented: "he views the

The homoeopathic remedy acts in this way by virtue of the natural law that "a weaker dynamic affection is permanently extinguished in the living organism by a stronger one if the latter (whilst differing in kind) is very similar to the former in its manifestations."[266] While morbific influences are by nature weak, affecting only subjects who are susceptible,[n] remedies are capable of affecting everyone to whom they are administered: the intrinsic power of the remedy is greater than that of the morbific cause.[267]

Cure by similars is hence identical in principle to observed instances of the cure of certain diseases (or their *sequelae*) by other stronger similar diseases.[o]

Hahnemann insisted that only one remedy be given at a time and continually belabored his allopathic colleagues for their multi-ingredient prescriptions:

> As though they were independent beings endowed with free volition, each ingredient in a complete prescription has its task allotted to it . . . something for the tendency to vomit, something else for the diarrhoea, something else for the evening-fever and night-sweats, and as the patient is so weak, tonic medicines must be added, and not one alone, but several, in order that what the one cannot do (which we don't know) the other may.[268]

This was illogical, in his opinion, since all the symptoms proceed from one cause.[269] Hence, if a single medicine meets all the requirements of cure by its homoeopathicity to the disease cause (i.e., to the disease symptoms), this one must be administered:[270]

> The nature acts according to eternal laws without asking your leave; she loves simplicity and effects *much* with one remedy, whilst you effect *little* with many. Seek to imitate the nature!

disease as *something material,* which, after the cure is completed, may still remain lurking in some corner in the interior of the body . . . So dreadful is still the blindness of the old pathology!" (*Organon,* Sec. 8, note 5).

[n]See below, pp. 409-411.

[o]See above, pp. 374-375.

> To write very composite recipes, and several of them in the course of the day, is the climax of parempiricism; to administer quite simple remedies, and not to give a second before the action of the first has expired—this and this alone is the direct way into the inner holy place of the art. Make your choice![271]

The prescription is based, as already noted, on the *propria* and not the *communia:* "the homoeopathist . . . judges of the prevailing disease according to its peculiarities and phenomena (its individuality) without suffering himself to be led astray to a wrong mode of treatment by any pathological systematic nomenclature; and by attention to the present state, complaints, and ailments of the patient he generally, by means of the suitable (specific) remedy, brings about the desired recovery."[272] And the *propria* of each remedy (as seen from the provings) differ from the *propria* of every other.[273] Only one remedy can be "most similar" to the *propria* of the patient, and this one must be prescribed.

An equally important reason for prescribing only the single remedy was that all provings were of single substances—not of mixtures.[p] Knowledge of the symptomatology of single substances could not be used to predict their combined effect when administered together.[274] Finally, Hahnemann notes, "it is wrong to attempt to employ complex means when simple means suffice . . . a simple medicinal substance when used in diseases, the totality of whose symptoms is accurately known, renders efficient aid by itself alone, if it be homoeopathically selected."[275]

Physicians have prescribed medical mixtures in the past because they "hold it beneath their dignity to prescribe one single simple medicament, and nothing more, in a disease, and would let the patient die and the medical art ever remain as a non-art, sooner than part with their learned prerogative of prescribing *artistically compounded recipes.*"[276] Also because it is more difficult to find the single indicated

[p]Chemical *compounds,* of course, were subjected to proving from the earliest days of homoeopathy and have been in constant use since that time.

remedy than to prescribe a mixture: "it would be inconvenient to search for such a one, [hence] we put in one prescription something to meet every indication, and thus we fulfil the requirements of the school."[277]

Neither of these motives was supposed to affect the homoeopathic physician.[q]

Hahnemann's distrust of causal speculation extended also to the exciting cause. While disease is a derangement of the vital force "by the dynamic influence upon it of a morbific agent inimical to life,"[278] he was more concerned with describing the derangement and finding the curative analog than with defining the nature of the dynamic exciting cause.[r]

At the same time, he was aware of epidemics and contagious diseases—which appear to depend upon an exciting cause affecting large numbers of persons in the same way. Hence his doctrine of disease is qualified by a special treatment of "miasmatic" diseases.

"Miasmatic" diseases are acute diseases that arise from a "miasm of constant character," are usually contagious, and often epidemic.

> We observe a few diseases that always arise from *one and the same* cause, e.g., the miasmatic maladies: hydrophobia, the venereal disease, the plague of the Levant, yellow fever, small-pox, cow-pox, the measles, and some

[q]See *Divided Legacy,* III, 328-401.

[r]He does, however, urge the physician to eliminate *material* exciting causes: "He will remove from the room strong-smelling flowers, which have a tendency to cause syncope and hysterical sufferings; extract from the cornea the foreign body that excites inflammation of the eye; loosen the over-tight bandage on a wounded limb that threatens to cause mortification, and apply a more suitable one; lay bare and put a ligature on the wounded artery that produces fainting; endeavor to promote the expulsion by vomiting of belladonna berries, etc. that may have been swallowed; extract foreign substances that may have got into the orifices of the body (the nose, gullet, ears, urethra, rectum, vagina); crush the vesical calculus; open the imperforate anus of the new-born infant, etc." (*Organon,* Sec. 7, note 3). On the homoeopathic attitude to microorganisms as exciting causes see below, pp. 412*k* and 679-680.

> others, which bear upon them the distinctive mark of always remaining diseases of a *peculiar character;* and because they arise from a contagious principle that always remains the same, they always retain the same character and pursue the same course, excepting as regards some accidental concomitant circumstances, which, however, do not alter their essential character.[279]
>
> As regards acute diseases, they are [sometimes] those diseases in which many persons are attacked with very similar sufferings from the same cause *(epidemically);* these diseases generally become infectious *(contagious)* when they prevail among thickly congregated masses of human beings. Thence arise fevers, in each instance of a peculiar nature, and, because the cases of disease have an identical origin, they set up in all those they affect an identical morbid process . . . sometimes they are peculiar *acute miasms* which recur in the same manner (hence known by some traditional name) which either attack persons but once in a lifetime, as the smallpox, measles, whooping cough, the ancient smooth bright red scarlet fever of Sydenham, the mumps, etc., or such as recur frequently in pretty much the same manner, the plague of the Levant, the yellow fever of the sea-coast, the Asiatic cholera, etc.[280]

"Miasmatic" disease thus presents certain recurring traits, from one victim to the next, which are a function of the causal "miasm." In this it differs from "all other cases of disease [which] are mere individualities, that is to say, all present themselves in nature with different combinations of symptoms, have never before occurred, and can never occur again in exactly the same manner."[281]

But Hahnemann warns against expecting any therapeutic assistance from this causal knowledge of miasms:

> It is very easy to say that we may attribute itch to the itch miasm, the venereal disease to the venereal miasm, variola to the variolous miasm, ague to the marsh miasm.

> By pronouncing these names not the slightest advance is made to obtaining a more accurate knowledge of these diseases, nor yet to their appropriate treatment. The morbific miasms are as thoroughly unknown to us as regards their internal nature as the diseases themselves they produce. Their essential nature is quite beyond the reach of our senses, and their true remedies will never be learned from what the books can teach us regarding their exciting causes.[282]

For the miasmatic disease does not appear in precisely the same form in every victim—even when it is epidemic: "in all these indescribable varieties occur, which often alter the whole affair."[283]

The miasmatic disease generated by a miasmatic cause is a phenomenon greater and more extensive than any one person sick with it, and the symptoms of the "disease" must be gathered by combining the symptoms of all those suffering from it:

> All those affected with the disease prevailing at a given time have certainly contracted it from one and the same source and hence are suffering from the *same* disease; but the whole extent of such an epidemic disease and the totality of its symptoms (the knowledge whereof, which is essential for enabling us to choose the most suitable homoeopathic remedy for this array of symptoms, is obtained by a complete survey of the morbid picture) cannot be learned from one single patient, but is only to be perfectly deduced (abstracted) and ascertained from the sufferings of several patients of different constitutions.[284]

> Thus, in the year 1813 one patient would be prostrated with only a few symptoms of this plague [typhus], a second patient showed only a few, but different, ailments; while a third, a fourth, etc., would complain of still other ailments belonging to this epidemic disease, while they were, nevertheless, all sick with one and the

> same pestilential fever, and the entire and complete image of the typhus fever reigning at the time could only be obtained by gathering together the symptoms of all, or at least of many of these patients.[285]

In this Hahnemann was obviously extrapolating his experience with the provings, where he found that each substance produced its full symptomatology only when administered to a number of persons:

> All the symptoms peculiar to a medicine do not appear in one person, nor all at once, nor in the same experiment, but some occur in one person chiefly at one time, others again during a second or third trial . . . The whole of the elements of disease a medicine is capable of producing can only be brought to anything like completeness by numerous observations on suitable persons of both sexes and of various constitutions.[286]

Thus the disease generated by a miasm (or a medicinal substance—in the proving), while specific to that exciting cause, has protean manifestations and varies from one sick person (or one prover) to the next.

Hence all those sick with a miasmatic disease cannot be treated by the same "specific" medicine: "there are peculiar specifics for the pure disease and others for its varieties."[287] Hahnemann's principle that each individual case of *any* disease has a curative analog in the materia medica applies equally to miasmatic diseases.

But this principle is now qualified in two ways.

In miasmatic diseases the symptoms of one patient alone may not be a sufficient guide to treatment but should be supplemented by the symptoms of others suffering from the same miasm. In the 1813 typhus epidemic:

> the one or two remedies found to be homoeopathic healed the epidemy, and therefore showed themselves specifically helpful with every patient, though the one might be suffering from symptoms differing from those of others, and almost all seemed to be suffering from different diseases.[288]

Furthermore, some miasms are more powerful than others and produce the disease more often in its relatively "pure" form—this being the form most amenable to treatment with the classic "specific" remedy.

Malaria and syphilis, for instance, appear quite often in their pure form:

> It is only the very great simplicity and constancy of [malaria] and syphilis that permitted remedies to be found for them, which appeared to many physicians to have specific qualities; for the variations in these diseases occur much more seldom, and are usually much less important than in others, consequently bark and mercury must be much more often serviceable than not so. But neither is bark specific in [malaria], in the most extended sense of the term; nor mercury in syphilis, in its most extended sense; they are, however, probably specific in both diseases when they occur simple, pure, and free from all complication.[289]

The same is true for smallpox, measles, and several others.[290]

Hahnemann's underlying principle, however, remains valid: each case of a miasmatic disease must be examined carefully by the physician to ascertain if the symptoms warrant prescription of the usual "specific". If not, he must look elsewhere for the similar remedy:

> Pity it was that it was not observed *why*, for example, of the seven-fifteenths of all the so-called agues in which bark was useless, three-fifteenths required *Nux vomica* or bitter almonds, another fifteenth opium, another fifteenth blood-letting, and still another fifteenth small doses of ipecac, for their cure! It was thought sufficient to say, "Bark was of no use, but *Ignatia* cured," the *why* was never satisfactorily answered. Were it a case of pure ague, bark must be of service; where there were complications, with excessive irritability, especially of the *primae viae,* however, it was no longer a pure case of ague, and it

> could not do good; here were now *reasons* for choosing as a remedy, or as an auxiliary means, *Ignatia, Nux vomica,* or bitter almonds, according to the different conditions of the system; and it could not, and should not have been wondered at that bark was not useful.[291]

Just as the miasm can be extended in space, so it can be extended in time, becoming the "chronic disease . . . produced by a miasm which continues the same through all generations."[292]

The existence of "chronic disease" gave rise to a second modification in Hahnemann's doctrine.

After several decades treating patients with homoeopathic remedies and finding that in certain cases cure was not permanent, Hahnemann concluded that failure was due to the presence of an underlying inherited chronic disease.[293] This chronic disease had to be treated first, with the remedies specific to it; when the patient had thrown off the chronic disease, subsequent acute illnesses, no longer complicated by this chronic one, were easier to treat with success.[294]

Hahnemann concluded that three principal chronic diseases exist: psora, syphilis, and gonorrhoea (which he called sycosis).[s]

Of these psora is by far the most widespread, accounting for seven-eights of all chronic diseases. It is an ancient miasm which has taken different forms at different stages in history, from leprosy in the Middle Ages through various forms of erysipelas to the less virulent, but still serious and even fatal, scabies.[t]

[s]Thus Hahnemann went against John Hunter's theory of the identity of syphilis and gonorrhoea (and against his own earlier view) and was the first to assert that they are different diseases (1828). Credit for this finding is usually attributed to Philippe Ricord (1799-1889) of the Paris School whose *Traite Pratique des Maladies Veneriennes* appeared in 1838. It is probable that this idea, like many others introduced into Paris medicine at this time, came from homoeopathy. Hahnemann's *Chronic Diseases* was translated into French in 1832 (*Doctrine et Traitement Homoeopathique des Maladies Chroniques.* Two Volumes. Paris: Bailliere, 1832).

[t]Scabies ("the itch," *die Kraetze, dartres, teigne, gale*), although often treated humorously in the literature, was not a jocular matter for those suffering from it.

Syphilis and gonorrhoea had appeared more recently, in the sixteenth century, taken root in the populations of Europe, and were now being passed on from generation to generation.[u]

These chronic diseases are perpetuated, in particular, by the incorrect (i.e., suppressive) treatment of their acute forms.[294] [v]

They assume an infinite variety of forms in different individuals, like the other miasmatic diseases whose full symptomatology is manifested only over a large group of victims, and Hahnemann wrote five volumes of their symptoms.[295]

While he suggested a number of internal medicines for treating these three chronic diseases, the major remedies were: sulphur (for psora), mercury (for syphilis), and *Arbor vitae* (for gonorrhoea).[w] He particularly rejected—as local suppressive treatment which only exacerbates the condition —sulphurous ointments in psora, mercurial ointments in syphilis, and surgical intervention to excise the skin growths (warts, chancres, bubos) associated with syphilis and gonorrhoea. He called these skin symptoms benign in the sense that they balance and contain the internal disease which—provided the skin is left undisturbed—will not progress or, at

J. F. Autenrieth estimated in 1807 that 15% of each generation (counted as 30 years) was sick with scabies at one time or another, while 1% of each generation died of it. Of the 1,200,000 persons in Wuerttemburg 6400 were sick with scabies—and 430 died—every year (*Versuche fuer die praktische Heilkunde* [Tuebingen: Cotta, 1807], 233-234). For further discussion of scabies, see below p. 468.

[u]For further discussion of venereal diseases, see below, pp. 417-418, 466.

[v]Another fruitful source of chronic disease, of course, was the incorrect (i.e., non-homoeopathic) treatment of acute diseases generally. These fell outside Hahnemann's theory of chronic diseases, since they came in such variety that it was impossible to investigate them, and Hahnemann professed himself unable to cure them properly (*Organon,* Sec. 74, 75. *Lesser Writings,* 736-752). See above, p. 368. The mercurial medicines, which Hahnemann in 1789 warned may "set the fibers into morbid irritable vibrations, the source of all sorts of chronic diseases that are difficult to cure," continued to be used liberally by the profession for decades, and in the United States for another century (*Lesser Writings,* 139. *Divided Legacy,* III, 245-246).

[w]Here some might see a parallel with Paracelsus' salt, sulphur, and mercury.

least, will progress less rapidly.[297] Inunctions, ointments, and excisions only accelerate the progress of the internal disease.[298] [x]

Hahnemann's ideas on chronic disease were presented to the world in his last work, *Die Chronischen Krankheiten, ihre Eigenthuemliche Natur und Homoeopathische Heilung* (1828).[299] It provoked a hurricane of opposition, outside the ranks of homoeopathy and within them. "Few books have stirred up more excitement in the medical world than Hahnemann's *Chronic Diseases.* His conception of these diseases and, in particular, his psora theory, aroused the criticism of friend and foe to a tremendous extent from the very moment of their publication. At this point many of his adherents and students refused to follow him any further. To his opponents these views of his seemed to be even more idiotic than the high dilution medicines of homoeopathy, and for nearly a century they have formed the target of their scornful ridicule."[300] The Central Congress of Homoeopathists, meeting in Frankfurt-am-Main in 1837, formally voted condemnation of the concept of chronic disease.[301] [y]

On doctrinal and historical grounds, however, this intense opposition was unjustified. Hahnemann's theory of chronic diseases was a logical development of his own ideas and reflected trends making themselves felt at this time in other areas of medicine.

[x] See below, pp. 418-419.

[y] Scabies was commonly regarded as a local disease of the skin (see, e.g., Cullen, *Synopsis of Methodical Nosology,* 176), and for decades Hahnemann's theory of chronic disease was regarded as a "fantasy"—with psora, especially, attributed to the itch-mite (*Acarus scabiei*) (see T. Puschmann, *Handbuch der Geschichte der Medizin* [Jena: Gustav Fischer, 1905], III, 433). This has been dutifully passed on by historians of medicine: "the more enlightened homoeopaths joined other enlightened physicians in ridiculing the whole doctrine, especially since the itch-mite, the accepted cause of scabies, was by this time well-known" (L. S. King, *The Medical World of the Eighteenth Century* [Chicago: University of Chicago Press, 1958], 185). But modern opinion supports Hahnemann in holding this disease to be genetically determined: "the one etiological factor universally agreed is heredity" (Editorial: "Psoriasis" in *British Medical Journal,* 16 November, 1974, 365). It afflicts up to 75 million persons in the world, and the 5 to 8 million in the United States alone spend up to $1 *billion* a year on treatments which are recognized as ineffective and often dangerous.

Reduction of the Dose. Dynamization. Poisons and Medicines

In his early years of practice Hahnemann used doses comparable to those of his colleagues: 5-50 grams of antimony, 20-70 grams of jalap root, ounces of hemlock juice, 12-15 grains of the powdered leaves and roots of *Belladonna,* and substantial amounts of quinine.[302] His 1796 "Essay" mentions "moderate" doses.[303] In 1799 he first announced the principle of the infinitesimal dose, and after 1800 his doses sizes were gradually reduced.[304] In 1800 he refers to a dose of arsenic "one ten-millionth the usual size."[305] In 1801 he was treating scarlet fever with one-drop doses of tincture of opium (each drop containing one five-millionth of a grain) and giving as a preventive 1/432,000 of a grain of dried juice of the *Belladonna* berry.[306]

This reduction was apparently due to Hahnemann's observation that medicines administered in substantial amounts according to the law of similars caused severe aggravation of the symptoms.[307] Once he had embarked on this course, his natural curiosity led him to seek its limit. He claimed that medicinal effect is based on quality, not quantity, and that it remains present however small the amount of medicine prescribed.[308] [z] The use of infinitesimals was justified ultimately by experience.[309]

> Has perchance Nature given us a law that we regard a scruple or a grain as the smallest and most suitable dose of all medicines—even of the most powerful? Has she not put knowledge and means into our hands so that we can arrange the more powerful and most powerful substances into smaller and smaller doses, some of them to a tenth

[z]Hahnemann perhaps owes the distinction between "quantity" and "quality" to John Hunter who observed that infection with venereal disease depends on the quality of the poison, not its quantity (*Works,* II, 142). A certain General von Korsakoff in Russia, who was active in the homoeopathic movement there, suggested in 1832 that the power of the high dilution results from "a kind of infection or communication of the medicinal power . . . to the non-medicinal vehicle," and this is the explanation accepted today (*Lesser Writings,* 763, note; *Divided Legacy,* III, 493-494).

> of a grain, the more powerful to a hundredth or a thousandth of a grain, the highly powerful ones to a millionth, billionth, or even to a trillionth, quadrillionth, and quintillionth of a grain? . . .[310]

All doses yield primary symptoms, while perceptible secondary symptoms are produced only by relatively large doses.[311] Smaller doses yield no perceptible secondary symptoms but only the gradual restoration of health.[312]

The appropriate dose of medicine for any given case of disease is determined "not by fine-spun reasoning, not by specious sophistry," but by "pure experiment, careful observation of the sensitiveness of each patient, and accurate experience."[313]

The second volume of the *Reine Arzneimittellehre* (1816) gave detailed directions for preparing doses as small as the decillionth part of a grain.[314] Hahnemann's technique was to mix one part of the medicine with 99 parts of milk sugar (if the medicine was dry) or 99 parts of alcohol (if the medicine was a liquid) and then triturate it (if dry) or shake it (if liquid) for some time until the mass was uniformly mixed. This formed the "first centesimal dilution" (if the ratio of medicinal substance to vehicle was 1:9, this was the "first decimal dilution"). When one part of this dilution was thereupon mixed with another 99 parts of milk sugar or alcohol, and again triturated or succussed, the "second centesimal dilution" was produced. And so on down (or up) to the thirtieth centesimal which Hahnemann generally recommended (although exceeding it at times) as the furthest limit of the dilution of medicines.[315]

Since the Avogadro limit (the point at which no trace of the original medicinal substance can statistically be expected to remain in the dilution) is reached at the twelfth centesimal or 24th decimal dilution, this aspect of the Hahnemannian doctrine caused hilarity outside the ranks of the faithful and some consternation within. Hahnemann's more enthusiastic followers, moreover, continued to dilute the drugs beyond the thirtieth centesimal. General von Korsakoff in Russia went as far as the 1500th centesimal, while Equerry Jenichen of Wismar carried dilution to the 2500th, 8000th, and even 16,000th.[316][a] Hahnemann responded in a letter to a follower in Lemberg: "I do not approve of your potentizing medicines higher than [the thirtieth centesimal]—there must be some end to the thing. It cannot go on to infinity."[317]

He proposed, in this same letter, that the thirtieth centesimal dilution be made the standard dose: then "a homogeneous process arises in the cures of all homoeopaths, and if they describe a cure, we are able to work after them in the same degree, since they are operating with the same tools as we are. Then our enemies cannot reproach us with having nothing definite, no fixed standard."[318] But this proposal never caught the fancy of his followers, and doses well beyond the thirtieth centesimal have been used in homoeopathy since Hahnemann's time.[b]

The problem of dose size was complicated further by the associated doctrine of "dynamization," i.e., that the trituration (of dry substances) and succussion (of liquids) practiced at each stage of preparation actually *enhanced* the power of the remedy—so that the second centesimal was more powerful than the first, and the tenth, twentieth, or thirtieth centesimals more powerful still.[319][c] In one writing Hahnemann explained this in terms of the finer comminution of the medicinal substance increasing its area of contact with the patient's organism.[320] In the *Organon,* however, he stated that trituration and succussion release the "spirit-like power" of the medicine—which is compatible with his assumption

[a]R. E. Dudgeon remarks that fortunately Jenichen shot himself when he reached the 16,000th or there is no telling what heights he might have reached (*Theory and Practice of Homoeopathy* [London: Leath and Ross, 1854], 355.)

[b]This question was a cause of discord among homoeopathic physicians in the late nineteenth century (*Divided Legacy,* III, 328-401).

[c]Hahnemann stated: "This development of the spiritual power of medicines to such a height by means of the multiplied and continued *trituration* and *succussion* of a small portion of medicinal substance with ever more and more dry or fluid unmedicinal substances, deserves incontestably to be reckoned *among the greatest discoveries* of this age" (*Lesser Writings,* 729-730). But both Stahl and Paracelsus had alluded to the possibility of heightening the spiritual power of a medicine (*Theoria Medica Vera,* II, 39; *Divided Legacy,* I, 421 ff.).

that medicines act through their spiritual (*geistlich*) or dynamic impact upon the organism.[321 d]

When critics observed that one of the typical "high" dilutions required adding to the medicinal substance an amount of diluent equivalent to the water in Lake Geneva, or perhaps the Baltic Sea, Hahnemann retorted that the process involved more than the mere mixing of medicine with diluent: "by the *succussion* and *trituration* there ensues not only the most intimate mixture, but at the same time—and this is the most important circumstance—there ensues such a great and hitherto unknown and undreamt of change, by the development and liberation of the dynamic powers of the medicinal substance so treated, as to excite astonishment."[322]

An interesting by-product of the doctrine of dynamization was that substances inert in their natural state—such as gold, silver, silica, etc.—were seen to develop medicinal powers when triturated with milk sugar.[323] Hahnemann recommended a potentization of metallic gold as an antidote for suicidal tendencies.[324]

Hahnemann's dose reduction made possible the systematic use of poisons in medicine. While this had been recommended by von Stoerck and others,[e] it could not be practiced as long as large doses were considered necessary. With dilution and dynamization, however, poisons could now be examined for their curative powers. Hahnemann concludes that a "poison" is merely a medicinal substance used in the

[d]For this reason Hahnemann warned against shipping the liquid remedies over long distances, since they receive "an enormous number of additional succussions during the transport, and they are so highly potentized during a long journey that on their arrival they are scarcely fit for use, at least not for susceptible patients, on account of their excessive strength, as many observations go to prove" (*Lesser Writings,* 736). Fortunately for suffering humanity, the dry pills were not affected in this way (*ibid.,* 766).

[e]See, for example, Melchior Frick, *Tractatus Medicus de Virtute Veneniorum Medica* (Ulm, 1701), and the writings of Anton von Stoerck (collected in H. Piedvache, *Etudes de Therapeutique Experimentale* [Paris: Bailliere, 1887]).

wrong way, i.e., prescribed in too large a dose: "extravagance of dose, unsuitable form of administration, and wrong place of application render harmful not only some but all medicinal substances. Improper selection, wrong form, and exorbitant quantity of all medicines, though they may be but slightly potent, make them destructive, make them what the public calls poisons. Medicines become poisons simply by imperfect use; in themselves no medicines are poisonous."[325] Since "poisons" are "substances of which the effect on the human organism is notorious, and of which, therefore, the medicinal value is beyond doubt," no reasonable man should neglect "those treasures of therapeutic value." "A time is coming when a wiser generation will pity or even laugh at our simplicity, in so stigmatising the very strongest remedies." "Where the public sees only objects of abhorrence, the wise man beholds objects worthy of the deepest veneration and avails himself of them whilst adoring the eternal fountain of love. *Sapere aude!*"[326]

The homoeopathic pharmacopoeia later used dozens of the most powerful poisons: *Belladonna,* aconite, arsenic, strychnine, rattlesnake poison, viper poison, various spider poisons, the saliva of rabid dogs, etc.[f]

The Physis in Homoeopathic Doctrine

Much allopathic criticism of homoeopathy in the nineteenth century stressed its supposed denial of the inherent

[f]Hahnemann notes that "the patrons of new medicines generally commit the error of carefully but injudiciously concealing the disagreeable effects of the medicines they take under their protection," and that these effects ("side-effects," poisonous effects) are precisely the guides which the physician needs for the correct administration of these remedies: "were it not for this suppression of the truth we might, for instance, from the morbific effects the bark of the horse-chestnut *(Aesculus hippocastanum)* is able to produce, form a just estimate of its medicinal powers" (*Lesser Writings,* 297-298). Thus in homoeopathic theory the medicine's "side effects" are the clearest guides to its therapeutic use.

The history of the homoeopathic materia medica in the nineteenth century is discussed in Harris L. Coulter, *Homoeopathic Influences in Nineteenth-Century Allopathic Therapeutics* (Washington, D.C.: American Institute of Homeopathy, 1973).

healing capacity of the organism.[327] As late as 1910 a professor of pharmacology at Halle University wrote: "When Hahnemann was trying to found the so-called homoeopathic theory a century ago, he quoted as a fundamental principle this statement: 'There is no such thing as natural healing. The physician is the only one who can heal with his homoeopathic remedies.' A more nonsensical utterance has seldom been spoken."[328]

Such an utterance, although never uttered by Hahnemann, would indeed have been nonsensical. But it is true that his opponents, and even many of his followers, were confused by his attitude toward the *physis* (*die Natur*).

The Empirical tradition, of course, accepted the *physis* and interpreted the patient's symptoms as the effort of the *physis* to overcome the disease. Symptoms were thus beneficial, and treatment aimed to intensify and further their development.

Hahnemann's approach differed from the above in that, while accepting the existence of a vital force in the organism, he interpreted the symptoms in part as the onslaught of the disease and in part as the curative efforts of the vital force: "in no given case can we ascertain which of the morbid symptoms are caused by the primary action of the morbific agent, which by the reaction of the vital force for its own relief. Both are inextricably mixed up together before our eyes."[329] [g]

The remainder of his views on the *physis* flow from this initial position.

In principle, the inherent healing power is rather weak, incapable of cure by its own efforts: "for were it possessed of such a model ability, it would never have allowed the

[g]Here he seems to divide disease symptoms (like those from provings) into "primary" and "secondary"—the first being the symptoms of the morbific influence and the second being the reaction of the organism. This aspect of homoeopathic doctrine was never developed, and all the symptoms were taken to represent the organism's reaction (see below, p. 409*h*).

Van Helmont had also maintained that part of the *Archeus* is infected, while the rest struggles against the infection (*Oriatrike,* 531: see above, p. 34).

organism to get sick."[330] The "disease" is an impairment of the vital force itself:

> The efforts of the organism for its own preservation . . . are in reality the disease itself, and the morbidly affected vital force is the producer of the visible disease![331]

> Everything that the crude nature does to relieve itself in diseases, in those of an acute, but especially those of a chronic kind, is extremely imperfect and even *actual disease.*[332]

> The natural disease is . . . one produced by an inimical spirit-like agency which, like a kind of infection, disturbs in its instinctive existence the spirit-like principle of life within the organism, torturing it as an evil spirit and compelling it to produce certain ailments and disorders in the regular course of its life.[333]

Therefore, the *physis* cannot be relied upon as an effective agent of cure:

> For purposes of cure, the morbidly depressed vital energy possesses so little ability worthy of imitation, since all changes and symptoms produced by it in the organism are the disease itself. What intelligent physician would want to imitate it with the intention to heal if he did not thereby sacrifice his patients?[334]

When it does effect a cure, the process is lengthy and wasteful, exhausts the patient, does further damage to the organism, and gives rise to new sufferings:

> The nature . . . cannot, like an intelligent surgeon, bring together the gaping lips of a wound and by their union effect a cure . . . knows not how to straighten and adjust the broken ends of a bone lying far apart and exuding much (often an excess of) new osseous matter . . . cannot put a ligature on a wounded artery, but in its energy causes the patient to bleed to death . . . does not understand how to replace a dislocated shoulder, but by the swelling it occasions around it soon presents an obstacle

> to reduction . . . in order to remove a foreign body from the cornea, destroys the whole eye by suppuration . . . with all its efforts can only liberate a strangulated hernia by gangrene of the bowel and death, and . . . by the metaschematisms it produces in dynamic diseases, often renders them much worse than they were originally.[335]

In particular, the vital force cannot resist chronic disease:

> This *irrational vital force receives into our body without hesitation* the greatest plagues of our terrestrial existence, the spark that kindles the countless diseases beneath which tortured mankind has groaned for hundreds and thousands of years, the chronic miasms—psora, syphilis, sycosis—not one of which can it diminish in the slightest degree, far less expel single-handed from the organism; on the contrary, it allows them to rankle therein until, often after a long life of misery, death at last closes the eyes of the sufferer.[336]

Hence, although accepting cure by the *physis*, with its coction, crisis, and evacuation,[337] Hahnemann regards it as an inferior mode. Even more important (and this is the motive behind his severe treatment of the *physis* in the Introduction to the *Organon*), the efforts of the physician to imitate the *physis* are not the equivalent of the same procedures when they are spontaneous: "we cannot imitate her critical sweat, her critical diuresis, her critical abscesses of the parotid and inguinal glands, her critical epistaxis . . . I am therefore astonished that the art of medicine has so seldom raised itself above a servile imitation of these crude processes . . . Just as if these imperfect and forced imitations were the same thing as what the nature effects in the hidden recesses of vitality, by her own spontaneous efforts, in the form of crises! Or as if such crises were the best possible method for overcoming the disease, and were not rather proofs of the (designed) imperfection and therapeutic powerlessness of our unaided nature!"[338]

> The allopathy of the Old School not only greatly overrated these efforts of the crude automatic power of the nature, but completely misjudged them, falsely considered them to be truly curative, and endeavored to increase and promote them, vainly imagining that thereby they might perhaps succeed in annihilating and radically curing the whole disease . . . In almost all cases in which the diseased vital force endeavored to subdue the violence of a dangerous internal malady by evacuating blood by means of vomiting, coughing, etc., the Old School physician, *duce natura,* made haste to assist these supposed salutary efforts of the nature, and performed a copious venesection, which was invariably productive of injurious consequences and palpable weakening of the body. In cases of frequently recurring chronic nausea, he produced, with the view of furthering the intentions of the nature, copious evacuations of the stomach by means of powerful emetics—never with a good result, often with bad, not infrequently dangerous and even fatal consequences.[339]

Most important of all, however, is Hahnemann's feeling that the physician's mission is higher than mere imitation of the imperfect efforts of the *physis:* "[God] does not permit us to make use of the so-called crisis, like the nature, for the cure of a number of fevers . . . but he enables the investigator to discover remedies wherewith he may cure the fever more rapidly than the corporeal organism is capable of producing crises, and to cure them more certainly, more easily, and with less suffering, with less danger to life, and fewer after-sufferings than the unassisted nature can do by means of crises."[340] "*No! the true healing art is that reflective work, the attribute of the higher powers of human intellect, of unfettered judgment and of reason selecting and determining on principle in order to effect an alteration in the instinctive, irrational, and unintelligent, but energetic automatic vital force, when it has been diverted by disease into abnormal action.*"[341]

But after assisting the *physis* out the front door, Hahnemann lets it back in through the window—*via* his doctrine of primary and secondary symptoms. The secondary symptoms of drugs represent the reaction of the vital force: "By giving a remedy which resembles the disease the instinctive vital force is compelled to increase its vital energy until it becomes stronger than the disease which, in turn, is vanquished. Then, by interruption of the medication, health follows . . ."[342 h]

Thus homoeopathy was merely a new variant of the traditional Empirical reliance on the *physis* as the principal instrument of cure. Instead of permitting the *physis* to cope with disease through coction, crisis, and evacuation, the homoeopathic physician reinforced and guided it by the secondary symptoms of his remedies.

Idiosyncrasy. Susceptibility. Immunity

That the vital force reacts to the similar medicine, thus overcoming the morbific cause, seems logically defective, for how can the vital force react to the medicine when it was too weak to withstand the morbific stimulus?

This kind of speculation did not interest Hahnemann greatly:

> As this natural law of cure manifests itself in every pure experiment and every true observation in the world, the fact is consequently established: it matters little what may be the scientific explanation of *how it takes place,* and I do not attach much importance to the attempts made to explain it.[343]

but he guessed that morbific influences affect only susceptible persons, while medicines, on the contrary, affect everyone:

[h]Here, therefore, Hahnemann interprets *all* the symptoms of the disease as the reaction of the vital force. Whether or not it was his ultimate position, it is the interpretation accepted by later homoeopathic physicians.

> The inimical forces, partly psychical, partly physical, to which our terrestrial existence is exposed, which are termed morbific noxious agents, do not possess the power of morbidly deranging the health of man unconditionally; but we are made ill by them only when our organism is sufficiently disposed and susceptible to the attack of the morbific cause that may be present, and to be altered in its health, deranged, and made to undergo abnormal sensations and functions–hence they do not produce disease in every one nor at all times.
>
> But it is quite otherwise with the artificial morbific agents which we term medicines. Every real medicine, namely, acts at *all* times, under *all* circumstances, on *every* living human being, and produces in him its peculiar symptoms.[344]

Thus the vital power of the person falling ill of a disease is *a priori* incapable of reacting vigorously to this particular morbific influence: if it had been capable of reacting, the person would not have fallen ill in the first place.

Here Hahnemann incorporates into homoeopathic doctrine the very pregnant concept of susceptibility to disease which, although rooted in antiquity, was to come into prominence later in the nineteenth century.[i] He identifies it with idiosyncrasy: "a peculiar corporeal constitution which, although otherwise healthy, possesses a disposition to be brought into a more or less morbid state by certain things which *seem* to produce no impression and no change in many other individuals."[345]

Susceptibility has another aspect as well: the diseased organism is far more susceptible to the action of the medicine than is the healthy one:

> There are patients whose impressionability, compared to that of unsusceptible ones, is in the ratio 1000 to 1.[346]

[i] See below, p. 466. Later in the century many homoeopaths viewed the chronic miasms as types of inherited susceptibility or predisposition (Haehl, *Hahnemann,* I, 150).

> None but a careful observer can have any idea of the height to which the sensitiveness of the body to medicinal irritations is increased in a state of disease. It exceeds all belief when the disease has attained a great intensity.[347]

Implicit in susceptibility is its opposite—immunity—which Hahnemann calls toughening, hardening, or habituation. He probably came to an appreciation of these two conditions by observing the varying effects of epidemics. He notes that physicians and clergymen called upon to visit persons sick with contagious diseases should accustom themselves gradually to the infection: *"by very gradually approaching and accustoming ourselves to the inflammatory material of the contagion [we may] blunt by degrees our nerves to the impression of the miasm* (morbid exhalation) *otherwise so easily communicable."*[348] Physicians and nurses "gradually accustom themselves to the exhalations of the most infectious diseases, and their system in the course of time becomes quite insensible to them."[349] In the beginning of an epidemic the physician should see his patients "more frequently, but each time stay beside them as short a time as possible."[350] The "most compassionate, young physicians" who neglect this precaution are in epidemics soonest carried off, while "the hard-hearted sort of everyday doctors who love to make a sensation by the large number of patients they visit daily, and who love to measure the greatness of their medical skill by the agility of their limbs and their rapidity, most certainly escape infection."[351] By the same token, "there are some layers-out of dead bodies in large cities who attain a great age, and have breathed the exhalations from thousands of corpses that have died of infectious diseases. There have also been grave-diggers who in the time of a pestilence have buried the last inhabitant of their district."[352]

The appropropriate homoeopathic remedy for any disease condition should have a prophylactic effect when administered to the healthy, since the cure and prevention of disease are achieved in the same way—by arousing the organism's defences.[353] Hahnemann describes a case of chronic asthma aggravated by cold weather where the appropriate remedy cured the patient by heightening his "capacity of resisting inclement weather."[354]

He advocates hardening children to changes in weather by exposing them gradually to increasingly severe temperatures, quoting Hippocrates against the prevailing custom of exposing them suddenly to extreme cold: "changes from one extreme to another cannot be undertaken without danger and caution, and I cannot too strenuously insist upon the truth of this observation."[355] [j]

His understanding of immunity made him aware of the role of disease carriers ("healthy miasm-bearers") in epidemics.[356] In 1831 he argued that the Asiatic Cholera was propagated not through the air but by contact between persons.[357] And those primarily responsible were the physicians and nurses who, through repeated exposure to the cholera *contagium,*[k] are "at last . . . completely hardened against even the most poisonous cholera miasm at the bedside and rendered quite uninfectible by this pestilence."[358]

> *Thus the cholera physicians and nurses are the most certain and frequent propagators and communicators of contagion far and wide;* and yet amazement is expressed, even in the public journals, how the infection can spread so rapidly the very first day, from the first cholera patient at the one end of the town to persons at the other end of the town who had not come near the patient![359]

This accusation was only one additional reason for the medical profession's hostility toward homoeopathy.

[j]See *Aphorisms* II, li: "Excess and suddenness in evacuating the body, or in replenishing, warming, cooling, or in any other way disturbing it, is dangerous; in fact, all excess is hostile to the *physis.* But 'little by little' is a safe rule, especially in cases of change from one thing to another."

[k]He suggests that the "contagious matter of the cholera most probably consists . . . [of an] enormous brood of . . . excessively minute, invisible, living creatures" (*Lesser Writings,* 758).

Isopathy

Isopathy was a trend in homoeopathy which ran its course in the 1830's. Meaning cure through "equals" (Greek: *isos;* Latin: *aequale*), this idea was expressed by one writer as: "all infectious diseases contain in their own infectious material the means of their cure."[360]

Cure *per aequale* is a logical development of cure *per simile.* The initial impetus for this line of investigation was provided by the work of Constantine Hering (1800-1880) on the pathogenetic effects of snake venoms.[l] While on a zoological expedition to Surinam in 1831 Hering extracted the poison of the *Lachesis trigonocephalus* (bushmaster), mixed it with sugar, and potentized it to the first centesimal dilution. This he proved on himself, observing a series of symptoms similar to those of the bite of this snake but milder.[361]

He concluded that the saliva of a rabid dog, the morbific matter of smallpox scabs, and other venoms and disease products might be prepared in the same way and used to treat disease.[362]

He was particularly interested in discovering a substitute for Jenner's cowpox inoculation, as the existing technique was too dangerous. Many died from the inoculation which infected them with excessively severe cases of cowpox as well as with other diseases, especially syphilis, acquired from the serum or the unsanitary instruments used in the procedure.[363] [m]

He did not regard the treatment of a disease with its morbid product as "treatment *per aequale,*" however, hold-

[l]Constantine Hering, who was born in Saxony and emigrated to the United States, becoming the "father of American homoeopathy," is discussed in *Divided Legacy,* III, *passim.*

[m]Prior to Jenner's discovery smallpox inoculation was done by applying pustular matter to the tip of a lancet and scratching the skin with it until it bled (Benjamin Bell, *A System of Surgery* [Edinburgh: Elliot, 1789-1790], IV, 388). Jenner used lymph from humans with cowpox and inserted it beneath the skin with ivory points. With both procedures there was extreme danger of contracting other diseases from the donor.

ing that the potentized substance could only be regarded as a "similar." Its characteristics are changed during transformation into a homoeopathic medicine, and, furthermore, matter from a diseased organism is no longer an *aequale* when used to treat diseases of a different organism. Nevertheless, Hering had high hopes for this mode of treatment and claimed that "regardless of whatever scourge arrives from the Orient, the remedy will reach us at the same time."[364]

Like other physicians, homoeopaths were not immune to the temptation to oversimplify, and to minds of lesser stature than Hering's isopathy seemed to offer a simple and direct connection between disease and remedy. The isopathic idea hence stimulated a flood of books and articles. One of the most important was Johan Joseph Lux's *Isopathik der Contagionen* (1833) which claimed that "if we potentize every *contagium* and use it in the same way as a homoeopathic medicine, we will be able to heal all these diseases." He specifically called for potentization of a drop of blood from a cow infected with anthrax, or a drop of nasal mucus from a cow with rinderpest, for the treatment of these diseases but noted that he had not performed such experiments himself.[365]

Lux was followed by another homoeopathic veterinarian, Georg Adolph Weber, who in 1836 published an account of his treatment of anthrax along the lines suggested by Lux.[366] Weber extracted the liquid from the spleen of a cow dead of anthrax, potentized it to the 30th centesimal, and used it to prevent and treat anthrax.[367] He held that the prophylactic administration of four or five of these pills to cattle every day during an epidemic held them immune. The curative dose was ten to twenty of the pills every hour or so until fifteen or twenty doses had been administered.[368] In trials supervised by the county health authorities Weber claimed a recovery rate of 80%, as against 20% recovery under the normal treatment of the time.[369]

He noted that this medicine cost virtually nothing to prepare, making it popular with the peasants.[370]

A third pioneer of isopathy was Gustav Wilhelm Gross (1794-1847) who in 1832 reported using potentized matter from scabious eruptions in treating psora.[371] Hering did the same for tuberculosis and syphilis, producing remedies which he called *Phthisinum* and *Syphilinum.*[372]

These investigations raised the doctrinal issue of the relationship between the *simile* and the *aequale.* Gross for a while claimed that the *aequale* was the true law of cure, the *simile* only an approximation of this law.[373] Hahnemann was nonplussed by the isopathic trend and wrote in the *Organon:* "to attempt to cure by means of the very same morbific potency *(per idem)* contradicts all normal human understanding and hence all experience . . . To use a human morbific matter (a *psorin* taken from the itch in man) as a remedy for the same human itch or for evils arisen therefrom is —? Nothing can result from this but trouble and aggravation of the disease."[374]

He suggested that "in this way, undoubtedly, certain diseases peculiar to animals may give us remedies and medicinal potencies for very similar important human diseases and thus happily enlarge our stock of homoeopathic remedies,"[375] and this was the conclusion ultimately accepted by the homoeopathic profession. These substances, which came to be known as "nosodes," were regarded as valuable supplements to the materia medica but not as automatically curative in the diseases from which they were derived.[376] For one thing, they were seen to be often ineffective when employed in this way.[377] For another, the provings of these substances often yielded symptoms quite different from those commonly associated with the diseases from which they had been taken.[378]

A principal use of the nosode was to stimulate a suppressed disease to manifest all its symptoms: Hering activated latent syphilis with *Syphilinum.*[379] Lux administered five pills of *Psorinum* to a patient with latent psora: after two months his whole body erupted in a rash which was then amenable to treatment.[380] Others reported using *Vaccininum* in diseases from badly performed vaccinations.

Despite its doctrinal tribulations isopathy was a fruitful concept, and the use of nosodes became very common in homoeopathic practice. In 1835 a physician in Istanbul reported successful treatment of bubonic plague with the 30th centesimal dilution of matter from a bubo.[381] A Hungarian landowner in 1845 potentized the saliva from cattle sick with cattle typhus, introduced it under the skin of healthy cattle, and reported that it seemed to confer immunity.[382] This technique was commonly used in cattle and sheep anthrax.[383] An American physician potentized the saliva from a rabid dog and proved it on himself in 1854.[384][n] Another used potentized copper to treat diarrhoea from noodles cooked in a copper pot.[385] He prescribed the same remedy to a child ill from candy containing a copper-based coloring additive.[386] Homoeopaths treated various iatrogenic diseases with potentizations of the allopathic medicine which had caused the disease.[387]

The work done later in the century on immunization and antitoxins by Pasteur, Koch, Behring, and others owed much to the isopathic movement in homoeopathy and to the steady use of nosodes in this school from the 1830's onward.[o]

Hering's Law

The only significant addition to homoeopathic doctrine was made by Constantine Hering. Known as "Hering's Law,"

[n]The Editor of an American medical journal (allopathic) commented on this proving: "the fact is, he has made out a case of hydrophobia, and it is presumed that the homoeopathic remedy for the poisonous effects of bites from rabid animals will henceforth be to have the suffering patient again bitten by the same or some other rabid animal. If any of our readers have any doubts as to the efficacy of homoeopathic remedies, or the *science* which is displayed by the practitioners of that absurd doctrine, we recommend to them a careful perusal of the two articles in the journal alluded to" (*Boston Medical and Surgical Journal* LI [1854-1855], 144). This is a fair sample of the attitude of medical orthodoxy to the isopathic principle before it was legitimized by Pasteur.

[o] Pasteur's claims to originality were sharply disputed by the French homoeopaths (see J. P. Tessier, "Les Precurseurs de M. Pasteur," *Bulletin de la Societe Medicale Homoeopathique de France* XXVI [1884-1885], 97-107, 177-192).

this is a guide to the diagnosis and treatment of chronic and other diseases.

Hering held that as disease passes from acute to chronic the symptoms move from the surface to the interior, from the lower part of the body to the upper, and from the less vital organs to the more vital.[388] Under correct homoeopathic treatment the symptoms of a chronic disease disappear in the reverse order of their appearance, that is, the disease moves "backwards" through its stages of development and into its acute form, whereupon the patient can be restored to health.

> In all chronic and lingering cases the symptoms appearing last, even though they may appear insignificant, are always the most important in regard to the selection of a drug; the oldest are the least important; all symptoms between them have to be arranged according to the order of their appearance. Only such patients remain well and are really cured who have been rid of their symptoms in the reverse order of their development.[389]

Hering's Law is rooted in certain of Hahnemann's observations and dicta about the relationship between "local" and "constitutional" disease manifestations, specifically, in his warnings against suppressing the external manifestations of psora, syphilis, and sycosis.

The development of Hahnemann's thought is seen most clearly in his writings on syphilis. His early book on the venereal disease agreed with Hunter that the constitutional form of the disease arises through continual "inoculation" from the chancre. By 1816, however, he had reversed himself, holding that the constitutional form *precedes* the chancre: "It is very probable that the infection during impure coitus takes place in the first seconds, and then no washing or cleansing of the genitals is of any avail; the nature from that time proceeds uninterruptedly in her course, altering the whole internal organism in the manner peculiar to this disease."[390] Appearance of the chancre some days later is proof of the complete occupation of the organism by the syphilis miasm.

The chancre serves as an outlet for the constitutional disease, relieving the pressure on the vital force: "this chancre, the evidence of the now internal affection, is designed by the nature to assume, as it were, the palliative office of substitution, relieving and keeping in subjection the latter."[391] Hence it should not be excised or burnt off with acids: "when the indwelling venereal disease is completely destroyed and cured by the sole internal employment of the best mercurial preparation, then the chancre heals up of itself without the aid of the slightest external remedy; if, however, it is driven off by external means, without curing the internal malady, the latter inevitably bursts forth in the form of syphilis."[392] "It then *invariably* happens that either an inguinal bubo soon occurs, or after a few months the general venereal disease (syphilis) breaks out."[393]

The medical profession, therefore, was treating syphilis in the wrong way: "almost all the physicians and surgeons of the habitable globe have gone on regarding [the chancre] as a purely local and at first insignificant ulcer confined to the outer surface of the skin, and have exerted themselves to dry it up and destroy it by local means as rapidly as possible, and have even considered this destruction of the chancre as the chief object of their treatment, just as though the venereal disease proceeded from it (the chancre) as its source."[394]

In the other two chronic diseases treatment of the skin symptoms is equally harmful: "old ulcers on the legs get worse as long as the internal psora is uncured . . . the fig warts increase and grow while the sycosis is not cured."[395] When the external manifestations are excised or removed, "the nature makes up for its loss by rousing the internal malady . . . when this occurs it is usual to say, although *incorrectly,* that the local affection has been *driven back* into the system or upon the nerves by the external remedies."[396] [p] "Driving off the skin the psoric eruption by

[p]See, for instance, Ph. J. Desault, *Cours Theorique et Pratique de Clinique Externe* (Paris: Delaplace, 1803), I, 4-19, against the danger of applications to the skin in psoriasis (*la gale*), causing *repercution* (a driving inward) of the disease.

all sorts of ointments, burning away the chancre by caustics, and destroying the condylomata on their seat by the knife, the ligature, or the actual cautery [red-hot iron]; this pernicious external mode of treatment hitherto so universally practiced has been the most prolific source of all the innumerable named or unnamed chronic maladies under which mankind groans; it is one of the most criminal procedures the medical world can be guilty of, and yet it has hitherto been the one generally adopted and taught from the professional chairs as the only one."[397] [q]

In the *Chronic Diseases* he extended this observation to miasmatic and other diseases:

> All such miasms become first internal maladies of the whole system before their external assuaging symptoms appear on the skin.[398]
>
> Not infrequently phthisis passes over into insanity; dried-up ulcers into dropsy or apoplexy; intermittent fever into asthma; affections of the abdomen into pains in the joints or paralysis; pains in the limbs into hemorrhage, etc., and it was not difficult to discover that the later diseases must also have their foundation in the original malady and can only be a part of a far greater whole.[399]

In these comments Hahnemann was only extending and giving form to the Hippocratic concept of disease as a dynamic process with certain necessary stages.

The *physis* is not strong enough to overcome such diseases as syphilis and scabies but can offset the impact of the morbific cause by developing external (skin) lesions. If these are treated improperly and suppressed, the consequence is an intensification of the internal disease. Thus disappearance of the skin lesions, without concomitant cure of the internal disease, augurs ill for the patient's future.

[q]But Hahnemann states that wiser physicians had always regarded psora as a constitutional disease and treated it only with internal (not topical) remedies (*Chronic Diseases,* 46-48). Autenrieth in 1807 inveighed against treating scabies with salves, noting that they perpetuate the scabies and gave rise to numerous *sequelae* (*Versuche fuer die praktische Heilkunde,* 229-232).

In the light of these observations Hahnemann came to realize that certain categories of symptoms are intrinsically more significant than others, since they indicate the stage reached by the disease process. He saw, in particular, that mental and emotional symptoms are always the leading indicators of the remedy and by the second (1835) edition of the *Chronic Diseases* had started rearranging symptoms in the light of this principle, placing the mental and emotional symptoms at the forefront of the discussion of each remedy.[400]

Hering's three principles only completed the systematization of symptomatology which Hahnemann had already commenced. While relating primarily to the transition from acute to chronic disease, they are applicable in part to the treatment of the stages of acute disease. Hering's Law shows Hahnemann's stress on mental and emotional symptoms to have been entirely justified, as their locus, the brain, is at the same time a major organ, one of the innermost organs, and the uppermost part of the body.[401]

NOTES

[1] *Annalen der gesammten Medicin* II (1810), 31.

[2] *Journal der praktischen Heilkunde* XLIX (1819), st. VI, 8-9.

[3] Samuel Hahnemann, *Lesser Writings* (New York: William Radde, 1852), 420.

[4] All biographical information on Hahnemann is from Richard Haehl, *Samuel Hahnemann, His Life and Work* (London: Homoeopathic Publishing Co., 1922).

[5] *Ibid.*, II, 6.

[6] *Loc. cit.*

[7] *Ibid.*, I, 10.

[8] William Windelband, *A History of Philosophy* (New York: Harper, 1958), II, 526.

[9] Linn J. Boyd, *A Study of the Simile in Medicine* (Philadelphia: Boericke and Tafel, 1936), 32 (quoting *Anleitung alte Schaeden und faeule Geschwuere gruendlich zu heilen* [Leipzig, 1784]).

[10] Haehl, *Hahnemann,* I, 1.

[11] *Ibid.*, II, 383: "I have not lived in vain."

[12] Hahnemann, *Lesser Writings,* 512.

[13] *Loc. cit.*

[14] *Ibid.*, 249-303.

[15] Two Parts (Leipzig: Barth, 1805). Revised and expanded as the *Reine Arzneimittellehre.* Six volumes in four (Dresden: Arnold, 1811-1821). This work went through more editions and was later translated into Latin by Ernst Stapf and issued as the *Materia Medica Pura.* Two volumes (Dresden: Arnold, 1826, 1828).

[16] Dresden: Arnold, 1810. This work went through five editions in Hahnemann's lifetime. A sixth edition, revised by him before his death, was not released by his widow and was finally published only in 1921 (all references in the following pages are to this sixth edition).

[17] Parts I to III (Dresden: Arnold, 1828). Part IV (Dresden: Arnold, 1830). A second edition, including a new Part V, was published 1835-1839.

[18] S. Hahnemann, *Dissertatio historico-medica de Helleborismo veterum* (Leipzig Dissertation, 1812). Translated and printed in S. Hahnemann, *Lesser Writings,* 569-617.

[19] See his "View of Professional Liberality at the Commencement of the Nineteenth Century" (1801), *Lesser Writings,* 362-368.

[20] *Allgemeine homoeopathische Zeitung* XXVI (1844), 182 (translated in Haehl, *Hahnemann,* II, 98).

[21] Haehl, *Hahnemann*, I, 100.

[22] See "The Treatment of the Typhus or Hospital Fever at Present Prevailing" (1801), "Observations on the Scarlet Fever" (1808), "Treatment of the *Purpura Miliaris*" (1821), "Cure and Prevention of Asiatic Cholera" (1831), "Appeal to Thinking Philanthropists Respecting the Mode of Propagation of the Asiatic Cholera" (1831) in *Lesser Writings*, 369-385, 479-483, 695-696, 753-756, 756-763.

[23] Hahnemann, *Organon*, Introduction, 39.

[24] *Ibid.*, Introduction, 40.

[25] Hahnemann, *Lesser Writings*, 538.

[26] Haehl, *Hahnemann*, I, 35.

[27] Sprengel, *Histoire de la Medecine*, VI, 235.

[28] Haehl, *Hahnemann*, I, 112.

[29] *Ibid.*, I, 108.

[30] Hahnemann, *Lesser Writings*, 439.

[31] *Ibid.*, 492-493.

[32] *Ibid.*, 424.

[33] *Ibid.*, 423.

[34] *Ibid.*, 493.

[35] *Ibid.*, 423.

[36] *Ibid.*, 420.

[37] *Ibid.*, 422, 690.

[38] Hahnemann, *Organon*, Introduction, 32.

[39] Hahnemann, *Lesser Writings*, 737-738.

[40] *Ibid.*, 522.

[41] Hahnemann, *Organon*, Sec. 7, note 4.

[42] Hahnemann, *Lesser Writings*, 738.

[43] Hahnemann, *Lesser Writings*, 536-538.

[44] Hahnemann, *Organon*, Introduction, 36.

[45] *Ibid.*, Introduction, 43.

[46] *Ibid.*, Introduction, 47 and note 12.

[47] Hahnemann, *Lesser Writings*, 476-479.

[48] *Ibid.*, 501, 673ff.

[49] *Ibid.*, 252-255.

[50] *Ibid.*, 255.

[51] *Ibid.*, 254-255.

[52] *Ibid.*, 478, 670-671.

[53] *Ibid.*, 501.

[54] *Ibid.*, 253, 673ff., 722.

[55] *Ibid.*, 678.

[56] *Ibid.*, 253.

[57] *Ibid.*, 255.

[58] *Ibid.*, 502 note.

[59] *Ibid.*, 687-690.

[60] *Ibid.*, 500.

[61] *Ibid.*, 490.

[62] *Loc. cit.*

[63] *Ibid.*, 422.

[64] Hahnemann, *Organon*, Introduction, 30-31.

[65] Hahnemann, *Lesser Writings*, 520.

[66] Hahnemann, *Organon,* Introduction, 34.
[67] Hahnemann, *Lesser Writings,* 237-238.
[68] Hahnemann, *Organon,* Introduction, 44.
[69] Hahnemann, *Lesser Writings,* 739.
[70] *Ibid.,* 555.
[71] Hahnemann, *Organon,* Sec. 104, note 90.
[72] Hahnemann, *Lesser Writings,* 714.
[73] *Loc. cit.* See, also, *ibid.,* 718.
[74] Hahnemann, *Organon,* Author's Preface to the Sixth Edition, 16, note 1.
[75] Hahnemann, *Lesser Writings,* 399, 744.
[76] *Ibid.,* 238.
[77] *Ibid.,* 545.
[78] *Ibid.,* 551.
[79] *Ibid.,* 501, note.
[80] *Ibid.,* 346-349.
[81] *Ibid.,* 685-686.
[82] *Ibid.,* 499.
[83] *Ibid.,* 433.
[84] *Ibid.,* 533.
[85] Hahnemann, *Organon,* Introduction, 43.
[86] *Ibid.,* 44.
[87] Hahnemann, *Lesser Writings,* 554.
[88] *Ibid.,* 527.
[89] *Ibid.,* 528.
[90] *Ibid.,* 547.
[91] *Ibid.,* 513.
[92] *Ibid.,* 419.
[93] Hahnemann, *Organon,* Introduction, 71.
[94] Hahnemann, *Lesser Writings,* 310.
[95] *Ibid.,* 248, note.
[96] Hahnemann, *Organon,* Sec. 228, note 125.
[97] Hahnemann, *Lesser Writings,* 727.
[98] *Ibid.,* 532.
[99] *Ibid.,* 497.
[100] *Loc. cit.*
[101] *Ibid.,* 487.
[102] *Ibid.,* 186.
[103] *Ibid.,* 241.
[104] *Ibid.,* 202.
[105] Hahnemann, *Organon,* Sec. 60, note 66.
[106] Hahnemann, *Lesser Writings,* 488.
[107] *Ibid.,* 517, 619.
[108] Hahnemann, *Organon,* Introduction, 45.
[109] Hahnemann, *Lesser Writings,* 261.
[110] Hahnemann, *Organon,* Introduction, 47.
[111] *Ibid.,* Introduction, 68. *Lesser Writings,* 350, 412, 556, 739, 748.
[112] Hahnemann, *Lesser Writings,* 748.
[113] Hahnemann, *Organon,* Introduction, 36, note 5.
[114] *Ibid.,* Introduction, 45.
[115] *Ibid.,* Introduction, 66.

[116] Hahnemann, *Lesser Writings,* 435.
[117] *Ibid.,* 184.
[118] *Ibid.,* 376.
[119] *Ibid.,* 388.
[120] *Ibid.,* 412.
[121] Hahnemann, *Organon,* Introduction, 55, note 18.
[122] Hahnemann, *Lesser Writings,* 491.
[123] *Ibid.,* 618.
[124] *Ibid.,* 489.
[125] *Ibid.,* 513-514.
[126] *Ibid.,* 439.
[127] Hahnemann, *Organon,* Sec. 7.
[128] Hahnemann, *Lesser Writings,* 420.
[129] Samuel Hahnemann, *The Chronic Diseases, their Peculiar Nature and their Homoeopathic Cure.* Translated from the second enlarged German edition of 1835 by Professor Louis H. Tafel (Philadelphia: Boericke and Tafel, 1904), 11.
[130] Hahnemann, *Lesser Writings,* 496.
[131] *Loc. cit.*
[132] *Ibid.,* 435.
[133] *Ibid.,* 720.
[134] *Ibid.,* 439.
[135] Hahnemann, *Organon,* Sec. 25.
[136] *Ibid.,* Introduction, 89.
[137] *Ibid.,* Sec. 1.
[138] *Ibid.,* Introduction, 31.
[139] Hahnemann, *Lesser Writings,* 617.
[140] *Ibid.,* 687.
[141] *Ibid.,* 688.
[142] *Loc. cit.*
[143] *Loc. cit.*
[144] *Ibid.,* 689.
[145] *Loc. cit.*
[146] *Ibid.,* 687.
[147] *Ibid.,* 691.
[148] *Loc. cit.*
[149] *Ibid.,* 436.
[150] *Loc. cit.*
[151] *Ibid.,* 259.
[152] *Loc. cit.*
[153] *Ibid.,* 1-153.
[154] John Hunter, "A Treatise on the Venereal Disease," *Works* (London: Longman, 1837), II, 131-488.
[155] All biographical information on Hunter is from the *Dictionary of National Biography.*
[156] Hunter, *Works,* II, 143, 417-419.
[157] *Ibid.,* II, 131.
[158] *Ibid.,* II, 131-132.
[159] *Ibid.,* II, 131, 153, 192, 381.
[160] *Ibid.,* II, 140.
[161] *Ibid.,* II, 154, 405.
[162] *Ibid.,* II, 150.

[163] *Ibid.*, II, 194, 200, 342, 430, 455, 459, 472.
[164] *Ibid.*, II, 455.
[165] *Ibid.*, II, 436.
[166] *Loc. cit.*
[167] Hahnemann, *Lesser Writings*, 87-88.
[168] *Ibid.*, 89.
[169] *Ibid.*, 62, 80, 103.
[170] *Ibid.*, 127.
[171] *Ibid.*, 99-100.
[172] *Ibid.*, 62.
[173] *Ibid.*, 99.
[174] *Ibid.*, 133.
[175] *Ibid.*, 134.
[176] *Ibid.*, 135.
[177] *William Cullen's Abhandlung ueber die Materia Medica* (Leipzig: im Schwickertsten Verlage, 1790), II, 108-109.
[178] Hahnemann, *Lesser Writings*, 265.
[179] [S. Hahnemann], *Defence of the Organon* (Philadelphia: Boericke and Tafel, 1896), 76.
[180] Hahnemann, *Organon*, Sec. 20.
[181] *Ibid.*, Sec. 108.
[182] *Ibid.*, Sec. 108, note 91.
[183] Hahnemann's medicine chest, at the time of his death, contained 202 remedies (Haehl, *Hahnemann*, II, 424).
[184] Hahnemann, *Lesser Writings*, 266-267. See, also, *ibid.*, 453-454.
[185] *Ibid.*, 624.
[186] See Cullen, *First Lines of the Practice of Physic*, I, 106. E. A. Ackerknecht, "Aspects of the History of Therapeutics," *Bulletin of the History of Medicine* XXXVI (1962), 389-419, at 414.
[187] Hahnemann, *Organon*, Sec. 63-68.
[188] Hahnemann, *Lesser Writings*, 454.
[189] Hahnemann, *Organon*, Sec. 157, 158, 282.
[190] Hahnemann, *Organon*, Sec. 23.
[191] Hahnemann, *Lesser Writings*, 518. See, also, *Organon*, Sec. 60.
[192] Hahnemann, *Organon*, Sec. 59.
[193] Hahnemann, *Lesser Writings*, 519.
[194] *Ibid.*, 506.
[195] *Ibid.*, 529: "He sees only what is in front of him."
[196] *Ibid.*, 749.
[197] *Ibid.*, 485-486.
[198] *Ibid.*, 751.
[199] *Ibid.*, 746.
[200] *Loc. cit.*
[201] Quoted in Haehl, *Hahnemann*, I, 258.
[202] *Annalen der gesammten Medicin* II (1810), 31-75 and 193-256, at 49.
[203] Quoted in Ameke, *History of Homoeopathy*, 269.
[204] Hahnemann, *Lesser Writings*, 745.
[205] Hahnemann, *Organon*, Introduction, 80.
[206] *Ibid.*, Introduction, 90, note 38.

[207]Freiherr Anton von Stoerck, *Libellus quo demonstratur: stramonium, hyosciamum, aconitum non solum tuto posse exhiberi usu interno hominibus, verum et ea esse remedia in multis morbis maxime salutifera* (Vienna, 1762) and others. These works were collected and translated into French by H. Piedvache, *Etudes de Therapie Experimentale: Stramoine, Jusquiame, Aconit, Fraxinelle, Pulsatille* (Paris: Bailliere, 1887).

[208]Hahnemann, *Organon*, Introduction, 82, note 31.

[209]*Ibid.*, Introduction, 85-87.

[210]*Ibid.*, Introduction, 87, notes 33, 34.

[211]*Ibid.*, Introduction, 87, note 35.

[212]*Ibid.*, Introduction, 88, note 35.

[213]*Ibid.*, Sec. 36.

[214]*Ibid.*, Sec. 38, 40.

[215]*Ibid.*, Sec. 38.

[216]*Ibid.*, Sec. 46.

[217]*Loc. cit.*

[218]*Loc. cit.*

[219]*Ibid.*, Sec. 46, note 47.

[220]Hahnemann, *Lesser Writings*, 718.

[221]*Ibid.*, 691.

[222]*Ibid.*, 727.

[223]Hahnemann, *Organon*, Sec. 84 (stress added).

[224]*Ibid.*, Sec. 104, note 90.

[225]Hahnemann, *Lesser Writings*, 724.

[226]*Ibid.*, 725.

[227]*Loc. cit.*

[228]*Ibid.*, 726.

[229]*Ibid.*, 727.

[230]*Ibid.*, 444.

[231]Hahnemann, *Organon*, Sec. 153. See, also, Sec. 128.

[232]*Ibid.*, Sec. 154.

[233]*Ibid.*, Sec. 165.

[234]*Ibid.*, Sec. 235.

[235]Hahnemann, *Lesser Writings*, 769-770.

[236]*Ibid.*, 713.

[237]*Ibid.*, 525.

[238]*Ibid.*, 442, note.

[239]*Ibid.*, 504.

[240]*Ibid.*, 507.

[241]*Ibid.*, 329.

[242]*Ibid.*, 442.

[243]*Ibid.*, 690.

[244]*Ibid.*, 523.

[245]*Ibid.*, 713.

[246]Hahnemann, *Organon*, Sec. 73, note 71 and Sec. 81, note 79.

[247]*Ibid.*, Sec. 185.

[248]*Ibid.*, Sec. 189.

[249]*Ibid.*, Sec. 193.

[250]Hahnemann, *Lesser Writings*, 272-303. *Organon*, Sec. 212.

[251] *Ibid.*, Sec. 210.
[252] *Ibid.*, Sec. 145.
[253] *Ibid.*, Sec. 147.
[254] *Loc. cit.* and p. 35, note 4.
[255] Hahnemann, *Lesser Writings*, 260-261.
[256] *Ibid.*, 515, note.
[257] *Ibid.*, 415.
[258] *Ibid.*, 515, note.
[259] *Ibid.*, 451-452.
[260] *Ibid.*, 478.
[261] *Ibid.*, 484.
[262] *Ibid.*, 466.
[263] Hahnemann, *Organon*, Sec. 147.
[264] *Ibid.*, Sec. 17.
[265] *Ibid.*, Sec. 8.
[266] *Ibid.*, Sec. 26.
[267] *Ibid.*, Sec. 30-33.
[268] Hahnemann, *Lesser Writings*, 348.
[269] *Loc. cit.*
[270] *Loc. cit.*
[271] *Ibid.*, 350.
[272] *Ibid.*, 741.
[273] *Ibid.*, 509.
[274] *Ibid.*, 320, 499.
[275] Hahnemann, *Organon*, Sec. 274.
[276] Hahnemann, *Lesser Writings*, 501.
[277] *Ibid.* 348-349.
[278] Hahnemann, *Organon*, Sec. 11, 73.
[279] Hahnemann, *Lesser Writings*, 440.
[280] Hahnemann, *Organon*, Sec. 73.
[281] Hahnemann, *Lesser Writings*, 622, note.
[282] *Ibid.*, 534.
[283] *Ibid.*, 525.
[284] Hahnemann, *Organon*, Sec. 102.
[285] Hahnemann, *Chronic Diseases*, 33-34.
[286] Hahnemann, *Organon*, Sec. 134-135.
[287] Hahnemann, *Lesser Writings*, 260.
[288] Hahnemann, *Chronic Diseases*, 33-34. See, also, *Organon*, Sec. 102. Constantine Hering later wrote: "In all zymotic diseases we have, as in other epidemics, to sum up all the symptoms of as many cases as we can examine properly, and concentrate their symptoms into one image, from which to select that remedy really 'specific' to the zymosis" (*Analytical Therapeutics* [N.Y. and Philadelphia: Boericke and Tafel, 1875], 25).
[289] Hahnemann, *Lesser Writings*, 260.
[290] Hahnemann, *Organon*, Sec. 100.
[291] Hahnemann, *Lesser Writings*, 260 note.
[292] *Ibid.*, 689.
[293] Hahnemann, *Chronic Diseases*, 28.
[294] *Ibid.*, 31 ff.

[295] Hahnemann, *Lesser Writings,* 646-649.
[296] Hahnemann, *Chronic Diseases,* 36. *Organon,* Sec. 103.
[297] Hahnemann, *Lesser Writings,* 652. *Chronic Diseases,* 83.
[298] Hahnemann, *Lesser Writings,* 652-659.
[299] Four Volumes. Dresden: Arnold, 1828, 1830. Second Edition (Five Volumes), Duesseldorf: Schaub, 1838, 1839.
[300] Haehl, *Hahnemann,* I, 137.
[301] Ameke, *History of Homoeopathy,* 138.
[302] Haehl, *Hahnemann,* I, 311.
[303] Hahnemann, *Lesser Writings,* 249-303 *passim.*
[304] Haehl, *Hahnemann,* I, 312ff.
[305] *Ibid.,* I, 312.
[306] Hahnemann, *Lesser Writings,* 369-385.
[307] This is the assumption of Hahnemann's biographer (Haehl, *Hahnemann,* I, 312), and Hahnemann discusses the aggravation of symptoms from too large doses (*Lesser Writings,* 453-455). See, also, Boyd, *A Study of the Simile in Medicine,* 93.
[308] Hahnemann, *Lesser Writings,* 630, 763.
[309] Hahnemann, *Organon,* Sec. 279.
[310] Haehl, *Hahnemann,* I, 314.
[311] Hahnemann, *Organon,* Sec. 63, 112, 160.
[312] *Ibid.,* Sec. 66, 112, 160. *Lesser Writings,* 454.
[313] *Ibid.,* Sec. 278.
[314] Samuel Hahnemann, *Reine Arzneimittellehre,* II (Dresden: Arnold, 1816), 23-27.
[315] Haehl, *Hahnemann,* I, 328.
[316] *Ibid.,* I, 321-322.
[317] *Ibid.,* I, 322.
[318] *Loc. cit.*
[319] Hahnemann, *Organon,* Sec. 269, 270. *Lesser Writings,* 728-734.
[320] Hahnemann, *Lesser Writings,* 386.
[321] Hahnemann, *Organon,* Sec. 269, 270.
[322] Hahnemann, *Lesser Writings,* 728-729.
[323] Hahnemann, *Organon,* Sec. 269.
[324] Hahnemann, *Lesser Writings,* 695, 732.
[325] Haehl, *Hahnemann,* I, 75.
[326] *Ibid.,* I, 76.
[327] H. Haeser, *Lehrbuch der Geschichte der Medicin* (Jena: Mauke, 1868), 825. Haehl, *Hahnemann,* I, 282-283. Ameke, *History of Homoeopathy,* 297-300.
[328] Haehl, *Hahnemann,* I, 283.
[329] Hahnemann, *Organon,* Introduction, 54, note 18, and Sec. 63.
[330] *Ibid.,* Sec. 22, note 12.
[331] *Ibid.,* Introduction, 66.
[332] *Ibid.,* Introduction, 65.
[333] *Ibid.,* Sec. 148.
[334] *Ibid.,* Sec. 22, note 12.
[335] *Ibid.,* Introduction, 56.
[336] *Loc. cit.*
[337] Hahnemann, *Chronic Diseases,* 75. *Lesser Writings,* 437.

338 Hahnemann, *Lesser Writings,* 437-438.
339 Hahnemann, *Organon,* Introduction, 60-63.
340 Hahnemann, *Lesser Writings,* 437.
341 Hahnemann, *Organon,* Introduction, 67.
342 Hahnemann, *Die Chronische Krankheiten,* Second Edition, 1828, IV, 4 (quoted in Boyd, *The Simile in Medicine,* 59).
343 Hahnemann, *Organon,* Sec. 28.
344 *Ibid.,* Sec. 31, 32.
345 *Ibid.,* Sec. 117.
346 *Ibid.,* Sec. 281.
347 Hahnemann, *Lesser Writings,* 464; cf. *ibid.,* 388, 552.
348 *Ibid.,* 170.
349 *Ibid.,* 166.
350 *Ibid.,* 169.
351 *Loc. cit.*
352 *Ibid.,* 167.
353 *Ibid.,* 390.
354 *Ibid.,* 319.
355 *Ibid.,* 193.
356 *Ibid.,* 761.
357 *Ibid.,* 756 ff.
358 *Ibid.,* 760.
359 *Loc. cit.*
360 Johan Joseph Lux, *Die Isopathik der Contagionen* (Leipzig: Kollmann, 1833), 3.
361 *Bibliotheque Homoeopathique* II (1833), 42 ff.
362 *Ibid.,* 101 ff.
363 *Ibid.,* 105 ff.
364 *Ibid.,* 107.
365 Lux, *Isopathik der Contagionen,* 10.
366 Weber, *Der Milzbrand und deren sicherstes Heilmittel.*
367 *Ibid.,* 92. Weber observes that the sixth centesimal was ineffective.
368 *Ibid.,* 85.
369 *Ibid.,* 93.
370 *Loc. cit.*
371 Lux, *Isopathik der Contagionen,* 12.
372 *Bibliotheque Homoeopathique* III (1834), 257-270, 348-362. R. Tischner, *Geschichte der Homoeopathie* (Leipzig: W. Schwabe, 1932), III, 602.
373 *British Journal of Homoeopathy* VII (1849), 336. Tischner, *Geschichte der Homoeopathie,* III, 602.
374 Hahnemann, *Organon,* Sec. 56, note 63. See, also, *Lesser Writings,* 629, note.
375 *Loc. cit.*
376 Tischner, *Geschichte der Homoeopathie* (Leipzig: Schwabe, 1932-1939), III, 602. *Bibliotheque Homoeopathique* IV (1835), 297. Auguste Rapou, *Histoire de la Doctrine Medicale Homoeopathique* (Paris: Bailliere, 1847), II, 190.
377 Rapou, *Histoire de la Doctrine Homoeopathique,* II, 202. *British Journal of Homoeopathy* XII (1854), 262.
378 *Bibliotheque Homoeopathique* III (1834), 272.

[379] *Ibid.*, IV (1835), 295.

[380] Lux, *Isopathik der Contagionen*, 12.

[381] *Bibliotheque Homoeopathique* VII (1836), 102-109.

[382] J. P. Tessier, "Les Precurseurs de M. Pasteur," *Bulletin de la Societe Medicale Homoeopathique de France* XXVI (1884-1885), 186.

[383] *Ibid.*, 106 ff. *Bibliotheque Homoeopathique* VIII (1837), 280 ff. *British Journal of Homoeopathy* XII (1854), 260 ff.

[384] *Philadelphia Journal of Homoeopathy* III (1854-1855), 262-274.

[385] *Hygeia* (Karlsruhe) IV (1836), 486-487.

[386] *Loc. cit.*

[387] Lux, *Isopathik der Contagionen*, 13. Tischner, *Geschichte der Homoeopathie*, III, 602.

[388] Constantine Hering, "Hahnemann's Three Rules Concerning the Rank of Symptoms," *Hahnemannian Monthly* I (1865), 5-12.

[389] C. Hering, *Analytical Therapeutics* (New York and Philadelphia: Boericke and Tafel, 1875), I, 24.

[390] Hahnemann, *Lesser Writings*, 650.

[391] *Ibid.*, 651.

[392] *Ibid.*, 652

[393] *Ibid.*, 653.

[394] *Loc. cit.*

[395] Hahnemann, *Organon*, Sec. 201.

[396] *Ibid.*, Sec. 202.

[397] *Ibid.*, Sec. 203.

[398] Hahnemann, *Chronic Diseases*, 70.

[399] *Ibid.*, 30.

[400] S. Hahnemann, *Die chronischen Krankheiten, ihre eigenthuemliche Natur und homoeopathische Heilung*. Zweite auflage (Dresden and Leipzig: Arnold, 1835-1839). Five volumes.

[401] Hering, "Hahnemann's Three Rules," 10 ff.

CHAPTER VII

EMPIRICAL REACTIONS (2): THE PARIS SCHOOL FROM CABANIS TO TROUSSEAU

Homoeopathy was the discovery of a single man, but in Paris after 1789 the whole medical profession was shocked into a review of accepted ideas. Caught up in the political and social transformations of the epoch, it responded with a series of new therapeutic formulations.

The complexity of the relationships makes this period difficult to describe. While the issues crystallized in Empirical and Rationalist patterns, the forcing-bed atmosphere of intellectual life, the feverish political excitement, the unending wars, the epidemic and endemic diseases which cut off so many of these physicians at an early age—all contributed to a short life-expectancy of medical ideas and the rapid succession of one therapeutic fashion upon another.

Professional discipline and control largely disappeared with the Revolution, and the field was open to new talent in an unprecedented way.

These years engendered the idea of "progress"—which affected physicians no less than others. The conviction that mankind had entered a new epoch of history imparted a pervasive urgency to medical investigations, and each coveted the honor of placing the coping-stone on the completed edifice.

From 1789 until the death of Claude Bernard in 1878 six periods can be distinguished in Paris therapeutics.

The years from 1789 to 1798 saw a rejection of the Rationalist orthodoxy of Boerhaave, Haller, and Hoffmann for the Hippocratic and neo-Empirical principles of Pierre Jean-Georges Cabanis (1757-1808). The existing medical schools and societies were replaced by three écoles de santé (schools of health)—in Paris, Montpellier, and Strasburg. All instruction was centered on the practical care of the sick—and especially of the wounded being gathered in from the rapidly multiplying battlefields. This utilitarianism attracted many Montpellier graduates to Paris where they assumed a dominant position. Medicine became closely aligned with surgery, and surgeons took leading roles in the Paris Ecole de Santé.

The second period is stamped with the spirit of the "French Hippocrates," Philippe Pinel (1745-1826), and runs from the appearance of his *Nosographie Philosophique* in 1798 until his death in 1826. The other eminent leader of Paris medicine during these decades was Rene Theophile Hyacinthe Laennec (1781-1826) whose great work, the *Auscultation Mediate,* appeared in 1819. Both accepted the Hippocratic reliance on symptoms, rejection of proximate causes, and preference for general treatment over local.

The third period was a response to the weakness of Pinelism—and of pre-Hahnemannian Empiricism generally—the absence of a clear and unambiguous relationship between diagnosis and therapy, thwarting the physician's desire to act decisively. Pinel's preference for expectancy and traditional remedies of the milder sort aroused the resistance of his colleagues, and the accumulated tensions found a spokesman in F. J. V. Broussais (1772-1838) whose 1816 *Examen de la Doctrine Medicale Generalement Acceptee et des Systemes Modernes de Nosologie* attacked him for ignoring internal pathology. Broussais hypothesized "irritation" of the gastrointestinal tract as the cause of all diseases and treated it only by withholding food and applying leeches. His system was wildly popular for a full decade and was phased out by the profession only with reluctance.

The reaction to Broussais, from the mid-1820's to the mid-1830's, was named "Eclecticism" by its founder, Gabriel Andral (1797-1876). A synthesis of Broussais' pathological orientation and the symptomatic preference of Pinel, it sanctioned the use, in moderation, of all existing therapeutic procedures. The eclectic period yielded many of the "specific diseases"—typhus, typhoid, diphtheria, and others—which have remained cornerstones of medical speculation to this day.

But all four periods were marked by a primitive understanding of pharmacology, and the mid-1830's reacted to this with the *Traite de Therapeutique et de Matiere Medicale* (1836) of Armand Trousseau (1801-1867). Passing through nine editions and translated into English, Spanish, and Italian, this work for decades gave guidance to physicians of all countries, but its principles (and many specific applications of medicines) were taken from homeopathy. Hence the Empirical origin of the Paris School led in a roundabout way to an Empirical conclusion as these physicians reached an uneasy compromise with Hahnemann.

Trousseau prided himself on being an "Empiric," but it was a confused and inconsistent Empiricism, as his doctrines were distorted by the political imperative to maintain independence from homoeopathy. By the time of their author's death Trousseauism was a morass of ad hoc and mutually incompatible pharmacological principles.

The reaction to be anticipated was, therefore, a cleansing of the Augean stables with a flood of pure Methodist theory, and this was the work of Claude Bernard (1813-1878). In him Broussais' search for a localized disease mechanism, as improved by Francois Magendie (1783-1855), issued in a reductionist and mechanistic physiology which remained the accepted theoretical model for the next hundred years.

Collapse and Reconstruction: 1789-1798

In the last years of the ancien régime French medicine was an incongruous mixture of Iatrochemistry, Iatromechanism, and the symptomatic descriptions of Sauvages and Barthez, organized in a Galenic-Hallerian framework and taught largely in Latin:[a] "in appearance . . . a small number

[a]An idea of eighteenth-century medical education in Paris may be obtained from Pierre Chirac, *Traite des Fievres Malignes, Pestilentielles, et Autres* (Paris: Vincent, 1742) or Pierre Fabre, *Essais sur Differents Points de Physiologie, de Pathologie, et de Therapeutique* (Paris: Didot, 1770). See, also, Rene Taton, *Enseignement et Diffusion des Sciences en France au XVIII Siecle* (Paris: Hermann, 1964). Part II. Chapter I: L'Enseignement Medico-Chirurgical. Chapter II: L'Enseignement des Sciences Pharmaceutiques.

of clear and easily grasped ideas which promised to unveil to all eyes the mechanism of our functions, the intimate nature of diseases, and the most impenetrable mysteries of life."[1]

A 1790 report to the National Assembly by Felix Vicq d'Azyr (1748-1794), permanent secretary to the Royal Society of Medicine, described the situation in vivid language:

> What benefit can there be from years of study spent in reading and copying out *Prolegomena Medicinae* made up entirely of definitions and sterile logical divisions? What good can come of schools which teach neither the complete human anatomy, nor the art of dissection, nor botany, nor medical chemistry in its full extent, nor pharmacy, nor the art of prescription writing, nor nosology, nor the history of medicine, nor the treatment of diseases? Where not a word is said of the physician's public duties and where no professor has ever practiced medicine at the bedside? From which the student emerges without having learned anything of what a practitioner must know?

At examinations "the thesis is defended by the professor, while the student remains silent: who would pay attention to him anyway?" The professors cannot afford to be strict, since they themselves know almost nothing; hence almost everyone passes, and a flood of inferior practitioners is loosed on the country to learn medicine only from their own mistakes.

Therefore, the public in many places relies on surgeons for the practice of medicine.

Vicq d'Azyr recommended that the schools of medicine and surgery be fused, with courses in anatomy, physiology, operative surgery, chemistry, physics, hygiene, and, finally, theoretical and practical medicine (semeiology, pathology, nosology, and therapeutics). While medical instruction previously had been verbal and divorced from experience, thereafter it was to be based on facts and observation.[b]

[b]*Societe Royale de Medecine, Nouveau Plan de Constitution pour la Medecine en France, Presente a l'Assemblee Nationale par la Societe Royale de Medecine, 1790.* Although unsigned, this was known to be from the pen of Vicq

The Revolution's leaders initially shared the popular view of medicine as an object of ridicule and decided that the Republic could dispense with a healing profession altogether.[2] The Faculté was dissolved by the Assembly in 1792 and the Royal Society of Medicine and the Academy of Surgery in 1793—together with 17 other medical facultés, 15 collèges de médecine, several collèges de chirurgie, and all the other scientific societies. But within eighteen months the French armies had lost upwards of 600 surgeons, and the Convention asked the chemist, Antoine Fourcroy (1755-1809), to submit a report on reorganizing the medical profession and reforming medical education. Based on Vicq d'Azyr's earlier effort and with the collaboration of Francois Chaussier (1746-1828), drawing also on a 1790 essay by Cabanis on the necessity of centering medical education in hospitals,[3] Fourcroy's 1794 report to the Convention established écoles de santé at Paris, Montpellier, and Strasburg, did away with the reading and memorizing of Galenic texts, accepted the theory of coction as the guide to treatment, introduced surgery into the curriculum, and involved the students in the work of hospitals and clinics.[4]

All instruction was now in French, the division between medicine and surgery was abolished, and the title of "physician" was replaced by "health officer" (officier de santé).[5] The Revolution's determination to return to Empirical principles in medicine is seen in Fourcroy's motto: "Read little, see much, and do much."[6]

Even though the écoles de santé were renamed facultés de médecine in 1808, a new Society of Medicine was founded in 1796, and the title of "physician" was restored in 1803 (as a higher degree than "health officer"), the change in the

d'Azyr—who died tragically a few years afterwards. The first and only secretary of the Royal Society of Medicine, brought into existence (over strenuous professional opposition) in 1776 to reform the Faculté, he spent a lifetime combating the excrescences of Boerhaavian medicine only to fall victim to the Revolution which pursued the same aims as himself. Becoming physician to Marie Antoinette in 1789, he witnessed her execution in 1793 together with that of his intimate friends, Condorcet and Lavoisier. Sensing that the guillottine awaited him also, and plunged into a profound melancholy by the Terror, he died a natural death at age 46.

pattern of instruction was definitive, setting the tone of Paris medicine for the next several decades.[7]

A number of factors had combined to discredit the pre-Revolutionary Rationalism and direct physicians' attention to the Empirical end of the spectrum.

The ideas of Jean-Jacques Rousseau, as set forth in the *Emile* and other writings on hygiene, medicine, and physicians, had been eagerly grasped by society: "A weak body enfeebles the mind: hence the rule of medicine, an art which is more pernicious to men than all the ills it claims to cure."[8] "Live naturally, be patient, and avoid physicians . . . their lying art, instead of prolonging your days, deprives you of their enjoyment . . . Do not go into this lottery where you have too many chances against you."[9] "I think the physicians who tended me did as much harm as the disease . . . Each treated me in his own way, gave me no relief, and weakened me considerably."[10] "I am continually told that the physician is at fault while medicine itself is infallible. That's all very well, but let medicine then come without the physician; when they come together, there is 100 times more to fear from the artist than to hope for from the art."[11]

He particularly detested bloodletting, treating his own attacks of *angine* (sore throat) with warm footbaths. He had a high opinion of hygiene, especially as it concerned infants and children, and his writings virtually created the specialty of pediatrics.[12]

The main source of Rousseau's ideas about child health and welfare was probably the *Traite de l'Education Corporelle des Enfants en Bas Age* by his close friend, Jean-Charles Desessartz (1729-1811),[13] a graduate of Montpellier and profound admirer of Bordeu.[c] This symbolizes the very powerful impact of the southern school on Paris. Barthez was the most prestigious medical thinker in France. Many of the leading Paris clinicians were Montpellier graduates. And Paris medicine in the early nineteenth century was ultimately an attempt to combine traditional Rationalist pathological anatomy with the Empirical vitalist postulates of Montpellier.

[c]See his "Eloge de Bordeu" (November 8, 1777) in *Memoires de la Faculte de Medecine de Montpellier,* Volume XIV.

The final influence on post-Revolutionary medicine was surgery, as seen in the adoption of a combined medical-surgical course by the écoles de santé. This was not only because surgeons were more trusted than physicians. Nor was it due only to the army's need for surgeons. The restoration of surgery to the medical curriculum represented the fusion of theory and practice.

The medieval separation of the two disciplines reflected the divorce of theory from practice, and the increasing abstraction of Rationalist medicine was its consequence. Paracelsus urged their fusion, and called himself a surgeon, precisely to emphasize that theory emerges from practice, that the physician must deal exclusively with the *visible.*[d]

This same *Zeitgeist* led Hahnemann–hundreds of miles away on the other side of the battlefront–to propose that therapeutic theory be based only on symptoms.

A leading surgeon of Lyons, Marc-Antoine Petit (1766-1811), wrote in 1806: "one must, as far as possible, make medicine ocular."[14] Two decades later Laennec stated the same: "in a word, I have tried, with regard to diagnosis, to put internal organic lesions on the same level as surgical diseases."[15] And even the Rationalist, Jean-Baptiste Bouillaud (1797-1881), stated some years later: "In heart and lung diseases the ear, if I may so express myself, *seeing* and *touching* these organs by means of an attentive examination, picks up signs which, as Laennec put it, render the diagnosis of most of the diseases in question as certain as that of some surgical diseases, such as fractures and dislocations."[16] [e]

The best-known medical figure of Revolutionary Paris was the surgeon, Pierre-Joseph Desault (1744-1795), the founder of French clinical surgery and surgical anatomy. A peasant's son who had learned from a master-surgeon of his village, Desault's courses in anatomy were based exclusively on cadavers and operations; he advised students to ignore books, charts, and theoretical explanations and to develop their powers of observation.[17] "Desault never explained

[d] *Divided Legacy,* I, 366, 464, 494.

[e] On Bouillaud see below, pp. 530-532.

anything, but as a faithful observer of the nature, spoke only her language."[18] He abandoned to physiology "the study of the minute structures where the empire of the senses ends and that of the imagination begins."[19] "Nearly everything was consideration of shape, magnitude, position, and direction. [His students] were to paint a picture rather than to acquire learning. They were to see the surface, not penetrate the depths."[20] [f]

And Desault, like all other surgeons of his time, was beholden for medical as well as surgical ideas to John Hunter's writings on the blood, inflammation, and venereal disease.

Thus, just as a large group of Paris clinicians came from Montpellier, so an equally sizable group came to medicine through surgery and had their initial training and practical experience in (usually military) surgery.[g]

More than half of the twenty-two professors first appointed to the Paris Ecole de Santé were surgeons (1794-1795 academic year), the most outstanding being Desault himself.[h] Anatomy was compulsory in each of the three years of study, physiology in the first two years, and operative surgery in the last two.[i] The remaining courses—

[f]Carl Wunderlich (1815-1877) wrote later: "the whole trend of recent French medicine comes from the surgical school. Desault has, without doubt, exercised the greatest influence as a paragon of precise observation and in relating surgery to its anatomical basis" (quoted in O. Temkin, "The Role of Surgery in the Rise of Modern Medical Thought," *Bulletin of the History of Medicine* XXV [1951], 248-259, at 257).

[g]Such were Corvisart, Bichat, Broussais, Recamier, Dupuytren, Richerand, Alibert, Laennec, and others.

[h]The first professor of internal diseases (*clinique interne*) was Jean-Nicolas Corvisart (1755-1821) who suffered from heart disease and thus took an interest in it. He revived Auenbrugger's method of percussion for heart disease and was a strong influence on Laennec (see below, pp. 486-487). He became Napoleon's physician and after the latter's fall retired from public functions. Napoleon once said of him: "an honest and able man but a little rude." Other than the works on heart disease we have by him: *Aphorismes de Medecine Clinique* (Paris: Masson, 1929).

[i]Surgical instruction was given at the Ecole Pratique, established in 1798 as part of the Ecole de Santé. It afforded a "wisely ordered collaboration between practice and theory" (*Journal de Medecine, Chirurgie, Pharmacie* I [1801], 70).

pathology, materia medica, hygiene, midwifery, chemistry, and pharmacy—were spread over the three years. The students were at all times expected to spend part of the day at one of the three Paris clinics (venereal diseases, maternity, and smallpox)—"to get used to seeing sick people and treating them."[21]

The collapse of the medical profession and its institutions had swept aside that bugbear of the medical mind, theories of internal pathology, and in Year III of the Republic (1794-1795) the Ecole de Santé called for a total return to Hippocratic principles, specifically, the coction doctrine. The course in "internal pathology" stressed, as first order of business, "the danger of false theories and the need to study the history of diseases in the writings of good observers, verifying them at the sickbed."[22] The student then studied the disease itself, described as "the effort of the nature" (*le travail de la nature*), with special emphasis on rare cases.[23] He went on to analyze possible patterns of disease onset, progress, and termination—requiring "a preliminary knowledge and study of coction which proceeds in different and various ways from one disease to the next; then of the pulse and excretions which are the indicators of coction; and then the history of true and false crises, the character of the cure, changes in disease, and true and false signs of death and their consequences."[24] Diseases were to be classified according to their modes of progression and a study made of the effects of various medicines; special attention was directed to the vital, curative, and palliative indications.[25]

The final year included the history of medicine from Hippocrates and the Egyptians through the eighteenth century with emphasis on the rules of correct observation and the biographies of famous physician-observers.[26] The history of veterinary medicine was included—not only because the "health officers" had to care for horses during their military duty but because the holistic medicine taught at the Ecole de Santé demanded attention to animal diseases as well.

The only significant philosophical influence on Paris medicine at this time was Cabanis who, in 1789, had been the first to urge that this subject be taught in hospitals and, in 1790, laid the doctrinal basis for the medical reform put through by the Revolution.

Cabanis has been rather slighted by historians because he did not discover some previously unknown organ, tissue, or disease. But what he did discover was far more important—the whole Hippocratic and Empirical tradition which he advanced as the foundation of medical education.

Initially a student of Greek and German literature and British Empirical philosophy, he became a physician in 1783—in part out of concern for his own poor health. During the final years of the ancien régime he frequented the salon of Mme. Helvetius where he met the philosophes, Diderot, D'Alembert, Holbach, and Condorcet. He married the latter's sister-in-law and was greatly under his influence.

He welcomed the Revolution, was a friend of the Girondins, and became personal physician to Mirabeau. He was appointed to the Council of 500 where in 1798 he presented a *Report on Medical Education* confirming and elaborating the 1794 ideas of Fourcroy.[27] His two major writings on medical philosophy were *Coup d'Oeuil sur les Revolutions et sur la Reforme de la Medecine* (1795) and *Du Degre de Certitude de la Medecine* (1798)[28] which discuss the reasons for the poor standing of physicians and the public's lack of respect for medicine: "some call medicine a scourge of humanity; physicians themselves treat it as charlatanism; on all sides one hears the reproaches of Moliere, Montaigne, and Rousseau—the only sure way to recovery is through one's own recuperative powers."[29]

Cabanis sought a remedy for this distressing situation by analyzing the revolutions through which medicine has passed and concluded that, amid the welter of conflicting facts and theories, salvation would be found in Hippocratic principles: practice must be based on observation of the *physis* and the physician's own therapeutic experience. Only by creating a reliable method will medicine be delivered from false systems.[30]

In 1798 he urged introduction of a special course on "general therapeutic method" in the Ecole de Santé.[31]

The Hippocratic principles of *Aphorisms, Epidemics, The Art,* and *Ancient Medicine* were perverted in ancient times by Empedocles and Aristotle (and in modern—through cultivation by a leisure class). Although improved by the elimination of priestly control, Greek medicine was made equally dogmatic by these philosophers. Galen proposed to restore Hippocratic medicine, but "in his hands it acquired more the trappings of Hippocratic medicine than its true wealth. The observations gathered by Hippocrates and the rules he extracted from them, while now more brilliant and systematic, lost much of their purity . . . the *physis,* which the physician of Cos had always grasped with such precision and reserve, was stifled and lost . . ."[32]

The Galenic tradition was continued by Boerhaave, while true Hippocratic medicine was developed by Akron of Agrigentum and Serapion of Alexandria and restored in modern times by Paracelsus, Van Helmont, Stahl, and the School of Montpellier: the latter is now "the most important doctrine and will soon be the dominant and only medical doctrine."[33] [j]

The solidism of Cullen and Hoffmann was only a revival of ancient Methodism.[34]

The Hippocratic therapeutic method assumes that the *physis* is always combating morbific influences, and the physician acquires his knowledge by observing these efforts of the *physis* as expressed in the patient's symptoms.[35] The method of the *physis* thus becomes the model for the physician, and a true medical theory is a compendium of observations of the *physis:* "the theoretical part of a science should be a simple enumeration of the sequence, the classification, and the relations among all the facts of which the science is composed—their summary expression, so to speak. If theory does not remain severely within these narrow limits, it will no longer be presenting methodical tables of real objects; they will be groups of results alien to the facts, vain fantoms."[36] The "method" of the *physis* is its theory,

[j] Both Serapion and Akron were reputed founders of the Empirical School (*Divided Legacy,* I, 73*j*, 199, 203, 258, 281).

and the profusion of "theories" and "facts" with which therapeutics is burdened can be evaluated by testing them against the curative method of the *physis*.[37] By following and perfecting the method of the *physis* therapeutics will become more certain and reliable.[38]

The role of the auxiliary sciences in medicine has been exaggerated—despite Bacon's warning against introducing into medicine theories developed outside it.[39] Scientific conceit leads the physician to premature application of anatomical, mathematical, physical, or chemical knowledge—yielding ridiculous results, especially in modern solidism.[40] "The more rigorous terminology of modern science leads to even more vicious results when it certifies the existence of relationships unverifiable by attentive observation."[41] "Nature is unaware of the fantasies invoked to explain her, and the living nature, in particular, has her own procedures which must be studied from the facts, not from vain conjectures or even more vain calculations."[42]

Medical knowledge is not gleaned from these sciences but emerges from therapeutic experience, from the curative process.[43] Medicine was practiced before physicians existed, and it must be taught at the bedside—in hospitals and clinics.[44]

The physician need not attempt to define the *physis* or understand its operations, as this knowledge is almost surely unattainable.[45] "For us there exist only facts presented either simultaneously or in succession . . . When we see one following upon another, we call the first the cause and the second the effect, but these names do not confer any new qualities. They only express the order of their succession."[46] The most one can say is that causal relationships are probably ascertained by the attentive examination and comparison of many diseased states.[47] This may be viewed as "clipping the wings of genius" in compelling physicians to act as simple copyists or compilers of tables of observations, but, as Bacon observed, rather than "give wings to genius," let us "attach lead to her feet."[48]

How, then, does the physician observe and understand diseased states?

Here Cabanis adopted the epistemology of modern Empiricism in support of the ancient. Locke had called knowledge a mixture of sensory data and preexisting ideas.[49] Condillac went further, denying preexisting ideas and reducing all knowledge to sensory percepts: ideas are put together out of such percepts and can be analyzed or broken down again into these very percepts (*composition des idees* and *decomposition des phenomenes*).[50] [k]

Applying this method to medicine, Cabanis held that diseases are not "entities" but only groups of symptoms, each observable symptom being the equivalent of one of Condillac's sensory percepts and the "disease" itself one of Condillac's "ideas."[51] [l] Hence medical practice can be improved by improving medical language.[52]

The symptoms are limited in number. Only their combinations are infinite—yielding the inexhaustible variety of diseased states.[53] Observed in the order of their appearance, the symptoms convey to the physician a correct understanding of the disease process, enabling him to cure in the same way as the *physis*—through vomiting, sweating, diuresis, etc.[54] [m] But the movements of the *physis* are not always beneficial and must sometimes be opposed: a copious bloodletting can cut short (*juguler*) a dangerous fever, and the art generally—by its swift and certain production of coction and crises—can replace the slow and uncertain processes of the *physis*.[55] [n]

Although he can effect these results, the physician is still ignorant of the intimate nature of his remedies and of the proximate causes of disease. Each medicine is a specific with its own peculiar power on the organism, one which can be

[k]This sceptical sensualism was called *"ideologie"* by Destutt de Tracy (1754-1836). It became the official philosophy of the Revolution.

[l]Cf. Van Helmont's "disease idea" and the Montpellier doctrine of "disease elements" (above, pp. 32 and 263).

[m]This analysis of the symptoms over time is called *"analyse historique"* (Cabanis, *Oeuvres Completes,* I, 227-228, 236-239).

[n]*Juguler*—literally, "cut the throat of," "throttle."

learned only through observation and not by *a priori* chemical analysis.[56] Since this power differs with the patient's pathological condition, one must repeat procedures hundreds of times to become a skilful prescriber.[57]

Medicines are often administered carelessly, in ignorance of their true curative powers.[58] Cabanis urged a return to botanicals.[59]

But he was more concerned with diet, disease prevention, and improving the patient's environment than with pharmacology: the treatment of disease is, in principle, no different from prescribing the correct diet in health.[60] He rejected abstract analysis of the digestive process in favor of a comparison of different diets for their effect on this process.[61]

His writings on hygiene and environmental influences on health led to establishment of a course in hygiene at the Ecole de Santé. He was professor there of legal medicine, clinics, and medical history from 1799 to 1808, even though a large practice, his own poor health, and steady involvement in politics limited his academic activity.[62]

In some respects he was far ahead of his time—as in urging governmental supervision of the medical profession or in advocating several small hospitals rather than a few large ones.[63]

He wanted medical knowledge to be accessible to everyone, and for a decade after the Revolution medical schools were free and open to all comers (but attendance at clinics was restricted to medical students).[64]

Cabanis had an equal interest in veterinary medicine.[65]

While he urged attention to the socio-economic dimension of medicine, this insight perished for lack of understanding and support by his colleagues. And Cabanis himself was indecisive on many doctrinal issues.

For instance, he attempted to efface the distinction between Empiricism and Rationalism despite his own clear preference for the former: while admitting that the "very name [the Empirics] bore, the terms they used, and their basic rules continually placed them in the true path of analysis, which must begin by observation,"[66] he concludes that their quarrel with the Rationalists was largely verbal: "the Empirics reasoned experience, while the Rationalists experimented their reasoning."[67] Both based treatment on the same facts, even though the Rationalists called these facts "causes."[68] What the physician must seek is, therefore, an *"experience raisonnee."*[69] If the science were made up of comprehensive collections of observations together with short inductions from them (aphorisms or *epilogismoi*[o]), i.e., the method of Bacon, this would reconcile the differences between the two schools.[70]

Not only was his indecisiveness historically inaccurate, it confused his perception and solution of the three major issues with which a medical philosophy must deal: (1) the relationship between pathological anatomy and symptoms, (2) the criteria of disease classification, and (3) the rules for administering medicines or prescribing treatment.

Thus he failed to provide clear guidance on the three issues of greatest concern to the Paris School in the decades to come.

On the relative importance of pathological lesions and symptoms Cabanis took two incompatible positions. On one hand, he wrote that the best pathology, that of the Ancients, is identical with semeiology.[71] He rejected anatomy in favor of "living anatomy"—the study of internal changes occurring during the disease process or at different stages of life.[72] While the physician needs some anatomical knowledge, the discipline is inherently unreliable, and its procedures are, at best, "painful and disgusting." The physician should guard against being led by them to incorrect conclusions.[73] [p]

But his 1798 *Report* to the Committee of 500 urged a chair of pathological anatomy in each école de santé, "that anatomy which, from the organic lesions observed after

[o]See *Divided Legacy,* I, 252g, 271-274. Baglivi had also urged that medical knowledge be accumulated in aphoristic form (*De Praxi Medica,* 86, 164-168, 181). An aphoristic structure of knowledge is, of course, the opposite of the analytical structure favored by Rationalism.

[p]Cf. the view of Celsus that the physician needs some knowledge of anatomy, but not too much (*Divided Legacy,* I, 253).

death, seeks to penetrate the history of the disease phenomena and to determine their true cause."[74] [q]

Cabanis' ambiguity on this point undermined his attempt at disease classification.

He decided that the nosologies of Cullen and Sauvages were inadequate and that a new one was needed: otherwise "medicine would often float to and fro without a compass on an unknown sea," as the facts are too numerous, and memory alone cannot encompass them all.[75] While the Empirics say that each patient is unique, they still use medicines boldly, showing that they have reached some conclusion about disease classes.[76] Similar traits can always be found among different patients: the point is to discover ones which are meaningful and meet the needs of therapy.[77]

Cabanis resolved this issue by dividing symptoms into *propria* and *communia* and giving precedence to the former as guides to treatment: his *Report* to the Council of 500 urged particular attention to rare and unusual cases,[78] and he noted the importance of strange symptoms: "disgusts or peculiar appetites, intensifications or fleeting weaknesses of vital functions; alterations which occur with a given periodicity or return at an indeterminate time are both the signs of internal changes and the instruments with which the *physis* effects the cure."[79]

But he was no more successful than Sydenham or Baglivi in proposing a method for distinguishing "peculiar" symptoms from mere "irregularities" or "complications" and could only exhort the physician to become a better observer and to intensify his "tact" and sympathy with the patient: "by identifying himself with the sufferer, associating himself with his sufferings, through the rapid play of his sensitive imagination, the physician perceives the disease at a single glance and grasps all its traits at once."[80]

The final problem—how to match remedies with diseases—was also referred to the physician's "tact" or intuition: "a

[q]His physiology and pathology were close to those of his pupil and friend, Anthelme Richerand (1779-1840), whose *Nouveaux Elements de Physiologie* (Paris: Crapard, 1802) was patterned on Haller's sensitivity and irritability.

happy instinct, rather than knowledge, leads to the first rules."[81] Almost everything depends on "*coup d'oeuil* and a happy instinct."[82] Just as the patient's instinct leads him to the correct foods, so the physician's instinct tells him the correct remedy.[83]

Cabanis was not the last physician of the Paris School to fall back on intuition when confronted with a knotty problem of analysis. His interest in diet, hygiene, public health, and disease prevention doubtless reflected dissatisfaction at his own inability to find better solutions to the traditional problems of therapeutics.

Born in 1757, Cabanis was a precise contemporary of Hahnemann, and the parallels between the two are striking. In the very same years both were seeking a way out of medicine's methodological labyrinth, and both did so by abandoning Rationalism for Empiricism.

The differences between the two are equally marked. While Cabanis remained at the level already reached by Sydenham, Baglivi, and Stahl, Hahnemann's chemical and pharmacological learning advanced the discussion to a new stage. The law of similars and its corollaries yielded solutions to all the problems which continued to plague Cabanis.

But the latter's formulations provided solid and useful ground for French medical speculation during the ensuing half-century, and the principal ideas developed and implemented in these decades are found in his works. At the same time, the problems which baffled Cabanis were equally baffling for his followers—until French medicine adopted some of the ideas of Hahnemann.

Pinelism: 1798-1826

In his *Coup d'Oeuil sur les Revolutions et sur la Reforme de la Medecine* Cabanis praised the work on disease classification being done by Philippe Pinel, whose *Nosographie Philosophique, ou la Methode de l'Analyse Appliquee a la Medecine* appeared in 1798 and was for more than twenty years a basic text and guide for Paris practitioners and medical students.[84]

The son of a rural physician, Pinel was first destined for the priesthood and then turned to mathematics, starting his medical studies at Montpellier only in 1774.[85] There he spent much of his time in hospitals, and his medical thought in later years was intimately bound up with clinical practice.[86]

After graduation he came to Paris where Cabanis introduced him to salon life.[87] Like his mentor, he was attracted by British Empirical philosophy and its French spokesman, the Baron de Condillac. In matters medical Pinel was very unsure of himself (even at age 46 admitting "extreme uncertainty" about the correct method to follow) and spent a number of years as professor of geometry.[88] He translated Cullen's *Synopsis of Methodical Nosology*, edited a journal of hygiene for several years, issued an edition of Baglivi's writings, and published several Iatromathematical articles of his own.[89]

He was finally stimulated to enter practice by the death of a friend who, in a fit of insanity, ran out of his house and was devoured by wolves.[90] In 1792 he took charge of the Bicetre insane asylum and immediately showed his intellectual independence by having the chains and fetters removed from the patients. In 1794 he became the first professor of hygiene at the Ecole de Santé and shortly afterwards assumed the chair of internal pathology.[r]

His *Nosographie Philosophique* in 1798 was followed in 1802 by the *Medecine Clinique Rendue plus Precise et Plus Exacte par l'Application de l'Analyse*—a compendium of clinical cases following the "*methode de l'analyse*" set forth in the *Nosographie*. The reason for their enormous success (the *Nosographie* had a sixth edition in 1818 and the *Medecine Clinique* a third edition in 1815) is given by Isidore Bricheteau (1789-1862), an early biographer of Pinel:

> One must imagine the state of medicine at the time. The system of Boerhaave had collapsed. An expiring humoralism was in conflict with the doctrine of spasms

[r]He was succeeded at the Bicetre by Jean Esquirol (1772-1849) who later wrote the first treatise on mental diseases.

imagined by Hoffmann and developed by Cullen. But this humoralism was still alive and popular in practice. The students were impregnated with it before they even entered the schools and could not shake it off. The only bases of public education in medicine were some obscure compilations in Latin. They had no elementary texts and had to take as models various traditions of the former Faculté de Médecine. Needed was an elementary work in which the most important facts would be analyzed and subjected to the crucible of experience and criticism, and classified according to a philosophic method. This was Pinel's *Nosographie Philosophique.*[91]

And Bricheteau does not even mention the Brunonianism which had by this time markedly confused medical thinking in France.[s]

Like Cabanis, Pinel sought a revival of the Hippocratic and Empirical vitalist principles represented by Van Helmont, Sydenham, Baglivi, Stahl, Sauvages, and Montpellier, with rejection of the proximate causes and mechanistic speculations of Galen, Cullen, and Boerhaave.[92] [t] "The only solid knowledge available to the human understanding" is that based on experience.[93]

This attitude owed much not only to Pinel's Montpellier training[u] and acquaintance with the writings of Baglivi but also to his passionate admiration for Rousseau: once, after a visit to the philosopher's grave, he was unable to sleep for five days and nights.[94] [v]

[s]Gabriel Andral, for instance, wrote in 1823 that the principal division in medical opinion in the 1790's was between those who were for Brown and those who were against him (*Clinique Medicale* [Paris: Gabon, 1823], I, xviii).

[t]He observes that Boerhaave's only useful writing was *De Commendando Studii Hippocratis:* "by what fatality, then, did he contradict himself—founding his system on the application of mechanics to the laws of the animal economy?" (*Nosographie Philosophique,* 1802, III, 476).

[u]As a medical student Pinel had made a long condensation of Stahl's *Theoria Medica Vera* (I. Bricheteau, "Discours sur Philippe Pinel," *Journal Complementaire des Sciences Medicales* XXIX [1827], 300).

[v]This did not prevent him from citing with approval Corvisart's retort to Rousseau's wish that "medicine should come without the physician"—"in that case, diseases would have to come without patients" ("Medecine" in *Dictionnaire*).

In Pinel's opinion the defect of Hippocratic doctrine was its lack of a disease classification (to which Sydenham had already called attention).[95] The problem posed by Pitcairn: "a disease once given, find the correct remedy," is too general; the only question medicine can pose itself in its present state is: "a disease once given, how do we determine its true character and the place it occupies in a nosological table."[96]

Pinel thus turned his mind to the problem which had baffled Sauvages, Bordeu, and Barthez: how to elaborate a nosology which would guide the physician through the maze of different forms in which diseases appear.[97]

In tackling it he accepted the traditional Empirical assumptions about the *physis,* coction, the proximate cause, and sense-perception.[98] The internal mechanisms of the organism, the interactions of the solids and fluids of the body, are an "inexhaustible object of vain reasonings, of frivolous discussion and explanation . . . should we not abide by the sense-perceptible phenomena, that is, the impressions received by the sight, the touch, the smell, the hearing? Have we any other way of recognizing internal lesions than by their external signs and the results of previous research on analogous objects?"[99] [w] Morgagni's attempt to classify diseases according to the organ affected was an error: the physician is guided not by the simple position of the parts but by their structure and associated vital functions.[100] The correct approach was that of Linnaeus and Antoine Jussieu (1686-1758) in describing the botanical world—entire reliance on visible attributes with "severe precision in description and exact and uniform definition."[101] This was also Condillac's prescription for acquiring reliable knowledge.[102]

Furthermore, Pinel accepted the assumption of Baglivi, Sauvages, and Barthez that the curative efforts of the *physis* are not infinite but finite: "aside from circumstances of age,

[w]Pinel is commonly called a "solidist," and he did aim to "dispose completely of the scientific jargon of humoral medicine." But while he holds the solids to be more important than the fluids, this knowledge is not needed for practice, and, in any case, the physician cannot be certain of it (*Nosographie Philosophique,* 1802, I, ii, ix, 106).

sex, climate, and way of life, all is reduced to a determinate number of entirely analogous acute or chronic diseases."[103] This assumption may also reflect his experience at the Bicetre, where he found that the mentally ill, if left undisturbed, tended to settle into a limited number of classes: mania, melancholy, dementia, and idiocy (following Condillac's division of the intellectual faculties).[104] Further evidence in favor of the constant nature of disease classes is the similarity between modern diseases and the descriptions given by the ancients.[105] [x]

It follows that if diseases are described with extreme accuracy, they will fall into a systematic and regular nosology which the physician can follow and thus avoid most of the errors of practice.[106]

Each disease is a process with a beginning, a middle, and an end.[107] While some are simple, others are complex—due to the superposition of two or more diseases one upon the other.[108] Further complications are introduced by the age, sex, and constitution of the patient, the climate, season, and locality, the exciting cause of the disease, and the prevailing "epidemic constitution."[109]

Complex states may be broken down following Condillac's rules for the *"decomposition des phenomenes,"* and disease species, genera, and classes can be built up again from these elemental states by comparing their symptoms—Condillac's *"composition des idees."*[110] [y] This same procedure is used in botanical classification.[111]

But not all symptoms are of equal value: "When one seeks these signs at the sickbed, some are very obvious, others more or less pronounced or equivocal, certain ones may have no value at all or even be misleading in very complex cases; one must know how to reject them and substitute new symptoms for them."[112] The disease history must be reduced to its "fundamental symptoms," the ones which are directly related to the "nature of the disease."[113]

[x]Baglivi had stated the same (see above, p. 203).

[y]Cf. with Baglivi's "primary diseases" (above, p. 204).

The physician must separate important symptoms from unimportant, and here Pinel again followed the lead of Baglivi and Sydenham, distinguishing the "specific" or "distinctive" symptoms from the "common or accidental" *and attaching them to the "disease" rather than to the individual patient.*[114] [z]

> I call the student's attention to the traits which may be regarded as specific to the disease, and then I can assign the disease the place it should occupy in my nosology . . . By this method the science of signs so assiduously cultivated by the ancients and so often reduced to general maxims, is linked to the specific character of diseases . . .[115]

In a "bilious-putrid fever," for example, he calls attention to the gastric symptoms (headache, a bitter taste in the mouth, thirst, sensitivity of the epigastrium) and the adynamic symptoms (the patient is supine with glazed eyes and a tense abdomen) but ignores the *symptomes communs* (tongue dry and dark brown in the center, sharp pains in the extremities, a fever with paroxysms in the evening, accelerated respiration, moaning).[116] In an "ataxic meningo-gastric fever" the ataxic symptoms are delirium, paroxysms of fever, and fainting at night; the gastric symptoms are suborbital headache, a desire for acid drinks, a full pulse, and epigastric pain; the *symptomes communs et accidentels* are: general lassitude, pain in the limbs, a dry tongue, burning heat of the skin, and epistaxis.[117] In a "gastro-adynamic pneumonia" the peripneumonia symptoms are: dull pain on the right side of the thorax, a flushed face, difficulty articulating words, bloody sputum, inability to sleep on the right side, red patches on the cheeks; the gastric symptoms are: bitter taste in the mouth, a heavy feeling in the epigastrium, frontal headache, extreme thirst, and burning heat of the skin; the adynamic symptoms are: extreme debility, a rough brown coating on the tongue, fetid sputum, dirty scum on the teeth, and an irregular pulse; the *symptomes communs et acciden-*

[z]See above, pp. 204-206.

tels are: headache, a hard rapid pulse, paroxysms in the evening, a tendency to faint, and abundant evacuation after taking an emetic.[118]

Etienne Pariset called Pinel's nosography a portrait gallery of diseases grouped according to family resemblance whose principal merit was extreme fidelity to nature; as such, it made a profound impression on students who were like blind men seeing for the first time.[119] And Pinel did indeed perform an earthshaking task in dividing the known universe of diseases into 100-odd species acceptable to his contemporaries. This must greatly have benefited treatment in promoting greater individualization, while elimination of the *symptomes communs* from diagnosis may have made practice milder, since these were precisely the symptoms the physician was accustomed to attack most energetically.

But the classification was still arbitrary to a degree—just as the classifications of Sydenham and Baglivi had been arbitrary. Once Pinel had accepted the existence of a given "disease," he selected certain symptoms as characteristic of that "disease" and called them "specific," "distinctive," etc. Other symptoms were classified as *"commun"* or *"accidentel,"* depending upon whether they were encountered more or less frequently.

It may be assumed that the arbitrariness of the classification was compounded when the "species" were combined into a "genus." Pinel resolved this problem seemingly by a play on words: *"on s'arrete seulement a certains symptomes fondamentaux qui leur sont communs* [i.e., to the species] *et qui, par leur reunion, sont propres a former l'histoire du genre."*[120] What are *communia* in the species become *propria* in the genus!! But this sort of speculation could not, in any case, affect practice, since for Pinel the genus had no metaphysical existence, being only a "complex and abstract idea."[121] "One must take care not to attribute reality to 'fever' in general, not to consider it as existing by itself, not to define it; it is a purely abstract term, like 'tree' or 'metal,' which covers several analogous objects. What are we then to make of so many grave dissertations, so much frivolous research, vainly repeated time and again from Galen's days to our own, on the essential character and definition of 'fever'?"[122] The physician's experience is with individual patients, not with disease entities, and even though observations must be generalized to some extent, he should display a "wise reserve" and avoid "attributing reality to abstract expressions."[123]

We have already discussed the origins of the "specific disease" in the writings of Sydenham and Baglivi.[a] With them the "specificity" consisted in an "exaltation" of the humors which recurred time after time in the same way. Pinel defines diseases as "fleeting changes of greater or lesser duration in the vital functions, manifested by external signs with a constant uniformity for their principal traits and an innumerable variety as regards their accessory traits."[124]

For Pinel diseases were still only perversions of function: although falling into defined classes, they had no life, being, or substance of their own. But this was an unstable and ambiguous position, and in the early nineteenth century the "specifically affected person" became the "specific disease."

The early editions of Pinel's works divide diseases into "essential fevers" (inflammatory, bilious, mucous, putrid, malignant, and pestilential) and "phlegmasies" (of the mucous membranes, diaphanous membranes, glands, muscles, and skin).[125] The "fevers" were subdivided into 15 genera and 40 species, the "phlegmasies" into 22 genera and 77 species.

With later editions the classification was extended to include "hemorrhages," "neuroses" (nervous diseases), and "organic diseases"—these last again subdivided into "general organic lesions" (syphilis, scurvy, gangrene, cancer, tuberculosis, scrophula, yaws, etc.) and "particular organic lesions" (aneurysm of the heart, anasarca, hemorrhoidal tumors, etc.).[126]

The distinction between "neuroses" and "organic diseases" reflects the development of pathological anatomy by Bayle, Laennec, and others, their division of diseases into

[a]See above, pp. 196-197.

"vital" and "organic,"[b] but Pinel did not really accept the disease localization implicit in the concept of "organic disease." While the "phlegmasies" are ordered according to their seat in the body, the symptoms are still the dominant criteria of classification.[127] Botanists do not classify plants according to the regions in which they grow; most diseases are still of the whole organism, and Pinel warns against attempts at precise localization.[128]

Bricheteau wrote that Pinel attached little importance to pathological anatomy and disease localization, "regarding it more as an object of speculative curiosity, so that he seemed to fear taking the first steps in a career which he himself had opened to others."[129]

For him classification was the "scientific" part of medicine, therapeutics being determined by the disease class.[130] From his understanding of the disease process in any particular species and his skill in prognosis the physician makes one of three possible determinations: either the disease is self healing; or it is fatal; or it is one in which the physician can influence the *physis* in the direction of cure.[131]

Most diseases fall in the first group and are healed naturally—through coction, crisis, and evacuation.[132] The physician practices expectancy—not leaving the patient alone but regulating his diet and ensuring that his surroundings are hygienic.[133] Stahl and Gideon Harvey have contributed much to a proper understanding of expectancy.[134]

Some diseases which are benign by nature become dangerous when interfered with.[135] Incorrect treatment can metastasize some into cancers.[136]

Many diseases, however, tend not to recovery but to death.[137] Acute diseases which the *physis* cannot concoct become chronic: instead of the anticipated salutary reaction there is torpidity of the functions, and the excretions do not bring about the natural critical solution.[138] In such cases the

[b]Thus Pinel holds that "neuroses," if sufficiently serious or extended in time, lead to organic diseases (*Nosographie Philosophique,* 1818, III, 294). See below, pp. 472-488.

physician can do no more than palliate the patient's sufferings.[139]

The final group are those diseases in which the physician's efforts can make a difference: the healing reaction is too weak and must be supported by the physician, or it takes a wrong direction—a "reversal of the laws which conserve the animal economy."[140]

To cure these the physician must understand the laws of the *physis*. Diseases have their periods which must be respected; the physician assists the disease through its proper stages.[141] Symptoms take on different meanings from one stage to another; hemorrhage, for example, is sometimes harmful but more often beneficial, and the same is true for fevers.[142] Pinel accepts the "sane and fruitful ideas of Van Helmont and Stahl" as revived by Bordeu, i.e., that hemorrhage is the nature's way of discharging excess blood.[143] He holds that Boerhaave misunderstood this point and was thus responsible for the excessive bloodletting since his time; nor did Boerhaave understand Stahl's views on the beneficial effect of inflammation, leading physicians to think in terms of "obstruction, thickening of the blood; they want to combat everything in fever as if the *physis* was inert . . . they let blood as if it were a destructive element which must be removed from the body."[144] [c]

Pinel criticizes his colleagues who, misunderstanding the disease process, prescribe purely symptomatically.[145] This only deranges the *physis* and introduces complications.[146]

Active intervention should support the *physis* and remove obstacles from its path.[147] The physician should strive, above all, to avoid errors, "i.e., not to make victims."[148] Sometimes a serious disease can be transformed into a less serious variety.[149]

Practice is founded on ability to recognize the particular disease process and experience in prescribing; it cannot be based on assumed knowledge of proximate causes, as such knowledge is forever foreclosed to the human mind.[150]

[c]The early years of the century were a time of popular antagonism to bloodletting (see *Bibliotheque Medicale* LIII [1816], 225, discussing an 1802 scarlet fever epidemic).

Chemistry, in particular, regardless of how much progress it may have made, cannot be a guide to diagnosis and therapeutics.[151]

Pinel's own treatment was mild and expectant, with much use of oxymel (honey and vinegar), hydromel (honey and water), barley water, *tisanes* of various kinds, etc.[152] He occasionally used opium and blistering, very rarely bloodletting.[153] He employed about 80 simple remedies, opposed polypharmacy ("I pass on the long prescriptions to those who believe in their omnipotence"),[154] and advised physicians to employ medicines indigenous to the country.[155] He urged abandonment of the voluminous pharmacopoeias inherited from previous ages.[156]

His contemporaries accused him both of excessive expectancy and of overactive medication.[157] [d]

The class of "organic lesions" in the last edition of Pinel's *Nosographie Philosophique* was a concession to work being done at the time in pathological anatomy, but otherwise he relied entirely on the symptoms for diagnosis and treatment. This line of analysis was carried even further by his contemporaries, Francois-Joseph Double (1771-1842) and A. J. Landre-Beauvais (1772-1840), both products of Montpellier who imported the pure southern doctrine to Paris.

Double's *Semeiologie Generale, ou Traite des Signes et de leur Valeur dans les Maladies* (1811) resembles Pinel's analysis in attempting to establish criteria for evaluating symptoms; he divides them into the same three classes as Pinel: "those belonging essentially to the disease," "accidental symptoms," and the "general or common ones which occur in almost all diseases and consequently are not to be associated with any one in particular."[158] Landre-Beauvais does the same: symptoms are "characteristic," "common," or "accidental."[159] Both reject the use of pathological-

[d]For the often fatal "acute croup" (diphtheria) in children Pinel used: potassium-antimonium tartrate as an emetic, camphorated liniments to provoke inflammation of the skin, inhalation of sulfuric ether, irritant clysters, sternutatories, purgatives, and bloodletting (C.J.A. Schwilgue, *Dissertation sur le Croup Aigu des Enfants.* Paris Dissertation, an X [1802]).

anatomical criteria to determine the importance of symptoms; both reject the proximate cause.

But here they fell into the same morass as the Montpellier School itself, with its thousands of unintelligible pages devoted to disease "elements." Symptoms could not be classified without invoking some additional criterion, and the force of circumstances at length compelled Paris physicians to look inside the body.

The impetus for this new departure was supplied by a young and tremendously hard-working genius who, in a very short life, switched the focus of medical interest from symptoms to underlying pathology. Xavier Bichat (1771-1802) studied surgery under Marc-Antoine Petit in Lyons and Pierre-Joseph Desault in Paris and was for a while regimental surgeon in the French armies. He collaborated with Desault until the latter's death in 1795, married his widow, and edited a posthumous edition of his works.

Bichat was not a medical practitioner but an anatomist—one of the most zealous ever known. He spent days and weeks without leaving the dissecting theater and in one peak winter cut up 700 bodies. The strain of this life, a predisposition to tuberculosis, and the effects of a bad fall brought his life to an end at the early age of 31—by which time his nine published works had transformed pathological anatomy.

Cabanis left three problems unresolved: the classification of diseases, the connection between symptoms and internal pathology, and the relationship between remedies and diseases. Pinel was wrestling with the first, and Bichat devoted himself to the other two, convinced that solutions would be found through knowledge of the alterations occurring in the body in disease and health. "What good is observation if the seat of the disease is unknown?"[160] "You can take notes at the bedside for twenty years and still be confused; open a few bodies, and all the obscurity will disappear."[161]

But Bichat was no mechanist. He praised Montpellier for rejecting the theories of Boerhaave. In abandoning this wrong road, however, they took another with so many twists and turns that they will never discover the exit.[162] He thus renounced the effort to cognize and classify diseases by their symptoms alone, to reduce the vital force to Montpellier's "elements" or to the "characteristic," "common," and "accidental" symptoms of Pinel, Double, and Landre-Beauvais.[163] The vital principle or *Anima,* defined by Bichat as the "group of functions which resist death,"[164] must be analyzed in a different way to be serviceable to medicine.[165]

Barthez had held the vital force to be a unity, but Bichat rejected this: in the physical sciences not all the phenomena are due to a single principle. Some can be ascribed to gravity, others to electricity, etc.; and the same approach must be taken in medicine.[166] Bordeu wanted to localize life in the organ, but "the idea of a separate life can no longer be applied to the individual organ. Since most of the organs are composed of very different simple tissues, the idea of life can only be applied to the tissues."[167]

The ultimate repositories of the vital force, therefore, are the tissues. Nature produces many effects from few causes, and in the living body these causes are the properties of the tissues.[168] In a clear parallel to Lavoisier's table of the chemical elements Bichat isolated 21 different tissues in the body—each with its own set of properties—and posited them as the fundamental building blocks of organic nature.[169] [e]

Bichat admired Haller: his sensitivity and irritability first pointed the way to a correct physiological analysis, but he erred in limiting these properties to nerves and muscles.[170] Francois Chaussier (1746-1828) advanced further, attaching these properties to the organs and thus developing Bordeu's original insights.[171] But Bichat regarded his own tissue-oriented approach as the best, allying the broad philosophical views of Bordeu with the experimental method of Haller and thereby improving on Pinel's attempt to establish a "judicious rapprochement" between the different membrane structures and their typical diseases.[172]

Bichat first analyzed each tissue for its vital properties (differing from physical or chemical properties and interpreted in terms of Haller's sensitivity and irritability), and

[e]Bichat's method also parallels Condillac's *"methode de l'analyse."*

then he analyzed each organ into its component tissues.[173] Disease is disturbed function due to excess or deficiency of one or several tissue properties, and cure is equivalent to restoring the tissue to its normal sensitivity or irritability (which Bichat called "contractility").[174]

In this way medicine and physiology were to become "exact sciences."[175]

He found that the nerves possess "animal sensitivity," the voluntary muscles "animal contractility," the involuntary muscles "sensitive organic contractility," "insensitive sensitivity" (*sensibilite insensible!!*), etc., but complications arose when he realized that the properties of any given tissue vary from one organ to the next: while bone and muscle retain the same properties wherever in the body they are located, the skin and mucous membranes alter their properties according to the organ, and glandular tissue, in particular, displays a very broad range of variation.[176]

The same problems beset his attempt to analyze function in terms of the tissue composition of the organ or organ system generating the function. Capillary circulation, the secretions, exhalations, and nutrition are governed, in principle, by the "organic sensitivity" and the "insensitive contractility."[177] The digestion, circulation, and urinary secretion are all functions of the "sensitive organic contractility" and the "organic sensitivity."[178] The voluntary movements and the voice fall under the "animal contractility."[179] But while some functions are effected by a single system, others result from a combination of systems, and Bichat found their analysis excessively complex.[180]

His pathology required a division of physiological functions into two groups: one pertaining to the "organic life" and the other to the "animal life." The first represents man's common heritage with the vegetable kingdom and includes nutrition, respiration, secretion, and metabolic processes—all centered on the heart and circulation.[181] The second includes the voluntary functions possessed only by animals—involving the reception of stimuli through the senses by the brain and the reaction from the brain through the nerves to the voluntary muscles; these functions are centered in the brain.[182] The "organic life" is located primarily in the fluids, the "animal life" in the solids. The body's vital properties are "mainly" attributes of the solids, while the fluids play the role of excitants; Bichat, however, admitted that the fluids are not completely inert.[183]

Diseases fall into four groups: one affecting the "organic life" and three the "animal life." The first are "fevers" and "nervous diseases" which seem to have no anatomical localization and are cured by crisis and evacuation–i.e., Pinel's "essential fevers" which Bichat ascribed to the liquids and the solids.[184] The other three disease groups are: (1) general or common alterations affecting a whole system of the body (here Bichat allowed only cancer and "inflammation"), (2) alterations peculiar to a given organ, and (3) diseases of a single tissue of an organ.[f] None of the diseases of these three groups–convulsions, spasms, epilepsy, "nervous diseases," etc.–are cured by crisis and evacuation.[185]

But these carefully delineated categories are upset by "sympathy" which causes the body's solids to interact in unpredictable ways.[186] "Sympathy" is undefinable, an aberration of the vital properties.[187] When one tissue of an organ has been diseased a long time, the whole organ is affected through sympathy.[188] "How easy it would be to study diseases if the phenomenon of sympathy did not exist."[189] "The *physis* fits only with difficulty into many of the categories to which men strive to subject her."[190]

Bichat's classificatory urge led him to attack this problem by subdividing "sympathy" into *"sympathie de sensibilite," "sympathie de tonicite," "sympathie d'irritabilite,"* etc., but more than this was needed to restore order to his analysis.[191]

He wrote little on therapeutics but reduced it (like Brown) to stimulation or pacification of the disordered sensitivities and contractilities.[192] In inflammation the exaltation of the "organic sensitivity" and the "insensitive contractility" are reduced by cataplasms, fomentations, and

[f]The division between "general" or "common" alterations which affect a whole system of the body and those peculiar to a single organ seems to be Bichat's formulation of the contrast between *communia* and *propria*.

bathing; depressed "organic sensitivity" is revived by drinking wine.[193] Emetics heighten the "sensitive organic contractility"; purgatives also, since they contract the intestines; at times the physician wants to calm the "sensitive organic contractility" with medicines which prevent vomiting, oppose intestinal irritation, etc.[194]

The medicine was not supposed to "fortify" or "debilitate" the body as a whole but only the particular tissue to which it was directed.[195] Toward the end of his life Bichat was testing medicines on healthy persons to ascertain the specific tissues affected by each.[196] [g]

Despite its apparent vitalism, Bichat's doctrine was reductionist in denying the autonomy of the vital force and attempting to subject it to *a priori* rules. Its impact on Paris thought was Rationalizing.

He was a Rationalist in assuming that reliable knowledge can be acquired of the body's tissues (even though he states elsewhere that primary causes cannot be known and that observation yields only knowledge of effects).[197] He was a Rationalist in attributing priority to pathological alterations rather than to symptoms: "diseases, or rather the symptoms which characterize them, should be distinguished according to the principles which cause or maintain them."[198] The symptoms which indicate the nature of the anatomical alteration are more important for treatment than those which only reveal change in function.[199] And he was a Rationalist in treating by contraries.

Significant is his denigration of coction: only one of his four disease groups is healed through coction.

The specifics of Bichat's anatomical and physiological views had little impact on his contemporaries, since his various sensitivities and contractilities were too complex and cumbersome,[200] but his overall approach to medicine left a

[g]Thus he was testing drugs on the healthy at precisely the same time as Hahnemann, but there is no reason to assume any relationship between them. The Zurich Medizingeschichtliches Institut possesses the notes of a German student who attended Bichat's lectures on this subject, but they have not yet been published.

permanent mark on the Paris School. His determinate and analytical vitalism was now in competition with the spontaneous and autonomous vitalism of Pinel, and the Rationalist corollaries of his method of analysis—the priority of internal pathology over symptoms, the need to pinpoint disease causes in the tissues, and cure through contraries—were long-lived and vigorous.

An influential and long-lived contribution of the Paris School to medicine was its broadening and deepening of the concept of "specific disease."

Physicians had long known that certain diseases repeat themselves time after time, reappearing always in the same form. Of these the most common were syphilis, smallpox, measles, and scabies (Hahnemann's "miasmatic diseases"), but others, such as rabies and the effects of snakebites, could be added. The Paris School isolated certain characteristics of these traditional diseases and combined them to form other "specific diseases" which have remained a part of medical thought and doctrine.

According to this developing view the "specific disease" should: (1) be common to a number of persons, (2) always take the same form, (3) possess some peculiar quality or attribute distinguishing it clearly from other diseases, and (4) be endowed with materiality—some dimension added to the healthy body when it is infected with the "specific disease."

Major support for the "specific disease" doctrine came from the increasingly frequent epidemics of this period—miasmatic diseases extended in space rather than over time.

In the Hippocratic Corpus such crowd diseases were ascribed to a particular quality of the atmosphere, and this explanation remained acceptable until the nineteenth century.[h]

An alternative explanation of crowd diseases, "contagion" or passage of the disease by contact, entered medical thought with the *Syphilis, sive Morbus Gallicus* (1530) of

[h]See *Divided Legacy*, I, 55.

Hieronymus Fracastorius (1483-1553)—an account of the syphilis pandemic which appeared shortly after the return of Columbus from the New World. Popularly regarded as an import from the West Indies, syphilis raged in Europe for decades and left an imprint on the public mind comparable to that of the Black Death 200 years earlier or the Asiatic Cholera 300 years later.

Fracastorius denied that syphilis was introduced by Columbus, since it appeared simultaneously in all the countries of Europe (and, in fact, last of all in Spain and Portugal), but he was vague about its origins. It is carried by "disease seeds" (*semina morbum*), is transmitted by contact (*contages*) or contagion, but is due ultimately to malign or poisonous astrological influences—the same combination of Mars and Saturn which had earlier brought the Black Death.[i]

In the early nineteenth century astrological explanations of disease had fallen out of fashion, but the other concepts popularized by Fracastorius—the "poisonous exhalation" (*le virus*), the disease "seed" (*le germe*), and the idea of transmission by contact—remained alternative ways to explain the propagation of crowd diseases.[201] [j]

While traditional speculation about epidemics yielded the idea that a single "disease" could be common to a number of persons, two further components—specificity and materiality—were needed.

As already discussed above, "specificity" of the *remedy* was a Paracelsan contribution, descended from the Galenic remedy which cured "by its whole substance" and from the medieval *remedia appropriata.* "Specificity" was attached to the patient's *disease* by Sydenham's "specific exaltation" of the humors.

[i]Disease "seeds," a neo-Platonic concept (see above, p. 29), figured prominently in Paracelsus' philosophy (*Divided Legacy,* I, 440, 449; Jolande Jacobi, ed., *Paracelsus: Selected Writings* [New York: Bollingen, 1958], *passim*).

[j]See "Infection," in *Dictionnaire,* which distinguishes "infection" by particles in the air from "contagion" by touch. In the seventeenth century "virus" (*le virus*) meant a poison of atmospheric or animal (snake, insect) origin. In the eighteenth century it acquired the meaning of poisonous disease product (of rabies, smallpox, etc.) which could generate the same disease when inoculated into another organism.

But this vague expression left the disease in a metaphysical limbo—more than a function of the organism's humoral balance but not yet an independent being.[k] To attain metaphysical respectability it needed the attribute of materiality.

This was acquired through further speculation about syphilis. John Hunter states that the local venereal lesion resulting from contact with a diseased person eventually, by "absorption," gives rise to a venereal "disposition" in the subject, a "constitutional disease."[202] This "disposition" or "constitutional disease," moreover, is "specific"—"a peculiar mode of action . . . different from all other actions attending inflammation; and it is this specific mode of action which produces the specific quality in the matter."[203] The relationship between the acute form of syphilis (i.e., the local lesion) and this "disposition" parallels the traditional relationship between acute and chronic disease.[204]

Syphilis was thus removed some metaphysical distance away from Sydenham's mere "specific exaltation" of the humors. A final attribute of the "disease entity" was heritability: although Hunter himself rejected congenital syphilis, by the early nineteenth century it was an accepted fact.[205]

Another illness whose analysis contributed to the new doctrine of specific diseases was smallpox.

Since at least the sixteenth century the folk medicine of Greece and Turkey had employed inoculation against smallpox, the peasants realizing that the inoculated variety of the disease was usually less serious than the natural form.[206] [l]

[k]The French *"maladie"* means both "functional disturbance of a single person" and "discrete disease common to many," reflecting the unstable relationship between the two concepts. While the English "disease" originally meant the former (i.e., "dis-ease"), it has come to mean the latter.

Viscount Bolingbroke (1678-1751) made fun of this medical confusion with the epigram that diseases are "beings, bare and empty of all substance, treated scientifically."

[l]The practice may have originated in Circassia from a desire to preserve the faces of the women, renowned for their beauty and constituting the area's major export (to the harems of the Ottoman Empire).

A better technique than inoculation—insertion of a moist smallpox scab into the nostrils—which avoided the complications and side-effects of inoculation as

The practice was introduced into England in 1721 by Lady Mary Wortley Montagu, wife of the British ambassador to thc Sublime Porte.

That any major medical improvement should come from the lay public rather than the profession, that the disease "seed" (*le germe*) existed in the pustular matter, that the coction process could be bypassed, and that inoculation conferred immunity against a later attack—were all unsettling ideas, and the medical profession resisted inoculation for many decades.[207] But eventually immunity (or habituation) became part of the fabric of medical thought—to be attached, as a possible attribute, to other specific diseases.[m]

Hunter noted in 1786 that a person recently cured of gonorrhoea is, for a time, more difficult to reinfect.[208]

The mirror-image of immunity is susceptibility, and Hunter states that not everyone is infected equally easily with the venereal disease. Some are more susceptible than others: "every animal may be said to have natural tendencies to morbid actions, which may be considered as predisposing causes, and these may be called into action whenever the immediate cause takes place."[209] Differences in the manifestations of syphilis from one person to another reflect "the different dispositions which the solids are in at the time; for I can easily conceive that a peculiarity of constitution may make a very material difference in the appearance of the same specific complaint."[210]

His use of the words, "disposition" and "constitution," points to the origin of "susceptibility."

Galenic medicine had assumed that one of the four humors in the normal healthy body could be in excess, predisposing the subject to the diseases associated with that humor. This particular "temperament," "diathesis," or "constitution" could be passed from parent to child and was

well as the transmission of other diseases associated with this practice, had earlier been reported by Francois Xavier Dentrecolles (1664-1741) and other Jesuit missionaries from China but had not made a profound impression on European popular or professional medical thought (Sprengel, *Histoire de la Medecine,* VI, 33 ff.).

[m]At first the word, "habituation," was used. "Immunity" was introduced into the medical vocabulary only in 1833. See below, p. 517.

called, in technical language, the "proegumenal" (predisposing) cause of the disease.

In the eighteenth century the proegumenal cause underwent a change in meaning. Just as (with Sydenham) the "specific disease" became separated from its humoral background, so the proegumenal cause became separated from the mixture of humors in the body and came to mean a condition qualitatively different from any mixture of the four humors.

This occurred through a change in the meaning of "diathesis" (the Greek word for "disposition," "state," "condition," etc.). Originally synonymous with "temperament" or "constitution," after the mid-eighteenth century it lost this neutral denotation and became synonymous with "cachexie" or "cachexia"—"an evil disposition of the body when all the nutriment turns into evil humors."[211] [n]

C. F. Daniel in 1781 contrasts the four traditional Galenic temperaments, which are "natural," with the "hereditary diathesis" which is "preternatural."[212] Cullen invokes the *"diathesis phlogistica"* as an element which exacerbates a fever.[213] The *Encyclopedie* accepts this "inflammatory diathesis," the "scorbutic diathesis," and others.[214] Jean-Charles Grimaud (1750-1789), a leader of the Montpellier School, adds to the four Galenic diatheses the "putrid bilious," "putrid mucous," and others; he attributes rickets and phthisis to a "hereditary disposition."[215] The editor of the 1815 edition of his writings calls "hereditary disease" one of the "predisposing causes" of disease, likening it to a "morbific seed" or disease "germ" in the subject's constitution which, when sufficiently developed, emerges as a true "disease."[216]

Etienne Pariset in 1814 called attention to the change in meaning of "diathesis." The neutral term is now "temperament" or "disposition." When one of these is *carried to an*

[n]Willis defined "diathesis" as "affection or disposition" (*Pharmaceutice Rationalis* [London: Dring, 1679], *A Table of all the Hard Words Derived from Greek and Latin.* In 1741 the *Chambers Cyclopedia* defined "diathesis" as "a term used by some writers in the same sense with constitution" (E. Chambers, *Cyclopedia,* Fifth Edition, 1741).

extreme, it turns into a "diathesis." And the "diathesis," in turn, is related to the "cachexia" as cause to effect.[217]

One of the diseases in which the concept of diathesis figured prominently was scabies. While Cullen and Wichmann regarded scabies as a local disease of the skin caused by the itch-mite,[218] more profound thinkers treated it with greater respect. Autenrieth in 1807 called it a constitutional disease associated with a "virus" which could be inherited or transferred by contact and was often complicated by gout, rheumatism, and syphilis.[219] The 1812 *Dictionnaire* states that it can be inherited, or contracted by contact if the individual is predisposed. It can also be provoked by some supervening disease: "the common people then say that the master seed was in the skin." Syphilis, in particular, can bring to the surface a hereditary "scabious taint."[220]

John Brown assimilated his "sthenic" and "asthenic" states of the body to "diatheses," thus upholding the idea of the disease as an entity apart from the normal physiology of the organism.[221] "Specificity," however, was quite alien to his system.

Cullen employed the concepts: "taint," "depraved state of the fluids," "hereditary disease," "phlogistic diathesis," "rachitic" or "scrophulous" "disposition," etc. as variables generating diseases or complicating them.[222] He attributed a whole class of diseases to "cachexies."[223]

Barthez assimilated the miasms of contagious diseases to poisons which attack the life principle directly. Syphilis, for instance, can be contracted in this way, without any local lesion.[224] [o] The "susceptibility" of the organism is an important factor in poisonings, and each poison or morbific virus acts by introducing a particular *"maniere d'etre"* into the life principle—"like Van Helmont's disease idea." Hence men with rabies walk on all fours, bark and snap like dogs, etc.[225] Gout is from a "specific gouty state of the humors" or "gouty diathesis" which is not just a "disposition of the constitution" but a "special disease."[226]

[o]Hunter had hypothesized that one case of syphilis in 10,000 could pass from the initial contact to the constitutional form without manifesting any local lesion (*Works,* II, 382).

These examples show how some eighteenth-century thinkers moved from the idea of disease as a mere function of the physiology to a somewhat different view—that disease is an entity with life or being of its own. This materialization of disease, while promoted by medical awareness of specificity, immunity, and the contagiousness of epidemic diseases, was also generated by the inner tension of the Rationalist definition of disease: disease and health, while "opposites," were still the product of the same combinations of elements or chemicals, the same hydraulic system in the body. But how could they be "opposite" one another if derived from the same source? This metaphysical ambiguity was laid to rest by making disease physical and stressing its independence of the body's humors or chemical elements.

Pinel reported on all of these trends in medical thought without allowing his system to be altered by them. Scabies (*dartres*) is both a local and a constitutional disease ("to use an expression of Hunter's") resulting from a scabious taint (*vice dartreux*).[227] Improper local applications can transform it into an even more serious chronic illness, and local treatment must therefore be combined with constitutional.[228] Scrophula is from a "scrophulous taint,"[229] and the first stage of phthisis is a "proximate disposition to phthisis."[230]

His discussion of syphilis is in the same vein. Calling Hunter's book on the subject "one of the most original and profound to have appeared in many years," he states that the venereal "poison" (*virus*) is contagious and is communicated "by a sort of inoculation beneath the epidermis" upon contact of the genitals.[231] Thence it is propagated through the body *via* the lymphatic system and becomes a "general disease, so to speak, constitutional."[232] "In order that the poison introduced into the system of the liquids should affect certain glands, these must be amenable [*sensibles*] to its action; hence it can rest more or less hidden and develop subsequently as a result of other external circumstances or predisposing causes such as overeating, pregnancy, etc."[233]

He concludes that recent discoveries about the lymphatic system have made it possible to distinguish local diseases from "constitutional" ones and that what Hunter has done for venereal diseases may perhaps be extended to others.[234]

Pinel's hint that diseases may be introduced from the outside and take possession of the organism, thus becoming "constitutional," ran counter to his definition of disease as a "fleeting change . . . in the vital functions" and raised the possibility of disease an an entity apart from the mere changes in the *physis.* His recommendation that Hunter's analysis of syphilis be extended to other diseases was an invitation to invent new "specific diseases," to fill his own abstract symptom categories with new content.

The invitation was accepted only a few years later. The 1808 Paris Dissertation of an otherwise undistinguished student, one A. Darbefeuille, transformed Pinel's symptom-syndromes into a system of disease entities by materializing the diathesis in a far-reaching way.[235]

In addition to the four Galenic diatheses Darbefeuille accepted a "nervous diathesis," due to excess cerebral excitability, and "septic," "ataxic" and "virulent" diatheses caused by "more or less profound degeneration of the system of forces and humors due to miasms, viruses, etc."[236] The latter are responsible for syphilis, smallpox, measles, scarlet fever, zona, urticaria, cancer, and others.[237] Thus the diathesis is a "specific degeneration of the system effected by agents which we call viruses."[238] "The material cause of each species, its nature and *genie,* are determined with precision."[239] [p]

The promotion of the diathesis to the rank of "specific disease" is seen in Darbefeuille's calling it a "material state." "This name more faithfully characterizes the changes in the animal economy than those given by Pinel. The name of the disease should set forth its material state. What really medical information does the name, 'adeno-nervous,' convey to the student? Can it be the precise sign of the material state which

[p]The word, *"genie,"* denoting the *divinum quid* of a disease, was much favored in Montpellier.

constitutes plague? Are [Pinel's] other denominations more precise?"[240]

Being material states, the diatheses are superior in rank to the local or organic disease manifestations. They can "affect each system, each organ which modifies them, according to its tissue composition [*pace* Bichat] . . . according to its mode of vitality . . . from this result the forms of diseases, formal states, local affections, which are so numerous and which receive their names from the affected organ or from the nature of the essential symptoms—such as pleuritis, apoplexy, etc."[241] These latter conditions, which are "formal states," "determine the particular affections which, being secondary diseases, are not part of the general disease."[242] And many apparently dissimilar diseases could now be grouped together as derivatives of a smaller number of materialized diatheses; they "may appear essentially different to the vulgar physician [but] are necessarily dependent on an identical determining cause—which must be remedied to ensure the complete cure of the secondary disease."[243] The "mucous diathesis," for instance, yields rickets, scabies, scrophula, and worms.[244] Scurvy and typhus are the effects of a septic-ataxic diathesis.[245]

All nosography must proceed henceforth from an understanding of the diatheses, these "material states."[246] Therapeutics will be simplified, since knowledge of the "material state must give the first, most direct, and most curative indication, while the indication from the formal state is in general only secondary, accessory, and always subordinated to the first."[247]

Darbefeuille's thesis was immediately picked up and presented to the general public in Pariset's article on the "Diathesis." He observes that, beside the four Galenic diatheses, the moderns also recognize the scabious, cancerous,[q] scrophulous, and gouty diatheses—usually congenital, and the verminous, scorbutic, gangrenous, and syphilitic ones—usually acquired by contact.[248] Darbefeuille, however,

[q]Another article in the *Dictionnaire* discusses the cancerous diathesis. The existence of this "cancerous taint" (*vice cancereux*) makes it inadvisable to operate in cancer; an operation only drives the "taint" further into the organism where it assumes a more malignant form ("Cancer" in *Dictionnaire*).

has added to the list a number of diatheses associated with various infectious or contagious miasms, viruses, and emanations: for instance, the smallpox diathesis associated with the smallpox virus; thus he agrees with F. Hoffmann who held that the smallpox virus exists primitively in the organism and only waits for an opportunity to manifest itself.

The diathesis differs from the "disposition" and can coexist with it. An understanding of diatheses is indispensable to nosology, especially in connection with epidemic diseases. Finally, it is essential to an understanding of therapeutics: for example, one would never let blood in a disease generated by a bilious diathesis.

Another prominent Paris physician to incorporate the diathesis in his medical writings was Gaspard Laurent Bayle (1774-1816)—commonly regarded as a founder of pathological anatomy but who is more significant as a theoretician of vitalist therapeutics.

Like Pinel, Bayle was first destined for the cloth and then studied medicine at Montpellier. After two years in the medical service of the armies he came to Paris and wrote a dissertation on nosology under Cabanis.[249] He went as physician to the Charité, where he made a towering reputation, and finally became one of the medical attendants of Napoleon. He died at age 40 of tuberculosis—the disease upon which he had written his most famous work.

Bayle was particularly concerned with: 1) the classification of diseases and 2) the relationship between symptoms and pathology.

His dissertation in 1802 discussed the first question and concluded that, for the time being at least, no scientific nosology of diseases can be created.[250] While a few diseases such as measles, plague, rabies, and syphilis truly deserve the name of species, all other species, genera, and classes are only abstractions.[251]

His 1805 article on therapeutics adopted a Hippocratic approach: reliance on the *physis,* expectancy, an aphoristic method of describing diseases, and frequent invocation of experience as the source of knowledge.[252] Bayle notes, however, that constitutional syphilis can be treated directly with mercurial remedies, as can scabies: in the latter case the mercury [*sic*] kills the *Acarus scabiei.*[253]

His 1810 classic on pulmonary phthisis developed many of the ideas advanced by Darbefeuille. Bayle professed ignorance of internal pathology, having "never penetrated the secrets which the Almighty seems to have reserved to Himself," but the signs, symptoms, course, effects, transformations, and occasional causes of diseases can be observed by the physician.[254] [r] The cause of phthisis is a "tuberculous diathesis" of a "special nature" which can generate any one of six apparently different varieties of pulmonary phthisis: granulous phthisis, phthisis with melanoses, cancerous phthisis, and three others.[255] Moreover, this diathesis can be present without any pathognomic symptoms (such as cough or expectoration): patients often die of emaciation and a hectic fever without further symptoms.[256] And phthisis exists even prior to the stage of hectic fever and emaciation.[257] The lung lesions are the first visible pathology produced by the tuberculous diathesis.[258]

Treatment should always be directed against the diathesis.[259] While none of the known methods are effective, one possibility would be to reduce the "excitability" of the lungs (following Bichat? Brown?) with *Belladonna, Aconitum napellus, Hyoscyamus,* or *Conium.*[260]

In 1812 Bayle wrote an article, "Pathological Anatomy (General Considerations on the Assistance which Anatomy can Furnish to Medicine)," giving the results of his decade of reflection on some of medicine's fundamental philosophical issues.[261]

All pathological change commences with symptomatic changes which may be called "vital symptoms" or "vital lesions." When carried far enough, these give rise to organic changes which, in turn, generate "physical symptoms."[s] For

[r] The title page of this work contains a quotation from Baglivi on the impossibility of attaining knowledge of the proximate causes of diseases.

[s] Only the "germ" (*le germe*) of the disease exists prior to the appearance of these "physical symptoms" (Bayle, "Anatomie Pathologique" in *Dictionnaire*).

example, in phthisis the degeneration of the lungs causes difficult breathing, coughing, spitting of blood, etc.

The exciting cause of the "vital lesions" is unknown except where the disease is contagious (syphilis, plague, smallpox, etc.).

Diseases can thus be divided into three groups. The first are those which are not contagious and where the "vital lesions" or "vital symptoms" cause no organic change (typical would be apoplexy). Pathological anatomy is of no assistance to nosology here. The second are the contagious diseases: while pathological anatomy is of some value to their nosology, classification is primarily determined by the contagious principle. The third are non-contagious diseases in which the "vital lesions" or "vital symptoms" give rise to an organic lesion and thereupon to organic disease: here pathological anatomy is useful for nosology.

But symptom patterns often do not correspond to pathological changes. Patients succumbing to a chronic diarrhoea sometimes have ulcerated intestines and sometimes not. Some who die of emaciation with brown vomit have stomach cancer, others not. And, on the contrary, some with stomach cancer have brown vomit and epigastric pains, others not. Some with ulcerated lungs have the typical phthisis symptoms, others not, etc. Preference here must be given to the pathological alterations and the "physical symptoms" caused by these alterations, with the "vital" lesions and symptoms relegated to second place. The defect of Sauvages' nosology was to rely mainly on the "vital," and not the "physical," symptoms.

In evaluating the disease class, moreover, the type of pathological change (*mode d'alteration*) is very important.

But the physician must always remember that pathological anatomy shows only the effects of the disease without providing insight into its essential nature. Physical changes are the effects of preexisting changes in the vitality. Hence, while "physical symptoms" may be the best guides to classification, the "vital" symptoms and lesions are the best guides to treatment.[262]

Thus Bayle remained a Hippocratic. One need not know the nature of the disease to treat it properly, only characteristic symptoms and medicines whose use is supported by long experience.[263] In many cases expectancy is appropriate, "not that erroneous expectant treatment which, without rule and without lights, combats unimportant symptoms, but that enlightened and steady symptomatic treatment which sometimes remedies alarming or dangerous symptoms and sometimes treats the disease according to the symptoms which bring it closest to some other species."[264]

Treatment is always easier when the disease is still in its vital stage, prior to serious organic degeneration.[265] Once the organic lesion has become serious, the disease is usually incurable, and palliative remedies only may be employed.[266]

The major thinker during these years was, of course, Rene Laennec, a Breton from Quimper who was a close friend of Bayle's and carried his ideas through to their ultimate development.

He studied medicine at Nantes and, after a period in the army, came to Paris for further work under Bichat,[t] Corvisart, and Guillaume Dupuytren (1777-1835).[u] In 1803 he graduated from the Ecole de Santé with first prizes in medicine and surgery. After some years in private practice he was appointed in 1816 to the Hopital Necker where he elaborated the theory and practice of mediate auscultation, publishing his great work on the subject in 1819.[267] Poor health then compelled him to retire for three years to his native Brittany, but in 1822 he returned as professor at the Charité and the Collège de France and personal physician to the crown princess. At this time he led the campaign against Broussais. He died of tuberculosis in 1826 at the age of 46.[268]

[t]He called Bichat's *Anatomie Generale* an "anatomy for physicians" and a work of genius (*Laennec, Documents Inedits Publies a l'Occasion de Son Centenaire* [Paris: Masson, 1926], 26).

[u]Guillaume Dupuytren was the most successful surgeon of his time, leaving at his death 200,000 francs for a chair of pathological anatomy at the Faculté. He taught surgical clinics at the Hotel-Dieu and was surgeon-in-chief of that institution (M. C. Perdrix, *Notices Historiques et Biographiques sur Ambroise Pare et Guillaume Dupuytren* [Paris: Crapelet, 1836]).

Like Bayle, Laennec is known to history as a founder of pathological anatomy (and, to medical students, as the inventor of the stethoscope), but he was more important as a theoretician of medicine who devised new solutions to many of the traditional problems.

His two foci of interest were the criteria of disease classification and the relationship between symptoms and internal pathology.

Laennec was educated as a Hippocratic. As already mentioned, he was sponsored in medicine by his uncle, a Montpellier graduate, whom he called his "second father" and to whom his dissertation, *Propositions on the Hippocratic Doctrine as it Relates to Practical Medicine,* was dedicated.[269] The Hippocratic faith burned as brightly in the end of his life. His nephew wrote in 1831 that Laennec was a complete vitalist and followed the Montpellierien, Jean-Charles Grimaud, in viewing diseases as "to some extent accidental functions, or, in other words, the result of a reaction of the vital principle against something harmful; in a word, he was as warm a partisan as anyone of the *physis* of Hippocrates."[270 v]

But this classic Hippocratic view that disease is one (and, at the same time, infinitely varied) conflicted in Laennec's mind with the trend of contemporary medical thinking in favor of isolating a finite group of discrete "diseases," materializing them, and rooting them in some internal pathological alteration or contagious principle. The heightened frequency of contagious and epidemic diseases in these decades of war, revolution, and social upheaval strengthened the orientation of medical thinking toward the "disease" rather than the patient.

The dualism of Laennec's thinking can be seen in his dissertation which attempts to determine whether Hippocrates regarded all diseases as essentially one (and all the

[v]Ackerknecht writes that in the notes for his last lecture course Laennec was an "aggressive polemicist for Hippocratic medicine, more so than in his published [works]" (E. Ackerknecht, "Laennec und sein Vorlesungsmanuskript von 1822," *Gesnerus* XXI [1964], 142-153, at 152).

different symptom-patterns as epiphenomena of this one disease) or, on the contrary, divided them into classes. For instance, he wonders whether Hippocrates considered all "fevers" to be one or ranged them in the five classes accepted by the late eighteenth century: inflammatory, bilious, mucous, putrid, and malignant.[271] All his later medical speculation wrestles with this dichotomy. Are diseases finite in number or infinite, and what are the criteria distinguishing them from one another?

Bayle had begun incorporating the contagious principle and the diathesis into nosological theory, combining them with speculation about "physical" and "vital" lesions and symptoms. Laennec brought this line of thought to a culmination, fusing the contagious principle, the diathesis, the *propria* and *communia,* and pathological anatomy in a synthesis which was perhaps as far as Hippocratic thinking could proceed in the absence of an input from chemistry and pharmacology.

As his dissertation title indicates, he was oriented toward practice. The purpose of medicine is the cure of diseases, but "to cure diseases one must know them, [and] to know them one must study them from all angles, using observation to ascertain the facts, reasoning to compare them, to classify them in the memory, and to recognize similar cases."[272]

Laennec appears to suggest the need for a nosology, but his Hippocratic instincts block the way: "the nature of the science which we cultivate does not, it seems, permit us to hope for a solution to [the problem of nosology]. Zoological and botanical disease species are beings [*etres*], while diseases are only modifications in the texture of the organs of the animal economy, in the composition of its liquids, or in the order of its functions."[273]

So a nosology is not possible, but the physician must still distinguish among apparently similar cases.[274]

And on this knife-edge—rejecting the possibility of a nosology but accepting the need to distinguish among similar cases—Laennec erected his theoretical structure.

He assumes at the outset that proximate causes are unknowable: "the futility of this sort of investigation is sufficiently demonstrated by the profound oblivion into which all such theories have lapsed at the death of their authors."[275]

He therefore had to look elsewhere for the criteria distinguishing one sick person from another and found them in the other types of disease causes—occasional, predisposing, and exciting.

The principal occasional cause is interference with one of the body's natural functions either in health or during treatment. Bronchial hemorrhage is caused by suppression of some other habitual hemorrhage (menses, bleeding hemorrhoids, etc.); hemoptysis often replaces suppressed menses and with the same periodicity; suppression of hemorrhoids can lead to pulmonary apoplexy.[276] Phthisis is occasioned by suppression of the menses or by incorrect treatment of a skin disease, driving it inward toward the lungs.[277] Pleurisy can be caused by suppressing gout, rheumatism, scabies, some customary evacuation, or a skin disease.[278] Syphilis, whooping cough, scurvy, and eruptive fevers can all be occasional causes of an outbreak of phthisis.[279] Most serious heart diseases are due to neglecting a common cold.[280]

Next to be considered are the predisposing (proegumenal) causes upon which these occasional causes operate. They are, above all, the various inherited or acquired diatheses. The syphilitic diathesis, for example, is transmitted by a virus or poison which passes by physical contact.[281] But other predisposing causes are congenital, common to whole families, an example being the tubercular diathesis.[282] It is then a latent state which can be triggered by any one of a number of occasional or exciting causes.[283] For example, an inflammation can hasten the development of tubercles in the lungs

> to which the patient was predisposed by a cause as yet unknown to us, but one which is certainly different from the inflammation itself; the organic movements which constitute the inflammation cannot in themselves produce the tubercles, but the excess movement and nutrition of the inflammatory upsurge have accelerated the appearance of a quite different modification of the economy. Thus, to use an expression which is perhaps

> not as alien to the subject as it appears, in this way the earth which is heavily plowed after a long fallow period, or abandoned to itself after many years of working, causes the germination of [*fait germer*] a multitude of seeds which it has contained within itself for years.[284]

The form taken by the tubercles is different in a scrophulous patient than in one who does not have a scrophulous diathesis.[285]

Finally there are the exciting causes: "diseases are modifications in the animal economy which can be produced by all the physical and chemical agents and, what is more, by aberrations of the vital actions."[286] [w] Laennec includes as exciting causes: disease "constitutions," shocks, physical injuries, emotional disturbances, viruses, and poisons.[287]

He made a study of the "constitutions" of the years 1804-1814, concluding that each such "constitution" has a "peculiarity" or "specificity" (*genie*) which it imprints upon all the diseases occurring during its period of dominance.[288] But he carried this line of analysis even further: any exciting, occasional, or predisposing cause of disease imprints its own specificity upon the disease:

> The causes of diseases are unfortunately most often beyond our reach; but experience shows us every day that they establish greater differences, at least as regards therapeutics, than the *physis* itself and the species of local organic lesions . . .[289]

For example, skin inflammations caused by simple puncture with a pin, by inoculation with anthrax, or by inoculation with smallpox virus will differ considerably from one another.[290]

And all these factors affect the nature of the treatment: "many pleuresies and cases of peritonitis yield no better to bloodletting than a bubo or a venereal ulcer on the neck, or a tumor of the knee due to gout, or the inflammation preceding hospital gangrene."[291]

[w]Pinel had also suggested that disease species are determined by exciting causes (*Nosographie Philosophique,* 1802, I, liii).

The exciting, predisposing, and occasional causes, singly or in combination, give rise first to symptoms and then to organic changes. Following Bayle, Laennec divides diseases into two classes: those which are purely "vital" (called, as he notes, "nervous diseases" in the eighteenth century) and those in which alterations of the vitality have proceeded far enough to generate organic disease.[292] "Inflammation," a vital act involving an increase of blood in the capillaries, is the intermediate link between "vital" and "organic" diseases, causing alterations in the texture of the organs and the formation of accidental tissue.[293]

In purely "vital" diseases the first step is a careful analysis of the symptoms. Laennec had an assistant take a thorough anamnesis, setting down all information in writing. Then he examined the patient himself, "neglecting nothing as useless," and adding to what had already been recorded.[294] [x] To ensure that the description was graphic, and to aid the memory, all measurements were made in terms of familiar objects: "the thickness of an almond, a pea, or a grain of millet . . . these terms present to the mind something more positive and better suited to the immediate description of the object."[295] The physician also inquired about occasional, exciting, or predisposing causes: an example of the latter might be hereditary phthisis.[296]

Since these diseases, by definition, manifest no pathological-anatomical changes, one patient must be distinguished from another by symptoms alone. Here Laennec followed the lead of Sydenham, Baglivi, and Pinel in modifying the ancient doctrine of *propria* and *communia* to hold that the *propria* (Sydenham's "peculiar" and "constant" symptoms) reveal the "disease" type, and are hence the basis of classification, while the *communia* (Sydenham's "common" and "adventitious" symptoms) serve to distinguish among the patients suffering from the same "disease."[297] [y] Being determined by

[x] Laennec's colleagues seem to have felt that many of his symptomatic descriptions were excessively long (*Auscultation Mediate,* 1819, I, xxviii). This was certainly the opinion of Broussais and his followers (see below, p. 498).

[y] See above, p. 204. Laennec was a tremendous admirer of Sydenham and Baglivi (*Auscultation Mediate,* 1819, II, 89; 1831, II, 404. See, also, *Traite Inedit sur l'Anatomie Pathologique* [Paris: Alcan, 1884], Title Page and 19).

climate and geography, as well as by the patient's idiosyncrasy, the *communia* indicate the greater or lesser degree of commotion in the patient's organism and are hence valuable for prognosis and treatment.[298]

Experienced practitioners are interested mainly in the *communia*, being concerned primarily with treatment. Only the younger generation of physician, who are interested more in the nosological aspects of medicine than in treatment, seek to ascertain the *propria*.[299]

The diseases with the most clearly defined *propria* are the epidemic and contagious diseases which Laennec's colleagues were investigating: the exciting cause, equivalent to a virus or poison, always yields symptoms making it easy to recognize such a disease.[300] But other diseases as well can be diagnosed and recognized by an appropriate symptom analysis.

Sydenham had originated the idea of disease specificity with his "specific exaltation" of the humors, and it was only appropriate that Laennec should look to him for an appropriate resolution of the problems associated with this new idea. Carried away by enthusiasm, however, he attributed this view to Hippocrates himself, although there is no mention of *propria* and *communia* in the Hippocratic Corpus.[302] [z] Such a distinction among symptoms was seen first in the ancient Empirical writings and is discussed most comprehensively by Celsus.[a] Needless to say, the ancient theory of *propria* and *communia* was the precise opposite of Laennec's doctrine, as the *propria* served to distinguish one patient from another, while the *communia* were ignored

[z]Laennec eventually admits this, stating that Hippocrates "carefully removed" from his writings all discussion of *propria* and *communia* (*sic*) (*Propositions sur la Doctrine d'Hippocrate,* 16). He does, however, seek support in *Epidemics* I, cap. XXIII: "learning from the common nature [*koines physios*] of all and the particular [*idies*] nature of the individual," but, since Galen at least, this passage has been taken to mean the common and particular natures of all *men*, not of all *diseases.* Laennec disputes Galen's interpretation of this passage on grammatical grounds (*Propositions,* 12). It is discussed in *Divided Legacy,* I, 22, 32, 251.

[a]Laennec calls Celsus "one of the best interpreters of ancient medicine" (*Laennec, Documents Inedits.* 15).

entirely.[b] But when a new level of analysis (the "disease") was interposed between the "common nature of all" and the "particular nature of the individual," the ancient categories had to be rearranged.

Laennec goes on to the diseases characterized by organic alterations. If they depend on a contagious principle, this principle remains the criterion of classification and is more significant than the pathological changes.[303] But in the absence of such a principle the physician must determine the relative weight and importance of symptoms and pathological-anatomical findings.

He was, of course, a pioneer of pathological anatomy, but his ideas here were misinterpreted by later generations for, as always, he was torn in two different directions. His Hippocratic and vitalist instincts conflicted steadily with his own anatomical discoveries, and most of his professional career he spent puzzling over the correct relations between symptoms and pathology.

In the first place, pathological changes are not the causes but the effects of alterations in the symptoms. Laennec agreed with Bayle that "vital" symptoms and lesions precede "organic." Many organic changes are fleeting and variable; many come into existence only during the death agony.[304] Furthermore, and this is most important, they are less numerous than the diseases generated by the variety of occasional, predisposing, and exciting causes. These latter "establish greater differences . . . than the species of local organic lesions."[305]

Thus pathological anatomy has only a subsidiary role. It is less important than the symptoms, as these latter point to the occasional, predisposing, and exciting causes which confer upon each disease its specific quality:

> I am far from denying the utility of a study of the anatomical species of diseases. I have scarcely occupied myself with anything else . . . I think that this study is

[b]The correct interpretation of *propria* and *communia* is that of Cabanis (above, p. 446).

> the only basis of positive knowledge in medicine and that it should never be forgotten in etiological investigations—which will otherwise become a pursuit of chimeras and a creation of phantoms . . . But I believe equally that it is dangerous to concentrate so exclusively on local affections that one loses sight of the different [occasional, exciting, or predisposing] causes upon which they may depend or, if you will, their known or hidden specificity [*genie connu ou cache*]. The inevitable disadvantage of such a shortsighted approach is often to mistake effect for cause and to fall into the still more serious error of considering as identical, and treating by the same methods, diseases *whose only visible alterations are similar anatomical lesions.* This error is due to a mediocre study of pathological anatomy.[306]

How does the physician avoid distorting his understanding of diseases by forcing them into a set of pathological pigeonholes less numerous than the diseases themselves?

Laennec tackled this problem early in his career, proposing a doctrine of specific pathological alterations in place of Bichat's and Morgagni's classification of pathological lesions according to locus alone.[307] [c] He owed this to Bichat's "general affections" which are identical in whatever part of the body they appear and differ from one another by their specificity rather than according to locus. While Bichat had recognized only cancer and inflammation as such "general affections," Laennec held that other *modes de lesion* would be discovered, equally capable of affecting a number of tissues and organs simultaneously and each associated with a given exciting cause or diathesis.[308]

He held that Pinel's "essential fevers" were precisely these sorts of general diseases.[309]

As a start Laennec proposed that all organic alterations be reduced to: alterations of texture, alterations of the

[c]Dupuytren bitterly disputed Laennec's priority in this (see his "Observations sur la Note Relative aux Alterations Organiques Publiee par M. Laennec dans le Dernier Numero du *Journal de Medecine,*" *Journal de Medecine, Chirurgie, Pharmacie* IX [1804-1805], 441-446).

nutritive process, alterations of form and position, and alterations associated with the presence of animate foreign bodies (worms and insects)—a more lifelike reflection of the *physis* and more useful for practice than the purely anatomical divisions of Bichat and Morgagni.[310]

This doctrine of specific tissue alteration was to be developed further by Bretonneau.[d]

The other problem, however, still remained: specific tissue alterations are subsequent to the symptoms. Laennec, therefore, was ambiguous about the role of pathological anatomy in the diagnosis and recognition of diseases.

He agreed that the same symptom-pattern can arise from different exciting causes, and the true nature of the disorder can be recognized only by pathological investigation.[311] Anyone can diagnose peritonitis if he has been trained in pathological anatomy, but those used to relying only on symptoms will sometimes call it an ileus, sometimes a hepatic colic, sometimes puerperal fever.[312] And the same applies to other diseases.[313] Whether obtained from autopsies or from mediate auscultation,[e] pathological-anatomical knowledge lends brevity and clarity to symptomatic descriptions and helps elucidate their meaning.[314]

But this cannot be carried too far. First of all, pathological alterations are localized, while disease is a phenomenon affecting the whole organism.[315] Pathological categories are too crude and must be read in conjunction with the symptoms to be correctly understood.[316]

> Above all, in transporting pathological anatomy into practical medicine, one must follow Hoffmann's principle of never doing anything of importance out of mere conjecture or hypothesis and refrain from thinking that precise knowledge of the disease species and its seat dispenses the physician from studying its *genie propre* and its indications in the reigning epidemic as in the idiosyncrasy of the patient.[317]

[d]See below, pp. 508-511.

[e]See below, pp. 486-488.

And the *communia* reveal the idiosyncrasy of the patient—his personal reaction to the disease; they must determine the course of treatment.[318] Laennec advised physicians to make a careful study of these "general symptoms" (*communia*)—in particular, information from the pulse as set forth in the writings of James Nihell and Solano de Luques.[319]

At the same time, the *communia* serve to refine the disease categories, since precise knowledge of the nosological species is given ultimately by the success of treatment.[320 f]

Laennec concludes that perhaps the most useful information to be obtained from pathological research (including mediate auscultation) is whether or not the patient is curable.[321]

In a sense he inverted the traditional Rationalist doctrine of symptoms and pathology. Whereas this tradition formed its disease entities on a pathological basis, introducing symptoms only to differentiate diseased states within the given pathological category, Laennec formed his disease classes symptomatically and used pathological anatomy to differentiate within a given symptomatic class. Pathological anatomy is an independent body of descriptive knowledge, an independent input into the diagnosis of diseases. Pathological-anatomical alterations are not necessarily connected to changes in the symptoms. Laennec went so far as to urge that this knowledge be isolated from the symptoms, the locus of the alterations, and from practical medicine generally—in a separate category with its own rules based on "the nature of the objects themselves."[322]

> One must consider the consequences of a disease as no longer having any connection with the disease which has produced them; in pathological anatomy the lesions, being the principal objects of our research, should be classified according to their own characteristics and not according to their [occasional, predisposing, or exciting] causes.[323]

[f]Unfortunately, since the *Auscultation Mediate* was not a treatise of practice, but a guide to diagnosis, Laennec deliberately omitted discussion of the *"signes generaux, communs, et, par consequent, incertains"* (*Auscultation Mediate,* 1819, I, xxiii).

For all of these reasons Andral lamented that Laennec, "one of the most consummate masters [of pathological anatomy], was so often struck by the impotence of a science for which he had done so much that he is endlessly warning us against it and . . . even goes so far as to deny it where it is evident. Strange uncertainty of the opinions of men: the further Laennec advances in pathological anatomy, the more often he refuses to recognize it. Not content with taking from vitalism what it contains of truth, he refused the new teachings which, cleansing vitalism of its errors, thereby restrained its application, but even so left it as a part of the truth."[324]

Laennec's understanding of the role of mediate auscultation as a diagnostic technique becomes clear in the light of his views on pathological anatomy.

Of all areas of the body subject to pathological deterioration the thoracic cavity is the most important. As Bordeu noted, the lungs are one leg of the tripod of life and hence are involved in nearly every disease.[325] "One can even say that in all species of disease, wherever their seat, death hardly ever arrives without the thoracic organs being somehow affected."[326] But (as Baglivi pointed out) thoracic diseases all have the same symptoms: cough, dyspnoea, expectoration—which makes their differential diagnosis problematical.[327] Moreover, the symptomatic variations do not necessarily correspond to organic changes.[328]

Leopold Auenbrugger and Jean-Nicolas Corvisart had developed a technique of percussing the chest, the resulting echo telling the informed ear something about the pathological changes occurring in the thorax.[g] Laennec considered this an excellent technique: "it submits to the immediate judgment of the senses several diseases which up until then had been recognized only by general and equivocal signs; hence it made their diagnosis both certain and easy."[329] But

[g]See L. Auenbrugger, *Nouvelle Methode pour Reconnaitre les Maladies Internes de la Poitrine par la Percussion de Cette Cavite.* Translated from the Latin, with comments, by Jean-Nicolas Corvisart (Paris: Migneret, 1808). Also J. N. Corvisart, *Essai sur les Maladies et les Lesions Organiques du Coeur et des Gros Vaisseaux* (Paris: Migneret, 1806).

it had serious drawbacks: the sounds obtained were muffled and indistinct, requiring very great skill for their interpretation, and it could not be used at all to diagnose the condition of the heart.

Sometimes the sound obtained from percussion could be clarified by applying the ear to the chest, but with many (unwashed) hospital patients this would be a disgusting procedure, and it is "scarcely to be proposed with most women, while with certain ones the very size of the breasts is a physical obstacle."[330]

One day, confronted with this very problem in the case of a young lady, Laennec decided to employ a piece of rolled-up cardboard—the precursor of the stethoscope.[331]

He held information obtained from this "mediate auscultation" to be identical with the "signs" obtained from autopsies, i.e., with pathological-anatomical data, and qualitatively different from symptomatic knowledge.[332] The advantage of mediate auscultation was to make these "signs" perceptible to the senses: "it would be a mistake to think that the nosological species determined by pathological anatomy can be recognized only on autopsy. They are easier to recognize in the living person and even then present the mind something which is much clearer and more positive than any nosological distinction based only on symptoms."[333] Mediate auscultation was even more reliable than a hypothetical vivisection of the thorax, since the ear is a better judge than the eye; in heart disease, for instance, the ear can judge changes in beat and rhythm more accurately than the eye can see them.[334]

Mediate auscultation thus made it possible to decide rapidly on the anatomical basis of many diseases. A certain type of rale, and not depressed breathing, is the pathognomic sign of peripneumonia. Pectoriloquy is the true pathognomic sign of pulmonary phthisis, etc.[335]

Once the disease had been diagnosed, Laennec selected his therapeutic technique on the basis of experience.[336] He was entirely eclectic and, despite his professed Hippocraticism, borrowed methods of treatment from many other schools and currents of medical thought.[h] In emphysema he urged medicines such as alkalies, neutral salts, soap pills, and hydrogen sulfide which make the mucous secretions more liquid, promoting expectoration and facilitating breathing.[337] When these are supplemented by bloodletting and emetics against incipient suffocation, the organic lesion and functional disorder are corrected simultaneously.[338] In general, medicines should lessen the "viscosity" of the humors.[339]

In diphtheria he used leeches, bleeding, vesicatories, sinapisms, cataplasms with hydrochloric acid applied to the larynx, etc.[340]

He praised "specific" remedies such as mercury, antimony, quinine, and vaccination: "there are no medicines more powerful than those whose action cannot be explained satisfactorily."[341]

In principle, he favored symptomatic treatment (provided the main symptoms were attacked, not secondary ones). As Corvisart has noted, while the expression, "symptomatic treatment," is usually mentioned with contempt, it is actually the correct way of medicine.[342]

In the end of his life Laennec was experimenting with homoeopathy.[i]

Return to Methodism: F. J. V. Broussais

Laennec and Pinel were both contemptuous of John Brown. Pinel taunted him with "mutilating and truncating the history of diseases to subjugate them to his own system."[343] Laennec identified his sthenic and asthenic diseases with the *strictum* and *laxum* of the Methodists,[344]

[h]He held that Hippocratic medicine would be equally Hippocratic in the absence of a theory of coction. And "evacuation is rarely the path of the *physis,* since an evacuation rarely coincides with convalescence; the restoration of menses or of hemorrhoids is rather the effect of the cure than its cause. To attack [pulmonary phthisis] directly it is probably necessary to correct some unknown alteration in the assimilative or nutritive faculty, i.e., as it appears, some alteration of the liquids," etc. (see "Extrait du Discours," xvi; *Auscultation Mediate,* 1831, II, 190).

[i]See below, p. 542.

and both thinkers strove to substitute a subtle and complex nosology for the Scotsman's primitive dualism.

Their campaign, however, imposed too great a strain on the intellectual capacities of the average physician (who instinctively preferred the simpler doctrine) and eventually provoked a reaction. In 1816 Francois Joseph Victor Broussais erupted with an attack on Pinelism which soon polarized French medicine.

As Broussais had his headquarters at the Val-de-Grace Hospital, while Pinel's followers were ensconced in the Faculté, this conflict is usually given as one between the Ecole de Paris and the Val-de-Grace, but it actually represented a resurgence of the conflict between Empiricism and Methodism. Broussaisism was only Brunonian dualism turned upside down, with a majority of diseases now ascribed to excess energy rather than to its deficiency.[j]

According to one biographer Broussais "made as much noise in his life as a man could make."[345] Born in St. Malo, at age 20 he volunteered as a seaman on a privateer. In 1795 his parents were murdered by *chouants* (Catholic Royalist partisans from Brittany and the Vendee) which affected him profoundly and doubtless colored his feelings for the Catholic Royalist Laennec. He went to Paris in 1795 to study under Bichat. Graduating in 1803, he practiced two years in France and then spent three years with Napoleon's armies in Holland, Germany, Austria, Italy, and Spain, attaining the rank of *"medecin principal d'armees"* and crystallizing his therapeutic views in the military camps and hospitals.[346] "Some starting point had to be found for studying internal diseases. Well, I took it from surgery!"[347] After Waterloo he came as second physician to the Val-de-Grace.

Broussais' lifelong aim was to simplify therapeutics by simplifying medical theory, and he did this by a new application of Haller's "sensitivity" and "irritability." These two properties of healthy tissue give rise to disease as well,

[j]A Montpellier professor punned that Broussaisism *"n'est que le Brownisme retourne"*, taking advantage of the dual meaning of *retourner*—"to return" and "to turn upside down" (quoted in E. Ackerknecht, *Medicine at the Paris Hospital* [Baltimore: Johns Hopkins, 1967], 70).

and morbid processes are thus qualitatively identical with healthy ones.[348]

His dissertation, on "hectic fever," maintains that all processes in the healthy and diseased organism can be reduced to a few: "on this general law, that a large number of causes only produce a small number of effects, and on the regularity of these effects, is founded the possibility of classifying the functions in the healthy person and diseases in the sick person."[349]

He was still sufficiently under Pinel's influence (to whom the dissertation is dedicated) to admit that "hectic fever" is sometimes independent of a local lesion,[350] but within a few years he had regressed to the position that diseases are not only uniform and regular in their symptoms but also localized in the body. He selected the gastrointestinal tract as the site of all diseases and "irritation" as their generative mechanism.

In all of this Broussais was only the spokesman for a rising trend in Paris medicine, a reaction against the complexity and detail of Pinelism which burdened practice by forcing the physician to observe his patients carefully and give hard thought to the diagnosis. Physicians on the whole prefer *a priori* guidelines for diagnosis and treatment.

It was a commonplace of late eighteenth-century Rationalist theory that certain inflammatory diseases result from an "irritation."[351] P. A. Prost wrote an opus on this subject in 1804.[352] Dupuytren in 1807, through one of his degree candidates, proposed classifying diseases in terms of various "irritations"—defined as "exaltation of the organic vital forces resulting from the action of an external or *internal* [*sic*] agent."[353] These straws in the wind were ignited by the passionate, dogmatic, and eruptive personality of Broussais.

His first major production (1808), on "phlegmasies, or chronic inflammations," demonstrated tuberculosis to be merely a chronic inflammation of the lungs and the other chronic diseases to be the effects of a similar inflammation of the digestive tract.[354] "Inflammation" is rooted in the "sensitivity" of the tissues and can be successfully quelled by bleeding, sedative drugs, and abstention from food.[355]

In 1814 he started a private course whose "impact was immense: the apparent simplicity of the doctrine, the impassioned words of the master, excited an indescribable enthusiasm."[356] In this year of the great typhus epidemic physicians were looking desperately for guidance in treating the intestinal inflammation, diarrhoea, and dysentery associated with this disease.

Broussais' second major production appeared in 1816, the *Examen de la Doctrine Medicale Generalement Adoptee et des Systemes Modernes de Nosologie,* which definitively fixed on the intestinal tract as the seat of all acute fevers and diseases, great and small, and called for the same "rational" treatment as earlier advocated for chronic ones.[357] Since disease processes were identical with those in health, Broussais called his system "physiological medicine," giving this science a bad name which it took decades to live down.[358]

The devastating impact of "physiological medicine" on thought and practice is best appreciated by examining it in terms of the three problems posed by Cabanis.

His first was the criterion for classifying diseases.

Broussais simply eliminated this from consideration. He saw himself as following Haller and Bichat in viewing all tissues as possessing "sensitivity" and "contractility" or "irritability," with irritation of one leading by sympathy to the irritation of others.[359] The gastrointestinal tract, with its central location and pronounced vasculo nervous structure, is the most subject of all to such irritation—either by sympathy or from the food passing through it continually.[360] All seeming differences among diseases are due only to the unpredictable operations of sympathy.[361] The lungs or skin can be irritated by external stimuli, causing erysipelas, plague, typhus, yellow fever, etc. and then, by sympathy, local inflammation of the lungs, kidneys, or intestines.[362] Only a fool could believe in Pinel's "essential fevers" which are nothing more than general irritation of the vascular system caused by local irritation of the capillaries, obstructing the flow of blood.[363] Pinel's "mucous fever," "adynamic fever," "ataxic fever," muscular weakness," etc.—even yellow fever, cancer, scurvy, and phthisis—are only variations of the underlying gastric fever.[364]

Mental illness is only "irritation" of the brain.[365]

Broussais condemned the whole system of Hippocratic medicine.[366] The *physis* has no curative power; disease is not a reaction of the *physis* to a morbific cause; crises are dangerous and should be avoided; fever is not beneficial, etc.[367]

Infectious and contagious diseases usually affect the organism through their "harmful corpuscles or irritant vapors which develop inflammation in the aerial cavities." By irritating and filling the aerial vesicles in the lungs they "oppose the aeration of the blood and cause asphyxias as a result of which certain phlegmasies, which are very difficult to destroy, remain on the tracheobronchial surface."[368] [k]

He was outraged by the concepts of "taint" (*vice organique*), diathesis, or "disposition." "I cannot accept the reasoning of those physicians who maintain that no appreciable cause is necessary for such a degeneration merely because they cannot always understand the process of its formation. If I am offended, it is because this dialectic is false and opposed to the progress of the science of diseases."[369] The "disposition" or "taint" of an organ or part of the body is nothing more than a local inflammation there, and even cancer is due to an underlying inflammation.[370] Pinel attributes phthisis to a scrophulous taint (*vice scrophuleux*) without even explaining what this is! His school claims that the seed (*le germe*) of phthisis remains in a family for generations—pure fatalism!![371]

Broussais decried all nosology, or acceptance of "diseases," as "ontology"—the attribution of life to imaginary beings.[372] He called it illogical and empirical, leading to scientific stagnation.[373] Pinel's ignorance of anatomy led

[k]Thus typhus is not caused by a "miasm," as admitting the existence of a "particular miasm" would make typhus "a species of fever *sui generis,*" but merely by a poisonous principle in the air (*Examen,* 1816, 375; *Traite de Physiologie Appliquee a la Pathologie* [Paris: Delauney, 1822-1823], II, 75-76).

him to neglect the disease locus and its anatomical cause.[374] He should have followed Bichat's dictum: "What good is observation if the cause is unknown?"[375]

Cabanis' second problem was the relationship between symptoms and internal pathology and the criterion for distinguishing important symptoms from unimportant.

This one also disappeared when gastrointestinal inflammation was made all-important. Only the symptoms of the local inflammation were significant: all others were due to "sympathy"—hence, unimportant for diagnosis.[376] Excessive concern with the patient's symptoms imposes additional burdens on the mind which only wants "a clear idea of how to reach the sole desirable end—the best method of treatment."[377] To Broussais a "complete history" of the patient meant a complete autopsy—which would reveal definitively which symptoms had been important and which not.[378]

Since Pinel does not relate symptom pictures to proximate causes in the intestines, his syndromes are purely imaginary.[379]

Cabanis' final problem—the relationship between medicines and diseases—was the easiest of all for Broussais to solve. The inflammation is subdued by (1) removing blood from the patient and (2) reducing his intake of food (to eliminate the source of irritation in the intestines).[380] Broussais' favorite therapeutic technique was application of leeches to the stomach or anus, and his *Histoire des Phlegmasies* devoted fifteen pages to this procedure alone.[381] [1] In a recent inflammation the loss of blood may be continued until the patient falls unconscious, but it should then be promptly stanched (especially in small children).[382] A crisis, which is "not an entity expressly designed to terminate an irritative disease" but "the result of the cessation of irritation of the viscera, permitting a return of

[1]Broussais' "hirudomania" caused the importation into France of 41,500,000 leeches in 1833, with only 9 or 10 million being exported; in 1824 2-3 million had sufficed (E. Ackerknecht, "Broussais or a Forgotten Medical Revolution," *Bulletin of the History of Medicine* XXVII [1953], 320-343, at 323). According to J. Beclard they were often piled on by handfulls (*Gazette Medicale de Paris* II [1880], 399).

action toward the periphery," is dangerous and should be aborted by phlebotomy.[383]

Treatment need not be differentiated, since nearly all diseases are from the same cause and require the same remedies "whose indications I have developed and shown to be astonishingly simple."[384] For example, the different varieties of pulmonary phthisis need not be distinguished according to their exciting causes, since all such causes lead to the same result–chronic pulmonary inflammation.[385] The leading indication is to destroy the inflammation and thus prevent the development of tubercles.[386] The different varieties of lung inflammation are not separate diseases, and the physician need only "heed the appeal of the suffering organ."[387] "Adjusting treatment to the individual patient" means adjusting it to his lower intestine.[388]

All diseases were reduced to inflammation: there were no "specific" diseases and no "specific" remedies.[389]

John Brown was the greatest enemy of a sane therapeutics in ascribing most diseases to the asthenic (weakened) state, whereas they are actually caused by heightened excitement or inflammation (i.e., sthenic). Broussais forbade physicians to use stimulants such as emetics and quinine.[390] Because Pinel sometimes stimulated his patients, Broussais accused him of "disguised Brunonianism."[391] Pinel's therapeutics is "difficult and repulsive to the student, unintelligible to the man of sense, and dangerous for the practitioner."[392] It is an "insupportable empiricism," meaning devoid of any rational basis–the kind of medicine Broussais admitted having practiced himself before becoming enlightened.[393] "Rational" treatment means associating therapy with the internal lesion.[394] The school of Pinel never explains what it is doing or gives reasons.[395] It deals only in tautologies: if asked the difference between an acute and a chronic disease, these physicians say that the latter go on for a longer time or, if pressed, that the patient is weaker; they will not say *why* a patient recovered, only that he recovered because he recovered.[396] [m] Instead of proper explanations

[m]The proto-Empiric, Herophilos, in the third century B.C., also gave tautological definitions out of reluctance to engage in etiological speculation (*Divided Legacy,* I, 195).

they delve into minutiae of description which are of no practical use—Laennec's accounts of thoracic diseases being a prime example.[397]

They are sceptical and fatalistic, ascribing difficult cases to some *vice organique* and abandoning their patients to the *physis.*[398] They hold that each disease has a predestined course with which the physician cannot interfere.[399] They spend time trying to distinguish between the efforts of the *physis* and the effects of the medicine: "How can one not be disgusted at always hearing 'Are the obstructions caused by intermittent fever or by quinine? Are fevers not sometimes an effort of the *physis?* a salutary effort to resolve the accumulation of blood?' As if the *physis* is seeking to destroy some morbific matter, as if most intermittent fevers are cleansing, and as if a large number of paroxysms are needed to effect coction."[400]

They lack the self-confidence necessary to a physician.[401] They talk about "experience," but experience is always slow to yield results.[402] They would rather classify diseases than treat them.[403]

Isidore Poullain, a physician in a military hospital, wrote an account of his experience with the Broussaisian system.

The ordinary routine was to set aside thirty leeches for each new admission. They were taken along by the attending physician when making his rounds. Where they would be applied—to the stomach or anus—was decided by the nurse who preceded the physician and asked of each patient in turn: " 'Where does it hurt? . . . In the stomach? . . . That's enough, I know what you need.' A moment later he placed a towel under the patient's stomach, as he needed the leeches applied there. If the patient said he had diarrhoea, the cloth was placed between his legs to show that the leeches should be applied to the anus. The house surgeon would come up and question the patient, but it was rare for the towels to be moved."[404]

Diet was rigid. Poullain encountered a patient who had been deprived of food for five days and begged to have some bouillon slipped to him in secret.[405]

On autopsy the physician could always find some alteration in the intestines even if no one else could see a thing there; gastroenteritis became endemic. "Isn't this reverting to the times of Moliere, making the art ridiculous?"[406] "This is, however, the ordinary routine of most of these 'physiological physicians.' Their outlook is so narrow and their self-confidence so great that they never notice their mistakes. They blame their failures on the *physis,* as if the *physis* was not a thousand times wiser than they are."[407]

"Physiological medicine" remained at the pinnacle of fashion until the political climate changed with the Royalist restoration of 1822.[408] [n] Thereafter it was on the defensive, although yielding ground only reluctantly. A medical journal reported in 1824 that Broussais was losing almost twice as many patients as the three other physicians at the Val-de-Grace (Broussais retorted that the hospital assigned him all the serious cases).[409] The 1830 "bourgeois revolution" of Louis Philippe restored liberalism to political favor; Broussais was given the chair of general pathology and therapeutics at the Faculté, but his new prominence only "exposed the decadence and desertion of this man who had been so powerful an influence on medical opinion."[410] He turned to phrenology, and his courses, as usual, were wildly successful; he was starting to investigate homoeopathy in 1838 when he died of rectal cancer amid the ruins of his system.

How was it possible that the subtle and scientific ideas of Pinel and Laennec should have been overwhelmed by the barbarous theories of this army surgeon?[o] When Laennec died in 1826 the leading obituary in a French medical journal stated that his views were not always logical, that he made a number of simple errors unworthy of so enlightened a man, that his death was a greater loss to his followers than to science, and that "nothing would have been lacking to his glory if he had adopted the healthy physiological doctrines

[n]It had a remarkable offshoot (combined with Brunonianism) in the Italian school of "contrastimulism" identified with the names of Giovanni Rasori (1766-1837) and Giacomo Tommasini (1768-1846) (see above, p. 299).

[o]Ackerknecht notes "the surprising fact that its time fell so enthusiastically in step with it" ("Broussais or a Forgotten Medical Revolution," 334).

which are the honor of this century."[411] Thus one of the greatest physicians in French history was (momentarily) eclipsed by a pure imposter.

The reasons are varied. Broussais appealed by his simplicity,[p] his ability to answer any question the physician might ask, his activism, his materialism—which suited the intellectual ambiance of the early nineteenth century—and by his claim to represent the first truly French system of medicine: *"Jamais la medecine francaise n'avait eu sa couleur propre!!"*[412]

None of these had anything to do with his system's therapeutic efficacy. Indeed, contemporaries made the same comment about Broussais that Charles II had made about Willis: his theories cost the country more lives than all the enemy armies. But therapeutic efficacy is not the only, or even the most important, determinant of a medical theory's viability. On the contrary, the doctrinal simplicity which detracts from therapeutic efficacy is a great advantage in the competition among theories for survival, and here Broussais held the prize. After twenty years Pinelism had become wearisome with its proliferation of symptomatic descriptions and absence of a firm theoretical structure. A physician wrote in 1819 that "practitioners rarely found at the bedside those simple pictures, so well drawn in the books of nosography, whose authors seem to have forgotten the endless complications of morbid affections. The discredit into which the most recent and best of the pyretologies [i.e., Pinel's] is beginning to fall shows that we were hoping in vain to find one which would withstand criticism."[413] Therapeutic scepticism has been carried too far—the new works on materia medica seem designed more to undermine confidence in the powers of medicine than to instill it.[414]

The author expressed the hope that a new man would arise and recast theory and practice in a new form: this was the role of Broussais.[415]

[p]Hahnemann wrote about Broussais: "The physicians in Europe and elsewhere accepted this *convenient treatment of all diseases* according to a single rule, since it saved them from all further thinking (the most laborious of all work under the sun)" (*Organon,* Sec. 60).

Pinel and Laennec recognized the complexity of the phenomena. Like Hahnemann, Laennec assured the physician that curing people was hard work, and *"le travail repugne a tous les hommes."*[416] But Broussais thought to eliminate the variety of diseased states which makes medicine difficult, simplifying practice by cutting everyone down to size on the procrustean bed of his system. Hence he mocked Pinel's categories as "arbitrary groups of symptoms" and Laennec's reports of autopsies for their "subtle and arbitrary distinctions, the minutiae of the details"—"facts of pure curiosity and no utility to those who study them."[417] "The details of his autopsies are too numerous to remember; one soon loses sight of the lesion upon which he claims to fix the reader's attention; and it is impossible for the latter to associate the cadaveric details with the symptoms for whose interpretation so many minutiae have been provided. These serious faults make this book too diffuse and difficult to read, thus harmful to the progress of the medicine of observation which Laennec wants to enrichen."[418]

Cancers are caused by irritation and not by a *"vice cancereux"*—"that's all the physician has to know, and everything M. Laennec has written on his black cancers is purely imaginary, a somber novel which I had great difficulty reading through to the end."[419]

A follower of Broussais, Eusebe de Salles (1796-1873), wrote: "one needed the patience of a Chinaman and the life of a Methuselah to reduce [Laennec's] descriptions to a few constant types. Laennec had the patience of a Chinaman, and, while his life was short, his atrabilious and monomaniac imagination was capable of drilling an artesian well with the extremely narrow idea upon which it seized."[420]

Another physician defended Broussaisism as a doctrine in which "the vague, supernatural, and false ideas of empiricism and ontology yielded . . . to notions which were clear, natural, and precise."[421]

To this Laennec responded that the system of Broussais is "neither lengthy to learn nor difficult to remember, while my book takes more work and attention. But my black cancers are bodies whose dimensions, consistency, and other physical qualities can be appreciated by the senses, while the 'irritation' of M. Broussais, which he defines as 'exaltation of the vital properties,' is a pure logical entity [*etre de raison*] as well as a very improbable hypothesis in most of the cases to which he applies it . . . M. Broussais and I cultivate sciences which are entirely different from one another—if not in their aim, then at least in their immediate object."[422]

Broussais was seeking an analytical medicine based on the discovery of "proximate causes," while Laennec was applying remedies, shown to be effective by experience, to cases described in terms of their symptoms and signs. He stated that the intestinal lesions, which Broussais called the proximate causes of disease, were only their effects and no more their "cause" than the spots on the skin are the "cause" of smallpox.[423] He hit the mark precisely in characterizing Broussais, like John Brown, as a follower of Methodism who reduced all medical facts to two classes. Contrary instances were rejected or else called "aberrations which cannot be defined but are still the effects of the single principle." They all claim that "the art will no more be long, as they reduce it to one or two principles which can be learned and put into practice in a few days; life will no more be short, as their theories applied to the treatment of diseases will always cure infallibly."[424] Andral called Broussais a "modern Themison."[425] [q]

The social function of Broussaisism was identical with that of Methodism—to simplify practice. A. L. J. Bayle wrote in 1828: "the partisans of this system have only one genre of medicines to combat all diseases; thus one can easily imagine how simple their medicine is to learn and to practice."[426]

Broussais' activism appealed to a generation of physicians weary of Pinelian expectancy. This aspect of Laennec's practice was ferociously caricatured in Eusebe de Salles' novel, *Sakantala a Paris,* one of whose protagonists is the physician, "Lasinec":

> starchy, taciturn, with a repellent manner and dressed like Cassandra, glacial; his mentality knows neither

[q]On Themison of Laodicea and the Methodist School see *Divided Legacy,* I, 291-301.

> exaltation nor curiosity except for a single object—destruction. Curing is only a pretext for the right to observe the marvels of a science of the death agony and the cadaver. Such a one was Lasinec: he was more than a minister of death. One would have said that the grim reaper was present in his gaunt figure. He had thrown on a pair of trousers and a jacket, and the skeleton stood revealed bare when he had taken off his hat or his gloves. His face was as dry as his hand; a bald cranium, a pallid color, a short nose, and prominent cheekbones gave him a true death's head appearance. And to make the resemblance more frightening he wore a pair of glasses with tortoise-shell rims which completely darkened his eyes.[427]

Lasinec is depicted as making the diagnosis and being enraptured by a perfect case of tuberculosis: "one of the most beautiful facts I have ever collected." He is entirely uninterested in the cure or well-being of the patient. The tubercles are the *"beau-ideal du genre."* "What I have observed in the patient will demonstrate to you all the periods of development of this singular disease." He can only advise the patient to refrain from overeating, indulgence in sexual activity, and excess thought, to prevent the disease from worsening. After Lasinec leaves, the main character exclaims: "Adieu, old rat of the amphitheater . . . talkative carrion crow, noseless bloodhound who mistakes a wounded stag for carrion. Adieu! I hope your own chest will be as full of the same tubercles as those you saddle on your patients."[428]

Broussais enlisted in his cause the rampant French nationalism of these decades. He attacked Pinel for following the Englishmen (*sic*), Cullen and Brown—members of the nation which had killed Napoleon (whom Broussais assumed to have died of gastroenteritis). He identified Laennec with the anti-nationalist "medico-Jesuit party" and called his followers "vile Kanto-Platonians"—meaning spiritual Prussians.[429] All this emotion combined with the materialism and anti-vitalism which passed for medical progress in the early nineteenth century, and was indeed in tune with the liberal nationalism dominating thought in other areas, made Broussaisism "prestigious and fascinating, even to its enemies."[430]

One group which never accepted Broussais was the Montpellier physicians. Although he wanted to be regarded as a disciple of Bordeu, the most eminent French physician of the previous century (with whom he had nothing in common except an interest in the gastric region), the vitalism of Montpellier repelled him, and he expressed particular contempt for these "mournful votaries" with their "elements" and "diatheses."[431] The votaries reciprocated these feelings fully and in Paris were the spearhead of the anti-Broussais movement.[432]

Even after his death and the collapse of his theories Broussais was usually described as the "illustrious reformer" of French medicine, and historians of the period show lingering sympathy for this man who, despite an attractive personality, was the cause of many innocent deaths.[r]

The history of Broussais is useful in showing that the influence of hospital medicine can be both good and bad. Pinel had used the hospital to establish a ramified nosography; Broussais used it to lump all patients into a single class. Laennec had praised hospitals for offering a large variety of pathological conditions and training the physician to recognize them;[433] Broussais used this opportunity to determine that all pathological lesions are identical.[434]

Hospital practice can thus help the physician to do what he wants to do in the first place, but its overall effect seems to be one of routinizing practice. Laennec complains that in hospital he could rarely learn enough about the patient's

[r]Ackerknecht claims that in Broussais "a good clinician-observer and a blind dogmatist were obviously able to dwell in the same skull" and that his "physiological concept of disease" was "progressive" ("Broussais or a Forgotten medical Revolution," 339. *Medicine at the Paris Hospital,* 71). However, a member of the Faculté, in a funeral Eulogy of Broussais, stated: "No, we cannot admit that Broussais was a profound observer. Perhaps no generalizer has ever pushed further his audacity and contempt for the facts furnished by observation" ("Eloge de Broussais," *Archives Generales de Medecine* VI [1839], 510-516, at 510).

previous history,[435] while Broussais was not interested in this information anyway.[s]

In a militarized society like France during these decades a hospital practice which economized on governmental expenditures for medicines, and even for the patients' food, was bound to enjoy a measure of official favor. But the appeal of Broussaisism was more than merely economic. The medical profession was thirsting for a doctrine of proximate causes after decades of Pinelian self-restraint, and Broussais admirably met their need.

The Eclectic Period: 1823-1836

In the 1820's and early 1830's medical speculation drew back from the extremes of Broussais' Methodism, with thinkers attempting various syntheses of "physiological medicine" and the Pinelian legacy.

Gabriel Andral (1797-1876) best combined these two approaches in a single system, and his 1823 *Clinique Medicale* was the opening salvo of the new medical orthodoxy.[436]

He and the other Eclectics, however, suffered from pharmacological ignorance, and the period came to an end in 1836 with the appearance of Armand Trousseau's *Traite de Therapeutique*[437] which provided French medicine with a much needed pharmacological dimension and determined the course of thought and practice for the next several decades.

The Hippocratic Tradition and Specific Diseases

Auguste-Francois Chomel (1788-1858), Pierre Bretonneau (1771-1862), Etienne Pariset (1770-1847), and Pierre Louis (1787-1872) proceeded from Hippocratic principles and the associated concept of specificity to evolve a number of "specific diseases" which are still accepted coin in twentieth-century medicine.

[s]Actually, Broussais was not even interested in further autopsies, feeling that his doctrine had been proven correct for all time: "the physician . . . should have a different aim than to satisfy his curiosity through autopsies of cadavers" (*Examen,* 1821, II, 751).

The extreme Hippocratic position was occupied by Chomel, a student of Pinel and Landre-Beauvais, who was professor of clinical medicine at the Charité and the Hotel Dieu, member of the Academy of Medicine, and personal physician to Louis Philippe.

Sickness is an alteration in the structure or functioning of the healthy organism whose intimate nature is unknown to us.[438] Such alterations are infinite, or virtually infinite, in number.[439] The organism reacts to them by striving to restore health, and this struggle proceeds in the way outlined by Hippocrates—with coction, crisis, and discharge of the cocted matter as sweat, an evacuation, or a skin eruption.[440]

The primary source of information about diseases is observation of their symptoms. While Broussais had the temerity to remark: "how will we treat diseases without knowing their intimate causes?" the better guide is Sydenham who based therapeutics on observation and experience, not on knowledge of "primary causes."[441]

A symptom is "any sense-perceptible change in an organ or function"; when observed and interpreted by the physician it becomes a sign.[442] They are extremely numerous.[443] The pulse is an important source of symptomatic knowledge —especially its speed, magnitude, hardness, and frequency— although the variety of pulses presented by Solano de Luques and Bordeu are now recognized as to some extent the product of ingenious speculation.[444] The physician must be adept at eliciting information from the patient through questioning.[445]

Symptoms can be divided into "characteristic" (or "principal") and "accessory." As long as the patient's illness is not from the disorder of some one organ, the more striking or salient symptoms are the principal ones, and all other are accessory.[446] But if a single organ is disturbed, the symptoms revealing the disorder of that organ—however slight and difficult to observe—become the principal ones, and other general symptoms—however striking—are only accessory.[447] Thus, in peripneumonia a slight pain in the side and a little blood in the sputum are the principal symptoms, while a severe headache and blood in the urine are accessory.[448]

Those who have tried to substitute chemistry for observation and experience at the bedside have been led astray, as the organism is not an inert bowl of chemicals.[449] "Experiments" of this nature are not the equivalent of the physician's "experience," as the results of "experiments" only go to form a part of the physician's "experience."[450]

Since all do not observe equally well, all do not acquire experience at the same rate.

In addition to symptoms the physician must observe specific, predisposing, and exciting causes. Specific causes are contagions (producing contagious diseases) and also certain gases in the atmosphere (such as the sewer gas which overcomes workers in ditches, the metallic vapors in lead and copper smelting establishments, etc.).[451] "The invisible principle which causes contagion is usually enveloped in some visible substance such as mucus, pus, or sweat."[452] While Linnaeus tried to prove that all contagious diseases are caused by microorganisms (*animalcules*), this is true only of scabies, not of plague, smallpox, or measles.[453] Some epidemic diseases are due to contagia, but others are caused by changes in Sydenham's "constitutions."[454]

The "constitution" is thus a predisposing cause of disease; other predisposing causes are related to the age, sex, or heredity of the patient.[455] An important one is the diathesis—meaning the disposition of one or several organs of the body to be affected by a disease.[456] Persons who break out in a skin eruption after eating strawberries or shellfish have a diathesis or "morbific idiosyncrasy" of some sort.[457] Predisposing causes are thus both inside and outside the body. An epidemic occurs when the external predisposing cause is identical with the predispositions of many of the inhabitants of a place.[458] For example, when bilious fevers are very common, persons of bilious temperament or constitution are most commonly affected; those of sanguine or lymphatic temperament, on the contrary, "find in their very constitutions a sort of resistance [*resistance*]" to the external bilious constitution.[459]

The physician must also investigate occasional and exciting causes of disease: the patient's diet, changes in his mode of life, fluctuations in the weather, etc.[460]

To information about symptoms and the above causes the physician adds data from autopsies and anatomical investigation, but he must proceed carefully—especially today when "exaggerated importance is generally accorded to anatomical lesions."[461] All lesions do not possess equal value: some, such as tubercles in the lungs, precede the disease; others, such as ulcerations of the intestines in phthisis, occur during the course of the disease; still another group (blood clots in the heart and major vessels) arise during the death agony; and a final series (transudation of bile into the intestines, swelling of the serous tissues) occur after death. Some pathological lesions (certain encysted tumors, adhesions of the lungs to the thorax) do not give rise to any symptoms at all.[462]

The physician should guard especially against considering disease forms or species as fixed, and unusual cases as "deviations" from them. There are no "illegitimate" disease forms, as all are equally true and valid.[463] Nor can the patient suffer from two "diseases" simultaneously: "When he presents the phenomena of bilious fever at the same time as those of inflammatory fever, one should not perceive this as a 'complication' of either of them but as a disease which is as simple as each of those whose symptoms seem thus combined."[464]

For this reason many attempts at disease classification do violence to the facts, putting very different conditions together in the same class.[465] Physicians suffer from a tendency to convert their own systematic ideas into eternal laws of nature, blaming the *physis* for any irregularities rather than their system: "the physician is amazed at the play of the *physis*, her bizarre effects, while the system retains the admiration which it has inspired."[466]

Hence many illnesses must be outside any system of classification.[467] Those due to specific causes, such as intermittent fever or the bee-sting sickness, are classified in function of these causes.[468] Some are contagious, appearing only at intervals, with pronounced skin symptoms and high mortality, attacking many persons at once, and usually not affecting the same person a second time.[469] Typical of these are typhus, typhoid, plague, yellow fever, syphilis, smallpox, and the British sweating sickness.[470]

Diseases not due to a specific cause can usually be recognized by some typical organic lesion: phthisis, inflammation, erysipelas, cancer, etc.[471] Sometimes they involve animate or inanimate foreign bodies inside an organ (cysts, worms, calculi) or excess liquid there.[472]

When a disease is not associated with a specific cause and has no defined anatomical lesion, its genus and species can be established only from the symptoms.[473]

The physician integrates all of this information with the aim of defining the disease from which the patient is suffering. The number of diseases in the world is virtually infinite, and "the same illness has perhaps never arisen twice in precisely the same form," but the physician must still try to establish parallels among diseased states.[474] This is done by application of reason—which cannot be eliminated from medicine entirely, as a blind empiricism would desire, but, as Sydenham has noted, should be "the simple and natural kind based on good sense which arises directly from the observed phenomena. Whenever one acts in medicine according to a series of arguments strung together more or less ingeniously, one falls into errors which are as harmful for the physician as they are dangerous to the patient."[475]

Once the physician has defined the disease and established his prognosis, he can proceed to treatment—which is not, therefore, based on knowledge of the "proximate cause" but aims to promote the self-healing efforts of the organism.[476] Medicines do not act against the "disease" but stimulate the *physis.*[477]

They can be classified as strengthening or weakening, calming or stimulating, and evacuating; there are also a few specifics, such as mercury for syphilis, sulphur for scabies, and vaccine for smallpox.[478] Perhaps additional specifics will be found one day for rabies, scarlet fever, and measles.

Chomel's own treatment was rather expectant; he opposed violent forms of therapy and credited Pinel with having instituted a salutary reform of the polypharmacal prescribing habits of their contemporaries.[479] "Even the layman has come to realize how vain and ridiculous are these monstrous combinations of drugs of all kinds which are almost as dangerous for the patient as they are inimical to the progress of the art."[480] He urged administration of one remedy at a time in order to evaluate its effect properly.[481]

He made a special study of rheumatism, typhus, typhoid, and various infectious diseases, leaving valuable descriptions of them and information on his therapeutic method.[482]

Chomel was the highest ideal of the Hippocratic physician. "He interrogated the patient with extreme care, making skilful use of the physician's *coup d'oeuil.* He examined attentively all the organs, both those obviously sick and those which might appear healthy; he taught his students never to make a diagnosis before conducting this comprehensive examination which, more than once, disclosed lesions whose existence had been unsuspected. In this way Chomel imparted an excellent direction to clinical practice and trained a whole generation of good physicians."[483]

A student described him as "of firm and loyal character, of an austere probity, imbued in the highest degree with the religion of duty; devoted, courageous, faithful to friendship in misfortune; disinterested, benevolent, sympathetic to everything which is good and to all who suffer . . ."[484]

Clearly his medical views were Empirical, in the Montpellier tradition of his professors, Pinel and Landre-Beauvais. He defined "pathology," for instance, not as the "classification of diseases, their causes and signs," but as "everything which has to do with the patient," including treatment—since treatment is one of the sources of knowledge of the disease.[485] Physiology, in turn, is the body of knowledge relating to health.[486]

Chomel was an enemy of oversimplification and, together with Laennec, led the attack against Broussais.[487] This, together with his political and medical conservatism, made him unpopular with the more forward-looking members of the next generation. A biographer wrote that he was very unjust toward the "illustrious reformer" on the question of essential fevers. Chomel's pathology was "down to earth, without scope and without a single overarching view . . . This name and this glory are gradually waning. As a learned physician, he did not leave behind a single truly remarkable work."[488]

While Chomel accepted the "specific cause" in principle, and used it as a criterion of disease classification, Bretonneau and Louis gave it dimensionality by their work on diphtheria and typhoid, and particularly by incorporating into the "specific disease" the attribute of "immunity."

Pierre Bretonneau of Tours studied at the Paris Ecole de Santé but, when unfairly failed in a botany examination (his favorite subject) by Alexis Boyer (1757-1833), withdrew without taking the M.D. degree and returned to Tours as a simple officier de santé.[489] There he remained as director of the hospital until late in life when he finally settled in the capital for his declining years.[t]

His provincial isolation kept him aloof from the fashions, intrigues, and intellectual pressures of Paris, and he could pursue an original line of investigation. He spent the years 1799 to 1814 promoting the recently introduced technique of smallpox vaccination, making himself an apostle of Jenner's discovery and even devising a technique for storing the liquid in fine capillary tubes to impede its deterioration.[490] In 1814 the prefect of his département noted the disappearance of smallpox in Bretonneau's canton (Bléré) since 1807.[491]

He returned to Paris in 1814-1816 to obtain the M.D. degree and thus witnessed the great typhus-typhoid epidemic. In 1819 the Touraine was stricken with an epidemic of diphtheria. These two diseases became his principal objects of research, and on them he lavished the same single-mindedness and determination that had induced him to abandon his studies in 1799 out of indignation at unjust treatment. For ten years he collected information on symptoms, methods of

[t]A peculiar fact about Bretonneau was that his first wife was 35 years his senior, and, as a widower of 78, he married the 18-year old daughter of a colleague. Thus 150 years elapsed between the birth of his first wife and the death of his second (Raoul Mercier, "L'Extraordinaire Vie de Pierre-Fidele Bretonneau," *Progres Medical* XIV [1937], I, *Supplement,* 5-6).

treatment, and autopsies, publishing nothing despite the entreaties of his friends.

When his Touraine colleagues, with whom he was never on good terms,[u] claimed that his hospital data were not comparable to theirs from civil practice, he went to the graveyards at night with his student and colleague, the surgeon Armand Velpeau (1795-1867), to disinter the bodies of children recently dead of diphtheria, thus verifying the existence of the typical throat lesions.[492] Thirty-six such autopsies performed at night in the city cemeteries effectively disproved the contentions of his opponents.[v]

Bretonneau's medical views were obviously influenced by his experience with smallpox and the immunity conferred by cowpox.[w] He was discussing the concept of disease specificity with Armand Trousseau as early as 1818, approaching it from the point of view of specificity of treatment.[493]

After returning home from Paris in 1816 he had experimented with application of hydrochloric acid to the mucous membranes of the mouth and throat in croup and diphtheria.[494] Encouraged by success, he then applied silver nitrate to the skin in smallpox and other eruptive diseases, finding that it inhibited the development of the pustules and prevented the disease from spreading.[495] The procedure was not mild: solid pieces of silver nitrate were plunged into the center of the pustule ("a cruel but necessary treatment"), but its success led to the following theoretical generalization: "all diseases whose course is regular and generally the same when left to themselves, or at least a great many of them, have in nature an agent susceptible of modifying them beneficially,

[u]The word, *diphtherite,* coined by Bretonneau was never used at meetings of the Tours Medical Society, and this society was one of the first to adopt *fievre typhoide* instead of Bretonneau's name for typhoid: *dothienenterite.*

[v]The townspeople, not realizing who these grave-robbers might be, occasionally shot at them, and Velpeau claimed to carry pellets in his rump for the rest of his life.

[w]During an influenza epidemic in 1847 a friend wrote to Bretonneau: "If only you could find a vaccine for this disease" (Paul Triaire, *Bretonneau et ses Correspondants* [Paris: Alcan, 1892], II, 445).

and perhaps of arresting them, if applied in time and in the correct way."[496]

At the same time he was elaborating a different approach to disease specificity, taking as his point of departure the "specific" *mode de lesion* of an internal organ or tissue proposed by Bayle and Laennec. This he employed in his research on typhoid where the lesion was inside the body and could not be treated (like diphtheria) with topical applications.

Armand Trousseau—who was Bretonneau's student, assistant, and Paris spokesman—reported in 1826 that, while Broussais, Andral, and others had described alterations of the gastrointestinal membrane in a variety of diseases, these diseases have not yet been properly differentiated from one another. "But it is probable that the internal tegument, as well as the external, is subject to diverse and specific inflammations."[497] Bretonneau (he continues) has finally clarified the question, isolating a disease whose seat seems to be exclusively in Peyer's glands and calling it dothienenteritis or dothienentery.[498] [x] Its specific feature is that Peyer's glands become larger, rounder, softer, and redder; it is identical with Pinel's "mucous adynamic fever" and Broussais' "gastroenteritis" and possesses "the singular prerogative of affecting the same individual only once in his lifetime as well as, perhaps, of being contagious."[499]

Bretonneau wrote a treatise on specificity in the early 1820's in which he clarified his view of typhoid, calling it a disease of the whole organism with a special lesion of the intestine: "a disease accompanied by an intestinal eruption and not one caused by this eruption."[500] [y] It is also contagious.[501] Its reproductive agent is "a miasmatic being which attaches itself and adheres to the morbid secretions." The local lesion is only of secondary importance,[z] as "the

[x]Bretonneau preferred "dothienenteritis," while Trousseau opted for "dothienentery" to emphasize its existence as a "specific disease." In the event, Louis' "typhoid fever" won out.

[y]This work, which was only published in 1922, has not been available to me.

[z]In 1855 Bretonneau observed that some plague victims manifested no internal lesions at all ("Diathese" in *Dictionnaire Encyclopedique*).

patient succumbs to the hidden damage caused by the poison from the morbific being."[502] The "miasmatic being" is a disease seed (*germe*) comparable to the seed of a vegetable which can retain its ability to germinate over long periods: "this tenacious vitality is ordinarily encountered among the very smallest seeds."[503] [a]

In 1826 he published his work on diphtheria. While Pinel classified his phlegmasies according to the organ inflamed, this was an inadequate criterion: "the specificity of the inflammation, much more than its intensity or the nature of the tissue in which it is located, influences the functional disturbance caused by each inflammatory lesion."[504] Laennec was right to urge classification of diseases on this basis.[505] Diphtheria is a pellicular inflammation of the mucous tissue of the throat and respiratory passages, a redness without swelling but with an exudation.[506] It is probably contagious.[507] The local inflammation gradually extends to the whole body and can be treated most effectively while still in the local stage—with topical applications of hydrochloric acid which "substitute" another inflammation for the diphtheritic one.[508]

There is no essential difference between gangrene of the gums due to scurvy, severe sore throat (*angine maligne*), and croup; the symptomatic differences are due to differences in the organs affected, but the distinctive characteristic—the pellicular inflammation—is identical in all three.[509] The organism can become habituated to this disease, just as it can resist poisons, venoms, and smallpox.[510] "Perhaps the influence of this habituation contributes to the extinction of certain contagious epidemic diseases by wearing out the capacity to contract them. Perhaps, by the same token, the person who is sick with scurvy of the gums is the least likely to contract croup during an epidemic."[511]

Bretonneau introduced an idea which had not been mentioned by Velpeau: the inflammation of diphtheria is *almost* identical with that induced by application of extract of cantharides to the mucous membrane of the mouth (in

[a]Cf. with Laennec's remarks about disease "seeds" (above, p. 479).

dogs). Does this mean that diphtheria is a specific disease? Or does the slight difference between the two types of inflammation indicate that it can occur in a variety of nuances while remaining a normal physiological modification of the vital properties—i.e., non-specific? "This is one of the major questions of practical medicine."[512 b]

He gave his final opinion in 1855. The existence of specific diseases is proved by the possibility of simulating each disease through application of some caustic or acid to the skin, each of which "accomplishes its task in its own way, without much regard for the subject's individuality."[513] Each member of the family of cantharis insects secretes a specific liquid when agitated or touched; each such liquid causes a special secretion when touched to the human mucous membrane; and the diphtheria or smallpox virus also produces this effect when contacting an exposed mucous membrane or raw spot on the skin.[514] Each caustic, each snake poison, each topical irritant leaves the "imprint of its seal," and the same is true of "invisible and imponderable causes which are revealed only by the varied symptoms peculiar [*propres*] to each." "I repeat, a special seed [*germe*], peculiar to each contagion, gives birth to each contagious disease. The epidemic scourges are engendered and disseminated each by its reproductive seed."[515]

"The specificity [*specialite*] of contagious diseases and their therapeutics is a great medical truth revealed by clinical observation against which no prejudice can prevail."[516]

The "virus" is related to the seed of each specific disease and seems almost to be alive in the sense later suggested by Pasteur, Auguste Chauveau, and Emile Duclaux. Thus Bretonneau states, *a propos* the "smallpox virus," "I am certain that the habituation [*accoutumance*] which conquers wild animals tames viruses as well (as distinct from poisons and vaccines). Penetrating into the economy, the viruses multiply there, which does not prevent the amount of each dose of

[b]In a letter written at this time (1825) Trousseau assured Bretonneau that the possibility of modifying and "attenuating" a local inflammation by treatment in no way detracted from the specificity of the inflammation (Paul Triaire, *Bretonneau et ses Correspondants,* I, 531).

virus successively absorbed from exercising a decreasing influence on its action, so that in epidemics the physicians with a numerous clientele, hastening from one patient to another, absorb only fractional doses of the virus and thus acquire an immunity [*immunite*] which has often been noted but seldom understood."[517] [c]

This resembles the ability of certain persons to ingest increasing quantities of arsenic until it ceases being harmful to them and actually becomes beneficial.[518]

While Bretonneau's parallel between diphtheria and the inflammation due to topical application of cantharides, as well as his idea of cure by "substituting" one inflammation for another, seem similar to Hahnemann's provings and cure through similars,[d] the source of Bretonneau's ideas was actually the ubiquitous John Hunter.

The Englishman called syphilis a local disease which gradually assumes a constitutional form: Bretonneau states the same about diphtheria.[519] Hunter wrote that the genitalia become "habituated" to the gonorrhoeal poison and cannot then readily be reinfected: Bretonneau states that the organism seems to acquire "by habituation [*accoutumance*] the capacity to resist diseases" such as smallpox, and even gonorrhoea, "if we are to believe the assertions of John Hunter."[520] Hunter had held that mercurial medicines cause typical rheumatism symptoms, with administration of more medicine only worsening the patient's condition: Bretonneau states the same about ulcerous inflammations of the skin and mucous membranes caused by mercurial medicines.[521] Hunter wrote that mercury "counteracts the venereal irritation by producing another of a different kind," and Bretonneau holds that his topical applications of

[c]On the word, "immunity," see below, p. 516. See, also, Hahnemann's views on the immunity attained by physicians during epidemics, pp. 411-412 above.

[d]By 1826, moreover, homoeopathic ideas were being discussed in France (see below, pp. 541 ff). In that same year the first French thesis on homeopathy by a medical student cited Velpeau's article as evidence in favor of Hahnemann's principle of similars (Theodore Boeckel, *Exposition de la Doctrine Homoiopathique* [*sic*] *du Docteur Hahnemann et Reflexions sur Cette Doctrine* [Strasburg Dissertation, 1826], 31).

hydrochloric acid "substitute another inflammation" for the diphtheritic one.[522] When topical applications of mercury to the throat give good results, "is it by substituting another irritation, a mercurial irritation, for the morbid irritation that calomel causes exfoliation of the concretions and thus opposes reproduction of the false membrane?"[523]

Hunter was held in high esteem by Pinel and other leaders of the Paris School; his influence on the development of this school's doctrine of specific diseases should not be overlooked.

Even so, Bretonneau cannot be deprived of credit. The influence of predecessors is all well and good, but each thinker seeks out the influences most congenial to him. Bretonneau was a practiced and pertinacious observer as well as an original thinker. His decade of experience with smallpox, its waxing, waning, and interaction with other diseases, was probably the determining factor in his conclusion that discrete diseases are the proper objects of medical investigation.

Laennec mentioned Bretonneau's work on diphtheria in the second (1826) edition of his *Auscultation Mediate,* but he himself interpreted this disease differently, calling it constitutional, not local, caused by a "special alteration of the liquids," and infectious (through the air) but probably not contagious. About Bretonneau's topical treatment with silver nitrate Laennec only remarks: "it perhaps acts in croup otherwise than as a rubefaciant."[524]

In the early decades of the century the warmest defender of contagionism, other than Bretonneau, Velpeau, and Hahnemann, was the Hippocratic, Etienne Pariset (1770-1847).[e] No one at this time disputed the contagiousness of smallpox, measles, syphilis, and scabies; the argument was over plague, cholera, yellow fever, typhoid, and diphtheria.[525] Pariset in 1820 wrote that yellow fever was a "contagious miasm" consisting of seeds (*germes*) which enter the organism and

[e]See his "Coction" in *Dictionnaire.* Also "Etienne Pariset" in *Dictionnaire Encyclopedique.*

propagate there, being cured by a proper coction and evacuation of the "products of the morbific alteration."[526] In 1837 he ascribed plague, whose focus was in the Nile delta, to the mummies buried in the ground which give off "thousands of dangerous germs." These attach themselves to the clothes and are carried from place to place.[527]

Such arguments, however, seemed weakened by the apparent inability of contagionists to inoculate themselves with matter from diphtheria and other diseases, due perhaps to inherited or acquired immunity of the test subjects.[528] An even more important reason for the strength of anti-contagionism was that acceptance of this principle would have upset existing hospital arrangements in requiring isolation of patients with contagious diseases.[529] Implicit in contagionism also was the conclusion that physicians were responsible for the spread of epidemics (as stated by Hahnemann in 1831).[530]

Another prominent Hippocratic in these years was Pierre Charles Alexandre Louis who supported Chomel in the conflict with Broussais,[f] helped perfect Bretonneau's doctrine of disease specificity, and gave thought to the relationship between symptoms and organic lesions. He also performed the first statistical study of the therapeutic effect of bloodletting.

Louis graduated at the Paris Ecole de Santé and then spent seven years in Russia. He returned to a position in Chomel's clinic where he passed the rest of his life, treating patients and lecturing to students. His principal writings were on phthisis (1825), typhoid fever (1829), and bloodletting (1835).

His work on phthisis (which settled, once and for all, the description of this disease) was the first to discuss its typical pathological lesions before presenting case studies with their symptoms. Louis held that pathological anatomy is a more

[f]See his *Examen de l'Examen de M. Broussais Relativement a la Phthisie et l'Affection Typhoide* (Paris: Bailliere, 1834).

important criterion of the existence of phthisis than are the symptoms, since organs whose structures have been profoundly affected often manifest no symptoms at all.[531] He concludes that the "cause" of phthisis, while unknown, has nothing to do with Broussais' "irritation."[532]

His two-volume treatise on typhoid settled the description of this disease also.[533] All of Pinel's "essential fevers" (except plague) and Broussais' gastroenteritis were henceforth seen as variants of typhoid.[534] Its proximate cause in the body is unknown, like that of phthisis, but the intestinal lesions are primary and present from the first day.[535] Cases with typical typhoid symptoms but lacking these intestinal lesions Louis called "simulated typhoid."[536] [g] "Otherwise we would have two measures and substitute caprice for reason"[537]

Both typhoid and phthisis are specific diseases. Louis states that ulceration of the intestine is found only in those suffering from typhoid: "so that, in this connection, typhoid is to the other acute diseases what phthisis is to the chronic ones."[538]

Louis opposed Chomel and the Hippocratic tradition in holding anatomical lesions to be primary and symptoms secondary.[h] Where Chomel and Laennec had stressed the exciting cause as the disease determinant, Louis subordinated the exciting cause to the proximate cause (i.e., the anatomical lesion): while the exciting cause has a "certain role" in the mortality and the development of secondary lesions, this role should not be exaggerated "as, it seems to me, has been done by certain persons who have particularly fixed their attention on those cases where the alteration of the small intestine was slight and disproportionate to the violence of the symptoms."[539] "In the majority of cases" the *mouve-*

[g]Cf. with the "legitimate" and "illegitimate" fevers of Galen and Boerhaave, also with Chomel's comments on the same subject (*Divided Legacy,* I, 228, 232; above, p. 505, and below, p. 674).

[h]In 1834 Chomel reiterated his opinion that typhoid is a general disease of which the follicular lesions are only the local expression. He also rejected Louis' "simulated typhoid"—the disease is still typhoid even without the mesenteric lesions (A. F. Chomel, *Lecons de Clinique Medicale Faites a l'Hotel-Dieu de Paris* [Paris: Bailliere, 1834-1840], I, 523-529).

ment febrile is in the same proportion to the pathological lesion in typhoid as in erysipelas and other diseases.[540]

In so asserting, however, Louis was contradicting his own training and principles. In 1834, for instance, he wrote that the commencement of a disease may be either a lesion of an organ or "a general state of disease which cannot be referred to the alteration (I mean the appreciable alteration) of any organ in particular."[541] Often no lesion can be found to explain the symptoms, and the physician must look to the predisposing and exciting causes.[542] In any case, while the lesion tells the physician the nature of the disease, the symptoms reveal its prognosis and thus guide the treatment.[543]

By the second (1841) edition of his work on typhoid Louis had slightly modified his stand on the exciting cause in the light of new discoveries about the contagiousness of typhoid.

The 1829 edition had not mentioned contagion, and the Academy of Medicine resolved in that year that typhoid is probably not contagious (after hearing a lecture on the subject by Bretonneau).[544] But a decisive advance was made in 1834-1835 by a certain Dr. Gendron who described recurring typhoid epidemics in French villages.[545] He noted that, while everyone accepts the contagiousness of smallpox, measles, scarlet fever, and even dysentery, typhoid epidemics are invariably ascribed to climatic changes or to the "constitution"—i.e., to infection (through the air) rather than contagion.[546] But after observing a series of cases where families sleeping together in the same bed passed typhoid to one another, Gendron concluded that it spreads by contagion, "poisoning by un unknown and impalpable principle known as a miasm."[547] The typhoid symptoms and the internal lesions are both the effects of this "miasm."[548]

Gendron observed further that recurring epidemics spared those who had once contracted the disease: he introduced the word, "immunity" (*immunite*), to replace "habituation" (*accoutumance*).[549] He also used the expression, "incubation period."[550]

Louis made full use of Gendron's articles in the second (1841) edition of his work on typhoid. The contagiousness of typhoid is henceforth proved by the phenomenon of immunity, and the epidemic is due to contagion rather than infection.[551] Failure of previous attempts to prove the contagiousness of typhoid he attributed to the acquired immunity of the subjects.[552]

He allowed a slightly greater role to the exciting ("miasmatic") cause in the "mortality and the development of secondary lesions" but held to his earlier view that the internal lesion is primary and the symptoms secondary.[553] [i]

Despite these discoveries, however, the doctrine of contagion was resisted. As late as 1855 Bretonneau wrote in exasperation that while the "common people" are perfectly willing to accept homoeopathy, hypnotism, and spiritualist seances, it is impossible to convince them of the existence of "specific disease causes."[554] Only when Louis Pasteur and Robert Koch (1843-1910) revealed the existence of microorganisms associated with specific diseases—replacing the vague "miasm" with a palpable material entity—did the specific cause gain professional and public acceptance.

In 1835 Louis produced a statistical investigation of the effect of bloodletting in certain diseases. He was attempting to solve the perennial problem of medical history—how many times an event must be observed to become "experience," to qualify as reliable knowledge:[j]

> People are always talking about "the experience of the centuries" in medicine; but how can this experience be a reality when those who write on medicine state "I have often seen," "I have rarely seen," instead of "I have seen so and so many times." Then the experience of one man could be added to that of another. But how can the

[i]Louis gave a long argument justifying his conclusion that lesions are primary, symptoms secondary, and that "simulated typhoid" exists (*Fievre Typhoide,* 1841, II, 308-311). "We can only say that in simulated typhoid the appearances have been entirely deceptive, and that we must be more attentive in observing diseases to seek some hidden sign which will prevent us from falling into error" (*ibid.,* II, 310).

[j]See *Divided Legacy,* I, 275.

> experience of the one who says "more," "less," "rarely," or "frequently" be added to that of the one who says "more or less rarely or frequently." Imagine the thousands of authors who have followed this course. It is as if you only had one and, in many respects, as if you had none at all. *If, then, there is a way of gathering the experience of the centuries in therapeutics, it can only be through using the numerical method.*[555]

When "experience" has been transformed into "general facts," medicine will become "scientific," and it will be possible to dispense with the physician's intuition or "tact."[556]

But physicians at the time pointed out that Louis' method did not take into account the possibility of non-identity or non-uniformity of the cases enumerated: if the patients in the given class are not all suffering from the same condition, the induction drawn from experience with this class will be valueless.

Louis' answer is illuminating.

He states, in the first place, that if each patient were different from each other, no experience could ever be acquired in medicine: "it would never be possible to attain to a general fact, even in pathology."[557] This same objection—non-uniformity of the cases observed—could be brought against any other proposal for making medicine scientific.[558] *Patients must fall into discrete and finite categories because that is scientifically necessary!!*

Furthermore, everyday experience shows that patients can be classified in this way: "the same medicine administered for the same disease in individuals who differ greatly in age, strength, and temperament can be almost always effective."[559] If people were essentially different from one another, everyone would have to follow a different diet, whereas 99% of the population eat the same foods.[560] Slight differences among patients become insignificant when a "highly effective" therapeutic agent is used.[561] [k]

[k]Note Bretonneau's comment that a caustic medicine exerts its effect "without much regard for the patient's individuality" (above, p. 512).

Therefore, in an epidemic, if 500 are treated with one medicine and 500 with another, more dying in the first group than in the second, it must be concluded that the second medicine is more effective.[562] This method of comparative trials was employed in the 1832 Asiatic Cholera epidemic, and no one objected except perhaps the patient (*le principal interesse*).[563] [1]

Louis made the final point that in a comparative trial any non-uniformity will afflict both groups of patients equally, permitting this factor to be, as it were, cancelled out.[564]

Hence the statistical method must be employed. In any case, all others in use for centuries have failed, leaving therapeutics in its infancy.[565] If apparently identical cases do not react to medication in the same way, this only proves that they were not identical, and research must then be done to refine the categories.[566]

Louis, of course, was correct in recognizing that a scientific therapeutics must face the problem of individual differences among patients, but his own proposal was only a vast *petitio principii,* an attempt forcibly to eliminate these very differences because "science" so requires.

Louis' understanding of medical science was defective. His effort to find firm ground in the constancy of "specific diseases" was doomed to failure from the start. It was Hahnemann's genius to perceive that firm ground could be found only in a classification of patients according to the curative treatment.

Since Louis' "numerical method" provides the rationale for twentieth-century (allopathic) therapeutic theory, it has

[1]The London Board of Health attempted a comparative statistical evaluation of treatments for Asiatic Cholera during the 1855 epidemic. The "alterative treatment" (with opium and calomel) and the "astringent treatment" (with sulphuric acid, opium, and chalk) were found superior to the "stimulant treatment" (with ammonia, ether, and brandy) and the "eliminant treatment" (with castor oil, olive oil, and emetics). The homoeopaths, using camphor, *Veratrum album,* and copper sulphate, had a considerably better recovery rate than any of the allopaths, but their statistics were rejected by the Board on the ground that inclusion would "compromise the value and utility of their averages of cure as deduced from the operation of known remedies" (Coulter, *Homoeopathic Influences in Nineteenth-Century Allopathic Therapeutics,* 53-54).

received more attention today than it did at the time of its appearance, and Louis' specific conclusions about bloodletting have been obscured.

He is considered, in particular, to have demonstrated its inefficacy, thus initiating the movement which culminated in the decline of phlebotomy sixty years later.[m] But this is quite incorrect, as Louis had no intention of condemning this technique, only of guiding and regulating its use.

His book was an examination of the effect of bloodletting in pleuropneumonia, erysipelas of the face, and inflammation of the throat (*angine*).[567] The patients were all bled, some the first day of the illness, some the second, some the third, etc., and a comparison was made of the time needed for recovery in each case.[568] Louis concluded that phlebotomy is ineffective in mild inflammations but very necessary in severe ones: "despite the limitations on its utility, bloodletting *cannot be neglected in serious inflammatory diseases which have their seat in a major organ,* either because of its influence on the state of the diseased organ or because shortening the duration of the disease reduces the chance of development of secondary lesions" [stress in the original].[569]

He preferred "general" bloodletting (the lancet) to "local" (with leeches)–a shot at Broussais.[570] He also warned that excess bloodletting weakens the patient and that severe inflammations cannot be aborted (*jugulees*) by repeated extraction of the patient's blood.[571] [n]

The thrust of his book was to rationalize and standardize techniques of phlebotomy, not to eliminate it entirely. The practice remained fashionable for decades,[o] and J. H. Baas,

[m]"By a statistical proof that bloodletting is of little value in pneumonia [Louis] did away with its abuse in that disease" (Garrison, *History of Medicine.* Third Edition [Philadelphia: Saunders, 1914], 342). Louis "sounded . . . the death knell for a dangerous 1000-year-old medical rite" (Ackerknecht, *Medicine at the Paris Hospital,* 104), etc. etc.

[n]This remark was aimed at Bouillaud (see below, p. 531).

[o]The article on "Saignee" in the *Dictionnaire Encyclopedique* devotes 34 large pages of text to an account of contemporary techniques of bloodletting. The

writing in 1876, does not even hint that Louis started a decline in bloodletting: he "censured large bleedings, etc. but gives in pneumonia large doses of tartar emetic in addition to free bloodletting, etc."[572] William Osler (1849-1919) was advocating a "timely venesection" as the best treatment for pneumonia as late as 1912.[573]

In fact, Louis' book was quickly forgotten by his contemporaries and resurrected at a later date to explain the decline of bloodletting actually due to the influence of homoeopathy. The lancet was not set aside in 1880 or 1890 because Louis in 1835 had stated that: "bloodletting *cannot be neglected in serious inflammatory diseases which have their seat in a major organ,*" but because allopaths for fifty or sixty years could observe their homoeopathic colleagues treating patients successfully without this time-honored technique.

All of the above should not obscure Louis' own qualities. His *Essay on Clinical Instruction* is guided by the highest ideals of the Hippocratic physician, calling for close attention to the symptoms, urging prognosis on the basis of critical signs and the exciting and predisposing causes, and stating that only the "empirical" modes of treatment (in contrast to "rational" ones) are reliable.[574] But his therapeutics was rather standard. In phthisis he followed Bichat and Bayle, urging opium and belladonna for the cough, bleeding for the pleuritic pain and the hemoptysis, blisters for the dyspnoea;[575] in typhoid he rejected derivatives and revulsives in favor of bleeding and tonics, etc.[576] Thus he rejected

author goes into detail on bleeding from the jugular ("the clavicle is bandaged to compress the vein . . . a larger lancet should be used than for ordinary bleeding, and the incision must be larger and deeper, because the jugular, although larger in size, is farther from the surface than the veins in the arms. The blood rarely comes out in a spurt but escapes in a dribble [*en bavant*] and must be guided to the receptacle by a little metal funnel or a simple visiting card"). He notes that this technique can be weakening, especially to children and infants ("a child at the breast, if bled, will often be nervous and irritable for months"). Also the "morbid element" may resist phlebotomy. There is a "modern school" which employs "preventive" or "precautionary" bleeding of healthy persons to ward off disease (an "unfortunate prophylaxis"). This article was published in 1878, *forty-three years after the appearance of Louis' book* (which is listed in the bibliography, although Louis' name does not appear in the article).

Bretonneau's (and Laennec's) suggestion that one inflammation can be eliminated by inducing a second inflammation: "it is a law of our economy that one inflammation brings on a series of secondary lesions and usually another inflammation."[577]

Rationalism and the Rejection of Specific Diseases

The above thinkers represent one side of the Eclectic period—the abandonment of Broussais for Hippocrates and the emergence of a doctrine of specific diseases. Another group, however, accepted Broussais' Rationalist-Methodist postulates while discarding some of the trappings: Jean Cruveilhier (1791-1874), Leon Rostan (1790-1866), and Jean-Baptiste Bouillaud (1796-1881). While recognizing some specific diseases, especially the contagious ones, they endeavored to restrict their number. Associating specific diseases with Pinel's "ontology," they defined morbid phenomena as aberrations of normal physiological processes.

Cruveilhier, from a family of surgeons, studied this discipline under Dupuytren, in 1823 took the chair of pathological anatomy at the Faculté, and in 1836 became chief physician at the Maternité.

From an early age he had been impressed by the "illustrious reformer" who "substituted the simplicity of nature for the apparent but lethal simplicity of systems."[578] "Now my mind is free of that vagueness and uncertainty which used to torment me, which even sometimes led me to doubt the certainty of medicine when I saw diametrically opposed treatments succeed in diseases which I thought were identical."[579] Broussais has shown that "general diseases" do not exist: thus the "essential fevers" are "dying with the humoralism which assumed a foreign matter expelled by an aroused economy."[580] Henceforth physiology and pathology will be united and will explain all alterations of function by the lesion of an organ.[581] Even though Broussais may have exaggerated in ascribing all diseases to irritation of the intestinal tract alone, the concept of irritation is still fundamental to an understanding of pathology.[582]

Thus Cruveilhier worked on (1) the tie between symptoms and internal pathological changes and (2) the internal pathological criteria of disease classes.[583] "Let us stop listening to the Pyrrhonists who keep invoking Hippocrates, Galen, Stahl, and Sydenham to retard the progress of pathological anatomy, to whom the autopsy seems more a curiosity than a useful procedure."[584]

His doctrine reverted to the physiological dualism of Sauvages and Barthez: the organism consists of a material part–the organs, and a vital part–the force holding the organs together–which "struggles against the laws of the inorganic kingdom and for a certain time seizes from it a part of this matter."[585] While some diseases only affect the vital force, the majority cause a physical change in the body. They can be organic degenerations, whether cancerous, scrophulous, or from a chronic local irritation; or they can be organic lesions from an irritation settling in some part of the body, an atony, or the extinction of life.[586]

The concept of "essential inflammation," meaning a spontaneous local irritation, is "far preferable to all the vague ideas founded on physiological hypotheses to which time always does justice."[587]

General or systemic diseases arise from "sympathy" with the malfunctioning organ.[588] The symptoms are useful only in revealing the existence and seat of the local inflammation, as science has progressed beyond the point where diseases are classified by symptoms alone.[589] "Organic causes" are gradually driving "systemic" causes out of medicine.[590]

If an organic lesion cannot be found, it only means that the lesion or inflammation is latent in the organ.[591] [p]

On the issue of the priority of symptoms vs. that of pathological lesions Cruveilhier in 1816 was undecided; he accepted two classes, one in which the vital lesion is primary and one in which the organic lesion is primary.[592] By 1849 his thinking had become more Rationalized: even though the

[p]Cf. Laennec's "*modes de lesion*" which would be revealed with the increasing progress of pathological anatomy (above, p. 483). See also below, p. 528.

local lesion is the effect of a "general cause" acting on the whole economy, it is "the most elevated cause to which we can attain, and even the point of departure, since it, so to speak, governs the entire disease and its intensity."[593] The "essence" of a disease is always unknown.[594] "The idea of the vital force is as vague as that of the mainspring of a watch [*sic*], and it is a palpable error to claim to explain the facts by this force."[595] Thus anatomical investigations and autopsies are the best sources of knowledge of disease causes.[596] We started using the word, "meningitis," for "cerebral fever" as soon as we realized that this fever was localized in the meninges; and we will soon say "follicular enteritis," instead of "typhoid fever," for the same reason.[597]

Without pathological localization we would be left with nothing but Sauvages' hundreds of symptomatic species which confuse sympathetic symptoms with idiopathic and offer the physician merely a choice between vague generalities and an infinity of particulars.[598] Even the so-called neuroses or nervous diseases will benefit from pathological anatomy, as in the case of idiocy due to a cyst, a cancer, or ossification of the brain.[599]

Organic chemistry, giving us a positive analysis of the body's morbid products, promises great benefit.[600]

These anatomical and chemical findings permit correct disease classification, and the "clinical characteristics"—symptoms, etiology, aspects of therapeutics—must be subordinated to them.[601] Diseases are grouped according to the nature of the pathological lesion.[602] Differences due to the texture of the organ, etc. determine the subspecies.[603] Nearly all lesions are common to all tissues: special lesions—encountered in one tissue only—are rare.[604]

Morbid species do not vary or transform themselves into other species, and the number of such species is limited: "much more so than has generally been thought."[605]

Cruveilhier called himself an "organo-vitalist."[606] While hoping to reconcile vitalism with the emerging reductionist biology, he was entirely a Rationalist, and even a Methodist.

He was very respectful of Magendie[607 q] and in the 1830's concluded that interference with the flow of blood in the capillaries (identical with the ancient Methodist *status strictus*) was the cause of inflammation and the root of all pathological change: "phlebitis, in a way, rules the whole of pathology."[608 r]

He thus increased greatly the use of phlebotomy—to remove the obstruction causing the phlebitis. Whereas in 1821 he had urged it in a few diseases, such as croup:

> repeated bloodletting until the face becomes completely pale, while at the same time emptying the inflamed parts by local bleeding . . . use the most energetic revulsives administered in such a way as to destroy the congestion at its origin or abort [*juguler*] it.[609]

in 1849 he was urging this sort of treatment for every disease known to medicine.[610]

Fortunately for his patients, Cruveilhier abandoned therapeutics to spend his declining decades on an illustrated anatomy. The pursuit of proximate causes with the newly developed microscope was continued by Hermann Lebert (1813-1878).[611]

The system of Leon Rostan resembles that of Cruveilhier and was likewise inspired by Broussais and Magendie.[612]

He studied at Paris and graduated in 1812. By 1814 he had become Pinel's deputy at the Salpetriere where for eight months he administered a 2000-bed ward for Napoleon's army returning from Russia. Four years later he was appointed physician at the same hospital where for the next fifteen years he gave heavily attended courses in "organicism."[613] A Zurich student noted in 1831 that Rostan's clinic was the most enlightening of all, being the only one given at the sickbed.[614]

[q]On Magendie, see below pp. 606 ff.

[r]John Hunter had actually been the one to introduce phlebitis into medicine but gave it a vitalist interpretation (*Observations on the Inflammation of the Internal Coats of Veins* [London: Johnson, 1793]).

In 1833 he acceded to the chair of internal clinics at the Faculté and from this rostrum was able to influence another generation of students.[s]

Rostan's discovery of "organicism" was originally motivated by dislike for Broussais: "the simplicity, the facility of [physiological] medicine flattered the laziness of some and the intellectual weakness of the majority."[615] "Our nephews will have difficulty believing that these propositions took us so much trouble to overthrow."[616] Broussais' "exclusive doctrine of irritation" aroused in him the desire to find a substitute, but after this promising start he was only able to offer a modified and expanded "physiological medicine," Broussaisism writ large.[617]

Broussais had allowed only the stomach and intestines to be inflamed: Rostan permitted each organ in the body to be an autonomous and spontaneous generator of disease.[618] Otherwise his "organicism" was identical with Broussaisism, as was charged by his contemporaries.[619]

He rejected "vital properties": Dupuytren and Magendie have shown life to consist only in the molecular organization of matter.[620] The human organism is a mechanism like a clock.[621] "Does it explain anything to say that an organ is *sensitive* because endowed with *sensitivity*, or *contractile* because endowed with *contractility?* Is this kind of reasoning different from that which tells us that opium puts a man to sleep *quia est in eo virtus dormitiva?* My heavens! do they think they explain anything by these *vital forces?*"[622]

Organicism was materialistic.[623] "Life" does not exist independently of some living organism, i.e., matter, and the manifestations of life are hence determined by the organization and structure of living matter.[624] [t] "Vital properties"

[s]Carl Wunderlich wrote in 1841 that Rostan's classes were always overcrowded (*Wien und Paris* [Stuttgart: Ebner and Seubert, 1841], 122).

[t]This idea is taken from Magendie (see below, p. 615). Rostan expressly denies that "life" is prior to the structure and organization of living matter: "thus there do not exist vital properties considered as the cause of organization, as independent of this organization" (*Exposition des Principes de l'Organicisme* [Paris: Labe, 1846], 126).

are only "the aptitude or disposition of the organs to act."[625] "Life" is the "organic disposition necessary for movement," a particular arrangement of the molecules.[626]

The organism is composed of organs which perform functions, one function per organ; there can be no lesion of a function, or of the "vital forces," without a corresponding organic lesion.[627] Each organ can be "primitively ill," and the fluids can also be "primitively ill."[628] If, in a given disease, the physician cannot find an organic malfunction, this means only that science has not yet advanced far enough: "Is our inability to explain them a reason to admit the existence of beings which are in no way demonstrated, or to reject logically irreproachable principles? Could not nature have available, to fulfill a function, resources of which we are still ignorant?"[629] A "disease" cause is always an abnormal state of an organ, not an "alteration of some pretended vital property."[630]

Rostan's whole medical edifice thus rested on the hypothesis of organic lesions.[631] Symptoms were significant only in pointing to the existence of lesions; the symptoms of the lesion were distinguished from those of the rest of the body—brought into play through "sympathy."[632] As several organs could be diseased simultaneously, a person could suffer from more than one "disease" at a time.[633]

Dropsy and jaundice, which used to be considered "functional," were now recognized as "symptomatic"—"with certain exceptions into the details of which it is impossible to enter here."[634] Asthma, which Laennec attributed to a lesion of the pulmonary tissue, was really due to a lesion of the heart.[635] Brain diseases were no longer ascribed to changes in the sensitivity and contractility of this organ but rather to "congestion, inflammation, hemorrhage, softening, cancer, fungoid tumors, tuberculous tumors, osseous tumors, acephalocysts, and sometimes to unperceived lesions."[636] "These diseases, formerly almost unknown, become, so to say, immediately as clear as the thoracic and abdominal ones."[637] Treatment was thereby greatly improved: "it is known to what degree of clarity we have attained in this scientific question."[638] Therapeutics, in a word, became "rational."[639]

The characteristic features of an Empirical doctrine were thus belittled by Rostan. The concept of "idiosyncrasy" virtually disappeared, dissolved into the molecules: genuine idiosyncrasies are few and far between and can be understood by any second-year medical student.[640] Certain diseases which he called "special"–meaning "always presenting the same characteristics" but not contagious–were ascribed to the capacity of an organ to be sick in a variety of different ways and were thus not "specific diseases."[641] Such were urticaria, prurigo, impetigo, tuberculosis, scrophula, some cancers, and others.[642]

Scrophula was due not to a "taint" (*vice scrofuleux*), but only to an exaggerated lymphatic constitution.[643]

He did recognize the existence of some "specific" diseases–the "special" diseases which were also contagious: syphilis, yellow fever, scabies, scarlet fever, and others.[644] But their number has greatly diminished under the influence of "physiological medicine."[645]

He admitted that the organic lesion is subsequent to the illness of the whole organism but maintained, even so, that, "although not constituting the whole disease, [it] is still the most certain guide to knowledge of its cause."[646]

He rejected prognosis in favor of diagnosis: "all of medicine resides in diagnosis alone; prognosis and therapeutic indications are all derived from it."[647] He rejected "empirical" modes of treatment and distrusted specific medicines: a "small number" of truly specific medicines have emerged from "this filthy mass of absurd formulas, these disgusting errors of the human mind."[648] [u]

He extolled organicism as ending the "vagueness of former doctrines, the metaphysical entities engendered by the imaginations of our forebears."[649]

A signal advantage of the new doctrine was to permit rapid examination of the patient. While some physicians interrogate the patient at length, gaining his confidence and thus contributing to a predisposition in favor of cure, this can

[u]By "empiricism" he meant the pharmacological therapeutics of Trousseau (see below, pp. 568 ff).

have deleterious effects: in a respiratory disease, for example, the patient is exhausted by lengthy questioning. It can worsen a mental illness also: "does not the man of art–whose ministry it is to comfort, to reduce pain, in a word, to cure–thereby himself become a deplorable cause of pain and even of death?"[650] No, it is far preferable to make the interview short: "in most cases one must ask as few questions as possible and arrive as rapidly as possible at a diagnosis." The first question is thus: "Where are you sick?" This is better than asking: "What is wrong with you," since one patient will say he has "nerve trouble," another will say "bile," a third "blood," a fourth "the humors," etc. But if you ask him "where?" he will point to the suffering organ–a big step forward in the diagnosis.

"Despite the precision of this question, however, it is often difficult to prevent the patient from wandering around the subject and pouring forth all his fantasies." Hence, the next question must be: "For how long have you been sick?" which "prodigiously curtails the work involved in diagnosing the disease one is combating."[651] Once the physician has pinpointed the disturbed organ, he knows that the remaining morbid phenomena are the consequence of sympathy.

For all of these reasons organicism became popular. In the early 1840's Rostan wrote that all physicians practice it, even though all do not admit it.[652] No one talks any more about "vital properties" as "beings existing by themselves." Now they are all connected with some functional disturbance.[653] "Never at the sickbed do you hear them talk about vital properties, their exaltation, diminution, abolition, or perversion: such talk is good only for the books. In practice, they are all organicists."[654]

The Rationalizing tendency in Paris medicine started by Broussais and fed by the physiological researches of Magendie reached a culmination of sorts in the philosophy and therapeutics of Jean-Baptiste Bouillaud who was professor of clinical medicine at the Charité for almost fifty years, a member of the Academy of Medicine from 1825 and of the Academy of Sciences from 1868, and for decades professor of medical clinics at the Faculté.

His 1826 *Traite Clinique et Experimentel des Fievres Dites Essentielles* saluted the new era which began when Broussais tore the veil from the so-called "essential fevers."[655] Far from being "essential," they are all associated with some local lesion: ordinary "fever" with the sanguiniferous system, bilious fever with the digestive system, ataxic fever with an irritation of the brain, etc.[656] Medicine is truly a physico-chemical science. It is also a science of observation and will become perfected when man can observe the molecular phenomena.[657]

In 1840 Bouillaud produced a treatise on articular rheumatism, showing that it often leads to inflammatory disease of the heart: his suggested therapy was repeated bleeding, *"coup sur coup"* as he described it; thus he converted innumerable cases of rheumatism into heart disease and proved the existence of his law.[658]

> Therapeutics is a true war against diseases. We must, as far as possible formulate appropriate rules for this sort of war, correct tactics . . . In acute diseases, which rapidly and energetically attack the bases of life, our means must be proportionate to the *force* and *rapidity* of the attack. The means generally employed hitherto seemed to us well below what we should demand of the art . . . The fundamental principle of our *therapeutic tactics,* which dominates all the rest, has been, in acute diseases, to deploy rapidly, one after the other [*coup sur coup*], the various weapons in our therapeutic arsenal, attacking, so to speak, the enemy at all points at once, and particularly at the most exposed ones, charging him unceasingly, giving him no rest for recuperation, pursuing him to the end, until he abandons the field and the therapeutist has exhausted all the resources available for the given case.[659]

One is not surprised to find out that Bouillaud's uncle and mentor in medicine made a career as an army surgeon.

In 1836 Bouillaud put his ideas together into an *Essay on Medical Philosophy,* depicting Rationalist/Methodist therapeutics in its purest form.

Medicine must be made exact by applying the exact sciences, physics, mathematics, and chemistry.[660] From observation of the phenomena one deduces the forces governing them—called "general causes or properties," "primary causes," etc.[661] They follow the laws of statics, mechanics, hydraulics, and organic chemistry: if these sciences cannot yet explain all the phenomena, it is because they are still undeveloped.[662] Diseases are not general but local, and the mission of science is to pinpoint their locus as precisely as possible: "the investigation must be pushed to the organic molecules themselves. Molecular anatomy is the *nec plus ultra* of this sort of progress."[663]

Predisposing causes exist, but they cannot give rise to disease without a "determining cause." Physical agents are important here, but Bouillaud rejected "these viruses [*virus*], these taints [*vices*], these rheumatic, gouty, scrophulous, etc. *principles* whose existence is as chimeric as the astral and divine influences accepted by Paracelsus."[664] Belief in them is only the "crudest superstition."[665]

There is a "vital force" in the body, but its efficacy has been grossly exaggerated by Sydenham, Stahl, and others.[666] The physician should endeavor to treat "rationally," applying his "exact knowledge of the nature and mode of action of his instruments,"[667] and not "empirically"—meaning "crude knowledge of the curative virtue of a given medicine, of whose mechanism one is entirely ignorant."[668] "Therapeutics is really only a *deduction*, a *corollary*, of the ideas and doctrines the physician has evolved on the *nature* of diseases."[669]

Bouillaud devoted ninety pages of this book to an exposition of bloodletting *coup sur coup*, presumably the ultimate in mid-nineteenth-century therapeutic rationality.[670] He proved by statistical analysis that Louis' attempt to limit bloodletting was an error: Louis' results were inconclusive because he was too timid with the lancet. Bloodletting in really massive quantities is, on the contrary, highly effective and a cure for many diseases: "*voila mon dernier mot.*"[671]

Eclecticism in One Person: Gabriel Andral

The recognized leader of the Paris School in the 1830's and 1840's, the personification of "Eclecticism," was Gabriel Andral.

An accomplished practitioner (Laennec had a high opinion of him) and an excellent medical politician, but not a profound thinker, Andral always settled for an acceptable compromise among competing factions at the expense of scientific truth.[671] A banner of tolerance in the campaign against Broussais, "Eclecticism" was carried too far, Andral's hatred for doctrinaire views leading him to hedge on every issue and take positions which seemed judicious and reasonable to his contemporaries but inconsistent and vacillating to later generations.

For originality and trenchancy of thought he was not the equivalent of a Laennec or even a Pinel, and his name has been rightly forgotten by all but historians of medicine.

He justified his shifts of position by the progress of medicine: "it is less to my opinions, changing and progressive like the science itself, than to the facts themselves that I urge the attention of practitioners . . . The facts are the real treasure of the science."[673] He claimed in 1840 to have recommenced medicine three times: when he learned pathological anatomy, when he mastered Laennec's method of physical diagnosis, and when he started his research on the blood.[674] A fourth departure was his lecture course on medical history for which he abandoned pathology while in his fifties, perhaps in an effort to seek new bearings. But he carried it only up to Galen and then left medicine entirely for private life, caring for his ailing wife until her death in 1872 and following her to the grave some years later.

Andral's qualifications for political leadership were impeccable. His father had gone to Naples as personal physician to Murat, returning after the latter's death to Paris where he was taken on by Charles X. Andral's own career started under the tutelage of the prominent clinician, T. N. Lerminier, and shortly thereafter he published a *Clinique Medicale* in four volumes which saw several more editions and remained standard for decades.[675] He became professor of hygiene at the Faculté in 1828, of internal pathology in 1830, and of general pathology in 1839 when he inherited the position of Broussais.[676]

His career was greatly advanced by marriage to the daughter of P. P. Royer-Collard (1763-1845) who, together with Victor Cousin (1792-1867), founded the French school of philosophical "eclecticism." This was official doctrine after the 1830 revolution, and it is not hard to see why Andral adapted it to his own purposes; he used the word first in 1829.

His other major writings were a *Precis d'Anatomie Pathologique* (1829),[677] which helped shift medicine from a solidist to a neo-humoralist basis, an annotated edition of Laennec's *Auscultation Mediate* (1837),[678] and the fully humoralist *Essai d'Hematologie Pathologique* (1837)[679]–the first treatise on hematology. While not great works, these were competent texts and essential teaching materials for the Paris medicine of these decades. To the author, however, they were primarily stepping-stones in a political career conducted with a feel for the prevailing currents. At every stage Andral took the middle position, and no unified body of doctrine can be extracted from his writings.

A tendency to trim his sails to the wind can be seen from the beginning. His thesis for the M.D., *Expectoration in Various Chest Diseases,* followed Hippocratic principles, with coction and crisis, but held that some diseases are resolved when the sputum is still crude.[680] Generally, the existence of crises is "one of the most delicate points in medicine, requiring the severest impartiality on the part of the observer."[681] His thesis for the *aggregation,* three years later, again took up the question of crises. Diseases fall into two classes, those usually resolved by a crisis and those usually resolved without crisis: "hence we must take the middle course," waiting for the crisis in mild diseases but using bloodletting and other active remedies in violent ones.[682] The *Clinique Medicale* discussed crises but attributed minor importance to them.[683] Andral's edition of the *Auscultation Mediate* corrected Laennec's excessive admiration for Hippocraticism: spitting of blood is not caused by suppressed menses, pulmonary apoplexy is not due to the cauterization or excision of bleeding hemorrhoids, etc.[684] In the 1850's he accepted the existence of coction and crisis in measles, smallpox, and some other eruptive fevers (the morbific matter being concocted and excreted in the pustules), but this formed only a small part of his pathology.[685]

He followed a middle course in the dispute over symptoms and pathology, i.e., over whether diseases are general or local phenomena. His *Clinique Medicale,* attacking Broussais, held that fevers are "general diseases which can become complicated by different local ones"; the lesions of the intestines seem sometimes the cause of the fever and sometimes its effect.[686] Bordeu criticized those who want to make all serious fevers into local diseases.[687] Thus Broussais' doctrine is true for some cases but not for all: "let us go where the facts lead us and know enough to stop when the facts no longer light the way."[688]

In this work Andral also accepted the predisposing cause in pleuro-pneumonia and other diseases: "without which the occasional causes would remain without effect." "By virtue of this predisposition the same cause yields a sore throat [*angine*] in one, a simple bronchitis in another, a pleuro-pneumonia in a third, and a gastritis or peritonitis in a fourth."[689]

He taught in 1825 that the study of symptoms must be combined with that of pathological anatomy: "a lesion given, determine the symptoms which it causes; and, vice-versa, a group of symptoms being given, determine the lesion which causes them."[690]

By the third edition of his *Clinique Medicale* Andral's views on intestinal diseases had incorporated the discoveries of Bretonneau and Louis. Now he divided Broussais' gastro-enteritis into three classes: (1) the "typhoid fever" of Bretonneau and Louis, marked by follicular lesions of the intestine; (2) a similar disease but with simple inflammation of the intestinal mucous membrane—Broussais' "gastro-enteritis"; and (3) a disease with typhoid symptoms, but no intestinal lesions, originating in the "nervous centers" of the body—Louis' "simulated typhoid."[691]

His edition of the *Auscultation Mediate* took the same middle course. Andral was largely responsible for popularizing Laennec's technique and made himself thoroughly proficient in it—rescuing it from Eusebe de Salles and others with their comments about the "patience of a Chinaman and the life of a Mathuselah," etc.[692] [v] He denied that Laennec had entered into excessive symptomatic detail and called for an even more elaborate classification of chest diseases.[693] Phthisis is a "general affection of the economy of which the pulmonary lesion is only a fraction or, if you will, an effect."[694] Symptomatic catarrh, "like many others," is only the "entirely secondary consequence of a general morbific cause which exerts its influence over the whole economy."[695] But he also urged full attention to the pathology: "is there any disease whose symptoms do not become clearer and, to some extent, more rational, to the person who knows the accompanying anatomical lesions?"[696] And he ended up in the middle:

> Disturbance of function can be the consequence of many factors other than a lesion in the arrangement of the molecules of the organ. Gravel, for instance, due to the presence of excess nitrogen in the blood, is not the product of a change in the texture of the kidneys, etc. But from failure to find appreciable alterations in the organ from which to explain a functional disorder one should not too quickly or too easily conclude that this alteration does not exist and immediately, as does

[v]But he ignored Laennec himself who, for political reasons, was not in public favor. Laennec was greatly offended, as both were, after all, teaching in the same school. He wrote that Andral "sought to place himself in the hypothesis of the author's death immediately after the publication of his work" (*Auscultation Mediate,* 1831, I, xi). Andral played a similar trick on his first benefactor, Lerminier, who had paid the costs of publication of *Clinique Medicale,* agreed to put his name on the title page, and written a short introduction, all of this contributing to the success of the enterprise. As the first volume was selling well, and Andral's course in pathological anatomy was very successful, he suddenly changed the title page, substituting a new one with only his own name as author, and thereafter they met only in consultations (Fauconneau-Dufresne, "Souvenirs des Commencements de la Carriere du Professeur Andral," *L'Union Medicale* XXIII [1877], 921-927).

> Laennec, attribute these symptoms to an alteration of the liquids or of the nervous system. Because the progress of pathological anatomy may reveal, in the very organ whose functions are disturbed, a lesion which had long remained unnoticed. Has not Laennec himself found in a pulmonary emphysema the cause of certain asthmas which, before his elegant researches, had been regarded as of nervous origin.[697]

He offered an attractive verbal resolution of the symptom/pathology conflict: while the individual patient displays symptoms first and pathology later, the general description of a "disease" must commence with the pathology and conclude with the symptoms.[698]

Another debate of the times was between humoralism and solidism. In 1823 Andral stated that Pinel's "essential fevers" can originate "equally in the solids and the fluids."[699] His 1829 *Precis d'Anatomie Pathologique* aimed to fuse the two strands of thought in the molecular exchange between the blood and the solids which takes place in the capillaries; he elaborated a complex disease classification on the basis of this primordial physiological function.[700] His final treatment of the subject came in his 1843 *Essai d'Hematologie Pathologique* which located pathological causes in the fluids alone, initiating the neo-humoralism which was thereafter official doctrine in the Paris School.[w]

He complains that physicians have studied only the physical properties of the blood, while this liquid should be analyzed chemically.[701] His own research revealed the blood's major components to be fibrin, globuli, and albuminous matter; when these are within certain limits (2-4 parts/1000 of fibrin, 110-140/1000 of globuli, and 80/1000 of albumen), the blood is healthy, while beyond them it is diseased.[702]

[w]It appeared a year after Magendie's essay on the blood in diseases (the fourth volume of his *Phenomenes Physiques de la Vie* [Paris: Bailliere, 1842]), and Andral gives Magendie full credit (*Essai d'Hematologie Pathologique* [Paris: Fortin, 1843], 7, 9). See below, pp. 628-630.

In plethora, for instance, the blood contains more globuli, causing a more rapid metabolism, a faster heart beat, fever, and hemorrhage. In anemia the globuli are reduced in quantity. The other disease classes of his time (pyrexias, phlegmasies, hemorrhages, dropsies, "organic diseases," and "neuroses") were also distinguished by particular ratios of fibrin, globuli, and albumen in the blood.[703]

Andral thus resolved the humoralism/solidism conflict in favor of the humors—as improved by chemistry: "there where anatomy can no longer reveal an alteration, chemistry shows us one."[704] This yielded a new solution to the symptom/pathology conflict: disease symptoms must be subordinated to hematological findings. Pneumonia, erysipelas, tonsillitis, bronchitis, and peritonitis—despite their symptomatic differences—require the same therapy, since all are marked by increased fibrin in the blood.[705] By the same token, diseases with quite identical symptoms may have a different hematology and require different treatment.[706]

Andral's contemporaries regarded this book as a "veritable event . . . which banished a time-honored error and enthroned a truth, showing by precise chemical analysis the alterations of the blood hitherto regarded as possible or probable and making a place for humoral lesions side by side with organic ones."[707]

This reflected their satisfaction at being presented with a whole new class of proximate causes upon which therapy could be based.

Andral held these changes in the blood to "intervene as causes in the production of a fairly considerable number of diseases."[708] "In plethora, as in anemia, the particular state of the blood is the appreciable cause of the general modification of the organism. Here, for us at least, is the primitive fact beyond which we cannot go and to which we have the right to relate all the others."[709] Even though certain (prior) forces in the patient's organism may have brought about this "constitution" of the blood, "once produced, this constitution is still the only discernible [*constatable*] fact, the only one which can be grasped by observation and be made the experimental cause of the phenomena."[710] [x]

Andral's conclusion that the whole "disease" is incorporated in the hematological changes reflected the impact of Magendie's experiments injecting chemicals in the veins of dogs to ascertain their effect (the Rationalist parallel to Hahnemann's provings). Andral observes that Magendie has thus proved the possibility of creating diseases artificially.[711] Alkalies dissolve the blood and yield a syndrome identical with typhus.[712] From these experiments one can draw conclusions about the possible influence of such modifications in the blood when they occur "spontaneously."[713]

Andral gave the profession a new solvent of medical facts and observations. Much of the older luggage could now be jettisoned. For instance, one of the sounds (*le bruit de souffle*) which Laennec distinguished upon auscultation was now seen to be caused by a globuli level lower than 80/1000.[714] Hemorrhages were no longer considered positive signs (as in Hippocratic medicine) but only signs of a low fibrin level.[715] "Idiosyncrasy" henceforth meant only that the fibrin, globuli, or albumen were at the limits of normality.[716] The production of fibrin was affected only by the acuteness of the phlegmasic state, not by any differences of constitution, temperament, age, or sex.[717]

Lesions of the organs were consequent upon some change in the blood, and the symptoms provoked by organic changes were no longer important, only those due to the state of the blood.[718]

Broussais' followers grieved at this restoration of humoralism, feeling that the "illustrious reformer" had been finally defeated, but a more profound analysis reveals that Andral himself was the defeated party: his new hematological doctrine was merely an updating of Broussais' Methodist dualism. Only two classes of disease exist: the blood is either

[x]In one passage, however, he states that the lower proportion of globuli in the blood of phthisis patients is not the disease cause but only a "sign" (*Essai d'Hematologie Pathologique,* 172. See, Also, *ibid.,* 68). "Experimental cause" was the new name for "proximate cause."

too thick (and coagulates) or too thin (and flows too easily).[719] Andral noted a certain parallel with Italian "contrastimulism," but the resemblance was even greater to Methodism in its pristine form.[720]

Andral, indeed, admitted a debt to the modern Methodist, Sylvius de le Boe, a "truly superior man," who was held back only by the primitive chemistry of the seventeenth century.[721] He noted the connection between Sylvius' acid and alkali experiments and those being performed by Magendie.[722]

Therapeutics was based on the symptoms of the state of the blood,[723] and, while Andral did not discuss treatment in the *Essai d'Hematologie Pathologique,* there were suggestions of a system based on acids, alkalis, and phlebotomy (Methodism had made copious use of bloodletting to eliminate obstructions in the circulation). Excessive fibrin must be reduced by "revulsives" and alkaline remedies.[724] Acid medicines must be used in typhoid, where the blood is thin and needs coagulation.[725] The globuli in the blood are lessened by a short hemorrhage or bloodletting, the fibrin by a longer one.[726] Phlegmasies are shortened by extensive bloodletting.[727] Cruveilhier's "phlebitis" came into its own as "stasis"—due both to excess and to insufficient fibrin.[728]

In his *Precis d'Anatomie Pathologique* Andral suggested diluting the blood with water as the best treatment for diseases in which the fibrin content is high: hence the utility of having the patient drink much water in diphtheria.[729] He cited with approval Magendie's injection of water into the veins of a patient with meningitis.[730]

The fate of specific diseases in Eclecticism was thus to be dissolved in hematological theory. Snake venoms and mineral poisons such as mercury all have their effect on the blood, and contagious diseases such as measles, smallpox, and scarlet fever also take the form of an alteration of the blood.[731] "Thus it has been concluded that the blood should alter, and that this alteration should be the point of departure of the disease, when the cause of the alteration is absorption of a miasm, a virus, or a poison."[732]

Trousseau and Homoeopathy

The Paris School in its early decades was far more concerned with pathological and physiological theory than with therapeutics. Pharmacology, especially, was an abandoned discipline, as the rationale for the use of many drugs had disappeared with the collapse of ancien régime medicine in 1789.[733] This pharmacological wasteland was further devastated by Brown, with his division of medicines into two classes and disregard for the therapeutics of the past, and by Broussais, restricting all therapeutics to the application of leeches at the anus. A. L. J. Bayle wrote in 1828 that while pathology and anatomy had advanced since the Revolution, therapeutics "has actually regressed; a number of substances and agents formerly regarded as salutary have fallen into oblivion or been proscribed; the numerous works on the virtues of medicines are no longer consulted, and there is so much scepticism and uncertainty that doubt has been cast on the efficacy of the most heroic substances."[734] He blamed this on Broussais, but the chief culprit was still the pathological-anatomical approach to medicine which sought disease causes in the lesions disclosed by autopsy: "since these structural disorders are reducible to a small number of species, the accepted medicinal agents have been reduced to a similarly small number."[735]

Bayle's own *Bibliotheque de Therapeutique* was one effort to dispel the darkness surrounding pharmacology. Others were Magendie's *Formulaire pour la Preparation et l'Emploi de Plusieurs Nouveaux Medicaments*,[736] J. G. Barbier's *Traite Elementaire de Matiere Medicale*,[737] and J. L. M. Alibert's *Nouveaux Elements de Therapeutique et de Matiere Medicale*.[738] Cullen's *Treatise of the Materia Medica* was still in use. But, as Trousseau later wrote, these works "were employed less by physicians than by medical students preparing for their examinations . . . there was scarcely any materia medica in existence, therapeutics being reduced almost entirely to leeches, some emollients, a few revulsives, and a little opium."[739] Even such a renowned clinician as Lerminier, known as a moderate, extracted quarts of blood from his patients,[740] and all the famous figures of Paris medicine employed savagely primitive techniques (except ones like Pinel who abandoned active treatment for expectancy).

Broussais was only the culmination of existing trends, appealing by his therapeutic simplicity but proposing essentially the same methods as those already in use.

The reaction of patients to being treated as raw material for the development of pathological theory, while not recorded in the literature, was seen in the instant popularity of homoeopathy which appeared in France in the 1820's and, in the following decade, provoked a split in the medical profession.

The Introduction of Homoeopathy

The first French homoeopath was J. Mabit, a former military surgeon who became a professor at the medical school of Bordeaux. He discovered the *Organon* in 1826 and by the 1832 cholera epidemic was in the full practice of the new system.[741]

He was a friend of Laennec and persuaded him to undertake trials of these new medicines in the last months of his life.[742]

In the same year Theodore Boeckel, a medical student at Strasburg (where French culture was in contact with German), wrote a dissertation on the New School which saw promise in its use of specific medicines and its pharmacological trials on healthy persons; he called for further investigation of homoeopathy by the medical profession.[743]

In 1828 Count Sebastian Des Guidi, fleeing his native Naples after leading an unsuccessful revolution against Ferdinand I, took a medical degree at Strasburg, became converted to homoeopathic practice, and settled in Lyons. In a short time he had spread the doctrine to 25 of his colleagues there and in Geneva–including such future leaders of French homoeopathy as Charles Peschier, Pierre and Edouard Dufresne, Auguste Rapou, and C. A. Gueyrard.

The first homoeopath in Paris was the Englishman, Frederick F. H. Quin, who had studied with Hahnemann in

Koethen and with his pupils in Leipzig.[y] He made a great reputation in aristocratic and diplomatic circles but soon returned to London as the pioneer of homoeopathy (at first called "Quinism") in that city. He was extraordinarily effective, and a segment of the British aristocracy have been homoeopathic adherents ever since.

Quin was followed in Paris by Paul Curie, grandfather of Pierre Curie, who had first encountered homoeopathy in Alsace in 1832. He eventually removed to London also, where he spent most of his life. Other leading Paris homoeopaths were Leon Simon, C. Croserio, Antoine Petroz (member of the Academy of Medicine), and Benoit Mure (who later pioneered homoeopathy in Brazil).

A. J. L. Jourdan of the Academy of Medicine, while not a practitioner of homoeopathy himself, translated all of Hahnemann's writings into French, starting in 1832 with the *Organon* (fourth German edition) and the *Chronic Diseases.*

The *Societe Homoeopathique Gallicane* was founded by the Lyons and Geneva homoeopaths in 1835 and the *Societe Homoeopathique de Paris* by the Paris ones in 1834. The first homoeopathic periodical was the *Bibliotheque Homoeopathique* which appeared in Geneva from 1833 to 1837. The *Journal de la Medicine Homoeopathique* and the *Archives de la Medecine Homoeopathique* were issued in Paris in the 1830's. In the latter decades of the century seventeen other homoeopathic periodicals in the French language were published in France, Belgium, and Switzerland.

The 1830's were a time of medical crisis in Europe, with the New School offering an intellectual and scientific challenge to thought-patterns taken for granted since ancient times. The crisis reached the United States in the 1840's: the founding of the American Institute of Homoeopathy in

[y]Quin was born in 1799 of uncertain parentage but may have been the illegitimate son of the Duchess of Devonshire (see G. Ruthven Mitchell, *Homoeopathy: The First Authoritative Study of its Place in Medicine Today* [London: W. H. Allen, 1975], 91). He was one of the leading dandies of his time and a member of the D'Orsay set (Ellen Moers, *The Dandy: Brummell to Beerbohm* [New York: Viking Press, 1960], 158). See his *Du Traitement Homoeopathique du Cholera* (Paris: Bailliere, 1832).

1844, and of the American Medical Association in 1846, caused a political and institutional division of the medical profession which has lasted, in some respects, to this very day. In Europe the division, while not so politically long-lasting, was equally profound.

All the later history of French medicine was affected by the introduction of homoeopathy in Bordeaux, Lyons, and Paris.

A major catalyst of opinion was the Asiatic Cholera—epidemic in 1832 and endemic for years thereafter. Hahnemann had written extensively on it and recommended three medicines for its treatment—camphor, copper sulphate, and *Veratrum album*—which were eventually adopted by the allopathic profession.[z] Camphor became especially popular in non-professional circles and found its way into nearly every cholera preparation. Hence, a prominent feature of the allopathic attack on homoeopathy was criticism of the homoeopathic treatment of cholera.[744]

Another factor in the spread of homoeopathy was Hahnemann's arrival in Paris in 1835, together with his young and well-connected French wife.[a] Her influence at Court was sufficient to extract a decree from the Minister of Public Instruction, F. P. G. Guizot, within six weeks of their arrival, permitting Hahnemann to practice medicine in Paris. The instinctive preference of the aristocratic and well-educated for homoeopathy was reinforced by Hahnemann's personal contact with exalted circles of French society.

The history of the allopathic-homoeopathic dispute was complicated by the virtual impossibility of formulating the issues in language which both sides could accept. And the intense political and economic antagonism between the two parties intensified the problem.

[z]See *Divided Legacy,* III, 267-269. Coulter, *Homoeopathic Influences in Nineteenth-Century Allopathic Therapeutics,* 46-55.

[a]A variety of jokes circulated in allopathic circles about the marital problems supposedly caused by the great age difference between husband and wife (e.g., *"Nous esperons que Madame ne se contente pas du decillionieme," Bulletin General de Therapeutique* VIII [1835], 320).

Thus it was a rare allopath who even understood the homoeopathic arguments (the homoeopaths, who were all converts, understood the allopathic arguments much better). They felt only that homoeopathy was an antagonist to be opposed and contended with at every turn.[b] Thus their arguments, seen in historical perspective, appear irrational, as they rejected in some forums principles and tenets which in others they were willing to accept. Underlying the whole dispute, however, was an inchoate allopathic awareness that accepting the homoeopathic principles meant revising the political and economic bases of medical practice.[c]

The Crystallization of Allopathic Hostility

The progress of homoeopathy in France was typified by Mabit's experience in Bordeaux. He used the new medicines during the 1832 cholera epidemic and reported good results to the Bordeaux Medical Society.[745] His reputation was made, and in 1834 he was called as physician to one of the town's prominent merchants.[746] A year later a Bordeaux allopath complained in the medical press:

> Thus, when I wrote you before that the new German doctrine was propagating slowly in Bordeaux, I was correct. But what a difference in the last month! Some of our leading citizens give an envious example of absolute confidence in the pleasant and agreeable rules of homoeopathy, and serious, studious, enlightened men—exempt hitherto from the prejudices and blind belief of the vulgar—no longer disdain recourse to a singular therapeutics, one contrary to all the ideas acquired by reason, knowledge, and experience; the very sight of the homoeopathic doctor who comes periodically to deposit gravely the precious globule on the organ of speech fails to shake

[b]Homoeopathy is a new system which "naturally seeks a quarrel with everyone" (*Gazette Medicale de Paris* II [1834], 1). "A doctrine which aims at nothing less than to overturn, from top to bottom, the medical edifice upon which so many skilled hands have worked for centuries" (*Bulletin General de Therapeutique* VI [1834], 107; see, also, *ibid.*, 358).

[c]See *Divided Legacy,* III, 376-382.

> their faith and no longer serves as a cause for hilarity, dominated as they are by a true magnetic fascination. All of this is so, but let us admit that it is truly extraordinary! How long will this rare credulity last? I do not know. But let us await patiently the fulfillment of the promise of the homoeopaths, and HE WILL LAUGH BEST WHO LAUGHS LAST.[747]

The gradual desertion of traditional medicine by such "leading citizens" cast a chill over allopathy. A journal observed in 1834 that "the sectators of Hahnemann, despite their small numbers, are, it is said, making a generous harvest at this moment in Paris," attributing it to "the love of high society for the marvellous."[748] "Everyone is now preoccupied with homoeopathy."[749] Trousseau wrote later that scarcely any physician had not lost some patients to the homoeopaths.[750] And the high fees the latter could charge also rankled. For example, Hahnemann treated the Marquess of Anglesea for a *tic douleureux* of many years' standing caused by the loss of a leg at Waterloo and charged 200 francs monthly, payable in advance, for once weekly visits; the Marquess' eventual cure caused a sensation, as he had been treated unsuccessfully by other physicians for two decades.[751]

The open conflict undermined the public's confidence in medicine and the medical profession. Bouillaud in 1836 complained of "people in society, and even some colleagues, who whisper in your ear, in all good faith, asking if you believe in therapeutics. According to them medicine should be to some extent assimilated to the science of those astrologers who could not look at one another without laughing. Certainly a true physician is upset when he hears people talking that way about medicine today. We should not be surprised if homoeopathy, which is certainly not worth more than the science of soothsaying, should be exploiting the credulity of the uninformed."[752] Ten years later Rostan wrote (in an article "On Disbelief in Medicine"): "Men of the cloth, of the sword, of all ages and sexes and all conditions of life, educated and uneducated," profess disbelief in medicine, but at the same time they believe in homoeopathy.[753]

The homoeopaths' insistence on treating patients by a new set of rules—and actually giving satisfaction—was unforgivable, and the allopaths soon ceased being patronizing.[754] While in 1834 Trousseau could still call the homoeopaths "honorable men, friends in whose good faith we have confidence," even though they practice a system which is "speculative" and "against scientific principles," the members of the Academy of Medicine in 1835 called the New School "dishonorable" knaves, ignoramuses, charlatans, and quacks.[755]

This attitude was justified, in a debate which continued for decades, by the typical arguments which Rationalists have adduced against medical Empiricism. Proximate causes are knowable: "it is incontestable that pathological anatomy has perfectly revealed to us the nature and seat of a number of diseases."[756] "The anatomical lesions of nearly all diseases are known, and the science of diagnosis consists precisely in progressing from the observed symptoms to the organic alteration; therapeutics, in turn, is directed at this real basis and not at mere appearances."[757] Disappearance of the symptoms is not equivalent to disappearance of the disease.[758] The rejection of nosology is unscientific, as is the individualization of treatment.[759] Homoeopathy is "illogical": "this doctrine is unbelievable—it runs against the known rules of medical logic."[760] Bouillaud called it "antirational."[761] The Academy of Medicine wrote to Guizot:

> First we subjected homoeopathy to the rigorous methods of logic, and logic immediately revealed in this system a series of those formal oppositions to the best-established truths, a number of those shocking contradictions, many of those palpable absurdities which inevitably ruin all false systems in the eyes of enlightened men even though they are not always a sufficient obstacle to the credulity of the multitude.[762] [d]

[d]To this the homoeopaths retorted: How can the Academy talk about "severe logic"? this "heterogeneous mixture of men and doctrines continually at odds with one another; the principles of one academician are his alone; each has his own diseases and consequently his own logic . . . The logic of some is not that of

Another group of arguments was aimed more particularly at the Hahnemannian adaptation of Empiricism. The infinitesimal doses came in for their share of ridicule.[763] The doctrine of chronic diseases was repugnant to allopathy, and the *Acarus scabiei* was resurrected as the true cause of psora (although the existence of this insect had been known for almost two hundred years).[764] [e] Isopathy seemed particularly vile and disgusting:

> To treat all the chronic diseases reputed of psoric origin it was imagined to *dynamize* the liquid in the itch vesicles (*psorin*); and some thought, for this purpose, to collect the *psorin* from the very person who was to be treated (*autopsorin*). Against pulmonary phthisis they *dynamized* the parenchyma of lungs affected by this disease. What can one say to all this? Good God! Once launched on the rails of a fantastic idea, how far do men allow themselves to be carried away by their imaginations!![765]

And the homoeopathic use of snake poisons provoked endless amazement.[766]

The law of similars was held to be "an illusion, pure and simple."[767] At best, the use of similars will intensify the

others, and what is an absurdity to some is truth for others. The most unfortunate and deplorable spectacle of scientific anarchy" (*Archives de la Medecine Homoeopathique* III [1835], 355). "What will any sensible man think of our science when he sees this justly celebrated school divided not only over theory but even over the most capital points of practice? What can be more scandalous than to see some professing eclecticism (with considerable talent, by the way), others numerical medicine with heavy bloodletting, and still others humoral medicine which they call 'Hippocratic.' And I will spare the reader all the sub-varieties such as 'physiological medicine,' 'organicism,' etc. One may hope that this anarchy in the School of Paris which is clearly undermining the medical confidence of the most enlightened persons will powerfully aid the propagation of homoeopathy" (*Ibid.*, VIII [1838], 437).

[e]The itch mite was first mentioned by an Italian physician in 1683 who had observed the slaves and poor people of Leghorn removing them from one another's skin with needles. Attention was again called to these parasites by Linnaeus and Wichmann in the mid- and late eighteenth century (Ameke, *History of Homoeopathy,* 69). G. L. Bayle in 1805 held that psora is caused by the *Acarus* and cured by mercurial ointments which kill the *Acarus* (G. L. Bayle, "Idee Generale de la Therapeutique" in *Bibliotheque Medicale* [Paris: Gabon, 1805], Vol. X). But the *Acarus* was presented as new discovery in the 1830's, proof that the homoeopathic theory of chronic diseases was incorrect.

disease.[768] "The axiom of the ancients, *contraria contraribus curantur,* cannot err; it is an eternal truth of common sense; it is the unshakeable principle of rational medicine."[769] [f]

Hahnemann's provings were denounced. Double stated that as early as 1801 he had dosed himself with quinine over a period of four months at Montpellier without arousing any sort of fever.[770] Andral claimed to have taken quinine in doses ranging from the infinitesimal up to 24 grains without being seized with intermittent fever; some associates who participated in the proving suffered a little headache and indigestion, but that was all; he claimed to have proved aconite, arnica, sulphur, and "a number of other medicines" in the same way without detecting any symptoms.[771] [g] "It is hence inexact to state that remedies give rise to diseases similar to those they cure."[772] Trousseau denied that quinine (eight grams of the powder) will give rise to any symptoms in a healthy person.[773] The chemist, P. J. Pelletier, announced that he had been ingesting small quantities of medicinal substances all his working life without detecting any symptoms: "at least on a healthy person the homoeopathic medicines have no effect."[774]

All homoeopathic cures were than ascribed to suggestion, to the alleged ascendancy of homoeopathic physicians over their patients, or to the natural healing power of the body.[775] One allopath told his patient: "Yes, I have seen some homoeopathic cures, but the patients are rarely alive a year later."[776] Other cures were said to be from their use of allopathic medicines in secret.[777] Andral called homoeopathy a medicine for hypochondriacs and nervous females, but, even if confined to these two classes, it "would still do good business."[778] "Neuropaths, full of a lively faith, have

[f] But this author went on to observe: "the point at which the medicine and the disease are contraries is still inaccessible to the limited grasp of our means of investigation" (Achille-Pierre Requin, *Homoeopathie* [Paris: Martinet, 1851], 15).

[g] This and other opinions of Andral were quoted extensively as evidence against homoeopathy, e.g., "Andral took quina in the requisite quantity but without acquiring intermittent fever" (Jonathan Pereira, *Elements of Materia Medica.* Fourth Edition [London: Longmans, 1854], I, 127).

conceived the consoling hope of a radical cure through the delicate contact between a microscopic globule and the tongue of every *believing* person."[799] The St. Petersburg Society of Medicine offered a prize for the best essay on the subject: all supposed homoeopathic cures are only the effect of the *vis medicatrix naturae.*[780 h]

Behind these doctrinal criticisms were serious reasons for opposing homoeopathy. The New School was new, and accepting it meant relearning medicine from the beginning. One homoeopath scoffed: "It would be cruel, we understand, to fall from the academician's chair to the school bench, to become a student after having been a teacher, to admit that one was in error and to see condemned to oblivion a fair number of the books which were one's claim to glory."[781]

The stress on symptoms and disregard of internal pathology meant that much of the standard medical education was pointless—and that a layman who could memorize lists and patterns of symptoms could practice homoeopathy almost as well as a physician.[782] At a stroke the new doctrine abolished much of the arcane and obscurantist paraphernalia with which medicine has always been loaded, but this paraphernalia constituted the physician's chief claim to social deference, and its loss was a serious blow to professional pride and confidence.

When the homoeopaths went further and appealed for support to the *lay public against other physicians,* every instinct of professional solidarity was aroused.

Accepting homoeopathy meant admitting that the physician until then had only maltreated his patients. While one maintained that he had switched easily to homoeopathy even after 24 years in allopathy, this was the exception.[783] A young physician, recently returned from a visit to Hahne-

[h]The widespread use of homoeopathy in veterinary medicine at this time was ignored by allopaths (for a rare exception see *Journal de Medecine Pratique* I [1835], 245: cures of horses with glanders). To counter these psychosomatic interpretations the homoeopaths also cited cures of infants and small children (see *Arch. de la Med. Hom.* VII [1838], 146-160: successful treatment of cholera in six infants aged 11 months, 5 months, 12 months, 7 months, 16 months, and 8 months).

mann in Koethen, who "repeated complacently that he was happy to have forgotten everything he knew of medicine before (according to him, he had been an assassin up to the moment he entered on homoeopathic practice)," was promptly expelled from his position in a Lyons hospital.[784]

Finally, homoeopathy was extremely difficult to practice. All efforts of the Paris School to attach symptoms to a limited group of pathological-anatomical changes had now to be cast aside, and the physician commenced anew with pure symptoms. In a series of articles constituting the first (and only) serious discussion of homoeopathy in a French allopathic journal Trousseau called attention to the 890 symptoms the homoeopaths obtained from *Lycopodium* (Club Moss), a substance used by allopaths only as a packing for pills: "For more details we refer to the undigested *Materia Medica Pura* of Hahnemann any curious people who will not be frightened by the labyrinth they enter in studying homoeopathy."[785] Observing the symptoms is not enough (Trousseau continues), the age, sex, and temperament of the patient must also be borne in mind, as success is determined by the degree of analogy between the pathogenetic effect of the medicine and the symptoms from these other sources:

> If, to these initial difficulties, one adds the problem of the exact appreciation of the characteristic symptoms and of the modifications they can undergo in the course of the disease, one has an idea of what the practice of homoeopathy involves. This selection of the characteristic symptom and of the medicative miasm [*sic*] seems at first glance, if not impossible, then at least extremely difficult when one thinks that the pathogenetic effects of most medicines are counted in the hundreds. There are no fixed *a priori* rules [*regles fixes, tracees a l'avance*].[786]

Trousseau's last sentence was the key to the allopathic difficulties. By "fixed *a priori* rules" he meant a nosological table of "diseases," each with its associated treatment. He complained that in the absence of such rules the remedy would be chosen arbitrarily, and in a later writing he called the homoeopaths "improvisers" in medicine.[787] The prospect of having to start from the beginning with each new patient, guided only by one's skill in observing symptoms, was truly frightening.

The homoeopaths retorted that a name cannot be given in advance to every possible combination of symptoms. Nor can a remedy be prescribed in advance–finding this remedy in each individual case is precisely the task of the physician.[788]

The homoeopaths did have "fixed rules," but these rules were different from the ones Trousseau was seeking. The difference between the two sets of rules was the difference between Empiricism and Rationalism.

The outcome of this rudimentary effort at dialogue was failure, as could have been expected. Both sides came to realize that a reasonable discussion of the conflict was impossible, and they sought a different technique for resolving it.

The Problem of Clinical Trials

Trousseau wrote in 1833 that the issues could be clarified through clinical trials: "whatever the outcome, it will be a service rendered."[789] Bouillaud refused to "debase himself by attempting to determine experimentally such enormous absurdities as those advanced by Hahnemann,"[790] but others were willing, and several trials were conducted in the early 1830's. The outcome was inconclusive, however, with neither side satisfied. In a dispute over fundamentals, where there was no agreement on terms, definitions, or procedures, there could be no agreement on the outcome of a clinical trial.

The most important of these trials were the series of Leon Simon and Paul Curie at the Hotel Dieu (under the supervision of Victor Bally, a member of the Academy of Medicine), and of Andral at the Pitié.[791]

Simon and Curie treated patients for almost five months; Bally kept the records and later reported to the Academy of Medicine that not a single patient had been cured, although one man with typhoid recovered after three months. Furthermore, a woman with uterine cancer thought she was better and went home, since the pain was relieved, but some weeks later she came back to die.[792] Bally offered to produce the records for anyone who wanted to verify them. Simon and Curie, in turn, reported in the homoeopathic press that many patients had been benefited but that Bally claimed to have lost the records when reshelving the books in his library (*sic*).[793] This inconsistency was never clarified.[i]

In 1834 and 1835 Andral ran one trial with 54 patients and another with 35. Of the first group eight showed steady improvement, while seven improved after taking the medicine but relapsed.[794] In the second group—patients with gastritis, dysmenorrhoea, headaches, smallpox, and other conditions—Andral reported a number of recoveries but ascribed them to the *vis medicatrix naturae:* "Certainly the symptoms subsided in some of these persons, but the passage of time alone brings this about."[795] Other recoveries he ascribed to bleeding, leeches, and the "ordinary remedies"; homoeopathic quinine in intermittent fever, aconite in other "fevers" (more than forty cases), *Mercurius solubilis* and *Thuja* in syphilis, and *Bryonia* and *Colchicum* in rheumatism—had all been without effect.[796]

He later claimed to have run trials on a total of 150 patients but gave no further details.[797]

No one asked Andral how he knew the recoveries were not due to the homoeopathic medicines. While a *post hoc* was not necessarily a *propter hoc,* it could well have been. Indeed, this was precisely the point at issue, and it was up to Andral to clarify it rather than gratuitously to ascribe recoveries to other factors.

The homoeopaths claimed that Andral's poor success only showed his inability to prescribe homoeopathically.[798] One observed that Laennec's mediate auscultation at first encountered the same incredulity: his colleagues could not

[i]Trials conducted at this time in Germany also ended in conflicting accounts of the results obtained, disappearance of the records, etc. (Ameke, *History of Homoeopathy,* 310 ff.).

detect these various sounds before becoming practiced in the technique: *Quod licet Jovi non licet bovi!*[799] [j] The *Organon* and Hahnemann's principal writings on materia medica had not yet even been translated, while Andral could not read German.[800] They accused him of misunderstanding the homoeopathic method and prescribing against the "predominant symptom" alone.[801] [k]

Trousseau and his colleagues conducted trials with starch pills on the hypothesis that the homoeopathic medicines were only placebos. At first they found striking psychosomatic effects, but later series yielded inconclusive results: some patients reacted, but others did not, and the reactions were not uniform.[802] Trousseau concluded that homoeopathy would never deprive the healing art of its "ancient authority, based on the therapeutic experience of the centuries."[803]

The allopaths concluded that homoeopathy was a nullity, and Andral was cited to this effect for decades.[l] They accused the homoeopaths of misleading the popular masses and practicing homoeopathy only because it paid well: *"l'industrialisme medical."*[804] The homoeopaths, in turn,

[j]An allopathic editor joked that this should be a lesson to anyone who wanted to treat homoeopathically before reading the "seven or eight large volumes being translated from the German by M. Jourdan" (*Revue Medicale Francaise et Etrangere* II [1835], 259-260).

[k]This criticism was correct, as Andral did not attempt to obtain a complete picture of the symptoms. He wrote that Hahnemann does not recognize pneumonia but sees there only a group of symptoms "among which he selects the predominant to combat it. I did what he does, and among the group of pneumonia symptoms I combatted the predominant one, sometimes with aconite, sometimes with belladonna" (*Gaz. Med. de Paris* III [1835], 190). Typical records of Andral's cases read: "disease: gastritis. Predominant symptom: intense fever," or "disease: dysmenorrhoea and chronic gastritis. Predominant symptom: intense headache," etc. (*Bull. Gen. de Ther.* VI [1834], 320).

[l]Pereira wrote in 1839: "Homoeopathia has been fairly put to the test of experiment by some of the members of the *Academie de Medecine,* and the result was a failure. Andral tried the system on 130 or 140 patients, in the presence of the homoeopaths themselves, adopting every requisite care and precaution, yet in not one instance was he successful" (*Elements of Materia Medica* [London: Longmans, 1839-1840], I, 45).

accused the allopaths of bad faith and dishonesty, and there the matter rested.[805] [m]

Homoeopathy and the Academy of Medicine

Trousseau wrote in 1834: "as long as the experiments of the homoeopaths are not made public, consequently submitted to general verification, we cannot discuss them."[806] When attempts at comparative trials fell through, the homoeopaths decided to publicize their doctrine, and popularize it among the lower orders of society, by establishing a free dispensary.[807]

For reasons never made clear Guizot referred this question to the Academy of Medicine for an advisory opinion. The dispensary could have been opened without the assent of either the government or the Academy, and Guizot's move may have been designed merely to make these worthies look ridiculous, or, as some of them observed, to make publicity for homoeopathy.[808] In both respects it was successful.

The Academy took several meetings to make up its mind: all were crowded as never before or since, and all were emotional in the highest degree. Instead of welcoming the opportunity to have homoeopathy tested in the light of day (Guizot had proposed that members be present at the dispensary as observers), the Academicians were almost unanimously opposed. Andral objected that "humanity cannot be subjected to experimentation" and went on to a lengthy account of his own homoeopathic experiments,

[m]In these very years the Academy was involved in another "paradigm dispute"—over the scientific basis of hypnotism. The committee appointed to investigate "animal magnetism" reported favorably in 1833, but one member of the Academy, A. L. Castel, argued that endorsing the committee's report "would destroy half of physiology, and it would be dangerous to propagate such facts in the public press." The Academy was in a state of "confusion and uncertainty" until another member proposed that the report be neither approved nor rejected but merely initialed, and this was done (M. P. Foissac, *Rapports et Discussion de l'Academie de Medecine sur le Magnetisme Animal* [Paris: Bailliere, 1833], 209). Castel was one of the ringleaders of the Academy's assault on homoeopathy (*Gazette des Hopitaux* VIII [1835], 136).

concluding that the only recoveries had been those of a small number of malaria cases.[809] [n] Bally discussed his own supervision of the trials by Simon and Curie: the only positive result was the typhoid patient who got well after three months.[810] [o] Louis announced that even to discuss homoeopathy was honoring it beyond its deserts.[811] Bouillaud called the New School "truly homicidal" in its treatment of pneumonia and expressed the hope that they would take their own medicines when sick.[812] C. C. H. Marc stated that in Germany homoeopathy was held in complete contempt and that Berlin had only three homoeopaths left, "one rogue and two ignoramuses (general laughter)."[813] Gilbert Breschet added that German physicians refuse even to discuss the subject, as it is professed only by charlatans.[814] Andral's father protested "with emotion" against discussing it then and there.[815] P. A. Piorry charged that homoeopathy rests neither on experience nor on reason.[816]

Two members attempted a more moderate tone but were shouted down. Jean Itard protested that they could hardly judge the new doctrine without having some facts at their disposal and that, after all, Academicians could be present at the dispensary: "Let us be liberal in deed, Gentlemen, and not only in words."[817] N. P. Adelon argued that condemning homoeopathy outright was a discredit to the Academy and might make homoeopathic experimentation impossible in the future; furthermore, it was improper for members to censure their own colleagues.[818] Pelletier urged that the homoeopathic challenge be accepted.[819] But the report recommended unanimously against the dispensary on the ground that homoeopathy "gives no guarantee or proof of its principles."[820]

Trousseau's request that homoeopathy provide experimental evidence was thus transformed into a demand for *a priori* proof of its principles, meaning proof that its principles were congruent with those accepted by the Academy.

[n]The editor of the transcript was careful to add in a note: "All physicians know that a large number of cases of simple intermittent fever are cured by diet without medicines, and a few days after entering the hospital."

[o]The editor noted: "This means that the disease cured itself."

The profession's attitude toward the New School was set forth with clarity in an 1834 editorial in the *Bulletin General de Therapeutique:* success is generally considered to justify a therapeutic procedure, but "while this same success justifies the end, it does not always justify the means; for the end to be legitimate, the means must also be legitimate. We are not afraid to say this—this is our position." Homoeopathy, however great its therapeutic success, was not legitimate: "with its vague principles, its unfounded assertions, its more than doubtful experiments, its infinitesimal doses, its medical *nihilism.* With a doctrine which negates all medicine, action in a void, a true chimera, therapeutics is no longer possible."[821]

Thus the homoeopathic therapeutic results and comparative statistics were ultimately irrelevant, since the method was "illegitimate."[p] This remained the allopathic attitude from that time on.

The homoeopaths, flourishing "despite the bad faith of accepted truths and private interests," held the incipient split in the profession to be disastrous for humanity.[822] They regretted also being cut off from their colleagues: "we were nearing port, and now we are once again in the open sea exposed to the storms and the tempests."[823]

They kept trying to explain homoeopathy to the allopaths but without success:

> When we talk to them about medical doctrine, they ask us upon which physiological system we base it and which system of pathology we have adopted. When we reply that all nosological and pathological systems are false and erroneous and proclaim the principle of absolute individualization of diseases, they reply that we are on the wrong road, and that therapeutics is not its own justification, because its results must be verified and evaluated; that without physiology and pathology we have no measure for making this evaluation properly; that

[p] As Moliere had written 200 years earlier: "Better die according to the rules than recover against the rules" (*L'Amour Medecin,* Act II, Scene V).

> we may well be led astray with respect to our own powers and our own announced results. To these objections . . . we must give some answer other than a simple rejection.[824]

The only possible answer to the allopaths was the one urged by Hahnemann—that homoeopathy be judged strictly by its results, but this was unacceptable *a priori* to the allopaths, and after 1835 the French profession was divided.

The Spread of Homoeopathy

The dispensary was opened in 1838 and soon followed by two others, inaugurating a new chapter in French medicine. By 1840 there were fifty French homoeopaths and by 1850 over 200. The New School expanded steadily until the end of the century and beyond, provoking occasional expressions of concern by leading allopaths.

Magendie commenced his physiology course in the mid-1850's with the following:

> We are deliberating on the future of medicine, but should we not take care to ensure its very existence? . . . Medicine can exist only if the patients have faith in it and come to ask for its assistance; it does not live by theory but by its clientele. But one cannot conceal the fact today that a certain number abandon classical medicine which they ironically call the "old medicine," and the patients deliver themselves, body and goods, to what they call the "new medicine." Homoeopathy, as that is what I am referring to, plans nothing less than to overturn the whole edifice of medicine.[825]

An editorial in *L'Union Medicale* at this same time stated:

> My dear colleagues, homoeopathy is gaining ground. The wave is rising from moment to moment. There it is with the young and beautiful Empress [Eugenie] in Caesar's palace. From time to time our medical societies see members who were previously faithful resign from their midst. Just last month one of these societies was afflicted by a letter of resignation caused by desertion to

homoeopathy and addressed by a colleague who up until then had shown serious scientific promise. Where are we going? Where are we going? Only yesterday I was told that one of these new converts to Hahnemann's religion asks every new client: "How do you wish to be treated, by the old medicine or the new?" And the client inevitably replies: "Which is better?" To which he immediately responds: "The new, but it is more expensive." Oh, what sacrilege! Oh, medical dignity, what has happened to you?[826]

Students in the medical schools were writing theses in defence of homoeopathy, and this provoked reexaminations of the doctrine by their professors—mostly unfavorable but with some exceptions.[827]

A Montpellier M.D. candidate in 1858 wrote a critical analysis of homoeopathy prefaced by the comment that "this system has entered the domain of public discussion; while people are entirely ignorant on the subject of organicism, vitalism, eclecticism, and all other systems in medicine, one often finds a lady in society, or even a peasant, asking for explanations of Hahnemannian medicine and the *similia similibus.*"[828] An 1865 debate over homoeopathy in the French Senate revealed that the New School had the allegiance of one tenth of the population and one eighth of the eminent senators themselves.[829] Trousseau charged in 1862 that 20 members of the Academy of Sciences were attended by "charlatans," i.e., homoeopaths.[830]

Even though most of the intellectual lights of allopathy remained resolutely hostile (Bretonneau professed "absolute contempt" for homoeopathy),[831] there were some exceptions. Isidore Bourdon of the Academy of Medicine accepted homoeopathy as a true extension of Hippocratic medicine, and this was supported by F. A. Jaumes, professor of pharmacology at Montpellier.[832] Antoine Imbert-Gourbeyre, professor of medicine at Clermont-Ferrand, wrote and published on homoeopathy while retaining his university position.[833] One of the most forthright supporters of homoeopathy in university circles was also at Montpellier. Risueno de Amador (1802-1849), a Spaniard who had become doctor of philosophy at Salamanca by the age of eighteen, then studying medicine at Montpellier and becoming a professor there, publicly professed homoeopathy in 1839; he recognized its connection both with Hippocratic method and with the Paracelsan doctrine of specifics as explicated by Van Helmont and Stahl.[834] "Hahnemann thus extended the sphere of vitalism by providing this doctrine with a practical basis."[835] In 1843 he suggested in a public lecture that Hahnemann was one of the great discoverers who have been unrecognized and maltreated by their contemporaries.[836] In 1844 he created a "sensation" at a scientific congress with a paper on "The Action of Imperceptible Agents on the Living Body," pointing out that semen, the saliva of a rabid dog, *Rhus toxicodendron,* and certain poisons are active in minute quantities—explainable only by the existence of a formal property, similar to Van Helmont's "idea," which can be separated from the material substance.[837] Diseases grow like plants: "a seed [*germe*] in propitious circumstances, matures," a person is infected by some seed today, and the morbific product will appear fifteen days after germination.[838] No one can grasp the cholera miasm which acts on the body's vitality; hence medicines must act on the vitality also.

> A dynamic or vitalist therapeutics is grafted onto a dynamic toxicology, hygiene, or physiology, just as Hahnemann is grafted onto Montpellier, and Montpellier onto Hippocrates . . . the progress of vitalist therapeutics in the last sixty years is far from overturning Hippocratic medicine or the true vitalism of Montpellier. On the contrary, it confirms them, making them practical instead of abstract.[839]

Jacques Lordat, one of the eminences of Montpellier in these years, stated that Risueno's advocacy had made him open-minded on the subject of homoeopathy, and others of the Montpellier professors were perhaps marginally less hostile to the New School than their Paris colleagues, recognizing the common Hippocratic heritage.[840]

Homoeopathy in France enjoyed the same support from the non-medical press as it did in England and the United States during those years.[q]

An allopath summed up the situation in 1888 with the wistful remark that while Broussais' theories, "enjoying the enthusiastic support of the entire body of physicians, could not withstand the force of the evidence," strangely enough the "vague and nebulous doctrine of Hahnemann, despite the opposition of the physicians of every country, has held a position up until the present day, without gaining, but without losing ground."[841]

The Allopathic Counterattack

The emergence of the New School, whose strength lay precisely in the area of the Old School's weakness, provoked a sense of panic in the profession, especially when it became clear that homoeopathy was not a transient phenomenon.

Two defensive measures were taken.

The first was administrative: the use of disciplinary action against physicians who practiced homoeopathy or consulted with homoeopaths, going as far as expulsion from medical societies.[r] The second was ideological: the elaboration of a competing doctrine which, by incorporating a small dose of Hahnemannism, conferred immunity against the more virulent form of this new medicinal disorder. This last was the work of Trousseau.

Thereafter physicians were protected against homoeopathy themselves and could announce to the public that they had done justice to the New School's ideas.

The first expulsion of a medical student for evincing an interest in homoeopathy, defined as "incompatible with the

[q]See, for example, the examination of homoeopathy published in *Gazette de France* (December 12, 1855) which concluded that it had been judged too severely by the medical profession and should be given a fair chance. See, also, *Divided Legacy*, III, 305-308.

[r]The American Medical Association, founded in 1846, took as its first order of business the adoption of a Code of Medical Ethics which enjoined the presence of homoeopathic M.D.'s in medical societies and forbade consultation with them (*Divided Legacy*, III, 179-206).

true principles of science," was in 1835.[842] By the late 1840's and early 1850's the district medical societies had adopted ethical rules prohibiting members from consulting with "a hypnotist, a homoeopath, or any other charlatan of this species"; the largest physicians' association of Paris at this time, with 1700 members, contained not a single homoeopath.[843] In 1856 the Anatomical Society, with Cruveilhier in the chair, unanimously expelled Jean-Paul Tessier (1811-1862) and three others for publishing reports in homoeopathic journals.[844] [s]

The allopathic journals either ignored homoeopathy entirely, leading these physicians to complain of a "conspiracy of silence," or they published spiteful and derogatory remarks without giving their opponents space to answer the accusations.[845] When *L'Union Medicale* featured a particularly defamatory article in 1858, the homoeopaths brought suit for libel, the journal being defended in court by Andral's son. They lost the case, but thereafter relations between the two groups were better.[846] The homoeopaths gained access to some public hospitals (especially in the South) but otherwise kept to themselves and avoided allopathic meetings.[847] Despite repeated allopathic assurances that the New School's principles were being undermined by "modern science," homoeopathy continued to flourish, and its relations with medical orthodoxy remained relatively even and non-polemical until the end of the century.[848] Homoeopathic popularity with the public and a considerable measure

[s]Tessier, who had been one of Andral's favorite students before deserting allopathy, was the recognized leader of French homoeopathy (see "Jean-Paul Tessier" in *Dictionnaire Encyclopedique*). In May, 1851, the Edinburgh College of Physicians expelled William Henderson, a professor of pathology at Edinburgh, who had formally espoused homoeopathy. It decreed that "no physician can, without derogation from his honor and that of his profession, consult with a homoeopath or cooperate with him in any medical act." The Provincial Medical Association in England at that time (including most of the practitioners of the country) resolved not to accept as members: (1) physicians practicing pure homoeopathy, (2) those practicing mixed homoeopathy and allopathy, and (3) those who consulted or had professional relations with homoeopaths (*L'Union Medicale* V [1851], 296, 490). On Henderson see *Divided Legacy,* III, 153, 155, 171.

of official support more than offset the hostility of allopathy.

The Infiltration of Homoeopathic Ideas into Allopathy

These same years saw gradual allopathic acceptance of many of the homoeopathic ideas.

The doctrine of similars, for example, was a traditional concept in medicine, Jenner's discovery of smallpox vaccination being only a recent instance. Boeckel's 1826 dissertation took for granted such applications of similars as *Rhus toxicodendron* in skin diseases, *Belladonna* in amblyopia, and the purgatives, rhubarb and *Gumma gutta,* in dysentery.[849] An 1834 allopathic attack on homoeopathy admitted that mercury gives rise to syphilis symptoms, *Dulcamara* to skin eruptions, *Belladonna* to symptoms of scarlet fever, and *Stramonium* to delirium and convulsions—these all being used in treating the same conditions.[850] [t] Philippe Ricord in 1838 urged that syphilis be treated by reinoculating the patient with pus from his own chancre.[851]

The ultramolecular dose, a standard object of allopathic ridicule, seemed to acquire respectability in an 1836 article in the *Bulletin* of the Academy of Medicine. One Dr. Lafargue experimented to ascertain how far an aqueous solution of morphine could be diluted without losing its capacity to provoke a skin rash. He dissolved a drop of laudanum in 25 drops of water and inserted a little under his skin, causing a blister to arise: "such a result should surprise us, as the liquid is made up of one part opium and 500 parts water." He obtained the same result with a drop of laudanum dissolved in 50 drops of water, and again with a drop dissolved in 100 drops of water. Lafargue decided not to carry the dilution further.[852]

Risueno knew of this experiment and reported it as evidence of the efficacy of medicines in tiny doses.[853]

[t]The author was probably unaware that Hahnemann himself had introduced *Belladonna* for the prevention and treatment of scarlet fever (Coulter, *Homoeopathic Influences,* 35-41). See below, p. 579.

But the key homoeopathic principle—which was to renovate the whole of nineteenth-century allopathic pharmacology—was the proving of remedies on healthy persons.

Bichat had suggested in the end of his life that medicines be tested on the healthy, this appeal being repeated by his follower, C. J. A. Schwilgue.[854] The latter may even have performed some experiments along these lines, but they were neither extensive nor systematic.[855] In 1805 Hahnemann published the first edition of his *Fragmenta de Viribus Medicamentorum,* and thereafter this question was fairly before the medical profession.

Francois Magendie provides a good example of how this homoeopathic principle, and a leading homoeopathic remedy, became accepted by allopathy.

Nux vomica and St. Ignatius' Bean (*Ignatia amara*) were among the first remedies proved by Hahnemann and published in the *Fragmenta.*[856] He recommended them in paralytic states, and three years later a German physician published in *Hufelands Journal* a cure of paralysis of the lower extremities with *Nux vomica* following the "Hahnemannian principle."[857] In 1808 a French medical student wrote a dissertation on the use of *Nux vomica* by German physicians, mentioning that it seemed to affect the nervous system.[858]

In 1809 Magendie reported on the action of upas poison, *Nux vomica,* and St. Ignatius' Bean when injected into the muscle of a dog; he determined that they affect the spinal marrow and suggested their use in diseases of the spinal cord.[859] [u] Two years later a certain Professor Fouquier at the Charité was the first person in France to treat paralysis effectively with *Nux vomica,* and Bretonneau used it in the same way. Trousseau credited them with the discovery, despite Hahnemann's evident priority, and historians since

[u]*Hufelands Journal* was excerpted regularly in *Bibliotheque Medicale* from 1805 to 1822, and the German article on *Nux vomica* appeared there in a French condensation (with no mention of the "Hahnemannian principle") in the same year Magendie's own article was published there ("Guerison d'une Paralysie des Extremites Inferieures qui avait Dure Trois Ans, par le Dr. Becker, praticien a Leipsic," *Bibliotheque Medicale* XXV [1809], 103-104).

that time have maintained that Magendie was the first to investigate medicines by administering them to healthy organisms.[860] [v]

While Magendie's "healthy organisms" were dogs and other animals, Jan Evangelista Purkyne (1787-1869) of Prague University was the first allopath to conduct pharmacological trials on human subjects. He freely admitted his debt to homoeopathy, writing that in the third and fourth years of his medical studies, "stimulated by the books of Hahnemann," he took various drugs and medicines to ascertain their effect on himself.[861] He continued these investigations throughout his life and is considered the founder of "physiological pharmacology"—a word he invented.[862] Purkyne held that animal experiments yield data only on the vegetative and peripheral nervous systems; experiments on humans were needed to discover the effects of remedies on the perceptual and intellectual faculties.[863]

The next significant figure to experiment with pharmacological substances on the healthy was Johann Joerg (1779-1856) of Leipzig, who was motivated by the desire to disprove Hahnemann's findings.[864] He gathered together a group of provers in the early 1820's and with their help proved hydrocyanic acid, valerian, *Arnica montana,* camphor, musk, St. Ignatius' Bean, iodine, digitalis, opium, asafoetida, and seven or eight others, to ascertain their dynamic properties.[865] "In future people will wonder why it took physicians so long to realize this."[866] However, Joerg hoped to employ these substances as contraries, not as similars. The first volume of his provings was not followed by others, perhaps because he realized that the work had already been

[v]Thus J. M. D. Olmsted: Magendie's investigations "mark the beginning of experimental pharmacology. They were the first records of attempts to administer chemical substances to living organisms in a systematic way so that the effects of similar chemical agents from different sources might be compared . . . These are the lines along which experimental pharmacology has proceeded from the year 1809 to the present time, and Magendie may rightly be called the father of this branch of medicine"(*Francois Magendie: Pioneer in Experimental Physiology and Scientific Medicine in XIX Century France* [New York: Schuman, 1944], 44).

done by Hahnemann.[w] Such, at least, was the opinion of Boeckel: "Whatever Joerg may say, we find a great similarity (as to the major symptoms) between the results he obtained and those published by Hahnemann, and this speaks in favor of the latter's materia medica."[867]

All of this activity brought to the fore another of Hahnemann's principal tenets–the identity of poisons and medicines. His "What are Poisons? What are Medicines?" had appeared in *Hufelands Journal* in 1806, and the medical public was alerted to this question also.[868]

J. C. Reil wrote in 1815 that "a large number of medicines are medicines precisely because they have the power to incite diseases . . ."[869] He does not seem to have done experiments on himself, however, and his view was doubtless taken directly from Hahnemann.

One obstacle to research on the poisonous effects of medicines–the absence of a comprehensive study of the subject–was eliminated in 1815 with the appearance of M. P. Orfila's *Traite des Poisons.* It presented, *inter alia,* the symptomatology of a large number of poisonous substances –such as mercury, antimony, *Belladonna, Dulcamara,* cantharides, sulphur, *Digitalis, Stramonium, Nux vomica,* and others–which had been used in medicine for decades and even centuries.[870]

In 1829 Robert Christison published another treatise on poisons which remarked: "the science of toxicology aids the physician in his inquiries into the action of remedies. Many of the most valuable remedies for combating disease being in larger doses violent poisons, their action as poisons, in some instances though certainly not in all, throws light on their action as remedies."[871] "This knowledge is particularly

[w]On Joerg see *Divided Legacy,* III, 254. The homoeopathic objection to all such allopathic provings was that they employed excessively large doses and thus obtained only the common symptoms (*communia*) from these substances. Only provings with very small quantities of the substances yielded the peculiar and specific symptoms (*propria*) of each substance (Richard Hughes, *A Manual of Pharmacodynamics.* Sixth Edition [London: Leath and Ross, 1893], 48 ff). See above, pp. 380-381.

called for in regard to those remedies–probably not few in number–whose therapeutic effects are not developed till their physiological effects have begun to manifest themselves."[872]

The idea of systematically testing substances on healthy persons, however, had not yet made its way into the textbooks of materia medica. Barbier mentioned, *en passant,* the idea of administering medicines to animals to ascertain "the modifications thus provoked in the living tissues,"[873] but neither Bayle nor Alibert discussed it at all.

Andral was apparently the first allopath to realize the significance of this concept for therapeutic theory. In 1834, before the battle lines had been drawn by the decision of the Academy of Medicine, he wrote that the time had perhaps come to base disease diagnosis and classification on clinical experiment rather than pathological anatomy:

> Leaving aside the whole classes of diseases in which the scalpel reveals nothing, even in the diseases most elucidated by pathological anatomy we see, every day, cases proving unalterably that the whole disease is not in the lesion; in the cadaver one notes that, apart from the organic alterations, there are indeterminate morbid conditions which seem to take precedence over the lesions themselves. But if this is true, therapeutics henceforth cannot be despotically dominated by pathological anatomy.[874]

Clinical experimentation has been a failure in the past because disease descriptions are slipshod; most of those in the literature are quite worthless.[875] Physicians love to pigeonhole cases:

> We love analogies, perfect identity is ravishing; differences–which divide up the facts–compel us to make long and laborious analyses; hence it is but a short step to ignoring the observed differences and contenting ourselves with the first relationships which we have grasped.[876]

What, then, is the cure for inability to describe diseases carefully?

> One very important task today would be to conduct experiments with the principal agents of the materia medica on the organism in its physiologic state . . . this must be developed much more extensively than it has been up to now. The subjects should be divided into analogous groups of greater or lesser size according to temperament, sex, age, etc. . . . Without prejudging the issue which the homoeopaths have raised recently with respect to the property of curative agents to determine in the organism those diseases which these agents are used to treat in allopathy, we feel that this view is supported by certain incontestable facts and, *because of the immense consequences which could ensue,* at least merits the attention of observers. Supposing, as is quite probable, that Hahnemann exaggerated (as is so easy for theoreticians) the numerous facts cited in support of his opinions, some of them are still in perfect harmony with his thought. If these experiments were repeated, other equally authentic facts would probably emerge; if a vigorous mind were to meditate over these facts and compare them after exploring all their aspects, *who knows what the consequences would be?* . . . Once the mode of action of therapeutic agents on the healthy economy has been determined, they will be better able to represent the economy's morbid modifications [stress added].[877]

While the language is convoluted, Andral agrees with Hahnemann that the symptoms produced by provings on the healthy can serve as the criteria for classifying diseases and distinguishing among otherwise similar cases.[x]

His "without prejudging the issue which the homoeopaths have raised recently" seems odd in view of his own report, earlier that year, on the lack of efficacy of homoeo-

[x]Andral's suggestion was followed up by Alphonse Guerard who, in 1839, submitted a thesis on the physiological action of medicines in a competition for the chair of materia medica and therapeutics at the Faculté (*Des Inductions que la Therapeutique peut Tirer de l'Action Physiologique des Medicaments* [Paris: Faculté de Medecine, 1839]).

pathic remedies. Although the New School physicians in Paris did not question Andral's good faith, they called him an "enigma" and accused him (rightly) of lacking the strength of his convictions.[878]

Trousseau and the Reform of the Pharmacopoeia

While Andral only stood on Mt. Nebo and looked over into Canaan, Trousseau led his multitudes into the Promised Land, reformulating allopathic theory to make possible the appropriation of homoeopathic principles and many homoeopathic remedies while remaining true to "medical tradition."

He wrote later that the 1830's were a time of pharmacological ignorance: the texts contained little materia medica and almost no clinical observation. The waves of pathological anatomy and physiology had subsided, and physicians were seeking a different approach, represented by investigations of the pathogenetic action of medicines and their comparative therapeutics. "The reason for our success was not only that we met this need, but also that we were faithful to the Hippocratic tradition and the experience of the centuries."[879]

Trousseau was born in Tours and became a teacher of rhetoric. But he met Bretonneau, studied medicine with him, and came to Paris to receive the M.D. in 1825. In 1828 he went with Pierre Louis and Nicolas Chervin (1783-1843) to observe an outbreak of yellow fever in the south of France. In 1831 he was appointed assistant to J. C. A. Recamier (1774-1852)—one of the holdouts against Broussais—at the Hotel Dieu.[880] There he encountered Hermann Pidoux, a more retiring personality, who became his lifelong collaborator.

The 1832 cholera epidemic stimulated Trousseau's first pharmacological investigations.[881]

They brought out the *Traite de Therapeutique et de Matiere Medicale* in 1836, reissuing it in a new edition every four or five years thereafter until the ninth in 1875 (after Trousseau's death). It was the dominant force in French medicine during these years and powerfully influenced practice in other Western countries.

On the strength of it Trousseau was appointed to the Faculté in 1839 and in 1850 replaced Chomel as professor of clinics at the Hotel Dieu.[882] In 1856 he was elected to the Academy of Medicine.

He was a Hippocratic, a vitalist, and an Empiric.

He accepted the Hippocratic principles: disease is a reaction of the *physis* to a morbific cause, recovery comes through coction and crisis, fever is beneficial, suppression of disease symptoms is dangerous, etc.[883]

He was a vitalist: vital processes are "autonomous, specific, unexplained, inexplicable" and obey laws different from those governing inorganic matter.[884]

He agreed with the principles of Empiricism. Observation and experience are the only sources of medical knowledge; proximate causes in the organism cannot be known; the nature of the disease is discovered from its cure; therapeutics is not the consequence of the knowledge developed in the "auxiliary sciences" but is prior to this knowledge, etc. etc.[885] He was hostile to Boerhaave and warmly praised the Empirics—Van Helmont, Sydenham, Stahl, Bordeu, Barthez, and particularly John Hunter, whom he called "superior to all the physicians who have contributed to the medical reform in France."[886]

But he was, above all, obsessed by homoeopathy which he considered alien to the Empirical tradition.[887]

As noted earlier, Trousseau in 1833 and 1834 had provided his colleagues with the only businesslike account of homoeopathic principles to appear in the allopathic press.[888] Later in life he claimed to have treated patients homoeopathically for six months without any discernible benefit.[889] And one third of the pages in the long Introductions to the successive editions of his *Traite de Therapeutique* were devoted to a critique of homoeopathy.[y]

He had much good to say about the New School. It has advanced three new ideas which must be taken seriously: 1) a new interpretation of the medicine, 2) a new method of constituting the materia medica, and 3) a general therapeutics

[y] Thirty pages out of 102 in the sixth edition (1858).

deduced from the relationship between the nature of the disease and that of the medicine.[890] "Homoeopathy has been of use to pharmacology. Under its influence societies have been formed in Germany for revising the materia medica. All medicines have been proven on healthy persons by physicians who, acting themselves as the subjects of their experiments, have not always, to be sure, avoided systematic illusions, but, endowed with much patience and attention, and always employing only simple substances, have constituted their *Materia Medica Pura* whence have emerged many very valuable notions about the specific properties of medicines and a whole crowd of details about their action of which we have been too ignorant in France. This ignorance meant that we knew only the crudest general properties of therapeutic agents and, confronted with diseases presenting subtle varieties of indications, we only too frequently lacked modifiers appropriate to these nuances."[891] [z]

These have shown that medicines have both general and specific effects on the organism, the latter being developed when very small doses are administered.[892] They do not act physically or chemically but by some "specific property," by "impression."[893] These general and specific effects, taken together, constitute the medicine's "diathesis."[894]

But while accepting these homoeopathic premises, Trousseau rejected the conclusion that treatment must be by similars: "if it were possible to produce with a medicine a morbid action very similar to that of [the disease], it would only intensify [the disease]."[895] What appears to be treatment with similars is actually "substitution" of the medicinal "diathesis" for the patient's disease; the "diathesis" subsequently disappears by itself, and the patient is cured.[896]

And "substitutive" treatment is only a part of pharmacology. The therapeutic effects of some medicines cannot be

[z]Trousseau had in mind, particularly, Johann Joerg and his followers, whom he calls a group of "timid homoeopaths" but praises for their services to the materia medica and cites very frequently (*Traite de Therapeutique,* 1836, I, 24-25, 37, *et passim*).

determined from tests on the healthy.[897] The poisonous properties of medicines tell us nothing about their therapeutic properties.[898] Hahnemann's definition of "medicine" is more like that of a poison.[899] Many medicines act "heteropathically" (i.e., by contraries) rather than homoeopathically or by substitution.[900]

Trousseau finally calls Hahnemann an "ultravitalist" who rejected both Empiricism and Rationalism, "the head of a sect who was more concerned with the triumph of his system than with telling the truth." Homoeopathy is "German mysticism" which has "stayed aside from all progress in medicine. One need not be a physician to understand and practice it. Nothing could be more curious than to see this system, produced amidst the reform of medicine by modern anatomy and pathology, as independent of them and as little associated with them as if it had been conceived in China."[901]

Trousseau found authority for "substitutive" treatment in Hunter, Brown, Laennec, and Bretonneau.

The first had taught that one "irritation" displaces another, and the second had "rescued from the shipwreck of modern medicine" the notion that the "disease" is an entity or diathesis which occupies and fills the whole organism.[902] But Brown's idea of disease was non-specific: specificity was provided by Laennec (for chronic diseases) and Bretonneau (for acute).[903] Bretonneau's experiments with irritants showed that each gives rise to a specific type of inflammation: "Bretonneau proved the specificity of phlegmasies by that of their medications and founded the specificity of medications on the distinction of phlegmasies into determinate species."[904] "To the action of each modifier there corresponds a specific modification."[905] "We transported the idea of specificity, the idea of the diathesis, from diseases *with a material basis* (where it had been restored by Laennec and Bretonneau) to diseases *without matter,* to neuroses, neuralgias, fluxions, hemorrhages, where it had not yet penetrated."[906]

Thus Trousseau came to "substitution" from Bretonneau's experiments with topical application of caustics to the throats of children with diphtheria, and his detailed discussion limits "substitutive" treatment to topical medication. It is a subhead of "irritant medication" and involves plasters in skin diseases, silver nitrate in diseases of the nasal mucosa, hydrochloric acid in stomach disorders (i.e., applied to the stomach lining), cauterization of the laryngeal membrane in diphtheria and whooping cough, inhalation of arsenical vapors in diseases of the bronchia, calomel enemas in dysentery, injections of the urethra in gonorrhoea, etc.[907]

The true point at issue between Trousseau and the New School, however, was not the topical application of irritants to the skin and mucous membranes but the constitutional or systemic effect of a medicine administered internally—whether considered a "similar" or a "substitute"—and here Trousseau simply evaded the issue. In one passage he criticized Hahnemann for wanting to extend the law of similars to internal conditions, and in another he urged the necessity of so doing, but nowhere did he discuss this in detail.[a]

Furthermore, he was unable to define "disease," although this concept was the basis of his whole doctrine of "substitution." "Diseases are neither entities [*etres*] nor purely accidental modifications of the organism. The medical Rationalism of which Broussais was the supreme expression is thus a chimera, and the Empiricism which was Laennec's reaction is no less impossible."[908] Although writing at length about "disease," Trousseau ridiculed systems of nosology as artificial constructions.[909]

His biographer commented: "Trousseau realized that diseases are (following Broussais' contemptuous expression)

[a]"What was true for local diseases and topical remedies was certainly much less so for general diseases and remedies; but Hahnemann, blinded by the truth of an idea which he had glimpsed and formulated, soon exaggerated the importance of his discovery, like all innovators" (*Traite*, 1858, I, 470). "Substitution can be exercised mediately, that is, through the organs of absorption and on the tissues with which the irritant agents are not in direct contact" (*Ibid.*, 1858, I, 477). The homoeopaths derided him for this, calling his discussion of "substitution" in internal conditions scientifically dishonest (*Archives de la Medecine Homoeopathique* IV [1836], 452-466; V [1836], 218-230; VI [1837], 105-113; VII [1838], 108-120).

only intellectual constructions [*etres de raison*]; but he also realized that these units, however artificial, are nonetheless needed. The mind, without being fooled by its creations, can only conceive them by attributing to them objective reality."[910]

Trousseau resolved this issue by holding that each "disease" contains a "nosological element" which must be treated "empirically" or specifically and a "physiological element" which must be treated "rationally."[911]

The inherent confusion of his philosophy stemmed from his pursuit of two incompatible aims: 1) a genuinely "Empirical" medicine which should be 2) palatable to his colleagues, i.e., easy to practice.

The true Empiricism was that of Hahnemann who held each *individual patient* to differ from each other, requiring the remedy specific to his own illness. But this position was too extreme for the average physician, imposing on him the heavy moral burden of discovering the one medicine best suited to the needs of the given patient.[b] It caused difficulty not only between homoeopathy and allopathy but even within the homoeopathic movement itself.[c] Trousseau cut down on both the variety of the patients and that of medicines, presenting the profession with a therapeutic doctrine which was easier to practice and therefore had greater appeal. He limited the universality of Hahnemann's law of similars by confining it to "substitutive treatment," applicable, in principle, only to certain diseased states—not to all.[d] And he limited the variety of sick patients by adapting

[b]J. H. Baas clearly understood this aspect of homoeopathy: "there is no disease which can withstand homoeopathy [in Hahnemann's view] . . . Hence, occasional failures are due, not to homoeopathy itself, but to human short-sightedness, which overlooked the proper homoeopathic remedy" (*History of Medicine,* 872).

[c]See *Divided Legacy,* III, 328-401.

[d]A Montpellier professor in 1847 accepted the law of similars in principle but criticized Hahnemann for erecting it into a "general rule" (F. A. Jaumes, *Essai de Pharmacologie Therapeutique Generale,* 225). Trousseau wrote: "A medicine is any substance capable of producing morbid action. Let us add, immediately, that

to his own purposes the emerging theory of "specific diseases." Individualization henceforth had to be carried only as far as the "disease," not as far as the individual case.

His Empirical instincts prevented him from giving a pathological-anatomical definition of "disease," but his instinct for self-preservation and professional advancement prevented him from rejecting the "disease" concept altogether and defining each patient's illness, as Hahnemann did, in terms of the curative remedy.

Despite these vagaries Trousseau's writings popularized the principle of proving medicines on the healthy. His *Traite de Therapeutique* was the first allopathic work to commence the discussion of each article of materia medica with an account of its physiological effect on the healthy person. While he mentioned experiments with animals, human trials were primary; Trousseau subjected himself and Pidoux to provings of valerian, camphor, musk, sulphuric ether, potassium cyanide (*sic*), *Stramonium, Conium,* turpentine, *Nux vomica,* and many others.[912] He cites Orfila and Christison often and assimilates the toxicological properties of remedies to their physiological ones, calling their knowledge a good guide to the remedy's therapeutic application.[913]

He realized that this was a pioneering and controversial step and notes, in the Introduction to the first edition, that, while the classes of medicines are a matter of general agreement, the ascription of a given substance to its proper class is controversial: but "we have the same rights as anyone else and, in any case, regard the question as otiose provided this subject *incertae sedis* be included somewhere in our work, whether in its right place or not, and there discussed properly."[914]

His initiative was highly successful and gradually converted the medical profession from an exclusive enthusiasm

this is in no way absolute and that a rigorous definition of a medicine, drawn from its very nature, cannot be given without immediately falling into systematic thought. Let us leave pretentiously categorical definitions to Aristotle . . ." (*Traite de Therapeutique,* 1858, I, lvii).

for bloodletting, setons, quinine, and mercury to a more sophisticated awareness of the possibilities of pharmacology.

Pidoux later described the reaction of their colleagues:

> No one today can imagine the spectacle offered by this new clinic . . . which revived forgotten therapeutic agents and introduced new ones . . . The notion of nosological and therapeutic specificity, modestly rediscovered in the provinces by Bretonneau, entered Paris with *eclat* . . . You should have seen the interested curiosity of the students, and above all of the senior physicians, before whose eyes Trousseau, with imperturbable confidence, employed all the medicines so feared by this generation raised in the dread of irritants. To them it was like handling hot coals. When they saw insoluble iron preparations, together with quinine and aloes, administered to a chlorotic woman whose stomach was torn by frightful pain, with a palpitating heart, vibrating arteries, and a congested and dysmenorrhagic uterus, the next day one was sure to find this poor girl's bed surrounded by physicians disturbed at the fate of this gastritis, this cardio-arteritis, this metritis which should have been exacerbated by the incendiary medicines administered the day before. And when these practitioners saw the tonic and stimulating medicines restoring the patient's appetite, relieving the stomach pain, sedating the spasms of the heart and arteries . . . their faith in the agents of the materia medica was restored . . .[915]

The *Traite de Therapeutique* was translated into Spanish, Italian, and English (in 1842, 1871, and 1880). The *Clinique Medicale de l'Hotel Dieu de Paris,* published in 1861, had a seventh edition in 1885 and was translated into English and German (1868).[916]

Long before these translations appeared, however, Trousseau's influence had spread outside France. Jonathan Pereira, who started lecturing on materia medica in 1835 and 1836, publishing his *Elements of Materia Medica* in 1839 and 1840, makes frequent references to Trousseau, Joerg, Orfila, and Christison and starts the discussion of each medicine with an analysis of its physiological (toxicological) effects on a healthy person.[917] He was more forthright than Trousseau in crediting Hahnemann with the initial discovery of this idea:

> The homoeopathists assert, and with truth, that the study of the effects of medicines in the healthy state is the only way of ascertaining the *pure* or *pathogenetic* effects of medicines–since when we administer our remedies to invalids, "the symptoms of the natural disease, then existing, mingling with those which the medicinal agents are capable of producing, the latter can rarely be distinguished with any clearness or precision."[918 e]

This work, translated in 1846 by Rudolph Buchheim, was used in German medicine.[f]

In the United States Alfred Stille's 1860 *Therapeutics and Materia Medica* gave guarded approval to the testing of medicines on the healthy and commenced the discussion of each medicine with a description of its "action" on healthy animals and man.[919] This work had a fourth edition in 1874.

Horatio C. Wood, professor of therapeutics at the University of Pennsylvania and a powerful figure in American medicine, issued a *Treatise on Therapeutics, Comprising Materia Medica and Toxicology* in 1874 which had a twelfth edition in 1905.[920] It specified that "experiments made with medicaments upon the lower animals or upon healthy human beings [are the] only rational scientific groundwork for the treatment of disease . . . We must discover what influence a drug exerts when put into the body of a patient before we can use it rationally; and we can gain this coveted knowledge only in the method indicated."[921]

[e] The quoted passage is taken from the 1833 English translation of the *Organon* (*The Homoeopathic Medical Doctrine or "Organon of the Healing Art"; a New System of Physic,* tr. from the German of S. Hahnemann by Charles H. Devrient, esq. [Dublin: W. F. Wakeman, 1833]).

[f] But Buchheim himself did not agree that trials on the healthy were the best guide to the medicinal use of a drug. In a long Preface he observed that to have altered Pereira's work in line with his own convictions would have changed it beyond recognition (Jonathan Pereira, *Handbuch der Heilmittellehre. Bearbeitet von Rudolph Buchheim* [Leipzig: Voss, 1846-1848], I, xvii). For more on Buchheim see below, pp. 634-637.

Roberts Bartholow, professor of medicine at Jefferson Medical College in Philadelphia and another leading figure in American therapeutics, issued a *Practical Treatise on Materia Medica and Therapeutics* in 1876 (eleventh edition in 1904) which stated: "as respects the therapeutic applications of remedies I have, as far as practicable, based them on the physiological actions."[922] [g]

His 1880 *Treatise on the Practice of Medicine* had its eighth edition in 1895 and was translated into Japanese in 1887.[923]

Thus the principle of proving medicines on healthy persons remained accepted by world medicine, as a result of the work of Trousseau, for more than a century after its first enunciation by Hahnemann.

And adoption of this principle was followed by the annexation of many leading homoeopathic remedies.

It was hardly to be anticipated that the pharmacology-poor allopathy of the early nineteenth century should be uninterested in the tremendous volume of new medicinal knowledge being developed in the New School, and once the principle of proving on the healthy had been accepted, no major obstacle remained to the passage of these remedies into allopathic practice.

The process was complex and has been discussed by us in detail elsewhere.[h]

The homoeopathic expansion of the existing pharmacopoeia was along three lines: 1) an extension of the medicines in traditional use to new diseases and applications, 2) the introduction of new substances into medicine and the revival of ones which had fallen into disuse, 3) the proving and popularization of substances brought into medicine in the nineteenth century by the American Eclectic School and the botanical and Thomsonian practitioners. Thereupon, these new pharmacological techniques and applications were,

[g]H. C. Wood and Roberts Bartholow are discussed in *Divided Legacy*, III, 259, 414.

[h]H. L. Coulter, *Homoeopathic Influences in Nineteenth-Century Allopathic Therapeutics* (83 pages). See, also, *Divided Legacy*, III, 258-276.

in a number of cases, taken over by allopathic practitioners, leading to an expansion of the allopathic pharmacopoeia and a net increase in the number of remedies used by the average practitioner.

Rudolf Virchow in 1849 mentioned the "ever-increasing number of medications."[924] Trousseau in 1861 stated that "the great therapeutic system of *substitution* today dominates all of practice."[925] Another French physician in 1874 claimed that, whereas all the new medicines introduced into practice from 1830 to 1865 could be discussed within the confines of a relatively short book, those introduced since 1865 were so numerous that no single person could cope with this flood of information.[926]

Many of these new remedies, including some of the most popular, were taken from homoeopathic practice.

Medicines in traditional use which were extended by homoeopathy to new diseases and conditions were: *Aconitum napellus* in "fever" generally; *Belladonna* in scarlet fever; *Ipecacuanha* as a remedy for nausea and vomiting; various cathartics (such as calomel, gamboge, jalap, croton oil, and castor oil) as remedies for diarrhoea and dysentery; sulphuric acid in acid indigestion and alkaline medicines for excessive alkalinity; *Juniperus sabina* in threatened abortion; camphor, *Veratrum album,* and copper sulphate in Asiatic Cholera; *Thuja occidentalis* in warts; *Copaiba* in urticaria, psoriasis and other skin diseases; *Cantharides* in nephritis; *Chelidonium majus* in liver diseases; *Stramonium* in hydrophobia; *Nux vomica* in paralytic states, asthma, constipation, and headaches; *Capsicum annuum* for hemorrhoids; coffee in the treatment of migraine headaches; *Hyoscyamus niger* in typhus; *Arnica montana* for cuts and bruises; ergot for headaches and neuralgias; *Grindelia robusta* in iritis and bronchitis.

Of the new substances introduced into medicine (or resurrected from ancient practice) by homoeopathy the following may be mentioned: *Veratrum album, Bryonia alba, Rhus toxicodendron, Cocculus indicus, Calendula officinalis, Cannabis indica* and *Cannabis sativa, Pulsatilla nigricans,* phosphorus and phosphoric acid, *Conium maculatum, Cactus grandiflorus,* nitroglycerine, *Apis mellefica.*

The principal Eclectic remedies popularized by homoeopathy were *Podophyllum peltatum, Iris versicolor, Gelsemium sempervirens, Caulophyllum thalictroides, Rumex crispus, Berberis, Apocynum cannabinum, Euonymus atropurpureus, Cimicifuga racemosa, Lobelia inflata, Hydrastis canadensis, Baptisia tinctoria, Sanguinaria canadensis,* and *Chimaphila maculata.*

While Trousseau discussed many of these drugs,[927] he was significant more for introducing the principles of "substitution" and proving on the healthy. Those who followed him incorporated homoeopathic pharmacology in massive quantities. Stille, for instance, introduced these remedies into his *Therapeutics and Materia Medica* and into the *National Dispensatory* of which he was editor for many editions. H. C. Wood introduced them progressively into his *Treatise on Therapeutics* and the *United States Dispensatory* of which he was editor. Roberts Bartholow took much of his pharmacology from the Eclectic practitioners (closely associated with the homoeopaths) in his native Cincinnati.[i] Samuel Potter went even further, graduating from a homoeopathic college (and then from an allopathic one) and in 1887 issuing a handbook of practice full of homoeopathic remedies which had its twelfth edition in 1912.[928]

This process was no less striking in England. Sydney Ringer, professor of materia medica at University College, London, issued a *Handbook of Therapeutics* in 1870 which had its thirteenth edition in 1897 and was considered the

[i]His biographer wrote: "A man less balanced than Doctor Bartholow, after his fruitful investigations into the merits of drugs used by the Eclectics, would have joined the latter, and thus have nullified his potentiality for good. But he had the bravery to employ those remedies and by his influence to encourage their use, with the happy result that our knowledge of drugs became richer and our means of fighting disease fuller and more comprehensive . . . The regular school was made more regular—if that were possible—while the Eclectics, for example, were honored, in a way, by having their choice remedies taken over by the regular school because of the liberal and independent course of Doctor Bartholow" (George F. Butler, "Roberts Bartholow: A Great American Therapeutist," *American Journal of Clinical Medicine* XX [1913], 125-128).

leading therapeutic guide of the English-speaking world.[929] [j] C. D. F. Phillips was for years a homoeopathic physician and then issued a *Materia Medica and Therapeutics* in 1874 which could have been copied verbatim from a homoeopathic manual.[930] It was very favorably received by the regular profession, one review noting "the resuscitation, on the ground of recent physiological researches, of certain articles which had great repute in former times, but had recently been credited with scarcely any active properties."[931] This had two editions and, like Ringer's work, was published in the United States as well.

Thus, the Paris School moved dialectically from its Empirical origins to an Empirical conclusion. By the end of the century homoeopathy, in part as mediated through the Paris School and in part through the direct example of the homoeopathic practitioners themselves, had revolutionized medical practice in the Western countries.

[j] A review of the second edition stated: "This treatise on therapeutics at once assumed the first position on the subject in the English language" (*British and Foreign Medico-Chirurgical Review,* January, 1872, 166). The British homoeopaths were incensed at "the attempt of Ringer and Co. (Ltd.) to palm off homoeopathic therapeutic treasures upon the ignorant members of the profession as 'University College Therapeutics' . . ." (*Homoeopathic World* XVI [1881], 530). Ringer's *Handbook* was published simultaneously in London and New York.

NOTES

[1] "Galenisme" in *Dictionnaire des Sciences Medicales.* Sixty volumes (Paris: Rapart, 1812-1822). Henceforth cited as *Dictionnaire.*

[2] P. J. G. Cabanis, *Oeuvres Completes* (Paris: Bossange, 1823-1825), I, 506-507.

[3] *Ibid.*, I, 361-397; II, 307-362.

[4] *Moniteur, an* III (1794-1795), #71 and #80.

[5] "Clinique" in *Dictionnaire.* Paul Triaire, *Recamier et ses Contemporains* (Paris: J. B. Bailliere et Fils, 1899), 95.

[6] M. P. Crosland, *Science in France in the Revolutionary Era* (Cambridge and London: MIT Press and the Society for the History of Technology, 1969), 54. On this period generally see David M. Vess, *Medical Revolution in France* (Gainesville: Florida University Press, 1975).

[7] T. Puschmann, *History of Medical Education* (New York and London: Hafner, 1966), 539 ff.

[8] J. J. Rousseau, *Emile,* Bk. I.

[9] *Ibid.,* Bk. II.

[10] J. J. Rousseau, *Confessions,* Book II, liv, viii.

[11] J. J. Rousseau, *Emile,* Bk. I.

[12] A. Cabanes, "Le Scepticisme Therapeutique de Jean-Jacques Rousseau," *Bulletin General de Therapeutique* 158 (1909), 33-48. R. Semelaigne, "Jean-Jacques Rousseau Juge par Pinel," *Chronique Medicale* 19 (1912), 627-628.

[13] Laignel-Lavastine, "Sources des Idees Medicales de Jean-Jacques Rousseau," *Chronique Medicale* 26 (1919), 225-234. Also *ibid.,* 27 (1920), 59.

[14] Marc-Antoine Petit, *Essai sur la Medecine du Coeur* (Lyon: Garnier, 1806), 163 (quoted in M. Foucault, *Naissance de la Clinique* [Paris: Presses Universitaires de France, 1963], 88).

[15] R. Laennec, *Traite de l'Auscultation Mediate.* Third Edition (Paris: Chaude, 1831) I, xxiii.

[16] J. B. Bouillaud, *Essai sur la Philosophie Medicale et sur les Generalites de la Clinique Medicale* (Paris: Rouvier, 1836), 86. See the discussion in O. Temkin, "The Role of Surgery in the Rise of Medical Thought," *Bulletin of the History of Medicine* XXV (1951), 248-259.

[17] Marc-Antoine Petit, *Eloge de Pierre-Joseph Desault* (Lyon: La Grenette, 1795), 15 ff.

[18] *Ibid.,* 24.

[19] P. J. Desault, *Oeuvres Chirurgicales.* Third Edition (Paris: Bailliere, 1830), I, 11.

[20] *Loc. cit.*

[21] *Plan General de l'Enseignement Dans l'Ecole de Sante de Paris: Imprime par Ordre du Comite d'Instruction Publique de la Convention Nationale. An III de la Republique* [1795], 11.

[22] *Ibid.*, 29.
[23] *Ibid.*, 29, 37.
[24] *Ibid.*, 30.
[25] *Ibid.*, 39.
[26] *Ibid.*, 48-49.
[27] Cabanis, *Oeuvres Completes,* I, 361-397.
[28] *Ibid.*, I, 1-360, 403-531.
[29] *Ibid.*, I, 506-507, 515-517.
[30] *Ibid.*, I, 4-6, 8, 12-13, *et passim.*
[31] *Ibid.*, I, 382.
[32] *Ibid.*, 56-59, 64-65, 93.
[33] *Ibid.*, I, 58, 85, 94, 110-111, 120, 127-128, 144.
[34] *Ibid.*, I, 142.
[35] *Ibid.*, I, 12-13, 20, 66, 195, 224, 240, 252.
[36] *Ibid.*, I, 12-13, 19, 222, 224, 240, 437, 450.
[37] *Ibid.*, I, 1, 4, 176, 206, 225.
[38] *Ibid.*, I, 225.
[39] *Ibid.*, I, 194.
[40] *Ibid.*, I, 201, 204, 242, 263-268, 314.
[41] *Ibid.*, I, 270.
[42] *Ibid.*, I, 195.
[43] *Ibid.*, I, 7, 9, 194, 364, 437.
[44] *Ibid.*, I, 7, 19, 34-35, 40, 56, 176-177, 194, 252, 364, 413, 437.
[45] *Ibid.*, I, 11, 173, 263, 446, 459.
[46] *Ibid.*, I, 173.
[47] *Ibid.*, I, 175.
[48] *Ibid.*, I, 225 (*Novum Organum,* Book I, Aph. CIV).
[49] Locke, *An Essay Concerning Human Understanding,* Book II, Chapter I.
[50] Condillac, *Traite des Sensations,* Extrait Raisonne.
[51] Cabanis, *Oeuvres Completes,* I, 230-231, 456.
[52] *Ibid.*, I, 180.
[53] *Ibid.*, I, 170, 470-471.
[54] *Ibid.*, I, 13, 227-228, 236-239.
[55] *Ibid.*, I, 13, 364, 499.
[56] *Ibid.*, I, 169, 242, 248, 274, 290, 310-315, 474.
[57] *Ibid.*, I, 177, 310.
[58] *Ibid.*, I, 168.
[59] *Ibid.*, I, 323.
[60] *Ibid.*, I, 452-453.
[61] *Ibid.*, I, 449, 452.
[62] *Ibid.*, I, 14-15, 298 ff., 410. Triaire, *Recamier et ses Contemporains,* 119. See J. L. Alibert, *Nouveaux Elements de Therapeutique et de Matiere Medicale* (Paris: Crapart, Caille, et Ravier, *an* XII [1803-1804]), xxiv-xxv. Crosland, *Science in France in the Revolutionary Era,* 55.
[63] Cabanis, *Oeuvres Completes,* I, 25-27, 307-362.
[64] *Ibid.*, I, 288. Puschmann, *History of Medical Education,* 539.
[65] *Ibid.*, I, 327-329.
[66] *Ibid.*, I, 86.
[67] *Ibid.*, I, 86, 224.
[68] *Ibid.*, I, 458.
[69] *Ibid.*, I, 199.
[70] *Ibid.*, I, 159, 222, 224.

[71] *Ibid.*, I, 270, 285.
[72] *Ibid.*, I, 267.
[73] *Ibid.*, I, 263-267.
[74] *Ibid.*, I, 377.
[75] *Ibid.*, I, 284, 465, 470.
[76] *Ibid.*, I, 468.
[77] *Ibid.*, I, 206.
[78] *Ibid.*, I, 378.
[79] *Ibid.*, I, 13.
[80] *Ibid.*, I, 177, 240, 460, 469.
[81] *Ibid.*, I, 176, 460.
[82] *Ibid.*, I, 505.
[83] *Ibid.*, I, 160.
[84] *Ibid.*, I, 285.

[85] C. Pinel, "Biography of Pinel," *Journal of Psychological Medicine* XIII (1860), 184-205. "P. Pinel," in *Dictionnaire Encyclopedique des Sciences Medicales.* 100 volumes (Paris: Masson, 1869-1889). Henceforth referred to as *Dictionnaire Encyclopedique.* The most recent biography of Pinel is W. H. Lechler, *Philippe Pinel, seine Familie, seine Jugend- und Studienjahre, 1745-1778* (Munich, 1959 [privately printed]).

[86] P. Pinel, *Nosographie Philosophique, ou la Methode de l'Analyse Appliquee a la Medecine.* Sixth edition (Paris: Brosson, 1818), I, lxxiii.

[87] E. Pariset, "Eloge de Pinel," *Revue Medicale* XXVI (1827), 520-533, at 522.

[88] P. Pinel, *La Medecine Clinique Rendue Plus Precise et Plus Exacte par l'Application de l'Analyse.* Third Edition (Paris: Brosson, 1815), i.

[89] See *Georgii Baglivi Opera Omnia Medico-Practica et Anatomica* (Paris: Duplain, 1788). Pinel's iatromathematical writings are discussed in Lechler, *Philippe Pinel,* 124.

[90] Pariset, "Eloge de Pinel," 523-524.

[91] Isidore Bricheteau, "Discours sur Philippe Pinel. Son Ecole et l'Influence Qu'Elle a Exercee en Medecine, Prononce Devant la Societe Medicale d'Emulation de Paris, dans sa Seance Publique du 5 Decembre, 1827," *Journal Complementaire des Sciences Medicales* XXIX (1827), 289-304, at 292-293.

[92] *Ibid.*, 300. Philippe Pinel, *Nosographie Philosophique.* Second Edition (Paris: Brosson, *an* XI 1802), I, ix, xi, xv, xxxii, lxxiii, 3; III, 480-483, 488, 502, 509. Philippe Pinel, *La Medecine Clinique Rendue Plus Precise et Plus Exacte par l'Application de l'Analyse* (Paris: Brosson, *an* X [1802]), 6.

[93] "Agissante (Medecine)" in *Dictionnaire.*

[94] Pariset, "Eloge de Pinel," 532. Semelaigne, "Jean-Jacques Rousseau Juge par Pinel," 627-628.

[95] Pinel, *Nosographie Philosophique,* 1802, I, 199. "Chronique (Maladies Chroniques)" in *Dictionnaire.* "Classification des Maladies Internes" in *Dictionnaire.* Pinel, *Medecine Clinique,* 1802, xxxii, 10.

[96] Pinel, *Nosographie Philosophique,* 1802, I, v-vi.

[97] "Nosographie" in *Dictionnaire.*

[98] "Chronique (Maladies Chroniques), "Agissante (Medecine)," "Medecine" in *Dictionnaire.* Pinel, *Medecine Clinique,* 1802, 6-7.

[99] Pinel, *Medecine Clinique,* 1802, 6-7.

[100] Pinel, *Nosographie Philosophique,* 1802, I, xxvii-xxviii.

[101] *Ibid.,* I, vii, xxvi. "Classification des Maladies Internes" in *Dictionnaire.*

[102] Pinel, *Nosographie Philosophique,* 1802, I, xiii, xxiii, 5.
[103] "Classification des Maladies Internes" in *Dictionnaire.*
[104] "Clinique" in *Dictionnaire.* "Notice Necrologique sur Pinel," *Archives Generales de Medecine* XIII (1827), 623-628, at 626. Pariset, "Eloge de Pinel," 526. Pinel, *Nosographie Philosophique,* 1818, I, iii, vi, xx-xxi.
[105] Pinel, *Nosographie Philosophique,* 1818, I, vi.
[106] "Classification des Maladies Internes" in *Dictionnaire.*
[107] Pinel, *Nosographie Philosophique,* 1818, I, vii.
[108] *Ibid.,* 1802, I, xxiv.
[109] *Ibid.,* 1802, I, ii, Pinel, *Medecine Clinique,* 1802, 269 ff., 294, 302, 432.
[110] Pinel, *Medecine Clinique,* 1802, xvi. Pariset, "Eloge de Pinel," 527-528.
[111] Pinel, *Nosographie Philosophique,* 1818, I, xix-xx.
[112] *Ibid.,* 1818, I, v.
[113] Pinel, *Medecine Clinique,* 1802, 14, 248.
[114] *Ibid.,* 1802, xi-xiii. Pinel, *Nosographie Philosophique,* 1802, I, xiii. "Classification des Maladies Internes" in *Dictionnaire.*
[115] Pinel, *Medecine Clinique,* 1802, xi.
[116] Pinel, *Medecine Clinique,* 1802, 67-68.
[117] *Ibid.,* 1802, 103.
[118] *Ibid.,* 1802, 189.
[119] Pariset, "Eloge de Pinel," 529.
[120] Pinel, *Nosographie Philosophique,* 1818, I, x.
[121] *Ibid.,* 1802, I, lvi.
[122] *Ibid.,* 1802, I, xxii.
[123] *Ibid.,* 1802, I, iv.
[124] *Ibid.,* 1802, I, vii. See, also, "Analyse Appliquee a la Medecine" in *Dictionnaire.*
[125] Pinel, *Medecine Clinique,* 1802 (disease table inside front cover).
[126] Pinel, *Nosographie Philosophique,* 1818, III, 573 ff.
[127] "Nosographie" in *Dictionnaire.*
[128] *Loc. cit.* Pinel, *Medecine Clinique,* 1815, 391.
[129] Bricheteau, "Discours sur Philippe Pinel," 295
[130] Pinel, *Medecine Clinique,* 1802, xxxix.
[131] *Ibid.,* 1802, 4-6. Pinel, *Nosographie Philosophique,* 1802, I, xxxv. "Classification des Maladies Internes" in *Dictionnaire.*
[132] "Chronique (Maladies Chroniques)" in *Dictionnaire.*
[133] Pinel, *Medecine Clinique,* 1802, 321-401. "Expectation" in *Dictionnaire.*
[134] "Expectation" in *Dictionnaire.*
[135] Pinel, *Medecine Clinique,* 1802, 2, 335, 367.
[136] *Ibid.,* 1802, xxxv.
[137] *Ibid.,* 1802, xxxii-xxxiii. "Agissante (Medecine)" in *Dictionnaire.*
[138] "Chronique (Maladies Chroniques)" in *Dictionnaire.*
[139] "Medecine" in *Dictionnaire.*
[140] "Agissante (Medecine)" in *Dictionnaire.* Pinel, *Medecine Clinique,* 1802, xxxiii, 335, 360.
[141] Pinel, *Nosographie Philosophique,* 1802, I, xxxv-xxxvi.
[142] "Chronique (Maladies Chroniques)" in *Dictionnaire.*
[143] Pinel, *Nosographie Philosophique,* 1802, I, xxxii, xl-xli.
[144] *Ibid.,* 1802, I, 52; III, 476.
[145] Pinel, *Medecine Clinique,* 1802, 391.
[146] Pinel, *Nosographie Philosophique,* 1802, I, 91, 93; III, 19.
[147] *Ibid.,* 1802, I, xxxviii.

[148] *Ibid.*, 1802, I, 1.

[149] Pinel, *Medecine Clinique*, 1802, 342.

[150] Pinel, *Nosographie Philosophique*, 1802, III, 509. "Agissante (Medecine)" in *Dictionnaire*.

[151] Pinel, *Nosographie Philosophique*, 1802, III, 516-517.

[152] Pinel, *Medecine Clinique*, 1802, *passim*.

[153] *Loc. cit.*

[154] *Ibid.*, 1802, xxxiii, 369, 387.

[155] *Ibid.*, 1802, 369.

[156] *Ibid.*, 1802, xxxiii.

[157] Bricheteau, "Discours sur Philippe Pinel," 300.

[158] F. J. Double, *Semeiologie Generale, ou Traite des Signes et de leur Valeur dans les Maladies* (Paris: Croullebois, 1811), I, 167.

[159] A. J. Landre-Beauvais, *Semeiotique, ou Traite des Signes des Maladies* (Paris: Brosson, 1809), 9.

[160] Xavier Bichat, *Anatomie Generale, Appliquee a la Physiologie et a la Medecine* (Paris: Brosson, *an* X [1801]), I, xcix.

[161] *Loc. cit.*

[162] *Ibid.*, I, lv.

[163] *Ibid.*, I, lxv.

[164] Xavier Bichat, *Recherches Physiologiques sur la Vie et la Mort* (Paris: Brosson, *an* VIII [1800]), 1.

[165] Bichat, *Anatomie Generale*, I, vii, xxxix, lv.

[166] *Ibid.*, I, xxxix.

[167] *Ibid.*, I, lxxx, lxxxiii.

[168] Xavier Bichat, *Traite des Membranes en General et de Diverses Membranes en Particulier* (Paris: Richard, *an* VIII [1800]), 183.

[169] Bichat, *Anatomie Generale*, I, vii, lxxix-lxxx.

[170] *Ibid.*, I, xxxix.

[171] Francois Chaussier, *Table Synoptique des Proprietes Caracteristiques et des Principaux Phenomenes de la Force Vitale* (Paris: Barrois, [*circa* 1815]).

[172] Bichat, *Recherches Physiologiques sur la Vie et la Mort*, ii. Bichat, *Anatomie Generale*, I, xcii. Bichat, *Traite des Membranes*, 3-4. "Classification des Maladies Internes" in *Dictionnaire*. Bricheteau, "Discours sur Philippe Pinel," 289.

[173] Bichat, *Recherches Physiologiques sur la Vie et la Mort*, 92-133.

[174] Bichat, *Anatomie Generale*, I, vii, xliv-xlv, xlvii.

[175] *Ibid.*, I, xcii, xcix.

[176] *Ibid.*, I, xciv.

[177] *Ibid.*, I, xliii-xliv.

[178] *Ibid.*, I, xliv-xlv.

[179] *Ibid.*, I, xlv.

[180] *Ibid.*, I, xcix.

[181] Bichat, *Recherches Physiologiques*, 7.

[182] *Ibid.*, 5-6. Bichat, *Anatomie Generale*, I, ci.

[183] Bichat, *Anatomie Generale*, I, lxii, lxiii, lxviii.

[184] *Ibid.*, I, lxvi.

[185] *Ibid.*, I, lxvi, xci-xcviii.

[186] *Ibid.*, I, lxvii.

[187] *Ibid.*, I, xc.

[188] *Ibid.*, I, xci.

[189] *Ibid.*, I, lix.

[190] *Ibid.*, I, xcviii.

[191] Bichat, *Traite des Membranes,* 66-67.

[192] Bichat, *Anatomie Generale,* I, vii, xlv, xlvii.

[193] *Ibid.,* I, xlvii.

[194] *Ibid.,* I, xlviii-xlix.

[195] *Ibid.,* I, 1.

[196] E. Ackerknecht, "Die Therapie der Pariser Kliniker zwischen 1795 und 1840," *Gesnerus* XV (1958), 151-163, at 156.

[197] Bichat, *Recherches Physiologiques,* 92-93.

[198] Bichat, *Anatomie Generale,* I, lxv.

[199] *Ibid.,* I, xciii.

[200] Jean Cruveilhier, *Essai sur l'Anatomie Pathologique en General* (Paris: Crochard, 1816), I, 19.

[201] "Contagion" in *Dictionnaire.*

[202] Hunter, *Works,* II, 153, 381, 404.

[203] *Ibid.,* II, 140.

[204] *Ibid.,* II, 139-140, 153.

[205] *Ibid.,* II, 383 ff. "Syphilis" in *Dictionnaire.*

[206] Sprengel, *Histoire de la Medecine,* VI, 33 ff. See *Lettres Edifiantes et Curieuses Ecrites des Missions Etrangeres par Quelques Missionaires de la Compagnie de Jesus* (Paris, 1731), XXI, 5 ff.

[207] Philippe Hecquet, *Observations sur la Saignee du Pied et sur la Purgation. Raisons de Doute Contre l'Inoculation de la Petite Verole* (Paris: Cavelier, 1724), 350 ff., 392 ff., 410 ff., 449 ff.

[208] Hunter, *Works,* II, 165.

[209] *Ibid.,* II, 155.

[210] *Ibid.,* II, 405.

[211] T. Willis, *Pharmaceutice Rationalis* (London: Dring, 1679), Table of All the Hard Words, etc. E. Chambers, *Cyclopedia.* Fifth Edition (London: Midwinter, 1741).

[212] Christian Frid. Daniel, *Systema Aegritudinum* (Lipsiae: Boehm, 1781), 40, 43.

[213] Cullen, *First Lines of the Practice of Physic,* I, 108-109, 297.

[214] "Disposition," in *Encyclopedie, ou Dictionnaire Raisonnee des Sciences, des Arts, et des Metiers,* IX (1782).

[215] Jean-Charles Grimaud, *Cours de Fievres* (Montpellier: Picot, 1815), II, 311; IV, 222, 301, 334.

[216] *Ibid.,* I, cxlvii.

[217] "Diathese" in *Dictionnaire.*

[218] Cullen, *A Synopsis of Methodical Nosology,* 176. Johann Ernst Wichmann, *Aetiologie der Kraetze* (Hannover: Koenigliche Hofbuchhandlung, 1791), 175.

[219] Autenrieth, *Versuche fuer die Praktische Heilkunde,* II, 229 ff.

[220] "Dartres" in *Dictionnaire.*

[221] Brown, *Elements of Medicine,* xii.

[222] Cullen, *First Lines,* IV, 212, 379 ff.

[223] *Ibid.,* IV, 199 ff.

[224] Barthez, *Nouveaux Elements,* II, 72.

[225] *Ibid.,* II, 72, 73, 87.

[226] Barthez, *Traite des Maladies Goutteuses,* I, ii ff.

[227] Pinel, *Nosographie Philosophique,* 1802, III, 300 ff., 337.

[228] *Ibid.,* 1802, III, 308.

[229] *Ibid.,* 1802, III, 344.

[230] *Ibid.*, 1802, III, 355.
[231] *Ibid.*, 1802, III, 364; 1818, III, 301, 303.
[232] *Ibid.*, 1802, III, 365.
[233] *Ibid.*, 1802, III, 366.
[234] *Ibid.*, 1802, III, 337.
[235] A. Darbefeuille, *Propositions sur la Medecine* (Paris Dissertation, 1808).
[236] *Ibid.*, 26.
[237] *Ibid.*, 26, 38.
[238] *Ibid.*, 38.
[239] *Loc. cit.*
[240] *Ibid.*, 32.
[241] *Loc. cit.*
[242] *Ibid.*, 40.
[243] *Ibid.*, 33.
[244] *Ibid.*, 34.
[245] *Ibid.*, 37.
[246] *Ibid.*, 31.
[247] *Ibid.*, 32.
[248] "Diathese" in *Dictionnaire.*
[249] For biographical information on Bayle, see "G. L. Bayle" in *Dictionnaire Encyclopedique.*
[250] G. L. Bayle, *Considerations sur la Nosologie, la Medecine d'Observation, et la Medecine Pratique* (Paris Dissertation, *an X* [1802]), 19, 21, 23.
[251] *Ibid.*, 10-11.
[252] G. L. Bayle, "Idee Generale de la Therapeutique" in J. N. Corvisart, *Essai sur les Maladies et les Lesions Organiques du Coeur* (Paris: Delahaye, 1855), 604-610, at 607-608.
[253] *Ibid.*, 609.
[254] G. L. Bayle, *Recherches sur la Phthisie Pulmonaire* (Paris: Gabon, 1810), xiii-xiv.
[255] *Ibid.*, xvi, 37, 69.
[256] *Ibid.*, 5.
[257] *Ibid.*, 6.
[258] *Ibid.*, 8.
[259] *Ibid.*, 86.
[260] *Ibid.*, 90, 109.
[261] G. L. Bayle, "Anatomie Pathologique (Considerations Generales sir les Secours que l'Anatomie Peut Fournir a la Medecine)" in *Dictionnaire.*
[262] Bayle, *Considerations sur la Nosologie,* 28.
[263] *Ibid.*, 52. Bayle, "Idee Generale de la Therapeutique," 609.
[264] *Ibid.*, 59. Bayle, "Idee General de la Therapeutique, 609.
[265] Bayle, "Idee Generale de la Therapeutique," 605-608.
[266] *Loc. cit.* Bayle, *Recherches sur la Phthisie Pulmonaire,* 86.
[267] Rene Laennec, *Auscultation Mediate, ou Traite du Diagnostic des Maladies des Poumons et du Coeur* (Paris: Brosson and Chaude, 1819).
[268] Biographical information on Laennec may be found in "Notice Necrologique sur Laennec," *Archives Generales de Medecine* XIII (1827), 620-625.
[269] R. Laennec, *Propositions sur la Doctrine d'Hippocrate Relativement a la Medecine-Pratique* (Paris Dissertation, *an* XII [1804]), Dedication.
[270] Rene Laennec, *Traite de l'Auscultation Mediate et des Maladies des Poumons et du Coeur.* Third Edition, with notes by Meriadec Laennec (Paris: Chaude, 1831), I, v-vi. On Laennec's Hippocraticism see also *Laennec, Documents*

Inedits Publies a l'Occasion de son Centenaire (Paris: Masson, 1926), 15-17 *et passim;* "Extrait du Discours Prononce par M. Laennec a l'Ouverture de son Cours de Medecine au College Royale de France," *Archives Generales de Medecine* I (1823), v-xx.

[271] Laennec, *Propositions sur la Doctrine d'Hippocrate,* 11-15, 18-27, 32.

[272] *Ibid.,* 34. Laennec, "Extrait du Discours," vi, xvi.

[273] Laennec, *Auscultation Mediate,* 1831, I, 123.

[274] Laennec, "Extrait du Discours," vii.

[275] Laennec, *Auscultation Mediate,* 1831, I, 123. For more on Laennec's rejection of proximate causes see *ibid.,* 1831, I, xix, xxi and II, 41, 57; "Extrait du Discours," vii.

[276] *Ibid.,* 1831, I, 247.

[277] *Ibid.,* 1831, II, 180.

[278] *Ibid.,* 1831, II, 326.

[279] *Ibid.,* 1831, II, 57.

[280] *Ibid.,* 1831, III, 102.

[281] R. Laennec, *Traite Inedit sur l'Anatomie Pathologique* (Paris: Alcan, 1884), 23.

[282] Laennec, *Auscultation Mediate,* 1831, II, 51, 55-57, 123.

[283] *Ibid.,* 1831, II, 51.

[284] *Ibid.,* 1831, II, 41.

[285] Laennec, "Anatomie Pathologique" in *Dictionnaire.*

[286] Laennec, *Auscultation Mediate,* 1831, I, xxix.

[287] Laennec, *Traite Inedit,* 23.

[288] Erwin Ackerknecht, "Laennec und sein Vorlesungsmanuskript von 1822," *Gesnerus* XXI (1964), 144. Laennec, *Auscultation Mediate,* 1819, II, 89.

[289] Laennec, *Auscultation Mediate,* 1819, I, 413. See, also, *Traite Inedit,* 76.

[290] Laennec, "Anatomie Pathologique" in *Dictionnaire.*

[291] Laennec, *Auscultation Mediate,* 1819, I, 413.

[292] *Ibid.,* 1831, I, 124, 438.

[293] Laennec, "Anatomie Pathologique" in *Dictionnaire.*

[294] Laennec, *Auscultation Mediate,* 1819, I, xxviii-xxix. *Laennec, Documents Inedits,* 16.

[295] Laennec, *Auscultation Mediate,* 1819, I, xxx.

[296] *Ibid.,* 1819, I, 19-20, 31.

[297] Laennec, *Propositions sur la Doctrine d'Hippocrate,* 11-15, 34.

[298] *Loc. cit.*

[299] *Ibid.,* 34.

[300] Laennec, *Traite Inedit,* 23.

[301] Laennec, *Auscultation Mediate,* 1819, I, 412-413.

[302] Laennec, *Propositions sur la Doctrine d'Hippocrate,* 11-16.

[303] Laennec, *Traite Inedit,* 23.

[304] Laennec, *Auscultation Mediate,* 1819, I, xxii, 2, 34; II, 359.

[305] *Ibid.,* 1819, I, 412.

[306] *Ibid.,* 1819, I, 412-413 (stress added).

[307] R. Laennec, "Note sur l'Anatomie Pathologique," *Journal de Medecine, Chirurgie, Pharmacie* IX (1804-1805), 360-378, at 364.

[308] *Ibid.,* 377. Laennec, "Anatomie Pathologique" in *Dictionnaire.* Laennec, *Traite Inedit,* 76.

[309] Laennec, *Auscultation Mediate,* 1831, I, 186.

[310] Laennec, "Note sur l'Anatomie Pathologique," 364. *Traite Inedit,* 50-51. "Anatomie Pathologique" in *Dictionnaire.*

[311] Laennec, *Auscultation Mediate,* 1819, I, xx-xxi. *Traite Inedit,* 20.

[312] Laennec, *Auscultation Mediate,* 1819, I, xxi.

[313] *Loc. cit.*

[314] *Ibid.,* 1819, I, xviii, xx.

[315] *Ibid.,* 1831, I, 186. Ackerknecht, "Laennec und sein Vorlesungsmanuskript," 149.

[316] Laennec, "Anatomie Pathologique" in *Dictionnaire.*

[317] Laennec, *Auscultation Mediate,* 1819, I, xxii.

[318] Laennec, *Propositions sur la Doctrine d'Hippocrate,* 12-15, 36.

[319] *Ibid.,* 36.

[320] Laennec, *Auscultation Mediate,* 1819, II, 86.

[321] *Ibid.,* 1819, I, xx.

[322] *Laennec, Documents Inedits,* 25. "Anatomie Pathologique" in *Dictionnaire.*

[323] *Laennec, Documents Inedits,* 25.

[324] R. Laennec, *Auscultation Mediate.* Fourth Edition, considerably enlarged by M. Andral (Paris: Chaude, 1837), I, viii.

[325] *Ibid.,* 1819, I, 1-2.

[326] *Ibid.,* 1819, I, 2.

[327] *Ibid.,* 1819, I, xx, 3.

[328] *Loc. cit.*

[329] *Ibid.,* 1819, I, 4.

[330] *Ibid.,* 1819, I, 7.

[331] *Ibid.,* 1819, I, 8.

[332] *Ibid.,* 1819, I, 14; 1831, I, xxii-xxiii.

[333] *Ibid.,* 1819, I, xxi; 1831, I, xxiii.

[334] *Ibid.,* 1819, II, 195.

[335] *Ibid.,* 1819, I, xxvi, 57.

[336] *Ibid.,* 1831, I, xxiii, 124.

[337] *Ibid.,* 1819, I, 223.

[338] *Loc. cit.*

[339] *Ibid.,* 1819, II, 86.

[340] *Ibid.,* 1831, I, 240 ff.

[341] "Extrait du Discours Prononce par M. Laennec," vii. *Propositions sur la Doctrine d'Hippocrate,* 35.

[342] Laennec, *Propositions sur la Doctrine d'Hippocrate,* 35-36.

[343] Pinel, *Nosographie Philosophique,* 1802, I, 56.

[344] Laennec, "Extrait du Discours," viii.

[345] E. Bouchut, *Histoire de la Medecine et des Doctrines Medicales* (Paris: Bailliere, 1873), II, 208.

[346] F. J. V. Broussais, *Examen de la Doctrine Medicale Generalement Adoptee et des Systemes Modernes de Nosologie* (Paris: Mequignon-Marvis, 1816), xi.

[347] Quoted in Erwin Ackerknecht, "Broussais or a Forgotten Medical Revolution," *Bulletin of the History of Medicine* XXVII (1953), 320-343, at 321 note 6.

[348] Chauffard, *Andral,* 16.

[349] F. J. V. Broussais, *Recherches sur la Fievre Hectique Consideree Comme Dependente d'une Lesion d'Action des Differents Systemes, Sans Vice Organique* (Paris Dissertation, *an* XI [1803]), 3.

[350] *Ibid.,* 2, 11.

[351] Pinel, *Nosographie Philosophique,* 1802, II, 1-16.

[352] P. A. Prost, *Medecine Eclairee par l'Observation et l'Ouverture des Corps* (Paris: Demonville, *an* XII [1804]), I, x ff.

[353] J. Marandel, *Considerations Generales sur les Irritations* (Paris Dissertation, 1807). Dupuytren was associated with this research (*ibid.*, v).

[354] F. J. V. Broussais, *Histoire des Phlegmasies ou Inflammations Chroniques, Fondee sur de Nouvelles Observations de Clinique et d'Anatomie Pathologique* (Paris: Gabon, 1808), I, xii-xix, 310-319; II, 546-549.

[355] *Ibid.*, II, 252, 548.

[356] "Broussais" in *Dictionnaire Encyclopedique.*

[357] Broussais, *Examen,* 1816, i-xix, 193.

[358] Almire Lepelletier de la Sarthe, *Histoire de la Revolution Medicale du XIX Siecle* (Paris: Bailliere, 1854), 416.

[359] Broussais, *Examen,* 1816, 420; also *ibid.*, second edition (Paris: Mequignon-Marvis, 1821), I, Propositions VIII ff. Broussais, *Histoire des Phlegmasies,* I, 139; II, 180, 548.

[360] Broussais, *Examen,* 1816, 421, 425. "Broussais" in *Dictionnaire Encyclopedique.*

[361] Broussais, *Examen,* 1821, I, vii.

[362] *Ibid.*, 1816, 423-425. F. J. V. Broussais, *Traite de Physiologie Appliquee a la Pathologie* (Paris: Delauncy, 1822-1823), II, 555.

[363] Broussais, *Examen,* 1816, 438, 454.

[364] Broussais, *Examen,* 1816, 188-193.

[365] F. J. V. Broussais, *De l'Irritation et de la Folie* (Paris: Delauney, 1828), *passim.*

[366] Broussais, *Examen,* 1816, 383.

[367] *Ibid.*, 1816, 195, 373, 375; *ibid.*, 1821, I, Proposition CCLXII.

[368] Broussais, *Traite de Physiologie,* II, 73-74.

[369] Broussais, *Examen,* 1816, 384, 406.

[370] *Ibid.*, 1816, 379, 387; *ibid.*, 1821, II, 733.

[371] *Ibid.*, 1821, II, 682.

[372] *Ibid.*, 1821, I, vii and II, 394.

[373] *Ibid.*, 1816, 370, 382.

[374] *Ibid.*, 1816, 406, 409.

[375] *Ibid.*, 1816, Title Page, 388. Broussais, *Traite de Physiologie,* I, 5.

[376] Broussais, *Examen,* 1816, 371. Chauffard, *Andral,* 16.

[377] Broussais, *Examen,* 1816, 273.

[378] Broussais, *Histoire des Phlegmasies,* I, iv-v.

[379] Broussais, *Examen,* 1816, ix, 410; *ibid.*, 1821, II, 394.

[380] Broussais, *Examen,* 1816, 216; *ibid.*, 1821, I, Propositions CCLXIII-CCLXXXIII. Broussais, *Histoire des Phlegmasies,* I, 148-151; II, 252.

[381] Broussais, *Histoire des Phlegmasies,* I, 520-535.

[382] Broussais, *Examen,* 1821, I, Proposition CCLXVI.

[383] *Ibid.*, 1816, 214.

[384] Broussais, *Histoire des Phlegmasies,* I, xviii.

[385] *Ibid.*, I, 515.

[386] *Loc. cit.*

[387] *Ibid.*, I, xiv. Chauffard, *Andral,* 15.

[388] Broussais, *Examen,* 1816, 214.

[389] *Ibid.*, 1816, 413. Chauffard, *Andral,* 38.

[390] Broussais, *Examen,* 1816, 222.

[391] Ackerknecht, "Broussais or a Forgotten Medical Revolution," 341.

[392] Broussais, *Examen,* 1816, 410.

[393] *Ibid.*, 1816, 195, 208.

[394] *Ibid.*, 1816, ix, 182, 383. Broussais, *Histoire des Phlegmasies,* I, v.

[395] Broussais, *Examen,* 1816, 379.

[396] *Loc. cit.* and 407.

[397] *Ibid.*, 1821, II, 711, 736, 750.

[398] *Ibid.*, 1816, 195, 376, 378, 383, 406-408.

[399] *Ibid.*, 1816, 372, 410. Chauffard, *Andral,* 17-18.

[400] *Ibid.*, 1816, 195.

[401] Broussais, *Examen,* Third Edition (Paris: Delauney, 1829), IV, 527, 554-555.

[402] *Ibid.*, 1829, IV, 555.

[403] *Ibid.*, 1816, 403.

[404] J. B. Isidore Poullain, *Des Medecins Physiologistes et de Leur Doctrine* (Paris Dissertation, 1826), 42-43.

[405] *Ibid.*, 45.

[406] *Ibid.*, viii, 38, 46.

[407] *Ibid.*, 46.

[408] Ackerknecht, "Broussais or a Forgotten Medical Revolution," 328.

[409] *Archives Generales de Medecine* V (1824), 305-307, 625.

[410] Chauffard, *Andral,* 33.

[411] *Archives Generales de Medecine* XIII (1827), 625.

[412] Broussais, *Examen,* 1821, I, xii.

[413] J. B. Regnault, *Considerations sur l'Etat de la Medecine en France Depuis la Revolution jusqu'a Nos Jours* (Paris: Mequignon-Marvis, 1819), 20.

[414] *Ibid.*, 29.

[415] *Ibid.*, 31.

[416] "Extrait du Discours Prononce par M. Laennec," vii.

[417] Broussais, *Examen,* 1821, II, 394, 674, 676, 733.

[418] *Ibid.*, 1821, II, 760.

[419] *Ibid.*, 1821, II, 734.

[420] Quoted in Chauffard, *Andral,* 35.

[421] Paul Delauney, "Un Medecin Broussaisien: le Docteur Beunaiche la Corbiere," *Bulletin de la Societe Francaise d'Histoire de la Medecine* XX (1926), 397-428, at 409.

[422] Laennec, *Auscultation Mediate,* 1831, I, xx-xxiii.

[423] *Ibid.*, 1831, I, 438.

[424] "Extrait du Discours Prononce par M. Laennec," xii. See, also, Laennec, *Auscultation Mediate,* 1831, I, xxix.

[425] Chauffard, *Andral,* 31.

[426] A. L. J. Bayle, *Bibliotheque de Therapeutique* (Paris: Gabon, 1828-1837), I, iv.

[427] Michel Malpart, *Un Medecin Romantique: Eusebe de Salles (1796-1873)* (Paris Dissertation, 1928), 30.

[428] *Ibid.*, 35.

[429] Ackerknecht, "Broussais or a Forgotten Medical Revolution," 340-341.

[430] Chauffard, *Andral,* 18.

[431] Chauffard, *Andral,* 19. Broussais, *Examen,* 1816, 388. "Theophile Bordeu," in *Dictionnaire Encyclopedique.*

[432] *Archives Generales de Medecine* V (1824), 305.

[433] Laennec, *Auscultation Mediate,* 1831, I, 12.

[434] Broussais, *Histoire des Phlegmasies,* I, ix.

[435] Laennec, *Auscultation Mediate,* 1831, III, 100.

436 Gabriel Andral [and T. N. Lerminier], *Clinique Medicale; ou, Choix d'Observations Receuillies a la Clinique de M. Lerminier* (Paris: Gabon, 1823-1827), Four Volumes.

437 Armand Trousseau and Hermann Pidoux, *Traite de Therapeutique et de Matiere Medicale* (Paris: Bechet Jeune, 1836-1839), Two Volumes in Three.

438 A. F. Chomel, *Lecons de Clinique Medicale* (Paris: Bailliere, 1834-1849), I, 538. A. F. Chomel, *Elements de Pathologie Generale.* Second edition (Paris: Crochard, 1824), 15, 18, 604.

439 Chomel, *Elements,* 3, 430.

440 *Ibid.,* 399-400. A. F. Chomel, *Des Fievres et des Maladies Pestilentielles* (Paris: Crochard, 1821), 29, 57.

441 Chomel, *Elements,* 130 ff., 602, 604.

442 *Ibid.,* 135.

443 *Ibid.,* 136.

444 *Ibid.,* 292.

445 *Ibid.,* 445-476.

446 *Ibid.,* 554

447 *Loc. cit.*

448 *Loc. cit.*

449 *Ibid.,* 537.

450 *Ibid.,* 533.

451 *Ibid.,* 46-49.

452 *Ibid.,* 55.

453 *Ibid.,* 61.

454 *Ibid.,* 123.

455 *Ibid.,* 69-98.

456 *Ibid.,* 110.

457 *Ibid.,* 111.

458 *Ibid.,* 112.

459 *Ibid.,* 113.

460 *Ibid.,* 98-101.

461 *Ibid.,* 527.

462 *Ibid.,* 525.

463 *Ibid.,* 437.

464 Chomel, *Des Fievres et des Maladies Pestilentielles,* 25. But cf. Chomel, *Elements,* 442, 451.

465 Chomel, *Elements,* 608.

466 *Ibid.,* 9.

467 *Ibid.,* 608.

468 *Ibid.,* 433.

469 Chomel, *Des Fievres et des Maladies Pestilentielles,* 451.

470 *Ibid.,* 455 ff. Chomel, *Lecons de Clinique Medicale,* 302.

471 Chomel, *Elements,* 431-432.

472 *Ibid.,* 526.

473 *Ibid.,* 433.

474 *Ibid.,* 430, 436.

475 *Ibid.,* 537.

476 *Ibid.,* 436, 529, 604.

477 *Ibid.,* 530.

478 *Ibid.,* 571-572.

479 Chomel, *Des Fievres et des Maladies Pestilentielles,* 29.

480 Chomel, *Elements,* 574.

[481] *Ibid.*, 575.

[482] "Auguste-Francois Chomel" in *Dictionnaire Encyclopedique.*

[483] *Loc. cit.*

[484] *Loc. cit.*

[485] Chomel, *Elements,* 1.

[486] *Loc. cit.*

[487] *Ibid.*, vii, 602.

[488] "Auguste-Francois Chomel" in *Dictionnaire Encyclopedique.*

[489] Raoul Mercier, "L'Extraordinaire Vie de Pierre-Fidele Bretonneau," *Progres Medical* XIV (1937), I, *Supplement,* 1-8, at 2. J. D. Rolleston, "Bretonneau: His Life and Work," *Proc. Royal Soc. of Medicine* XVIII (1924-1925), History of Medicine Section, 1-12, at 2.

[490] Jules Coquerelle, *Bretonneau (1778-1862): La Doctrine Specifique* (Paris Dissertation, 1892), 55.

[491] *Loc. cit.*

[492] Robert Debre, *Discours. Institut de France, Academie des Sciences. Celebration du Centenaire de la Mort de Pierre-Fidele Bretonneau, a Tours, dimanche, 18 fevrier, 1962,* 13.

[493] Rolleston, "Bretonneau: His Life and Work," 9.

[494] A. Velpeau, "Note sur l'Emploi des Caustiques, comme Moyen d'Arreter l'Eruption Varioleuse," *Archives Generales de Medecine* VIII (1825), 427-436, at 427.

[495] *Ibid.*, 428.

[496] Beatrice R. Lovett, "Pierre-Fidele Bretonneau," *Bulletin of the Society of Medical History of Chicago* IV (1928-1935), 54-70, at 61. Velpeau, "Note sur l'Emploi des Caustiques," 435.

[497] A. Trousseau, "De la Maladie a laquelle M. Bretonneau, medecin de l'Hopital de Tours, a Donne le Nom de Dothinenterie ou Dothinenterite," *Archives Generales de Medecine* X (1826), 67-78, 169-216, at 67.

[498] *Loc. cit.*

[499] *Ibid.*, 69-71.

[500] Quoted in E. Apert, "Bretonneau et la Specificite des Maladies," *Bulletin Medical* XXXVI (1922), 1083-1085, at 1084.

[501] *Loc. cit.*

[502] *Loc. cit.*

[503] Quoted in Debre, *Discours,* 18.

[504] Pierre Bretonneau, *Des Inflammations Speciales du Tissu Muqueux et en Particulier de la Diphtherite ou Inflammation Pelliculaire* (Paris: Crevot, 1826), 1.

[505] *Ibid.*, 5.

[506] *Ibid.*, 40.

[507] *Ibid.*, 85.

[508] *Ibid.*, 90-92.

[509] *Ibid.*, 47.

[510] *Ibid.*, 55.

[511] *Loc. cit.*

[512] *Ibid.*, 356, 366.

[513] Paul Triaire, *Bretonneau et ses Correspondants* (Paris: Alcan, 1892), II, 596.

[514] *Ibid.*, II, 575, 576, 596.

[515] *Ibid.*, II, 593, 595.

[516] *Loc. cit.*

[517] *Ibid.*, II, 599.

[518] *Ibid.*, II, 597.

[519] Hunter, *Works*, II, 139, 151, 153. Bretonneau, *Des Inflammations Speciales*, 42-45.

[520] Hunter, *Works*, II, 165. Bretonneau, *Des Inflammations Speciales*, 55.

[521] Hunter, *Works*, II, 422, 459, 470. Bretonneau, *Des Inflammations Speciales*, 196.

[522] Hunter, *Works*, II, 436. Bretonneau, *Des Inflammations Speciales*, 92, 94.

[523] Bretonneau, *Des Inflammations Speciales*, 94.

[524] Laennec, *Auscultation Mediate*, 1831, I, 230-231, 237, 240-241.

[525] On this see E. Ackerknecht, "Anticontagionism Between 1821 and 1867," *Bulletin of the History of Medicine* XXII (1948), 562-593.

[526] Pariset and Mazet, *Observations sur la Fievre Jaune Faites a Cadix en 1819* (Paris: Audot, 1820), ii, iv, v, 10, 11, 121.

[527] Etienne Pariset, *Memoire sur les Causes de la Peste et sur les Moyens de la Detruire* (Paris: Bailliere, 1837), 69, 97-104, 181, 182, 198.

[528] Robert Debre, *Discours*, 14.

[529] G. D. Rolleston, "Bretonneau: His Life and Work," 11. P. C. A. Louis, *Recherches Anatomiques, Pathologiques, et Therapeutiques sur la Maladie Connue sous les Noms de Gastro-Enterite, Fievre Putride, Adynamique, Ataxique, Typhoide, etc.* Second Edition (Paris: Bailliere, 1841), II, 371-372.

[530] Hahnemann, *Lesser Writings*, 756, 760.

[531] P. C. A. Louis, *Recherches Anatomico-Pathologiques sur la Phthisie* (Paris: Gabon, 1825), ix, xxi.

[532] *Ibid.*, 522.

[533] P. C. A. Louis, *Recherches Anatomiques, Pathologiques, et Therapeutiques sur la Maladie Connue sous les Noms de Gastro-Enterite, Fievre Putride, Adynamique, Ataxique, Typhoide, etc. etc.* (Paris: Bailliere, 1829). Two Volumes.

[534] *Ibid.*, 1841, xvii. "Typhoide" in *Dictionnaire Encyclopedique.*

[535] *Ibid.*, 1829, I, vii, viii, 11, 119-150; II, 318, 151.

[536] *Ibid.*, 1829, II, 431-433.

[537] *Ibid.*, 1829, II, 433.

[538] *Ibid.*, 1829, I, 452.

[539] *Ibid.*, 1829, II, 457-458.

[540] *Loc. cit.*

[541] P. C. A. Louis, *An Essay on Clinical Instruction* (London: Highley, 1834), 7.

[542] *Ibid.*, 12-13.

[543] *Ibid.*, 17.

[544] Robert Debre, *Discours*, 20.

[545] Dr. Gendron, "Recherches sur les Epidemies des Petites Localites," *Journal des Connaissances Medico-Chirurgicales* I (1833-1834), 193-198, 225-232, 295-302.

[546] *Ibid.*, 193-194.

[547] *Loc. cit.*

[548] *Loc. cit.*

[549] *Ibid.*, 195, 227, 232, 295, 296.

[550] *Loc. cit.*

[551] Louis, *Fievre Typhoide*, 1841, II, 313, 370-371, 376.

[552] *Ibid.*, 1841, II, 373.

[553] *Ibid.*, 1841, II, 377. Cf. with *ibid.*, 1829, II, 458.

[554] Triaire, *Bretonneau et ses Correspondants,* II, 595.

[555] P. C. A. Louis, *Recherches sur les Effets de la Saignee dans Quelques Maladies Inflammatoires et sur l'Action de l'Emetique et des Vesicatoires dans la Pneumonie* (Paris: Bailliere, 1835), 86.

[556] *Ibid.*, 72, 81, 87.

[557] *Ibid.*, 72.

[558] *Ibid.*, 76.

[559] *Ibid.*, 73-74.

[560] *Ibid.*, 74.

[561] *Loc. cit.*

[562] *Ibid.*, 75.

[563] *Ibid.*, 76.

[564] *Ibid.*, 80.

[565] *Ibid.*, 81.

[566] *Ibid.*, 84.

[567] *Ibid.*, 8.

[568] *Ibid.*, 70.

[569] *Ibid.*, 32.

[570] *Loc. cit.*

[571] *Loc. cit.*

[572] J. H. Baas, *History of Medicine,* 897.

[573] William Osler, *The Principles and Practice of Medicine.* Eighth Edition (New York: Appleton, 1912), 99.

[574] Louis, *Essay on Clinical Instruction, passim.*

[575] Louis, *Recherches Anatomico-Pathologiques sur la Phthisie,* 534-543.

[576] Louis, *Fievre Typhoide,* 1829, I, 453; II, 524.

[577] *Ibid.*, 1829, I, 453. Cf. Laennec, *Auscultation Mediate,* 1831, I, 241.

[578] Jean Cruveilhier, *Essai sur l'Anatomie Pathologique,* I, xxi.

[579] *Ibid.*, I, xix.

[580] Jean Cruveilhier, *Medecine Pratique Eclairee par l'Anatomie et la Physiologie Pathologiques* (Paris: Igonette, 1821), iii-iv.

[581] *Loc. cit.*

[582] *Ibid.*, I, iv-vi.

[583] Cruveilhier, *Essai sur l'Anatomie Pathologique,* I, xiv ff., 8, 13, 23.

[584] *Ibid.*, I, xiii.

[585] *Ibid.*, I, 1.

[586] *Ibid.*, I, 27, 76, 131-136.

[587] *Ibid.*, I, 105.

[588] J. Cruveilhier, *Traite d'Anatomie Pathologique Generale* (Paris: Bailliere, 1849-1864), I, 11-12, 25-26.

[589] *Ibid.*, I, 26-37, 55-58.

[590] *Ibid.*, I, 32.

[591] Cruveilhier, *Essai sur l'Anatomie Pathologique,* I, xvii.

[592] *Ibid.*, I, 21 ff., 131-136.

[593] Cruveilhier, *Traite d'Anatomie Pathologique,* I, 33-34.

[594] *Ibid.*, I, 29. Cruveilhier, *Essai sur l'Anatomie Pathologique,* I, 24.

[595] Cruveilhier, *Essai sur l'Anatomie Pathologique,* I, 2-3.

[596] Cruveilhier, *Traite d'Anatomie Pathologique,* I, 12, 25.

[597] *Ibid.*, I, 34.

[598] *Ibid.*, I, 26.

[599] Cruveilhier, *Essai sur l'Anatomie Pathologique,* I, 135.

[600] Cruveilhier, *Traite d'Anatomie Pathologique,* I, 13.

[601] *Ibid.,* I, 1, 43, 55-63.

[602] *Ibid.,* I, 39.

[603] *Ibid.,* I, 41.

[604] *Ibid.,* I, 41-42.

[605] *Ibid.,* I, 40, 51.

[606] *Ibid.,* I, 16.

[607] Cruveilhier, *Essai sur l'Anatomie Pathologique,* I, 113, 131; II, 350, 889; IV, 30, 245, 492, 523, 543.

[608] Jean Cruveilhier, "Phlebite," *Dictionnaire de Medecine et de Chirurgie Pratique,* II (Paris, 1834), 637-681, at 637.

[609] Cruveilhier, *Medecine Pratique Eclairee par l'Anatomie et la Physiologie Pathologiques,* xxv.

[610] Cruveilhier, *Traite d'Anatomie Pathologique,* I, 49.

[611] See his, *Physiologie Pathologique, ou Recherches Cliniques, Experimentales, et Microscopiques sur l'Inflammation, la Tuberculisation, les Tumeurs, la Formation du Cal* (Paris: Bailliere, 1845).

[612] Leon Rostan, *Cours de Medecine Clinique ou sont Exposes les Principes de la Medecine Organique* (Paris: Bechet Jeune, 1830), I, viii.

[613] "Leon-Louis Rostan (1791-1866)" in *Dictionnaire Encyclopedique.*

[614] Ackerknecht, *Medicine at the Paris Hospital,* 111-112.

[615] Rostan, *Cours de Medecine Clinique,* I, i.

[616] *Ibid.,* I, iii.

[617] Leon Rostan, *Exposition des Principes de l'Organicisme Precedee de Reflexions sur l'Incredulite en Matiere de Medecine* (Paris: Labe, 1846), 82.

[618] *Ibid.,* 167.

[619] *Ibid.,* xii, 166 ff.

[620] *Ibid.,* 94. Rostan, *Cours de Medecine Clinique,* I, viii.

[621] Rostan, *Exposition des Principes de l'Organicisme,* 97, 145.

[622] *Ibid.,* 136.

[623] *Ibid.,* 86 ff.

[624] *Ibid.,* 119-126.

[625] *Ibid.,* 126.

[626] *Ibid.,* 94-95, 116.

[627] *Ibid.,* 90-91.

[628] *Ibid.,* 85, 166-167. Rostan, *Cours de Medecine Clinique,* I, ix.

[629] Rostan, *Exposition des Principes de l'Organicisme,* 92.

[630] *Ibid.,* 145.

[631] Rostan, *Cours de Medecine Clinique,* I, 91.

[632] *Ibid.,* I, 112-113, 181.

[633] *Ibid.,* I, 182.

[634] Rostan, *Exposition des Principes de l'Organicisme,* 149.

[635] *Loc. cit.*

[636] *Ibid.,* 147.

[637] *Loc. cit.*

[638] *Loc. cit.*

[639] *Ibid.,* 149.

[640] *Ibid.,* 52-54.

[641] *Ibid.,* 154-155.

[642] *Loc. cit.*

[643] Rostan, *Cours de Medecine Clinique,* II, 702-703.

[644] Rostan, *Exposition des Principes de l'Organicisme,* 154-155.
[645] *Ibid.,* 155.
[646] *Ibid.,* 151.
[647] Rostan, *Cours de Medecine Clinique,* I, viii.
[648] *Ibid.,* I, 92, 101-102; III, 460 ff.
[649] *Ibid.,* I, viii.
[650] *Ibid.,* I, 179.
[651] *Ibid.,* I, 179-180.
[652] Rostan, *Exposition des Principes de l'Organicisme,* x-xiii.
[653] *Ibid.,* 82, 169.
[654] *Ibid.,* x-xi, 169.
[655] J. B. Bouillaud, *Traite Clinique et Experimental des Fievres Dites Essentielles* (Paris: Bailliere, 1826), i.
[656] *Ibid.,* iii-iv.
[657] *Ibid.,* vi-vii.
[658] J. B. Bouillaud, *Nouvelles Recherches sur le Rhumatisme Articulaire Aigu en General* (Paris: Bailliere, 1836).
[659] J. B. Bouillaud, *Essai sur la Philosophie Medicale et les Generalites de la Clinique Medicale* (Paris: De Just, 1836), 347.
[660] *Ibid.,* v-vii.
[661] *Ibid.,* vii-viii.
[662] *Ibid.,* 38-40.
[663] *Ibid.,* 260.
[664] *Ibid.,* 252-253.
[665] *Loc. cit.*
[666] *Ibid.,* 312-313.
[667] *Ibid.,* 309.
[668] *Ibid.,* 308.
[669] *Ibid.,* 302.
[670] *Ibid.,* 331-420.
[671] *Ibid.,* 420.
[672] Laennec, *Auscultation Mediate,* 1831, I, x ff.
[673] Gabriel Andral, *Clinique Medicale.* Third Edition (Paris: Deville Cavellin, 1834), I, vi-vii.
[674] Quoted in Emil Kratzmann, *Die neuere Medicin in Frankreich nach Theorie und Praxis* (Leipzig: Brockhaus, 1846), 108.
[675] "Andral," *Gazette des Hopitaux Civils et Militaires* XLIX (1876), 185-188.
[676] *France Medicale* XXIII (1876), 109.
[677] Paris: Gabon, 1829. See, also, second edition (Bruxelles: Societe Typographique Belge, 1837), Two Volumes.
[678] R. Laennec, *Auscultation Mediate.* Fourth edition, considerably expanded by M. Andral (Paris: Chaude, 1837), Two Volumes.
[679] G. Andral, *Essai d'Hematologie Pathologique* (Paris: Fortin, 1843).
[680] G. Andral, *Recherches sur l'Expectoration dans les Differentes Maladies de Poitrine* (Paris Dissertation, 1821), 15, 25.
[681] *Ibid.,* 25.
[682] G. Andral, *An Antiquorum Doctrina de Crisibus et Diebus Criticis Admittenda? an in Curandis Morbos et Praesertim Acutis Observanda?* (Paris Dissertation, 1824), 43-44, 50.
[683] Andral, *Clinique Medicale,* 1823, I, ii; III, 359-362, 365. *Ibid.,* 1834, I, 654; III, 540.
[684] Laennec, *Auscultation Mediate,* 1837, I, 308-309.

685 *L'Union Medicale* VII (1853), #26, 101.
686 Andral, *Clinique Medicale,* 1823, I, 495-500.
687 *Ibid.,* 1823, I, 501.
688 *Ibid.,* 1823, I, 503.
689 *Ibid.,* 1823, II, 320.
690 Chauffard, *Andral,* 36.
691 Andral, *Clinique Medicale,* 1834, I, 8-9.
692 Chauffard, *Andral,* 35.
693 Laennec, *Auscultation Mediate,* 1837, I, 40, 136.
694 *Ibid.,* 1837, II, 17.
695 *Ibid.,* 1837, I, 235.
696 *Ibid.,* 1837, I, 150.
697 *Ibid.,* 1837, I, 151.
698 *Ibid.,* 1837, I, 150.
699 Andral, *Clinique Medicale,* 1823, I, 495.
700 Andral, *Precis d'Anatomie Pathologique,* 1837, I, 306-320.
701 Andral, *Essai d'Hematologie Pathologique,* 7.
702 *Ibid.,* 28-38.
703 *Ibid.,* 45, 49, 57.
704 *Ibid.,* 10.
705 *Ibid.,* 74.
706 *Ibid.,* 134, 184.
707 "Andral," *Gazette des Hopitaux Civils et Militaires* XLIX (1876), 185-188.
708 Andral, *Essai d'Hematologie Pathologique,* 40.
709 *Ibid.,* 41.
710 *Ibid.,* 42.
711 *Ibid.,* 7.
712 *Ibid.,* 14.
713 *Ibid.,* 8.
714 *Ibid.,* 59.
715 *Ibid.,* 69, 132-135.
716 *Ibid.,* 29.
717 *Ibid.,* 79-81.
718 Andral, *Precis d'Anatomie Pathologique,* 1837, I, 308.
719 Andral, *Essai d'Hematologie Pathologique,* 140.
720 *Loc. cit.*
721 *Ibid.,* 15.
722 *Ibid.,* 14.
723 Andral, *Precis d'Anatomie Pathologique,* 1837, I, 308.
724 Andral, *Essai d'Hematologie Pathologique,* 124, 138.
725 *Ibid.,* 126.
726 *Ibid.,* 125.
727 *Ibid.,* 122-123.
728 *Ibid.,* 70-73.
729 Andral, *Precis d'Anatomie Pathologique,* 1837, I, 308.
730 *Loc. cit.*
731 *Ibid.,* 1837, I, 305-306, 310.
732 Andral, *Essai d'Hematologie Pathologique,* 9.
733 A. F. Chomel, *Elements de Pathologie Generale,* v.
734 A. L. J. Bayle, *Bibliotheque de Therapeutique,* I, i-ii.
735 *Ibid.,* I, ii.

[736] Third Edition (Paris: Mequignon-Marvis, 1822).

[737] Second Edition. Two Volumes (Paris: Mcquignon-Marvis, 1824).

[738] Fifth Edition. Three Volumes (Paris: Bechet-Jeune, 1826).

[739] A. Trousseau and H. Pidoux, *Traite de Therapeutique et de Matiere Medicale.* Eighth Edition (Paris: Bechet Jeune, 1868), I, v.

[740] Chauffard, *Andral,* 39.

[741] J. Mabit, *Observations sur l'Homoeopathie* (Bordeaux: Gassiot, 1835), 7-10.

[742] *Ibid.,* 8. *Archives de la Medecine Homoeopathique* III (1835), 73. Ludovic de Parseval, *Homoeopathie et Allopathie* (Paris: Bailliere, 1856), 43.

[743] Theodore Boeckel, *Exposition de la Doctrine Homoiopathique du Docteur Hahnemann et Reflexions sur Cette Doctrine* (Strasburg Dissertation, 1826), 29, 31, 44.

[744] *L'Union Medicale* III (1849), 170, 175-176. J. B. Bouillaud, *Traite Pratique, Theorique, et Statistique du Cholera-Morbus de Paris* (Paris: Bailliere, 1832), 179, 291.

[745] Mabit, *Observations sur l'Homoeopathie,* 10, 12.

[746] *Ibid.,* 17.

[747] *Journal de Medecine Pratique* (Bordeaux) I (1835), 196.

[748] *Bulletin General de Therapeutique* VI (1834), 318.

[749] *Ibid.,* VI (1834), 102.

[750] A. Trousseau and H. Pidoux, *Traite de Therapeutique et de Matiere Medicale* (Paris: Bechet Jeune, 1836), II (Part I), 22.

[751] *Bulletin General de Therapeutique* IX (1835), 298-300. Haehl, *Hahnemann,* II, 365.

[752] J. B. Bouillaud, *Essai sur la Philosophie Medicale et sur les Generalites de la Clinique Medicale,* 306.

[753] Rostan, *Exposition des Principes de l'Organicisme,* 4, 25.

[754] *Arch. de la Medecine Homoeopathique* II (1835), 477.

[755] *Journal des Connaissances Medico-Chirurgicales* I (1833-1834), 142. *Journal de Medecine Pratique* (Bordeaux) I (1835), 188-189.

[756] *Journal des Connaissances Medico-Chirurgicales* I (1833-1834), 236.

[757] "Homoeopathie" in *Dictionnaire Encyclopedique.*

[758] *Journal des Connaissances Medico-Chirurgicales* I (1833-1834), 236.

[759] Achille Requin, *Homoeopathie* (Paris: Martinet, 1851), 6.

[760] *Journal des Connaissances Medico-Chirurgicales* I (1833-1834), 239.

[761] J. B. Bouillaud, *Essai sur la Philosophie Medicale et sur les Generalites de la Clinique Medicale,* 310.

[762] *Arch. de la Medecine Homoeopathique* II (1835), 396.

[763] *Bull. Gen. de Ther.* IX (1835), 298. *Journ. des Conn. Medico-Chirurgicales* I (1833-1834), 239. Requin, *Homoeopathie,* 8. "Homoeopathie" in *Dict. Encycl.*

[764] *Bull. Gen. de Therapeutique* VII (1834), 135. Requin, *Homoeopathie,* 9. *Journ. des Conn. Medico-Chirurgicales* I (1833-1834), 238.

[765] Requin, *Homoeopathie,* 10.

[766] *L'Union Medicale* V (1851), 284.

[767] "Homoeopathie" in *Dictionnaire Encyclopedique.*

[768] F. A. Jaumes, *Essai de Pharmacologie Therapeutique Generale* (Montpellier: Castel, 1847), 225.

[769] Requin, *Homoeopathie,* 15.

[770] *Gazette Medicale de Paris* III (1835), 190.

[771] *Gazette des Hopitaux* IX (1835), 135.

[772] *Gazette Medicale de Paris* III (1835), 190.

[773] A. Trousseau and H. Pidoux, *Traite de Therapeutique et de Matiere Medicale.* Sixth Edition (Paris: Bechet Jeune, 1858), I, lix.

[774] *Gazette des Hopitaux* IX (1835), 136. See, also, Requin, *Homoeopathie,* 7. "Homoeopathie" in *Dict. Encycl.*

[775] *Journ. de Medecine Pratique* (Bordeaux) I (1835), 301-306. *Journ. des Conn. Medico-Chirurgicales* I (1833-1834), 237. "Homoeopathie" in *Dict. Encycl.*

[776] *Arch. de la Medecine Homoeopathique* I (1834), 38.

[777] "Homoeopathie" in *Dictionnaire Encyclopedique.*

[778] *Bulletin General de Therapeutique* VI (1834), 321.

[779] *Journal de Medecine Pratique* I (1835), 195.

[780] *Arch. de la Med. Hom.* IV (1836), 239-240.

[781] Parseval, *Homoeopathie et Allopathie,* 27.

[782] Trousseau, *Traite de Therapeutique,* 1858, I, lxv.

[783] *Arch. de la Med. Hom.* V (1836), 471-478.

[784] *Bulletin General de Therapeutique* VI (1834), 228.

[785] *Ibid.,* V (1833), 297.

[786] *Ibid.,* VI (1834), 102.

[787] *Loc. cit.* A. Trousseau, *Conferences sur l'Empirisme* (Paris: Delahaye, 1862), 20.

[788] *Archives de la Medecine Homoeopathique* I (1834), 40.

[789] *Journal des Connaissances Medico-Chirurgicales* I (1833-1834), 142.

[790] *Bulletin General de Therapeutique* VIII (1835), 158.

[791] Many other trials were reported: *Bull. Gen. de Ther.* V (1833), 235, 291-292; VI (1834), 104; *L'Union Medicale* III (1849), 182; *Revue Medicale Francaise et Etrangere* I (1834), 273-277; Jean-Paul Tessier, *De la Medecine Homoeopathique, suivi d'un Releve Comparatif des Malades Traites a l'Hopital Sainte Marguerite par la Methode de Hahnemann et par la Methode Ordinaire Pendant les Annees 1849, 1850, 1851; Reponse a la Lettre de Fredault* (Paris: Bailliere, 1852); *Montpellier Medical* II (1859), 478-481.

[792] *Gazette des Hopitaux* IX (1835), 136.

[793] *Arch. de la Medecine Homoeopathique* III (1835), 31-39.

[794] *Bull. Gen. de Therapeutique* VI (1834), 318-322.

[795] *Loc. cit. Gazette Medicale de Paris* III (1835), 190.

[796] *Gazette Medicale de Paris* III (1835), 190.

[797] *Arch. de la Med. Hom.* III (1835), 29.

[798] *Ibid.* I (1834), 39, 76-80; III (1835), 29.

[799] *Ibid.* III (1835), 350. *Revue Medicale Francaise et Etrangere* II (1835), 259-260.

[800] *Arch. de la Med. Hom.* I (1834), 76-80; II (1835), 400; III (1835), 351.

[801] *Loc. cit.*

[802] *Journal des Connaissances Medico-Chirurgicales* I (1833-1834), 238-241.

[803] *Bulletin General de Therapeutique* VI (1834), 128-131.

[804] Requin, *Homoeopathie,* 15. *La Medecine Traditionnelle et l'Homoeopathie. Proces Intente au Journal L'Union Medicale par Douze Homoeopathes. Plaidoirie de M. Andral* (Paris: Martinet, 1858), 41. *Bulletin General de Therapeutique* XI (1836), 392.

[805] *Arch. de la Med. Hom.* II (1835), 397.

[806] *Bulletin General de Ther.* VI (1834), 107.

[807] *Arch. de la Med. Hom.* II (1835), 400.

[808] *Gazette Medicale de Paris* III (1835), 190.

[809] *Gazette des Hopitaux* IX (1835), 135.

[810] *Ibid.,* IX (1835), 136.

[811] *Ibid.,* IX (1835) 148.

[812] *Ibid.*, IX (1835), 136, 148.
[813] *Journal de Medecine Pratique* I (1835), 188-189.
[814] *Loc. cit.*
[815] *Loc. cit.*
[816] *Gazette des Hopitaux* IX (1835), 136.
[817] *Gazette Medicale de Paris* III (1835), 189.
[818] *Gazette des Hopitaux* IX (1835), 148. *Bulletin General de Therapeutique* VIII (1835), 191.
[819] *Journal de Medecine Pratique* I (1835), 188.
[820] *Bulletin General de Therapeutique* VIII (1835), 158.
[821] *Ibid.*, VII (1834), 5-6.
[822] *Arch. de la Medecine Homoeopathique* II (1835), 397.
[823] *Ibid.*, IV (1836), 417, 420.
[824] *Arch. de la Medecine Homoeopathique* IV (1836), 424.
[825] Quoted in Parseval, *Homoeopathie et Allopathie,* 57.
[826] *L'Union Medicale* VII (1853), #5 (February 5).
[827] *Arch. de la Med. Hom.* VII (1838), 239; VIII (1838), 154. Cf. Requin, *Homoeopathie,* with Jean Kunzli, *Essai Critique sur l'Homoeopathie* (Paris: Bailliere, 1840).
[828] Henri Soules, *Essai d'un Examen de la Doctrine Homoeopathique de Hahnemann* (Montpellier Dissertation, 1858), 5.
[829] *L'Homoeopathie dans les Hopitaux. Memoire a Propos de la Petition des Ouvriers de Paris et de la Discussion au Senat* (*Seance du Premier Juillet, 1865*) (Paris: Bailliere, 1865), 2.
[830] A. Trousseau, *Conferences sur l'Empirisme,* 34.
[831] N. M. Chauvet, *L'Avenir de la Homoeopathie* (Tours: Ladeveze and Gilland-Verger, 1859), 2. See, also, Triaire, *Bretonneau et ses Correspondants,* II, 595.
[832] Parseval, *Homoeopathie et Allopathie,* 48. F. A. Jaumes, *Essai de Pharmacologie Generale,* 214.
[833] See his "Memoire sur les Proprietes Antinevralgiques de l'Aconit," *Gazette Medicale de Paris* IX (1854), 704-720.
[834] M. Rousset, "Notice sur M. le Professeur Risueno d'Amador," *Academie des Sciences de Montpellier, Section de Medecine. Memoires* I (1849-1853), 287, 301.
[835] *Ibid.*, 299.
[836] Risueno de Amador, *Des Decouvertes en Medecine* (Montpellier: Boehm, 1843).
[837] M. Rousset, "Notice sur M. le Professeur Risueno d'Amador," 303. Risueno de Amador, "Memoire sur l'Action des Agents Imperceptibles sur le Corps Vivant," *Bulletin de la Societe Medicale Homoeopathique de Paris* II (1846), 131-164, at 147.
[838] *Ibid.*, 149.
[839] *Ibid.*, 163.
[840] Chauvet, *L'Avenir de la Homoeopathie,* 6. Parseval, *Homoeopathie et Allopathie,* 40. F. A. Jaumes, *Traite de Pathologie et de Therapeutique Generales,* 1061-1063. J. B. Fonssagrives, *Traite de Matiere Medicale, ou Pharmacographie, Physiologie, et Technique des Agents Medicamenteux* (Paris: Delahaye and Lecrosnier, 1885), 954. *British Journal of Homoeopathy* XXVI (1868), 553-560.
[841] "Homoeopathie" in *Dictionnaire Encyclopedique.*
[842] *Gazette des Hopitaux* IX (1835), 76.
[843] *La Medecine Traditionnelle et l'Homoeopathie. Proces Intente au*

Journal L'Union Medicale par Douze Homoeopathes. Plaidoirie de M. Andral, 33, 37.

[844] Parseval, *Homoeopathie et Allopathie,* 30. Chauvet, *L'Avenir de la Homoeopathie,* 63.

[845] *L'Union Medicale* III (1849), 92, 170, 175-176, 182, 196, etc. "Homoeopathie" in *Dictionnaire Encyclopedique.*

[846] "Homoeopathie" in *Dictionnaire Encyclopedique. La Medecine Traditionnelle et l'Homoeopathie, passim.*

[847] "Homoeopathie" in *Dictionnaire Encyclopedique. L'Union Medicale* III (1849), 182, 581. *L'Homoeopathie dans les Hopitaux,* 2.

[848] "Homoeopathie" in *Dictionnaire Encyclopedique.*

[849] Boeckel, *Exposition de la Doctrine Homoiopathique du Docteur Hahnemann,* 42.

[850] *Journal des Connaissances Medico-Chirurgicales* I (1833-1834), 236-237.

[851] P. Ricord, *Traite Pratique des Maladies Veneriennes* (Brussels: Societe Typographique Belge, 1838), *passim.*

[852] *Bulletin de l'Academie Royale de Medecine* I (1836-1837), 40-42.

[853] *Bulletin de la Societe Medicale Homoeopathique de Paris* II (1846), 160.

[854] C. J. A. Schwilgue, *Traite de Matiere Medicale* (Paris: Brosson, *an* XIII [1805]), I, 127.

[855] Boeckel, *Exposition de la Doctrine Homoiopathique du Docteur Hahnemann,* 29.

[856] Hahnemann, *Fragmenta de Viribus Medicamentorum,* 1805, I, 150-161, 185-200.

[857] *Ibid.,* I, 193. G. W. Becker, "Heilung Einer dreijaehrigen Paralyse der untern Extremitaeten," *Journal der Practischen Heilkunde* XXVII (1808), st. III, 83-101.

[858] Eugene-Henri Desportes, *De la Noix Vomique* (Paris Dissertation, 1808), 33.

[859] F. Magendie, "Examen de l'Action de Quelques Vegetaux sur la Moelle Epiniere. Avril, 1809," *Bibliotheque Medicale* XXV (1809), 3-22. See, also, Alire Raffenau-Delile, *Dissertation sur les Effets d'un Poison de Java appele Upas Tieute* (Paris Dissertation, 1809).

[860] Trousseau, *Traite de Therapeutique,* 1836, I, 517.

[861] Jan Purkyne, "Rozprava o tom jak rozlicne veci lekarske na svem tele zkousel," *Casopis lekaruv Ceskych* V (1866), 12-14.

[862] "In memoriam J. Ev. Purkyne, 1787-1937," in *Purkynova Spolecnost* (Prague, 1937), 54-65, at 55.

[863] J. Ev. Purkinje, "Einige Beitraege zur physiologischen Pharmacologie," *Neue Breslauer Sammlungen aus dem Gebiete der Heilkunde* I (1829), 423-444, at 427.

[864] "Johann Joerg," *Monatsschrift fuer Geburtskunde* XI (1858), 439-441.

[865] J. C. G. Joerg, *Materialien zu einer kuenftigen Heilmittellehre durch Versuche der Arzneyen an gesunden Menschen. Erster Band* (Leipzig: Cnobloch, 1825).

[866] *Ibid.,* vii.

[867] Boeckel, *Exposition de la Doctrine Homoiopathique du Docteur Hahnemann,* 38.

[868] S. Hahnemann, "Was sind Gifte? Was sind Arzneien?" *Journal der practischen Heilkunde* XXIV (1806), st. III, 40-57.

[869] J. C. Reil, *Entwurf einer allgemeinen Pathologie* (Halle: Curt, 1815-1816), III, 190.

[870] M. P. Orfila, *Traite des Poisons tires des Regnes Mineral, Vegetal, et Animal, ou Toxicologie Generale* (Paris: Crochard, 1815). Two Volumes.

[871] Robert Christison, *A Treatise on Poisons* (Edinburgh: Adam Black, 1829), iv.

[872] *Ibid.*, v.

[873] Barbier, *Traite Elementaire de Matiere Medicale.* Second Edition, I, 168.

[874] *Bulletin General de Therapeutique* VII (1834), 10.

[875] *Ibid.*, VII (1834), 14.

[876] *Ibid.*, VII (1834), 13.

[877] *Ibid.*, VII (1834), 14.

[878] *Arch. de la Med. Hom.* III (1835), 361. Parseval, *Homoeopathie et Allopathie,* 25-26.

[879] Trousseau, *Traite de Therapeutique,* 1868, I, vi.

[880] On Recamier see: Henri Gouraud, *Eloge de M. Recamier* (Paris: Douniol, 1853); Paul Triaire, *Recamier et ses Contemporains, 1774-1852* (Paris: Bailliere, 1899); Louis Sauve, *Le Docteur Recamier* (Paris: Spes, 1938).

[881] H. Pidoux, "Trousseau. Eloge Prononce a la Societe de Therapeutique, dans sa seance du 5 Mars, 1869," *L'Union Medicale* VII (1869), 349.

[882] J. Beclard, "Trousseau," *Gazette Medicale de Paris* XXV (1870), 39.

[883] Trousseau, *Traite de Therapeutique,* 1836, I, 8-9, II (Part I), 53-54, (Part II), xii; *ibid.*, 1858, II, 674.

[884] A. Trousseau, *Clinique Medicale de l'Hotel Dieu.* Seventh Edition (Paris: Bailliere, 1885), I, 3-4.

[885] Trousseau, *Traite de Therapeutique,* 1836, II (Part II), vii; *ibid.*, 1868, I, ix.

[886] *Ibid.*, 1836, II (Part I), 303, 309, 324, 367, 401, 409; II (Part II), 154, 170; *ibid.*, 1858, I, ii-iii, xxxii-xxxiii, xlviii, l-li.

[887] *Ibid.*, 1858, I, liv.

[888] *Bulletin General de Therapeutique* IV (1833), 357-365; V (1833), 229-236 and 293-297; VI (1834), 101-107.

[889] Trousseau, *Conferences sur l'Empirisme,* 50.

[890] Trousseau, *Traite de Therapeutique,* 1858, I, liv, lvi.

[891] *Ibid.*, 1858, I, lxv.

[892] *Ibid.*, 1858, I, lxxxvi-lxxxviii.

[893] *Ibid.*, 1858, I, lxv.

[894] *Ibid.*, 1858, I, xv.

[895] *Ibid.*, 1858, I, lxi.

[896] *Ibid.*, 1858, I, lv, 470 ff.

[897] *Ibid.*, 1858, I, lviii-lix.

[898] *Ibid.*, 1858, I, lix.

[899] *Ibid.*, 1858, I, lvii.

[900] *Ibid.*, 1858, I, lviii.

[901] *Ibid.*, 1858, I, lvi, lxiv; *ibid.*, 1836, I, 351, II (Part I), 22.

[902] *Ibid.*, 1858, I, xii-xvi, xlviii, li.

[903] *Ibid.*, 1858, I, xxi-xxii, xliii, xlvii; *ibid.*, 1836, II (Part I), 24.

[904] *Ibid.*, 1858, I, xlii.

[905] *Ibid.*, 1836, II (Part I), 30.

[906] *Ibid.*, 1858, I, ci.

[907] *Ibid.*, 1858, I, 470-483.

[908] *Ibid.*, 1858, I, xxiv.

[909] *Ibid.*, 1858, I, xvii, xxi, xxiv, xxvi, xli.

[910] G. Beclard, "Trousseau," 29.

[911] Trousseau, *Traite de Therapeutique,* 1858, I, xv, xxix-xxxii, xliii.

[912] *Ibid.,* 1836, I, 2, 19, 24-25, 50, 71, 181, 207, 231, 268, 414-416.

[913] *Ibid.,* 1836, I, 53, 207, 267, 416, *et passim.*

[914] *Ibid.,* 1836, I, xxviii.

[915] H. Pidoux, "Trousseau. Eloge Prononce a la Societe de Therapeutique, dans sa Seance du 5 Mars, 1869," *L'Union Medicale* VII (1869), 349-350.

[916] Paris: Bailliere, 1861. Three Volumes.

[917] J. Pereira, *Elements of Materia Medica,* 1839, II, 601, 791-794, 855, 911, 1399, *et passim.*

[918] *Ibid.,* 1839, I, 7.

[919] Philadelphia: Blanchard and Lee, 1860. Two Volumes.

[920] Philadelphia: J. B. Lippencott, 1874.

[921] *Ibid.,* Ninth Edition (Philadelphia: Lippencott, 1894), ix (Preface to the First Edition).

[922] Tenth Edition (New York; Appleton, 1900), xii (Preface to the First Edition).

[923] New York: Appleton, 1880.

[924] R. Virchow, "Die Naturwissenschaftliche Methode und die Standpunkte in der Therapie," *Archiv fuer pathologische Anatomie und Physiologie* II (1849), 16.

[925] A. Trousseau, *Clinique Medicale de l'Hotel Dieu.* Seventh Edition (Paris: Bailliere, 1885), I, 16.

[926] E. Heckel, *Histoire Medicale et Pharmaceutique des Principaux Agents Medicamenteux Introduits en Therapeutique depuis ces dix Dernieres Annees* (Bruxelles: Manceaux, 1874), ii.

[927] Trousseau discusses the uses mentioned above of aconite, *Belladonna,* camphor, *Copaiba, Nux vomica,* coffee, and ergot, as well as *Veratrum album, Bryonia alba, Rhus toxicodendron,* and *Conium maculatum* (*Traite de Therapeutique,* 1858, I, 75, 113, 708, 776, 786, 801; II, 118, 271, 513, 651, 767).

[928] S. O. L. Potter, *A Handbook of Materia Medica, Pharmacy, and Therapeutics* (Philadelphia: Blakiston, 1887).

[929] New York: Wood, 1870.

[930] *Materia Medica and Therapeutics. The Vegetable Kingdom* (London: Churchill, 1874). *Organic Compounds. The Animal Kingdom* (London: Churchill, 1886). These were published in the United States in 1879 and 1886 respectively.

[931] *The Practitioner* XIII (1874), 204.

CHAPTER VIII

RELAPSE INTO METHODISM: MAGENDIE, VIRCHOW, BERNARD

The Empirical medicine of Pinel, Laennec, Bretonneau, Trousseau, and Hahnemann necessarily provoked a return to the Methodist pole of thought.

This was seen first in the career of Broussais, but his influence declined after ten or fifteen years. A more sustained Methodist effort was mounted by Francois Magendie (1783-1855), Rudolf Virchow (1821-1902), and Claude Bernard (1813-1878).

Aroused by the popularity of Empiricism, these thinkers sought a new point of departure for medical speculation in the molecular or corpuscular causal theories of Descartes—which they combined with the physiology of Brown and Broussais.

In this new Methodist synthesis Rationalism remained a potent force in medicine until the end of the nineteenth century and beyond.

Biographical

Francois Magendie was born in Bordeaux, the son of a surgeon who believed in Rousseau and absolute liberty and allowed the youngster to behave exactly as he pleased during the first ten years of his life.[1]

Thus he only learned to read and write in 1793, when the family moved to Paris; but he made up for lost time and four years later won a major competition with an essay on "Knowledge of the Rights of Man and the Constitution." His general education was cut short again, however, in 1799 when he was apprenticed as a surgeon to Alexis Boyer (1757-1833).

He defended a surgical thesis at the Ecole de Santé in 1808, and practiced surgery for some years thereafter, but abandoned it in 1813 for the infant science of physiology—apparently because Dupuytren, with whom his relations were intensely hostile, had a monopoly on the best practice and blocked the way to all rivals.

He was a founder of the revived Academy of Medicine in 1820 and in the same year was elected to the Academy of Sciences. In 1831 he succeeded to Recamier's chair as professor of medicine at the Collège de France and remained there until 1852. He died in 1855.

His principal writings: the *Precis Elementaire de Physiologie* (1816),[2] *Phenomenes Physiques de la Vie* (1842),[3] and *Lecons sur les Fonctions et les Maladies du Systeme Nerveux* (1839)[4] were all illustrations and exemplifications of the conviction, acquired in his youth, that the human physiology is best interpreted as a concourse of molecules. This, in turn, reflected his political liberalism and Revolutionary desire for a society of equals.

Rudolf Virchow, the inventor of "cellular pathology," was born to a peasant family in Pomerania, graduated at Berlin in 1845, founded the *Archiv fuer pathologische Anatomie* in 1847, joined the rebels in Berlin in 1848, and was installed as professor of pathological anatomy in that city in 1856—succeeding the eminent Johannes Mueller (1801-1858).[5]

He was more than a mere professor of physiology or pathology, however, making contributions also to epidemiology, sanitation, anthropology, and archeology. He had a deep interest in politics, joining the Prussian Lower House in 1862 as a deputy and serving in the Reichstag from 1880 to 1893.

In both medicine and politics he was (like Magendie) a profound liberal: society is a voluntary association of equal citizens, while the human organism is, in the same way, "a sort of social or societal gathering, where a mass of individual existences have been drawn to one another in such a way that each element retains its own special activity and contributes to the common effort when it feels so stimulated by the other parts."[6] Just as Virchow combated Bismarck in the Imperial Reichstag, so he fought against the idea that the human organism is dominated by a single force.

His contributions to medicine were made in the middle decades of the century, his major writings being *Die Cellularpathologie* (1858), the first volume of the *Handbuch der speciellen Pathologie und Therapie* (1854),[7] and a series of programmatic articles published in the *Archiv.*[8]

Claude Bernard was also a peasant's son, born in a village near Lyons. His first ambition was to be a tragic poet, but he was dissuaded from it and turned instead to medicine, graduating at the Faculté in 1839.[9] He never practiced this art, however, but went directly to Magendie's physiological laboratory at the Collège de France. In 1854 a chair of general pathology was established for him at the Faculté des Sciences. In 1855 he succeeded to Magendie's chair of medicine at the Collège de France. He was elected to the Academy of Sciences in 1854 and to the Académie in 1868. In 1869 he was created Senator by special Imperial decree.

His two major theoretical works were *Introduction a l'Etude de la Medecine Experimentale* (1865)[10] and *Principes de la Medecine Experimentale* (written between 1862 and 1877 but published only in 1947).[11]

The Decline of Medicine and the Medical Profession

While quarrels among physicians are as old as medicine itself, in the nineteenth century homoeopathy had exacerbated this tendency: the public was regaled with the spectacle of physicians assaulting one another verbally and in writing over the very foundations of medical theory and practice. The homoeopaths, furthermore, appealed for support to the lay public, involving non-professionals in medical disputes and forcing everyone to take sides.

The consequence was a drop in the prestige of (especially allopathic) physicians, a general loss of confidence in the efficacy of (especially allopathic) medicine.

Magendie noted in 1839 that medicine was in a "humiliating state of inferiority."[12] Virchow's early articles stated that confidence in therapeutics was at a low point, with most physicians convinced that "no genuine therapy exists,"[13] "an attitude of despair toward therapy . . . has spread more and more in recent years . . . among the laity also. The uncertainty of the pharmacopoeia and the lack of faith in medical skill are such current catchwords that hardly a novel seems to be written in which a physician does not play a deplorable role."[14] Bernard wrote some years later that faith in medicine was declining, with systems and doctrines losing their former credit.[15] Everyone asserts his own ideas and disputes those of the physician.[16] "Sorcerers, somnambulists, healers by virtue of some gift from heaven, are held the equals of physicians."[17]

And these thinkers to a great extent agreed with the public's estimate of medicine. Magendie called it "*une science a faire.*"[18] Hippocratic doctrine, in particular, he held to be a "blind cult of ancient errors."[19] Physicians are almost impotent to cure diseases.[20]

> A patient comes down with typhoid fever. Well, he will get a different treatment from one hospital to the next. The Pitié won't use the same remedies as the Charité or the Hotel Dieu. One practitioner praises purgatives, another bloodletting, a third extolls tonics, and a final group (to which I belong) allows the illness to pass more or less freely through its stages . . . Take twenty physicians belonging to the same school and professing apparently the same doctrines; will two of them, called to

> the sickbed, envisage the illness in the same way and prescribe the same treatment?[21]

Bernard held that while physicians, indeed, save lives, they also harm patients by their incorrect treatment; they cure some, but they kill more.[22]

These thinkers blamed medicine's poor image to some extent on homoeopathy but more on the "empiricism" of Trousseau and his school, which had opened up the field to "charlatans."[a] Many medical school graduates,

> scarcely out of the classroom, immediately put all their learning aside. They sincerely believe, and often persuade others to believe, that they know everything and can cure anything. Sometimes they make a brilliant career in this way, but it is at the expense of humanity and science. This method, which has only too many adherents, explains perfectly well the sort of discredit into which medicine has fallen these days and the great favor which charlatans enjoy with the public—whose ignorance and prejudices they exploit.[23]

They live in a state of "happy ignorance," knowing nothing, for instance, of the physical and chemical properties of the blood.[24] While "reputed to have a profound knowledge of *materia medica,* to be men of immense resources, etc.," to be "afraid of nothing, to find inexhaustible resources in their prescriptions, and to be *answerable* (that is the approved term) for their patients," this is only "blind routine."[25] [b] *They do not know what they are doing or why they are doing it:*

[a]Allopaths often used code language in referring to homoeopathy, and by "charlatan" Magendie and Bernard probably mean "homoeopath." Thus they blame Trousseau for making "empiricism" respectable and opening the door to homoeopathy. See Claude Bernard, *Principes de Medecine Experimentale* (Paris: Presses Universitaires de France, 1947), 28 and 250. For more on the "uncertainty of medicine" in the mid-nineteenth century and its connection with homoeopathy see *Divided Legacy,* III, 257-259 and Coulter, *Homoeopathic Influences in Nineteenth-Century Allopathic Therapeutics,* 20-22.

[b]Nothing equalled Magendie's contempt for the physician who was "answerable" for his patients!

> No doubt our organs, to function, are subject to a simple or multiple cause manifest in its effects, hidden in its essence. Call it the *Archeus,* the *praeses,* the vital force . . . the name is not important. What I want to know is the nature of this cause, its mode of action, its point of departure. How are you going to interpret it if you can neither define it nor understand it?[26]

Medicine, therefore, must be reconstructed on the basis of physiology.[27]

While Magendie advocated physiology *tout court,* Virchow urged "pathological physiology" as the new science which would provide medicine with the necessary causal knowledge.[28] "We define pathological physiology as the essential theoretical part of scientific medicine."[29]

> The natural-scientific method . . . presupposes an extended knowledge of the facts, and here we particularly include the continuous progress in diagnosis and prognosis generated by recent investigations into the nature and course of all kinds of disease processes. A sure development of therapy is only possible insofar as relations are established with these investigations. Of what use can it be to hear that some remedy or other has abolished a disease of the liver or an inflammation of the lung if there is no guarantee that liver disease was the essential difficulty, or that inflammation of the lung was really present?[30]

Claude Bernard's writings are replete with attacks on "empiricism." "Medicine is still in the shades of empiricism and suffers the consequences of its backward condition . . . Medical personality is placed above science by physicians themselves; they seek their authority in tradition, in doctrines, or in medical tact."[31] [c]

[c]"Tact," meaning the physician's intuitive grasp of the patient's condition, has been interpreted by Empirics as the distillation of lengthy experience (Laennec, *Auscultation Mediate,* 1831, II, 405; Bayle, *Considerations sur la Nosologie, la*

> Empiricists, with their faith in the efficacy of drugs as a means of changing the direction of diseases and curing them, content themselves with empirically noting medicinal effects without trying to understand their mechanism scientifically. They are never perplexed: when one remedy fails, they try another; they always have recipes or formulas at hand for any and every case because they draw on an immense therapeutic arsenal. Empirical medicine is certainly the most popular. People believe that through a kind of compensation nature provides a remedy for every ill, and that medicine consists in a collection of recipes for all ills, handed down to us, age after age, since the beginnings of the healing art.[32]

These physicians "dispense medicines in abundance and make a show of their so-called resources or therapeutic riches."[33] But basically it is all routine; these empirics do not know science and are thus only ignoramuses.[34] Trousseau's doctrine is the negation of science.[35] "In medicine . . . numerous discoveries are still to be made, because almost everywhere empiricism and obscurity prevail."[36]

The answer was "experimental medicine" which would make medicine scientific by founding it on physiology: "experimental analysis is our only means of going in search of truth in the natural sciences."[37] "Scientific medicine, like the other sciences, can be established only by experimental

Medecine d'Observation, et la Medecine Pratique, 63; Louis, *Recherches sur les Effets de la Saignee,* 87). Rationalists have based "tact" largely on the physician's rational faculty, his ability to perceive proximate causes, and this is attacked both by Hahnemann (see above, p. 332) and Trousseau: "the man of genius does not have second sight but more perfect sight . . . It is not an act of divination but the greater perfection of one of the senses, nothing more" (Trousseau, *Conferences sur l'Empirisme,* 17). To the extent that the Rationalist definition of "tact" also incorporated an experiential component it was rejected by the Methodist, Bernard: "the vague unconscious experience, which may be called medical tact," "I entirely understand a physician's saying that he cannot always rationally account for what he is doing . . . but if he goes on to proclaim his medical tact or his intuition as a criterion which he then means to impose on others without further proof, that is wholly unscientific" (Bernard, *Experimental Medicine,* 193, 210).

means."[38] "We can reach knowledge of definite elementary conditions of phenomena by only one road, viz., by experimental analysis."[39]

> When medicine becomes scientific, it must then be founded on physiology . . . knowledge of pathological or abnormal conditions cannot be gained without previous knowledge of normal states, just as the therapeutic action of abnormal agents, or medicines, on the organism cannot be scientifically understood without first studying the physiological action of the normal agents which maintain the phenomena of life.[40]

Physiology: the Definition of Life

The spearhead of the assault by Magendie, Virchow, and Bernard on Empiricism was directed at this doctrine's vitalism. They held that physiological processes are determinate—subject to analysis in terms of a body of cause-and-effect knowledge drawn from outside medical practice itself.

The Rationalist/Methodist mind finds unpalatable in vitalism the idea that the behavior of the living organism is autonomous, spontaneous, and purposive. Virchow notes that with the progress of physiology, "the notion of the spontaneity of vital actions, a notion still in force, must lose all significance."[41] Claude Bernard alluded frequently to this problem: "matter in living, as in inorganic bodies, can possess no spontaneity."[42] "The spontaneity of living bodies is simply an appearance and the result of a certain mechanism in completely determined environments . . . the behavior of living bodies, as well as the behavior of inorganic bodies, is dominated by a necessary determinism linking them with conditions of a purely physico-chemical order."[43] "Living matter is no more able than inorganic matter to get into activity or movement by itself."[44] [d]

[d]The determinism of vital processes was for Bernard an *a priori* principle which had to be taken on faith because without it no science of physiology was possible. See below, pp. 690-691.

In opposition to this spontaneity and autonomy of the organism Rationalism asserts a doctrine of "proximate causes"—conceived in chemical or mechanical terms—which are the substance of its physiology and the foundation of its pathology and therapeutics. But Methodism finds this all too complex and retreats to a higher order of abstraction, reducing the "proximate causes" (hence the body's autonomy and spontaneity) to a binary system. This is represented physiologically as the ebb and flow either of nervous force or of atoms and corpuscles.

The most visible manifestation of Methodism in Paris medicine was Broussais' 1816 *Examen de la Doctrine Medicale Generalement Acceptee,* but the "reformer" had been preceeded by several years in the theoretical realm. The whole program of the Methodist reaction was set forth by Magendie in his 1809 publication, "Some General Ideas on the Phenomena Peculiar to Human Bodies."[e]

A true science subsumes a variety of effects under a restricted group of general principles—physics and chemistry being good examples. But physiology is not yet a science.

"Observation" shows the body to be made up of "molecules" which have two modes of being: "nutrition"—the taking in of matter and its discharge to the outside, and "action"—the interplay among molecules which issues in some motion or the performance of some function.

These modes of being need not be ascribed to "sensitivity," "mobility," or any other property of the molecule;

[e]F. Magendie, "Quelques Idees Generales sur les Phenomenes Particuliers aux Corps Vivants," *Bulletin des Sciences Medicales* IV (1809), 145-170. Olmsted notes that this was Magendie's only publication not based on experimental research (*Francois Magendie* [New York, Schuman, 1944], 34). Temkin writes: "In other words, Magendie, outstanding throughout his life for his 'distrust of theory and firm faith in experiment,' conceived his program largely on theoretical grounds" ("The Philosophical Background of Magendie's Physiology," *Bulletin of the History of Medicine* XX [1946], 13). Molecular determinism was as much an *a priori* principle for Magendie as it was for Bernard, although he did not state it *expressis verbis.*

such words are used only because the mind has an irrepressible desire to assign "causes" to phenomena.[45]

Magendie limits himself to stating that molecular motion is the expression of "what will be called the vital force."[46]

Physiology has erred in the past by seeking the "causes" of phenomena when it should have been establishing their "general laws."[47] These laws are accessible to man's mind because the vital force does not behave arbitrarily. The molecular *structure* of each organ, tissue, or part of the body determines its *function,* each variation in structure leading to a different mode of manifestation of the vital force.[48] "I believe it possible to establish, even in the present state of the science, that whenever the vital force animates a body of such-and-such organization, it will produce such-and-such phenomena."[49]

While Magendie's program was patterned on the work of Baron Cuvier (1760-1832), who was analyzing the behavior of animals in terms of their bodily configuration and skeletel shape,[50] it owed even more to Descartes' *Treatise of Man* which had hypothesized the existence of corpuscular pro cesses invisible to the eye but accessible to reason. Magendie admitted that molecular processes are invisible, but "since we see matter displaced, it becomes certain for us that movement has taken place."[51] [f] "Does one see any better what occurs inside the heart during its contractions? Is this contraction not the result of the internal movement of the living molecules of which it is composed?"[52] While the digestion itself cannot be observed directly, to deny its existence would be an "exaggerated Pyrrhonism"—all parts of the body are continually casting off old molecules and taking on new ones.[53]

[f]Descartes had deduced the existence of corpuscles from observing the growth of plants and trees: "no one can doubt that there are bodies so small that they cannot be perceived by any of our senses, if only one considers what is being added each moment to those bodies which increase little by little" (see above, p. 123). In a later writing Magendie held the molecule to be visible under the microscope, with a diameter of 1/300th of a millimeter (Olmsted, *Francois Magendie,* 29, note).

Magendie had studied under Bichat at the Ecole de Santé, and his physiological research was an unremitting vendetta against the memory of this intellectually superior colleague who unfortunately died too early to be defeated personally in battle. The molecular hypothesis was designed to refute Bichat's complex series of "sensitivities" and "contractilities," showing them to be only the resultant of "nutrition" and "action" at the molecular level.[54] [g]

Magendie's mature thought continued his earlier preoccupation with the movement of molecules but interpreted it mechanically. The organism contains two groups of functions: one, associated with the heart and circulatory system, is governed by the principles of hydraulics; the other, centered on the nervous system, is the residue of the organism's vitality.[55] Bichat erred in holding that the "vital forces" in the body struggle against the drag and inertia of the "physical forces."[56] Although some phenomena fall under vital laws and others under physical laws, the two are not in conflict, as both are ultimately controlled by the nerves.[57] Moreover, the "truly vital phenomena are much fewer than we had thought," and their number will be further reduced with the progress of physiology.[58] The more one studies the phenomena of life, the more one is convinced that "all, or almost all, are influenced by the laws governing physical phenomena."[59]

Bichat's "tonic forces" are all reducible to elasticity.[60] Absorption and exhalation by the glands are due to the "property of *imbibition*" and that of "*exbibition,*" not to any "vital power" in the gland.[61] [h] The blood circulates as a

[g]In 1827 Magendie issued a new edition of Bichat's *Traite des Membranes,* holding that he had failed to distinguish the physico-chemical properties of tissues from their vital properties. "Bichat postulated wise and truly philosophical principles, and it is to be regretted that too often his active imagination led him to depart from them." "The author's mind was often carried well beyond the limits of a healthy logic." (X. Bichat, *Traite des Membranes.* New Edition, revised and annotated by M. Magendie [Paris: Gabon, 1827], viii-ix, 117).

[h]Magendie, who continually accused his colleagues of hypostatizing the functions of the body, was on dangerous ground with his *"imbibition"* and *"exbibition,"* and

system of pumps, tanks, and conduits, all set in motion by the heart.[62] [i] Laennec's heart sounds are explicable by the ordinary laws of acoustics.[63]

Magendie was especially intrigued by the capillaries, as the ultimate expression of the passage of molecules through pores. John Hunter and the physicians of Montpellier were mistaken in calling capillary action a vital phenomenon—due to some "harmony" between the capillaries and the blood—as this casts doubt upon Harvey's discovery of the circulation.[64] "Has anyone ever seen this action of the capillaries? Does it fall under the senses? No, no one has ever seen it, it is a supposition." If the capillaries were endowed with independent life, what would prevent them from directing the blood back into the arteries instead of the veins? Why should they not draw blood from the veins as well as from the arteries?[65] Attributing such a capacity to the capillaries is tantamount to holding that "each capillary is a sentinel whose vigilance never fails, and note that its intelligence is far superior to our own, since it never takes in materials harmful to the economy, whereas we, without realizing it, sometimes introduce deleterious substances into our stomachs."[66] Bichat thought that the blood was no longer under the control of the heart when it penetrated into the capillaries—a "purely gratuitous supposition."[67] The true cause of the movement of blood from the arteries to the pulmonary veins is the contraction of the right ventricle.[68] The circulation could be reactivated in a corpse if one could only start up the heart.[69] The role of the capillaries is entirely passive, in a word, and if blood will not pass through them, this can be due only to its excessive viscosity.[70] [j]

F. Dubois d'Amiens (1798-1873) had a good deal of fun with these terms ("Eloge de Magendie," *Memoires de l'Academie Imperiàle de Medecine* II [1858], ix).

[i] He did not even like the customary anatomical names for the parts of the heart, feeling that they smacked of vitalism. He proposed calling the auricles the "right pumps" and the ventricles the "left pumps"; the arteries and veins, in turn, could be called the "large pipes" and the "small pipes" ("Eloge de Magendie," xiii).

[j] Magendie knew of the experiments (in the early 1840's) of J. L. M. Poiseuille (1799-1869) demonstrating that no liquid could flow through a glass tube with

While the functions associated with the circulatory system were explicable in hydraulic or mechanical terms, nervous phenomena required a different mode of investigation. Magendie decided that they were outside the laws of physics, chemistry, and mechanics and could be understood only through vivisection.[71] "Magendie created his medicine in the amphitheater," undertaking the most comprehensive program of vivisection yet known to medicine.[72]

His course on the nervous system, professed year after year at the Collège de France, involved severing the nerves of a series of animals to show the effect of such operations on their general health and welfare. An American student who attended his lectures wrote that Magendie "has not only lost all feeling for the victims he tortures, but he really likes his business. When the animal squeaks a little, the operator grins; when loud screams are uttered, he sometimes laughs outright . . . in many cases the experiments are unnecessarily cruel and too frequently reiterated."[73] When Magendie presented the course in London, an Irish MP told the House of Commons that he had first nailed a medium-sized dog to the laboratory bench with spikes through its paws and ears, then

the diameter of a capillary, but he explained this away as "a question for hydraulics well worthy of our attention. Unfortunately, such is the perfection of the procedures employed by nature to solve this interesting problem that we can rather admire them than understand . . . It would be a serious error to apply to the passage of blood in the capillaries everything which has been learned from physical observation of the passage of liquids in inorganic capillary tubes. Some of the phenomena are common, some are different; each has to have its due" (F. Magendie, *Phenomenes Physiques de la Vie* [Paris: Bailliere, 1842], III, 138-142).

In 1920 August Krogh (1874-1919) received the Nobel Prize for demonstrating the independent contractility of the capillary walls.

The hypnotism controversy offers another instance where Magendie evaded an issue conflicting with his basic assumptions. He was appointed to the committee investigating "animal magnetism" but did not attend any of the meetings and on that ground refused to sign the report favorable to hypnotism (M. P. Foissac, *Rapports et Discussion de l'Academie de Medecine sur le Magnetisme Animal,* 208). Olmsted notes that Magendie "was inclined to take his appointments to [Academy of Medicine] committees very seriously," "the records of his attendance show that his absences were rare . . . there were three six-month semesters during which Magendie did not miss a single session and others which show only one absence" (*Francois Magendie,* 195, 225).

had proceeded to cut apart the nerves of the head and brain on one side, leaving the animal lying there until the next day when he performed the same procedures on the other side.[74]

These practices, and the brutality of Magendie's nature generally, made him an unpopular figure with the public and with his own colleagues.[k] While all would probably not have agreed with the British anti-vivisectionist who stated in 1879 that "the wretch, Magendie, was undoubtedly the most abandoned criminal that ever lived,"[75] Dubois d'Amiens reflected professional feeling when he observed that Magendie treated animal experiments precisely as though they were chemical ones: "the professor had his assistants, his equipment, and his reagents; there were animals, called 'subjects of the experiment,' and when one had to take out only half the brain, they were held over until the next class. The only difference was in the objects of the experiments: for the former it was inert and inorganic bodies, for the latter organized and living ones. The former produced effervescences and precipitates, the latter—movements, pain, and screams."[76] He told of an American Quaker who expostulated with Magendie that he did not have the right to make animals suffer, that it set a bad example, and that it accustomed the public to cruelty: "Magendie replied that his experiments had as their aim (which was true) and for their result (which was a little less so) to be useful to humanity."[77] Haller had limited vivisection to as few experiments as possible, and had performed them with great reluctance, while Magendie "was too attached to his experiments to feel these scruples."[78] Trousseau held information from vivisectionist experiments to be valueless, since the animals were in an unnatural state: "it is really deplorable to see physicians imagining themselves to be physiologists because they have killed a large number of animals."[79] Emile Littre

[k]Flourens wrote that Magendie was "rigorously honest in discussing his own efforts, criminally unjust and cruelly disdainful toward those of others, and ferociously intolerant of anyone who stood in his path" (*Eloge Historique de Francois Magendie* [Paris: Garnier], 17).

(1801-1881), the great French Hippocratic scholar, observed that while vivisection may be necessary, it should not be done capriciously or frivolously: "He who would interpret the mysteries of life, suffering, and death, should have an elevated mind, a pitying heart, and innocent hands."[80]

The chief benefit to humanity from Magendie's experiments on animals was his discovery of the distinction between the motor and sensory nerves, for which he shared credit with the Englishman, Charles Bell (1774-1842).[81]

He was not above experimenting on his own patients. In typhus and typhoid epidemics he liked to bleed the moribund cases, "less as a curative technique than as experimental research"–to ascertain the state of the blood.[82] He opened two arteries in an apoplectic woman to see if it would prolong her life, but she died in a few hours.[83] During an operation for cataract he probed the retina with his scalpel to see if it was sensitive.[84] To determine the effect of introducing air into the venous system he "on several occasions" injected air into his patients with (he claimed) no harmful consequences.[85] [1]

Magendie's research had a substantial impact on medical thought. His 1816 *Precis Elementaire de Physiologie,* embodying mechanical principles, eventually superseded Richerand's textbook based on Haller, Cabanis, and Bichat.[86] In 1842 he observed with satisfaction that the terms, "organic sensitivity" and "organic contractility," were passing out of fashion, being replaced by expressions from chemistry, physics, and mechanics.[87] Twenty years earlier, he commented, he would have been called an Iatromechanist, but in the meantime medical opinion had made notable progress.[88]

[1]Later that same year he injected air into the veins of a dog during an experiment, causing the formation of a clot and immediate death: "I was far, I admit, from suspecting such a result, since it is opposed to everything we know about the coagulability of this animal liquid in any system of vessels. You see, Gentlemen, we never perform an experiment without learning some new fact and without having our expectations in some way disappointed" (*Phenomenes Physiques,* III, 128).

Where Magendie had mapped and confined the vital force by limiting its expression to the movement of the molecules in one of the body's molecularly determined structures, Rudolf Virchow introduced a new factor by postulating the existence of "cells" as an intermediate layer of matter between the molecules and the body's organs and structural parts. "All our experience indicates that life can manifest itself only in a concrete form and that it is bound to certain substantial loci. These loci are cells and cell formations."[89] "Life is cell activity; its uniqueness is the uniqueness of the cell."[90] "The essential is to obtain recognition of the fact that the cell is really the ultimate morphological unit in which there is any manifestation of life, and that we must not transfer the locus of intrinsic action [*eigentliche Action*] to any point above the cell."[91]

This philosophical master-stroke, made possible by the microscopic investigations of Virchow's friend, Hermann Lebert, substituted a new microcosm (the cell) for the old (the whole organism) and thus yielded a series of new solutions to perennial philosophical problems: "all branches of biology find a common point in the cell doctrine; the idea of the unity of life in all living things finds its concrete representation in the cell . . . It is an organism in miniature; in itself it is already capable of carrying on a separate existence . . . for the cell is either the living individual itself or it contains–in outline at least–what we are accustomed to designate as such."[92]

Since it consists of both liquid and solid parts, the cell overcame and synthesized the conflict between solidism and humoralism.[93]

It was the playground for the free movement of the molecules–providing them with physical and metaphysical space but simultaneously restricting the purposiveness of the vital force to the sub-cellular level.[94] In this way Virchow produced a more determinist physiology than Magendie–who had allowed the *physis* to disport itself along all the pathways provided by the varied molecular structures of the body's tissues and organs.

According to Virchow's theory the cell forms and reproduces itself only in obedience to mechanical and chemical laws: "all physiological and pathological formation is only the repetition, the now more simple, now more complex reproduction of known, uniquely given patterns or types. The plan of organization within the species is unalterable."[95] "It cannot be said that cell formation is not mechanically determined simply because we are not yet able to express it in mechanical (that is, numerical and mathematical) terms, for with the same right an ignorant aborigine of New Holland would be entitled to say that a steam engine was not mechanically explicable."[96]

Furthermore, the cells interact with one another in obedience to the same mechanical and chemical laws:

> The particular performance of organic material appears peculiar to us, yet it does not take place otherwise than the activity and performance of the lifeless nature with which physics is familiar . . . as particular, as peculiar, and as much interiorized as life is, therefore, so little is it withdrawn from the rule of physical and chemical law . . . every peculiarity of life finds its explanation in peculiar arrangements of an anatomical or chemical character, in peculiar configurations of material whose universally occurring properties and powers are expressed in these configurations . . . This activity cannot be other than mechanical.[97]

Virchow could state with perfect justice: "You will see that I am more mechanical than anyone else when it comes to explaining the individual phenomena of life."[98]

He resembled Magendie in dividing physiological functions into two groups: (1) those relating to the vegetative nervous system (assimilation, nutrition, digestion) and (2) those depending on the autonomic nervous system. The former were capable of being reduced entirely to mechanical processes, while the latter also were gradually being explicated in physico-mechanical terms.[99]

All of these functions were derived from the "irritability" possessed by all cells—whether located in the muscles, the glands, the nerves, or any other part of the body.[100] "Irritability" was a sort of "latent life" endowed by the vital force, meaning the capacity to react to an external stimulant.[101] "Irritability is considered by us as the surest sign of life."[102]

By postulating that the cell reproduces and interacts with other cells only in accordance with mechanical laws Virchow had disposed effectively of the purposiveness of vital processes. "Irritability" did the same for their spontaneity: "if life itself were dependent on external stimuli . . . certain stimuli would in that case prove to be necessary conditions of vital activity, without which life could be carried on in a latent form only."[103]

He traced "irritability" to Glisson who had realized that each part of the body possesses its own *vita propria.*[104] [m] But Willis, Boerhaave, and Haller perverted the concept by identifying it with "contractility" and limiting it to muscular tissue alone.[105] "Irritability" in its pristine sense was restored to medicine by John Brown's "excitability" and "excitement"—an "earthquake" whose consequences (in Virchow's view) were very important for the development of physiology: "the impulse which it gave stimulated other men, by whom it was permanently applied to the true service of science."[106]

Thus Brown and Broussais, whose influence had started to decline, were resurrected and brought back *via* physiology.[n] By endowing Descartes' *petites parties* with "irritability" Virchow combined the two sources of modern

[m]The words, *vita propria,* were first employed by Hieronymus Gaub (1705-1780). Glisson himself had written: *"Quod vivit per se vivit vitam a nulla creatura praeter se ipsum dependentem. Hoc enim verba vivere per se sonant"* (R. Virchow, *Disease, Life, and Man* [Stanford: Stanford University Press, 1958], 160).

[n]Note the contrast with Trousseau, who had praised Brown for emphasizing the holism of disease. Virchow cites Brown as authority for a doctrine of localized disease and treatment. Magendie had also accepted "irritability": it is like the "x" in algebra—a name we give to a phenomenon to show that we cannot understand it (*Phenomenes Physiques,* II, 40).

Methodist speculation into a torrent which would sweep all before it.

Most of the phenomena attributable to the vitality could be explained by suitable adjustments of the "irritation" or "irritability" (which Virchow also called by Brown's name—"excitement"). Three types of "action" (*Action*) are provoked by an "irritant" (*Irritament*): nutrition, formation of a part, or the performance of a function.[108] "Nutritive irritation" is the power possessed by a part to take up matter and transform it when excited by an "irritant." If carried sufficiently far, this is converted into "formative irritation": the cells alter and divide, producing new cells.[109] And each element or part of the body performs its functions through innate "functional irritation."[110] [o]

The sources of "irritation" are the bloodstream, the nervous system, and simple physical contact among the cells.[111]

Claude Bernard limited the role of the vital force to the *creation* of "cells" or "histological units." "I should say: life is creation . . . what distinguishes a living machine is not the nature of its physico-chemical properties, complex as they may be, but rather the creation of the machine which develops under our eyes in conditions proper to itself and according to a definite idea."[112] "For physiologists the truly active elements are what we call anatomical or histological units . . . these are not chemically simple, but physiologically considered they are as simplified as possible in that their vital properties are the simplest that we know."[113] "Histological

[o]Chauffard thought this theory ridiculous: Virchow's "irritation" means that the growing child is actually sick, since irritation is a pathological fact. "What an abuse of words, and what a confused amalgam of sickness and health!! . . . Virchow aims to appropriate and Germanize Broussais' ideas by pushing them to an exaggeration which Broussais himself would not recognize" (Chauffard, *Andral*, 52).

Virchow's "nutrition" and "action" seem to be taken from Magendie's 1809 article (see above, p. 614).

units . . . are the only effective agents in vital phenomena."[114] "Anatomical units stand alone as organized living parts."[115] The ultimate autonomous unit is the cell.[116]

The *movement* and *action* of these "elements" or "cells" are not caused by the vital force but by the inherent "irritability" with which they are endowed at creation.[117] "The principle of action of every living thing is irritability . . . Without it the organ does not sense excitants and remains at rest."[118] Brown and Broussais were the first to understand the significance of irritability, although the latter erred in limiting it only to certain organs.[119] Actually it is responsible for the functioning of all organs and tissues; each possesses a different degree of irritability and thus reacts differently to identical stimuli.[120]

"Elements" and "cells" are not capable of spontaneous movement: "anatomical units, which are the most changeable and unstable of substances, are still inert, that is, they never break into vital activity unless some foreign influence invites them."[121] "Living parts have the power of being irritable, i.e., reacting under the influence of certain stimuli in a way specially characteristic of living tissues, such as muscular contraction, nervous transmission, glandular secretion, etc. But whatever the variety presented by the three classes of phenomena, whether the reaction be physico-chemical or vital, it is never in any way spontaneous. The phenomenon always results from the influence exerted on the reacting body by a physico-chemical stimulus outside itself."[122] "Each one of these bodies is inert, that is, it is incapable of putting itself into action; to do this, it must always enter into relation with another body, from which it receives a stimulus."[123]

In the lower animals a major source of such external stimuli is the circulating blood.[124] [p] In the higher animals, however, the situation is different. Here the major role

[p]Bichat had held that the fluids act as excitants of the solids (*Anatomie Generale* I, lxii, lxiii, lxviii). See above, p. 461.

belongs to the nervous system, created by the organism and, in turn, acting as its major stimulus.[125] [q] The blood is also a stimulus but—what is more important—acts as the "internal environment" (*milieu interieur*) through which the "elements" and "cells" interact with one another and through which all external stimuli are filtered.[126] "Two environments must be considered in physiology: the general macrocosmic environment and the microcosmic environment peculiar to living beings."[127] "Physiological phenomena in the higher animals take place in perfected internal organic environments endowed with constant physico-chemical properties."[128] "Vital phenomena are the result of contact of the organic units of the body with the inner physiological environment; this is the pivot of all experimental medicine."[129]

By postulating the existence of the *milieu interieur* Bernard was able to isolate the living organism from what he called the "macrocosmic" environment, with all its indeterminate and unpredictable influences, and convert it into a purely determinate entity: "if [physiologists] can go down into the inner environment of a living machine, they find absolute determinism that must become the real foundation of the science of living bodies."[130] "In the case of the complex higher organisms, physiologists and physicians must study the stimuli of vital phenomena, not in the relations of the whole organism with the general cosmic environment, but rather in the organic conditions of the inner environment. Considered in the general cosmic environment, the function of man and of the higher animals seem to us, indeed, free and independent of the physico-chemical conditions of the environment, because its actual stimuli are found in an inner, organic, liquid environment. What we see from the outside is

[q]This view of the nervous system resembles Hoffmann's interpretation of the heart as "the *perpetuum mobile* which has been sought for so long . . . by this mechanism the cause produces the effect which then reproduces the cause itself" (see above, p. 140).

merely the result of physico-chemical stimuli from the inner environment. That is where physiologists must build up the real determinism of vital functions."[131]

The living organism in its natural ("macrocosmic") environment was reduced to "cells" or "elements" in the *milieu interieur* where *absolute determinism prevails.* The living organism therefore functions as a mechanism or a chemical process. Bernard rejected any opposition between the vital force of the body and its physico-chemical forces: vitality is always expressed in physico-chemical terms.[132] "Observers who are enchanted to find that physical laws do not hold in the organism are poor thinkers. The problem must be posed physiologically, but then, the principle established, all vital acts must be reduced to mechanical movements (Descartes)."[133] "A living organism is nothing but a wonderful machine endowed with the most marvellous properties and set going by means of the most complex and delicate mechanism."[134] "Life, as it must in practice be regarded by the physiologist and the physician, is, in effect, only a mechanism."[135] "Physiologists should succeed in reducing all the vital manifestations of a complex organism to the play of certain organs, and the action of these organs to the properties of well-defined tissues or organic units. Anatomico-physiological experimental analysis, which dates from Galen, has just this meaning."[136]

Vital or organic phenomena differ from inorganic only in their greater complexity, not in their nature or essence.[137]

And the best way to elucidate the nature of such phenomena is through vivisection. "Zoological vivisection . . . is the most delicate and difficult branch of biological investigation, but I deem it the most fruitful and perhaps the most immediately useful for the advancement of experimental medicine."[138] "The scientific principle of vivisection is easy to grasp. It is always a question of separating or altering certain parts of the living machine, so as to study them and thus to decide how they function and for what."[139] "Vivisection of animals goes very far back. Galen may be considered its founder."[140] Those who reject vivisection reject "experimental medicine," i.e., they reject science itself.[141]

Pathology and Therapeutics

To these thinkers "disease" was not a specific being or entity added to the healthy organism but only an extension of normal physiological function—an outgrowth of physiology and understandable in purely physiological terms.

Magendie's classification of diseases thus followed his classification of healthy functions: one group is caused by alterations in the blood and is subject to the laws of hydraulics and physics, while the other arises in the solids and is explicable in terms of the vitality and the nervous system.[142] [r]

The blood is affected by heat, cold, food, drink, or miasms—all giving rise to changes in its coagulability.[143] It can also alter spontaneously or as a result of medication.[144]

While Magendie opposed the idea of contagion in principle, he recognized the existence of a few contagious diseases carried by a "reproductive germ."[145] Scabies is caused and transmitted by the *Acarus scabiei.*[146]

When the blood becomes too thick, it blocks the capillary circulation—Cruveilhier's phlebitis—giving rise to a series of phlegmasies and inflammations.[147] In the so-called red hepatization of the lung clots are formed in the areoles of the lungs.[148] If the blood, on the contrary, becomes too thin, it permeates the tissues around the capillaries and causes another series of diseases.[149] Peritonitis is an inflammation of the peritoneum generated in this way.[150] When sodium carbonate is given to neutralize the uric acid which would otherwise deposit and form stones in the kidneys, it

[r]He seems to assimilate this dichotomy to the traditional division of diseases into acute and chronic (*Phenomenes Physiques,* IV, 47). It will be noted that Andral took most of his discussion of the blood from Magendie (see above, pp. 537-538).

compounds with the fibrin in the blood, liquefying it and causing pneumonia.[151] [s]

Miasmatic diseases such as cholera, typhus, typhoid, and plague are all characterized by loss of coagulability.[152]

Magendie's interest in coagulability dated from the 1814 typhus epidemic when he observed that the blood remained fluid in patients who died but coagulated in those who recovered.[153] He decided that this was partly vital and partly a physical phenomenon.[154]

Cure was through reversing the process–restoring coagulability where it was lost and thickening the blood when it was too thin– but he was in a quandary over how this was to be done: the way in which drugs act on the organism is "one of the most obscure points in medicine."[155]

He attempted to investigate this by mixing acids and alkalis with guinea-pig blood in various proportions and combinations; he discovered that alkalis preserved the fluidity while acids caused clots but warned against extrapolating this information directly into therapeutics: "One should not pass judgment lightly on a matter so serious."[156] He tested bicarbonate of soda, potassium sulphate, iron sulphate, alum, lead acetate, silver nitrate, quinine, and digitalis but found that, while reducing the coagulability was relatively easy, restoring it when lost was more difficult.[157]

He did not reach any definite conclusions about the therapeutics of "nervous" diseases, although his course on the nervous system aimed to elucidate the relationship between diseases and injuries to the nerves.[158] He thought that by injuring the nervous system in various ways he could

[s]One American reviewer, at least, had a poor opinion of Magendie's ascription of all diseases to changes in the blood: "Ingenious and plausible as we are willing to confess his exposition of many of the pathological conditions of the organs and tissues to be, we cannot, however, admit that in all cases they are legitimate deductions from even those facts upon which he has based them, while, also, they run counter to all our experience in relation to the curative powers of most of the ordinary therapeutical agents" (*American Journal of the Medical Sciences* XXV [1839-1840], 171).

produce at will such diseases as typhus, yellow fever, and cholera—this being more precise and reliable information than that obtained at the sickbed.[159] He was tremendously excited by Bernard's discovery that puncturing the fourth ventricle of the brain heightened the sugar content of the blood and urine, feeling that this proved the influence of the nerves on nutritive processes. He immediately acquired the brain of a patient recently dead of diabetes and found that the corresponding spot on the fourth ventricle was slightly discolored.[160]

In diagnosis he held the state of the blood to be more important than the patient's symptoms.[161]

His treatment was largely expectant. Although the popularizer of many new medicines by his *Formulaire* and other works, he rarely used them himself—especially in his later years.[162] He opposed bloodletting, holding that the composition of the blood was more significant than its mere volume and that the composition was not affected by phlebotomy.[163] But he used this technique anyway in pneumonia and some other diseases.[164]

He treated renal calculi, caused by heightened uric acid content of the blood, with alkaline medicine.[165] He used Prussic Acid in the treatment of tuberculosis on the ground that it reduced the "sensitivity" of the lungs.[166]

He acquired brief notoriety by injecting two pints of warm water into the veins of man with rabies, bringing about a momentary recovery,[t] but the patient died two days later, apparently from septicemia.[167] Others attempted this treatment, but no one else had any luck with it.

For Virchow the cell was the starting point of pathological, as of physiological, processes, undergoing the same transformations in both cases. "Now if pathology is nothing

[t]This resembled the ancient method of treating for rabies by throwing the victim into a pond—a primitive application of the principle of contraries (*Divided Legacy,* I, 258).

but physiology with obstacles, and diseased life nothing but healthy life interfered with by all manner of external and internal influences, then pathology too must be referred back to the cell."[168] "Diseases are neither self-subsistent, circumscribed autonomous organisms, nor entities which have forced their way into the body, nor parasites rooted on it, but they represent only the course of physiological phenomena under altered conditions."[169]

The first stage in disease is an impaired relationship between the cell and its environment, giving rise to an "irritation" in the cell.[170] This "irritation" leads (as Broussais has noted) to an "inflammation."[171] Virchow defined this inflammatory stimulus as "some cause or other external to the part . . . and acting on it either directly or through the medium of the blood."[172] The changes occurring in an inflammation are identical with normal physiological changes—alterations of nutrition, function, or the formation of a part—but carried to an extreme.[173]

If the disease remains largely confined to the nutritional relationship between the cell and its environment, it is assimilated by Virchow to the traditional class of chronic afebrile diseases; if it spreads to the nervous system, he assimilates it to the class of acute diseases.[174] In any case, all diseases involve input from the cellular nutritional proccss and the nervous system.

If the inflamed cell is on the wall of a vein or artery, it causes a blood clot, i.e., Cruveilhier's phlebitis.[175] [u]

Most diseases are local, seemingly "general" diseases arising through "transport," to the rest of the body, of the particles and chemical substances given off by the local disturbance.[176] [v] Local diseases may be communicated to

[u]Thus Virchow rejected Cruveilhier's theory that phlebitis originates in the blood: the blood is always passive and incapable of being the point of origin of a disease (R. Virchow, *Die Cellularpathologie* [Berlin: Hirschwald, 1858], 177, 181).

[v]Cf. with John Hunter's theory of constitutional syphilis, above p. 358.

the rest of the body through the nervous system as well, or by direct contact among the cells.[177]

There is a true group of general diseases, however, which Virchow calls "general disturbances of nutrition."[178] When nutrition of the whole cellular system is inadequate, the consequence is atrophy–phthisis, consumption, emaciation, marasmus, etc.[179] When nutrition is in excess, the consequence is hypertrophy of some part and new formation–scrophula, tuberculosis, and cancers.[180]

"Fever" is caused by the involvement of the organism's regulatory centers, generating an abnormal "tension" (*Spannungsverhaeltnis*). While the *medulla oblongata* and the roots of the vagus nerve are apparently involved, Virchow felt that "spinal irritation" was the best explanation of "fever."[181] [w]

Another group of diseases is due to muscular weakness of the arterial and venous walls.[x] Virchow decided that there is a normal relationship between the volume of blood in the body, the pressure of the heart, and the muscular tension of the vascular walls: any change in the first two leads to distension or contraction of the veins and arteries.[182] When the vascular walls are distended, the blood passes through them and perfuses the surrounding tissues–a hyperemia which serves as a local irritant.[183] If the walls are constricted, there can be partial anemia, and the surrounding parts are deprived of necessary blood.[184] Blockage of the veins or arteries gives rise to an infarct or thrombosis.[185]

Sometimes the other fluids of the body perfuse the tissues or otherwise flow into some improper place–as in dropsy.[186]

Since the healing process is identical with the process of physiological regulation, Virchow's therapeutics is based on

[w]J. Legallois (1770-1814) had held that the spinal column is the locus of "life"–which is generated through "irritation" of the brain and spinal column by the blood (*Oeuvres de Legallois*, with notes by Pariset [Paris: Le Rouge, 1824], I, 141).

[x]In 1840 Jacob Henle (1809-1885) had demonstrated the existence of smooth muscle in the endothelial coats of the smaller arteries.

his pathological and physiological assumptions.[187] In fever the principal indication is to remove heat through cooling drinks and applications or by bloodletting (to reduce the irritation of the nervous system).[188] He employed "counter-irritation" and held that Broussais' theory of "irritation" as the source of disease had much to recommend it.[189] Digitalis, arsenic, quinine, metals, and plant alkaloids were used by him as febrifuges which acted on the regulatory centers: digitalis irritates the *medulla oblongata* and the roots of the vagus nerve, quinine acts hypersthenically on the sympathetic nervous system, etc.[190] He felt that they opposed the paralytic state which is the source of the fever and were thus to be distinguished from "tonic" methods which adjusted and regulated the process of cellular nutrition.[191]

The principal indication in inflammation was to destroy the irritation and thus restore the nutritive process.[192] Next was to rid the bloodstream of the noxious substance (*Noxe*) through vomitives, laxatives, or narcotics. Sometimes the *Noxe* could be neutralized chemically: acids in the digestive tract were treated with alkaline medicines. Proliferative (cancerous) processes could be eradicated with caustics.[193] Contagious matter (miasms) could be neutralized with chlorine or mercurial medicines.[194]

When the disease was from relaxation of the vascular walls, causing a local accumulation of blood which acted as an irritant, mild caustics, astringents, etheric oils, and ammonia preparations could be applied to the spot to constrict the walls and cut off the influx of blood.[195] Lateral pressure on the walls could be reduced "directly" by local bleeding or "indirectly" by blisters, plasters, the moxa, vesicants, fontanelles, etc.[196] General bleeding was also of use as well as antiphlogistic salts: these latter sometimes acted as alteratives, changing the composition of the blood, sometimes as counterirritants, substituting a new irritation for the old one (sulphur, magnesium, calomel, potassium–antimonium tartrate, etc.).[197]

When the vascular walls were contracted, warm applications were indicated.[198] If this was "passive congestion," i.e., the consequence of a sympathetic depression of the vascular nerves, reflecting an irritation of the corresponding cerebrospinal nerves, it was treated with excitants, vomitives, friction, the sharper ammonia preparations, etc.[199] If it was, however, an "active congestion," which was also sometimes a sympathetic reaction to cerebrospinal irritation, the physician had to use digitalis, hydrocyanic acid, cherry laurel water, etc.[200]

Intermittent fever (malaria), due to heightened sensitivity of the nerves, was best treated with quinine which decreases this sensitivity.[201]

Virchow actually had little interest in pharmacology, recommending hydrotherapy as the treatment of choice for many conditions. The leaders of Rationalist pharmacological investigation in Germany at this time were Rudolph Buchheim (1820-1879) and Carl Mitscherlich (1805-1871), relying on the new science of organic chemistry pioneered by Justus Liebig (1803-1873).

Hahnemann's pharmacology elaborated through provings on healthy persons had made a powerful impact on German medical thought. Virchow wrote: "Hahnemann exercised a beneficial influence; he was the first to test systematically the effects of medicaments on healthy people."[202] "Owing to the ever-increasing number of medications and a deficiency in the critical observation and study of their effects, doubt concerning their significance has by degrees grown so great that everyone who wants to accomplish something decisive for therapy in Germany applies himself to their investigation. The studies of Orfila in toxicology, as well as the experiments carried out by Hahnemann in the foundation of the homoeopathic system stimulated newer detailed investigations . . ."[203]

But he felt that "Hahnemann's test methods were so peculiar that no scientific pharmacologist could follow them."[204]

This same feeling motivated Buchheim, Mitscherlich, and Liebig to seek an alternative approach to the investigation of drugs. Rejecting Hahnemann's holistic Empirical paradigm, they sought to establish a Rationalist doctrine of proximate causes understood in chemical terms.

Hahnemann had maintained that the best guide to the administration of a drug (assuming the truth of the law of similars) was the pattern of symptoms it evoked in the healthy. Hence the first element of these scientists' attack on Hahnemann was to distinguish the symptoms of the drug (whether administered to a healthy prover or a sick person) from its "physiologic effect." Buchheim complained that researchers have merely noted down symptoms in provings without checking to ensure that they are "really essential for the effect of the drug."[205] If the physician had to rely on symptoms alone for his prescribing, this would hardly be scientific.[206] Mitscherlich also asserted that the "physiologic effect" of the drug has not been adequately distinguished from the symptoms which may be due to the prover's idiosyncrasy or other factors.[207]

The physician must know both the "physiologic effect" of the medicine and the symptoms.[208] "General pathology" is based on knowledge of "physiologic effects" and is scientific, while activities relying on symptomatic knowledge alone fall into "special pathology" and are not scientific.[209]

The first effect of a medicine on the human organism is chemical: it interacts chemically with the body's fluids and tissues, altering them and being altered in turn.[210] These chemical changes in the fluids then affect the body's organs and systems.[211] The patient's symptoms are thus only the ultimate effects of these other preceding changes and no longer possess primary importance.[212] They are the signs of a particular internal state. Observing the symptoms alone is not enough; one must ask *why* these symptoms have been produced.[213]

There is no direct or natural relationship between the medicine and the disease; its healing action is an "accidental" feature—the outcome of the chemical alterations which the remedy produces in the body's organs and systems.[214]

Buchheim wrote in 1846 that a purely empirical method in pharmacology is worthless both theoretically and practically; this discipline must be reorganized on a rational basis.[215] He and Mitscherlich were attempting to do for pharmacology what the French pathological anatomists had done for diagnosis: separate the "unimportant" symptoms from the "important" internal changes. By elaborating a group of pharmacologically understood "proximate causes" and applying them to a similar group of proximate causes derived from pathological anatomical investigation they hoped to make therapeutics scientific.[y]

These thinkers favored chemical analysis as one avenue to pharmacological knowledge but realized that this procedure can often be unreliable.[216] Hence they preferred experiments with animals. When humans are used, the drug must often be given in very small quantities (especially if it is poisonous), and then only symptoms are developed, not the "physiologic effect" which is the truly scientific knowledge.[217] Buchheim's career at the University of Dorpat was devoted to this sort of animal experimentation.[218]

[y]Virchow himself was unsympathetic to their efforts, holding that knowledge of the drug's "physiologic effect" gave little guidance to treatment: "it suffices for the practitioner to know that a specific effect follows administration of a drug in a specific pathological condition." Mitscherlich and Liebig betray "a lack of understanding of pathology—just as in the Iatrochemical school of the seventeenth century, derived from alchemy by pathologists, one notices a lack of security in chemistry" (Virchow, *Disease, Life, and Man,* 51-53). "Pathology is not a mere transcription or application of physiological laws . . . Therefore, no one can be allowed to claim that when we know the physiological effect of an agent, such knowledge suffices for its practical application in disease. Does knowledge of the physiological effects of strychnine suffice, after all, for a knowledge of the manner, the diseases, and the amounts in which it can be administered?" (*ibid.,* 52).

But Virchow's position here seems to contradict his principle of the identity of physiological and pathological processes, and Buchheim and Mitscherlich were more consistent (as was Magendie who held, after all, that knowledge of the physiologic effect of strychnine *did* provide guidance for its therapeutic use).

Mitscherlich held that the physician first discovers the "active ingredient" of the remedy and then determines whether it makes its way into the blood, what it does there, and how it affects the tissues; this is "scientific pharmacology."[219] In treatment the physician does not concern himself with a particular "disease form" (*eine bestimmte Krankheitsform*) but rather with the "primary disease" (*das primaere Leiden*): "When we know the effect of the medicine, the material changes and symptoms which it evokes, and when the disease is also broken down into symptoms and material changes; when we then find the inner connection between the effect which the medicine causes in the organism and the morbific change in the organism caused by the disease which this particular medicine cures, then we can grasp how the disease is healed."[220] But the application of the medicine to the particular "primary disease" must be guided by experience.[221]

Implicit in the approach of these physicians was rejection of the vitalist postulate that symptomatic changes precede pathological alterations and are thus a more subtle and delicate guide to the effects of medicines on the organism. The pharmacology of Buchheim and Mitscherlich necessarily emphasized the *communia* (the grosser effects of medicinal substances) which were displayed in the physiological and pathological changes produced by administration of medicinal substances in large doses; thus it was the opposite of Hahnemann's pharmacology, which aimed, above all, to bring out the *propria*—displayed in the prover's symptoms when only very small doses were employed.[z]

Bernard's pathology and therapeutics were affected by this emerging German school of pharmacology.

Like Magendie and Virchow he held pathological processes to be merely the exaggerated development of physiol-

[z]See the homoeopathic criticism of Johann Joerg, above, p. 566*w*.

ogical ones, differing "only because of the special conditions under which the vital laws manifest themselves."[222]

The "cause" of both physiological and pathological phenomena is the capacity of the tissue or cell to be aroused by an external stimulus, i.e., its "irritability."[223] When excited normally, the cell is nourished and reproduces itself; when excited abnormally, i.e., "irritated," it proliferates and alters, yielding heterologous tissue.[224]

Deviations of nutritive or functional irritability are the key to a number of diseases, and the nervous system plays a greater role in them than Virchow allowed.[225] Disease is a "dislocation or disturbance of the mechanism which regulates the contact of vital stimulants with organic units."[226]

Bernard allowed rather little space for viruses or contagion in his doctrines.[a] While bacteria and viruses do exist, and can attack the organism, the essential point is the organism's internal state, the irritability of its cells and elements—its "predisposition."[227] That is why everyone is not affected equally by these morbific agents.[228] Furthermore, viruses are often developed in the sick organism and are thus disease products rather than their causes.[229]

He believed that anthrax and rabies could develop spontaneously in the organism (without infection from the outside), the virus then possessing the capacity to transmit the disease to others.[230]

He attributed the effect of vaccines to the organism's power to become resistant to poisons.[231]

Therapeutics is based on pathology which, in turn, is generated by physiology.[232] It is a structure of "proximate causes," or, what is the same thing, "material conditions" of the phenomena.[233] "What we call the immediate cause of a phenomenon is nothing but the physical and material condition in which it exists or appears."[234]

[a]He wrote in his notebook: *"C'est bien etonnant, les contagions"* (Claude Bernard, *Cahier des Notes, 1850-1860* [Paris: Gallimard, 1965], 80).

"The object of science is everywhere the same, to learn the material conditions of phenomena . . . this goal is the same in the physico-chemical and in biological sciences."[235]

Therapeutics is the production of an artificial condition which promotes the organism's return to its normal state—by introducing some substance into the blood, by acting on the peripheral nervous system, or by placing the whole organism in a favorable environment.[236] Toxic and medicinal substances affect the cells and anatomical elements through the intermediary of the blood, producing alterations which affect the nutrition of the given element.[237 b]

In treating the patient the physician does not act on a "disease," since this does not exist, but on the conditions which favor the rise of the exaggerated physiological process which we identify as disease.[238] He affects these conditions by influencing the *milieu interieur;* upon his knowledge of this internal environment the physician "bases all his power."[239]

Therapeutics, however, is still in its infancy and will remain a purely empirical undertaking until knowledge of drug mechanisms can be acquired.[240] "It is not enough for experimenting physicians to know that quinine cures fever; but what is above all significant to them is knowing what fever is and accounting for the mechanisms by which quinine cures. All this is significant to experimenting physicians because, as soon as they know it, the fact of curing fever with quinine will no longer be an empirical isolated fact but a scientific fact."[241]

Knowledge of drug mechanisms can be obtained by testing poisons on animals: "*ubi virus, ibi virtus.* The only medicines are poisons."[242] "The physician who possesses modifiers of life strong enough to extinguish and kill it, can

[b]Liebig had characterized health as equilibrium between the supply of nutrition to the cells and their excretion of waste matter; disease is due to interruption either of the nutritional supply or of the discharge of waste matter (Justus Liebig, *Animal Chemistry* [Cambridge, Mass. Owen, 1843], 242-253).

modify it to any degree."[243] "Experimental medicine exists thanks to the fact that it can modify empirically the living organism of the human and of animals. You can kill, poison, living things with agents of a frightful energy; you can alter vital phenomena by reducing their doses or by employing less violent modifiers. . . . In striving to determine, using modifiers (poisons), the laws of the phenomena of life, we attack directly the problems of therapeutics."[244]

In 1845 Bernard undertook experiments with curare, a recently discovered South American poison, on frogs and other animals to determine the mechanism of death: he concluded that it destroyed the motor nerves without affecting the sensory ones.[245]

He discovered this information by killing the animals and autopsying them at various stages of poisoning, tracing the progressive alterations of tissues caused by curare: "by learning the ultimate cause of poisoning with curare we easily explain all secondary phenomena."[246] "To learn how man and animals live we cannot avoid seeing great numbers of them die, because the mechanisms of life can be unveiled and proved only by knowledge of the mechanisms of death."[247] [c]

This is because death by poisoning is only a *reproduction of the very process of life itself:* "what we call life is nothing other than the death of tissues, of organs, that is, their decomposition by exterior agents . . . one could say that disease is often from the beginning only an exaggeration of life and thus an exaggeration of the process of organic decomposition."[248] "Life" is manifested by the death of the body's organs: "the organs are continually being destroyed during life, as after death, and one could even say that no organ can function otherwise than by escaping momentarily from the vital force" (*sic*).[249] "Organic substance, once

[c]He rejected such experimentation on humans, since "neither the moral law nor that of the state permit making on man the experiments which the interests of science imperatively demand" (C. Bernard, *Experimental Medicine,* 123).

created, must be destroyed, and its destruction is what constitutes its vital manifestation" (*sic*).[250]

Bernard's thesis that life is actually death results from his understanding of "irritability." The life, activity, and action of the organism are all due to the impact of an irritant upon the "irritability" of the cells or elements. "Irritability is itself destruction . . . It uses up the living matter, and the more intense the irritability the more rapidly is the living matter consumed . . . Living matter does not fall into a state of chemical indifference with the ambiant environment only because the vital force incessantly creates new organs and new food for this minotaur which is called life and which should rather be called death."[251]

Bernard's philosophy is the mirror image of Hahnemann's. Where homoeopathy is oriented toward life and therapeutically optimistic, Bernard is oriented toward death and a therapeutic pessimist. Where Hahnemann assimilates poisons to medicines, Bernard assimilates medicines to poisons.[d] Where Hahnemann investigated pharmacology by proving medicinal substances in small quantities on himself, his children, and his friends, Bernard did the same by killing large numbers of animals.[e] Where Hahnemann had regarded medicine as divinely ordained and the noblest possible calling, Bernard calls the "science of life . . . a superb and dazzling lighted hall which may be reached only by passing through a long and ghastly kitchen."[252]

Since life is the equivalent of death in Bernard's physiology, medicines promote the tendency to life by

[d]When discussing the two, he usually mentions "poisons" first and "medicines" second, e.g. "through the organic environment modified by means of certain toxic or medicinal substances therapeutics enables us to act on the organic units" (Bernard, *Experimental Medicine,* 65). See, also, *ibid.,* 115, 159, 198.

[e]He denied that the symptomatic knowledge obtained from small doses is valid: "if a medicine which is a particular poison is given in a very light dose and produces some change, this change will have nothing to do with its nature. It is not a part of it, it is only fleeting" (C. Bernard, *Principes de Medecine Experimentale* [Paris: Presses Universitaires de France, 1947], 164).

promoting the tendency to death. This is what he means by the identity of medicines and poisons. "It seems to me that medicines must often act by depressing, thus arresting the organic destruction. This perhaps explains the effect of Bouillaud's bloodletting *coup sur coup*.[f] It means throttling the disease, i.e., preventing it from becoming exacerbated by placing the patient in the state of a cold-blooded animal."[253]

Diet must have the same effect. While some physicians believe in feeding their patients, diet really acts by depressing the organism.[254] "Dietetics must be founded on the study of inanition in health and disease."[255]

It is said that the patient's room should be well aired, but amputees actually recover faster in rooms where the air is stagnant. "It could be that when the air is not renewed, the individual declines little by little like a bird under a bell-jar and thus offers more resistance to the morbific cause which is exhausting him. In such a case good ventilation would be bad for the patient by activating the process of combustion."[256] Thus good ventilation is sometimes beneficial but not always. "If one puts a sick animal under a bell-jar, its nervous system declines, the animal becomes cold-blooded; one gives it just enough air to prevent it from dying, and then toxic agents have much less impact on it. In this way we create an idiosyncrasy which prevents the contraction of disease and promotes recovery . . . These are very important topics for research upon which all of experimental therapeutics must be based . . . Lowering or elevating the organism's physiologic state is like increasing or decreasing the dose of poison."[257]

Bernard concludes that suspension of physiologic function in this way does not affect the process of organic repair by the vital force (*sic*).[258] [g] The morbific process is inhibited, while the self-healing capacity is untouched: in this way the patient recovers!!

[f]See above. p. 531.

[g]How could he know that? On this supremely important point Bernard took a purely *a priori* position.

Bernard did not practice medicine and wrote comparatively little about it. But what he did write reflects his somber and pessimistic outlook.[h] Most physicians can do little for their patients and, in any case, treat medicine as a purely commercial undertaking. Moliere's words are still apposite: all is a question of fooling the patient, and the patient himself shops around until he finds a physician who will promise to cure him—preferring the one who diagnoses rapidly to the one who hesitates or takes a long time. Those physicians earn the largest salaries who can deceive their patients the most skillfully.[259]

He assumed that therapeutics must be guided by the principle of contraries—opposition to the physiological processes which are manifested as disease: "it was no longer merely a case of physicians guiding and helping nature in its fortunate tendencies . . . but also of combating and dominating nature in its evil tendencies: *medicus naturae superator.*"[260] "I think that functional lowering is one of the great principles of experimental therapeutics. Fever is only an exaggeration of destructive activity. Health is an equilibrium.

[h]His attitude toward physicians was surely colored by his own personal experiences with them. As a youth he worked for a while as a pharmacist's assistant and was amazed to find that all the spoiled drugs and remnants of prescriptions were thrown together in a jar to be sold as theriac: "often Claude Bernard told with a smile of his astonishment at how this nasty drug, fabricated from all the spoiled substances of the shop, was continually in demand, especially by the old women of the district, and cured them all the same. He couldn't get over it" (Georges Barral, *Claude Bernard* [Ververs: Gilon, 1889], 18). At age twenty he had a two-week illness diagnosed as "intestinal irritation" and treated with potions, mustard-plasters, and "all the terrors" of the pharmacy. And it should not be forgotten that his two sons, to whom he was deeply attached, both died in infancy, despite appropriate medical ministrations. He never felt at home in the Academy of Medicine and remarked to Pasteur, when the latter joined him there in 1873: "Haven't you noticed that when a doctor enters the room, he always seems on the point of saying, 'I have just saved the life of a fellow man.' " His successor at the Sorbonne, Paul Bert (1830-1886), wrote: "He who taught that medicine is or should be a science showed himself thoroughly sceptical about physicians, and when he talked of them, the shade of Sganarelle [a character in Moliere's *Le Medecin Malgre Lui*] always seemed to pass before him" (C. Bernard, *Experimental Medicine,* xviii).

It is necessary to act against the disease [*en sens inverse*], in fevers at least."[261] "We must often act against the tendencies of nature. If, for example, an artery is open, we clearly must not favor nature which makes the blood come out and leads to death. We must act in the opposite direction, stop the hemorrhage, and save a life. Just so, when a patient has an attack of septicemia, we must act against nature and stop the fever if we mean to cure our patient."[262]

A typical example of treatment by contraries was the use of sulphur in scabies: "we know the tick, and by it we explain the transmission of the itch, the skin changes, and the cure, which is only the tick's death through appropriate application of toxic agents. No further hypotheses need now be made about the metastasis of the itch, no further statistics collected about its treatment. We cure it *always,* without any exception, when we place ourselves in the known experimental conditions for reaching this goal."[263]

He disapproved of Hippocratic medicine. These physicians regard diseases as entities "which must be respected, or at least recognized, as spontaneous tendencies of nature."[264] Hence they know only how to treat expectantly:

> Observing physicians look on a living organism as a little world contained in the great world, like a kind of ephemeral living planet whose motions are ruled by laws which we discover by a simple observation, so as to foresee the progress and evolution of vital phenomena in health or disease, but without ever being able to alter their natural course in any way. This doctrine is found in Hippocrates in its purest form. Medicine of simple observation obviously excludes all manner of active medical intervention; for this reason it is also known as expectant medicine . . .[265]

The Hippocratic never wants to throttle the disease; when he deviates from expectancy, it is only to promote the tendency of the *physis* to run through the stipulated periods of the disease. The "experimental physician," on the other hand, wants to get right down to (*toucher aux*) the phenomena, dominate (*gouverner*) and arrest the disease, and master (*maitriser*) the *physis*.[266]

NOTES

[1] A comprehensive biography of Magendie is J. M. D. Olmsted, *Francois Magendie: Pioneer in Experimental Physiology and Scientific Medicine in XIX Century France* (New York: Schuman, 1944).

[2] Paris: Mequignon-Marvis, 1816. Two Volumes.

[3] Paris: Bailliere, 1842. Four Volumes. Volume IV was his "Essay on the Blood in Diseases."

[4] Paris: Ebrard, 1839. Two Volumes.

[5] On Virchow see E. Ackerknecht, *Rudolf Virchow: Doctor, Statesman, Anthropologist* (Madison: University of Wisconsin Press, 1953).

[6] R. Virchow, *Die Cellularpathologie in ihrer Begruendung auf physiologische und pathologische Gewebelehre. Zwanzig Vorlesungen gehalten waehrend der Monate Februar, Maerze, und April, 1858 im pathologischen Institute zu Berlin* (Berlin: August Hirschwald, 1858), 13.

[7] Erster Band. Allgemeine Stoerungen der Ernaehrung und des Blutes. Krankheiten des Bewebungsapparates (Erlangen: Enke, 1854).

[8] The most important of these have been translated and published as R. Virchow, *Disease, Life, and Man.* Selected essays, translated and with Introduction by Lelland J. Rather (Stanford: Stanford University Press, 1958).

[9] Biographical detail on Bernard can be found in the two works by J. M. D. Olmsted: *Claude Bernard, Physiologist* (New York and London: Harper, 1938) and *Claude Bernard and the Experimental Method in Medicine* (New York: Schuman, 1952).

[10] C. Bernard, *An Introduction to the Study of Experimental Medicine* (New York: Dover, 1957).

[11] Paris: Presses Universitaires de France, 1947.

[12] F. Magendie, *Systeme Nerveux*, I, 2.

[13] R. Virchow, *Disease, Life, and Man*, 49.

[14] *Ibid.*, 57.

[15] C. Bernard, *Principes*, 29.

[16] *Ibid.*, 252.

[17] C. Bernard, *Experimental Medicine*, 43.

[18] F. Magendie, *Systeme Nerveux*, I, 2. F. Dubois, "Eloge de Magendie," *Memoires de l'Academie Imperiale de Medecine* XX (1858), xxii. P. Flourens, *Eloge Historique de Francois Magendie* (Paris: Garnier, 1858), 25.

[19] F. Magendie, *Systeme Nerveux*, I, 3. *Phenomenes Physiques*, II, 44, 46.

[20] P. Flourens, *Eloge Historique de Francois Magendie*, 39-40.

[21] F. Magendie, *Phenomenes Physiques*, II, 5-6.

[22] C. Bernard, *Principes*, 68.

[23] F. Magendie, *Phenomenes Physiques,* IV, 12.

[24] *Ibid.,* I, 155. *Systeme Nerveux,* I, 9.

[25] F. Magendie, *Phenomenes Physiques,* I, 7; IV, 58. *Systeme Nerveux,* I, 9.

[26] F. Magendie, *Phenomenes Physiques,* II, 46.

[27] F. Dubois, "Eloge de Magendie," xxii. P. Flourens, *Eloge Historique de Francois Magendie,* 25.

[28] R. Virchow, *Disease, Life, and Man,* 36.

[29] *Loc. cit.*

[30] *Ibid.,* 56.

[31] C. Bernard, *Experimental Medicine,* 43.

[32] *Ibid.,* 209.

[33] C. Bernard, *Principes,* 31.

[34] *Ibid.,* 47.

[35] *Ibid.*. 51, 184.

[36] C. Bernard, *Experimental Medicine,* 191.

[37] *Ibid.,* 54.

[38] *Ibid.,* 2.

[39] *Ibid.,* 72.

[40] *Ibid.,* 2.

[41] R. Virchow, "The Position of Pathology among Biological Studies" in *Post-Mortem Examinations and the Position of Pathology Among Biological Studies.* New York Academy of Medicine, History of Medicine Series, No. 37 (Metuchen, N.J.: Scarecrow Reprint Corp., 1973), 126.

[42] C. Bernard, *Experimental Medicine,* 77.

[43] *Ibid,* 61.

[44] *Ibid.,* 79.

[45] F. Magendie, "Quelques Idees Generales sur les Phenomenes Particuliers aux Corps Vivants," *Bulletin des Sciences Medicales* IV (1809), 145-170, at 148, 150, 153, 154-155.

[46] *Ibid.,* 169.

[47] *Ibid.,* 153.

[48] *Ibid.,* 158-159.

[49] *Ibid.,* 159.

[50] See William R. Albury, "Physiological Explanation in Magendie's Manifesto of 1809," *Bulletin of the History of Medicine* XLVIII (1974), 90-99.

[51] Magendie, "Quelques Idees Generales," 149.

[52] *Ibid.,* 161.

[53] F. Magendie, *Precis Elementaire,* I, 20.

[54] F. Magendie, "Quelques Idees Generales," 163-165.

[55] F. Magendie, *Phenomenes Physiques,* IV, 37. *Systeme Nerveux,* I, 3, 40.

[56] F. Magendie, *Phenomenes Physiques,* I, 19.

[57] *Ibid.,* I, 16-19. *Systeme Nerveux,* I, 40.

[58] F. Magendie, *Systeme Nerveux,* I, 10.

[59] F. Magendie, *Phenomenes Physiques,* I, 309.

[60] X. Bichat, *Traite des Membranes,* 1827, 71.

[61] *Ibid.,* 109. F. Magendie, *Phenomenes Physiques,* I, 84-85.

[62] F. Magendie, *Phenomenes Physiques,* II, 126-128; III, 148.

[63] *Ibid.,* I, 9-10; IV, 78.

[64] *Ibid.,* II, 117, 120.

[65] F. Magendie, *Precis Elementaire,* II, 309-310.
[66] F. Magendie, *Phenomenes Physiques,* II, 120.
[67] *Ibid.,* II, 117.
[68] F. Magendie, *Precis Elementaire,* II, 310-311.
[69] F. Magendie, *Phenomenes Physiques,* II, 15.
[70] *Ibid.,* II, 123; III, 277.
[71] F. Magendie, *Systeme Nerveux,* I, 40; II, 5.
[72] F. Dubois, "Eloge de Magendie," xxvi.
[73] J. M. D. Olmsted, *Magendie,* 221.
[74] *Ibid.,* 140-141.
[75] *Ibid.,* 143.
[76] F. Dubois, "Eloge de Magendie," xxiii.
[77] *Ibid.,* xxiv.
[78] *Loc. cit.*
[79] A. Trousseau, *Dissertation sur les Generalites de la Physiologie* (Paris: Fournier, 1831), 18, 20.
[80] F. Dubois, "Eloge de Magendie," xxiv.
[81] See Charles Bell, *The Nervous System of the Human Body* (London: Longman, 1830).
[82] F. Magendie, *Phenomenes Physiques,* II, 198; III, 116.
[83] *Ibid.,* III, 29.
[84] J. M. D. Olmsted, *Magendie,* 146-147.
[85] F. Magendie, *Phenomenes Physiques,* I, 58.
[86] J. M. D. Olmsted, *Magendie,* 16. C. Bernard, *Francois Magendie: Lecon d'Ouverture du Cours de Medecine du College de France (29 Fevrier, 1856)* (Paris: Bailliere, 1856), 19.
[87] F. Magendie, *Phenomenes Physiques,* II, 28.
[88] *Loc. cit.*
[89] R. Virchow, *Disease, Life, and Man,* 84.
[90] *Ibid.,* 106.
[91] R. Virchow, *Die Cellularpathologie,* 3.
[92] R. Virchow, *Disease, Life, and Man,* 105.
[93] *Ibid.,* 81.
[94] *Ibid.,* 84.
[95] *Ibid.,* 117.
[96] *Ibid.,* 46.
[97] *Ibid.,* 106 107.
[98] R. Virchow, *Die Cellularpathologie,* 3.
[99] R. Virchow, *Disease, Life, and Man,* 46, 63.
[100] *Ibid.,* 86.
[101] R. Virchow, *Post-Mortem Examinations,* 126.
[102] *Loc. cit.*
[103] *Loc. cit.*
[104] *Ibid.,* 119-122.
[105] *Loc. cit.*
[106] *Ibid.,* 125-126.
[107] R. Virchow, *Die Cellularpathologie,* 346.
[108] *Ibid.,* 259, 346.
[109] *Ibid.,* 266, 276.
[110] *Ibid.,* 259.

[111] R. Virchow, *Handbuch der speciellen Pathologie,* 4.
[112] C. Bernard, *Experimental Medicine,* 93.
[113] *Ibid.,* 73.
[114] *Ibid.,* 76.
[115] *Ibid.,* 77.
[116] C. Bernard, *Principes,* 142.
[117] *Ibid.,* 149-154. *Experimental Medicine,* 77-78.
[118] C. Bernard, *Principes,* 149.
[119] *Ibid.,* 150.
[120] *Ibid.,* 150, 156.
[121] C. Bernard, *Experimental Medicine,* 78.
[122] *Loc. cit.*
[123] *Loc. cit.*
[124] *Ibid.,* C. Bernard, *Principes,* 150.
[125] *Ibid.,* 149.
[126] *Ibid.,* 148-149. *Experimental Medicine,* 63-64.
[127] C. Bernard, *Experimental Medicine,* 98.
[128] *Ibid.,* 62.
[129] *Ibid.,* 76.
[130] *Ibid.,* 80.
[131] *Ibid.,* 79.
[132] *Ibid.,* 61, 79.
[133] Claude Bernard, *Cahier des Notes, 1850-1860* (Paris: Gallimard, 1965), 154.
[134] C. Bernard, *Experimental Medicine,* 63.
[135] C. Bernard, *Principes,* 12.
[136] C. Bernard, *Experimental Medicine,* 72, 100.
[137] *Ibid.,* 86.
[138] *Ibid.,* 14.
[139] *Ibid.,* 104.
[140] *Ibid.,* 100.
[141] *Ibid.,* 101.
[142] F. Magendie, *Phenomenes Physiques,* IV (his "Essay on the Blood in Diseases"), 46-47. *Systeme Nerveux,* I, 3.
[143] F. Magendie, *Phenomenes Physiques,* IV, 45-46, 48.
[144] *Ibid.,* III, 12; IV, 48-49.
[145] *Ibid.,* I, 75.
[146] *Ibid.,* I, 78.
[147] *Ibid.,* II, 9; III, 441, 445. *L'Union Medicale* VI (1852), 236.
[148] *Ibid.,* IV, 48.
[149] *Ibid.,* IV, 57, 59.
[150] *Ibid.,* IV, 114-115.
[151] *Ibid.,* IV, 48-49.
[152] *Ibid.,* III, 9, 76; IV, 9, 48, 307. *Systeme Nerveux,* I, 7-8.
[153] F. Magendie, *Phenomenes Physiques,* II, 198.
[154] *Ibid.,* IV, 171, 382.
[155] *Ibid.,* IV, 218.
[156] *Ibid.,* III, 75-77; IV, 61.
[157] *Ibid.,* IV, 211-218.

[158] F. Magendie, *Systeme Nerveux,* I, 3, 31, 34, 35.

[159] F. Dubois, "Eloge de Magendie," xxvi.

[160] *L'Union Medicale* III (1849), 300. Academie des Sciences, *Comptes Rendues* XXVIII (1849), 393-394. C. Bernard, *Experimental Medicine,* 173-174.

[161] *L'Union Medicale* VI (1852), 236.

[162] F. Magendie, *Phenomenes Physiques,* II, 5. C. Bernard, *Francois Magendie,* 20. P. Flourens, *Eloge Historique de Francois Magendie,* 38-40.

[163] F. Magendie, *Phenomenes Physiques,* III, 33, 458.

[164] *Ibid.,* I, 146-147, 152.

[165] F. Magendie, *Recherches Physiologiques et Medicales sur les Causes, les Symptomes, et le Traitement de la Gravelle* (Paris: Mequignon-Marvis, 1818), 61.

[166] F. Magendie, *Physiological and Chemical Researches on the Use of the Prussic or Hydro-Cyanic Acid in the Treatment of Diseases of the Breast, and Particularly in Phthisis Pulmonalis* (New Haven: Howe and Spalding, 1820), 22.

[167] F. Magendie, *Phenomenes Physiques,* IV, 120.

[168] R. Virchow, *Disease, Life, and Man,* 81.

[169] *Ibid.,* 26.

[170] R. Virchow, *Post-Mortem Examinations,* 128. *Handbuch der speciellen Pathologie,* 47, 67, 71.

[171] R. Virchow, *Die Cellularpathologie,* 346.

[172] *Ibid.,* 347

[173] *Ibid.,* 283.

[174] R. Virchow, *Disease, Life, and Man,* 63-64.

[175] R. Virchow, *Die Cellularpathologie,* 177, 181.

[176] R. Virchow, *Handbuch der speciellen Pathologie,* 7. *Die Cellularpathologie,* 194.

[177] R. Virchow, *Handbuch der speciellen Pathologie,* 7.

[178] *Ibid.,* 271-371.

[179] *Ibid.,* 303.

[180] *Ibid.,* 326.

[181] *Ibid.,* 37.

[182] *Ibid.,* 98, 103.

[183] *Ibid.,* 82.

[184] *Ibid.,* 122.

[185] *Ibid.,* 128, 156.

[186] *Ibid.,* 182.

[187] R. Virchow, *Disease, Life, and Man,* 27, 149.

[188] R. Virchow, *Handbuch der speciellen Pathologie,* 43-44.

[189] *Ibid.,* 44.

[190] *Loc. cit.*

[191] *Ibid.,* 44-45.

[192] *Ibid.,* 81.

[193] *Loc. cit.*

[194] *Loc. cit.*

[195] *Ibid.,* 82.

[196] *Ibid.,* 82, 86.

[197] *Ibid.,* 88, 92.

[198] *Ibid.,* 128.

[199] *Loc. cit.*

[200] *Ibid.*, 141.
[201] R. Virchow, *Disease, Life, and Man,* 64-65.
[202] *Ibid.*, 181.
[203] *Ibid.*, 51.
[204] *Ibid.*, 181.
[205] Jonathan Pereira, *Handbuch der Heilmittellehre. Bearbeitet von Rudolph Buchheim* (Leipzig: Voss, 1846, 1848), I, vii.
[206] *Ibid.*, I, xvi.
[207] C. G. Mitscherlich, *Lehrbuch der Arzneimittellehre.* Second Edition (Berlin: Bethge, 1847-1851), I, 125.
[208] *Ibid.*, I, 3.
[209] J. Pereira, *Handbuch,* I, xvi-xvii.
[210] *Ibid.*, I, x-xi, xvi. Mitscherlich, *Lehrbuch,* I, viii. R. Buchheim, *Lehrbuch der Arzneimittellehre.* Third Edition (Leipzig: Voss, 1878), I, vi-vii. See, also, Justus Liebig, *Animal Chemistry, or Organic Chemistry in its Application to Physiology and Pathology.* Second Edition (Cambridge, Mass.: Owen, 1843), 161-162.
[211] C. G. Mitscherlich, *Lehrbuch,* I, vii-ix, 3.
[212] *Loc. cit.*
[213] J. Pereira, *Handbuch,* I, viii, xvi.
[214] *Ibid.*, I, x, xv-xvi. R. Buchheim, *Lehrbuch,* 67.
[215] J. Pereira, *Handbuch,* I, xvi.
[216] Mitscherlich, *Lehrbuch,* I, viii, xv. R. Buchheim, *Lehrbuch,* 68.
[217] C. G. Mitscherlich, *Lehrbuch,* I, 124-125.
[218] R. Buchheim, *Lehrbuch,* vi-vii. See Marianne Bruppacher-Cellier, *Rudolph Buchheim (1820-1879) und die Entwicklung einer experimentellen Pharmakologie,* Zuercher Medizingeschichtliche Abhandlungen. Neue Reihe, #88 (Zuerich: Juris Druck, 1971).
[219] C. G. Mitscherlich, *Lehrbuch,* I, viii.
[220] *Ibid.*, I, ix-x.
[221] *Ibid.*, I, x.
[222] C. Bernard, *Experimental Medicine,* 10.
[223] C. Bernard, *Principes,* 135, 141, 142, 147, 161.
[224] *Ibid.*, 150.
[225] *Loc. cit.*
[226] C. Bernard, *Experimental Medicine,* 76.
[227] C. Bernard, *Principes,* 160-163.
[228] *Ibid.*, 163.
[229] *Ibid.*, 141, 248.
[230] *Ibid.*, 163.
[231] *Ibid.*, 157. See, also, Claude Bernard, *Cahier des Notes, 1850-1860,* 80.
[232] C. Bernard, *Experimental Medicine,* 1-2.
[233] *Ibid.*, 193. *Principes,* 173.
[234] C. Bernard, *Experimental Medicine,* 65.
[235] *Ibid.*, 67.
[236] C. Bernard, *Principes,* 140.
[237] *Ibid.*, 153.
[238] *Ibid.*, 128, 140.
[239] *Ibid.*, 11, 98. *Experimental Medicine,* 65.

[240] C. Bernard, *Experimental Medicine,* 140, 194, 198, 216.
[241] *Ibid.,* 209.
[242] C. Bernard, *Principes,* 164.
[243] *Ibid.,* 7.
[244] *Ibid.,* 123.
[245] C. Bernard, *Experimental Medicine,* 88, 158.
[246] *Ibid.,* 216.
[247] *Ibid.,* 99.
[248] C. Bernard, *Principes,* 158.
[249] *Ibid.,* 158-159.
[250] *Ibid.,* 159.
[251] *Ibid.,* 151.
[252] C. Bernard, *Experimental Medicine,* 15.
[253] C. Bernard, *Principes,* 164.
[254] *Loc. cit.*
[255] *Loc. cit.*
[256] *Ibid.,* 165.
[257] *Loc. cit.*
[258] *Loc. cit.*
[259] *Ibid.,* 33, 181-183.
[260] C. Bernard, *Experimental Medicine,* 207.
[261] C. Bernard, *Principes,* 174.
[262] C. Bernard, *Experimental Medicine,* 213.
[263] *Ibid.,* 214. *Principes,* 73.
[264] C. Bernard, *Principes,* 15.
[265] C. Bernard, *Experimental Medicine,* 197.
[266] C. Bernard, *Principes,* 96.

CHAPTER IX

CONCLUSION: EMPIRICISM AND RATIONALISM IN THE HISTORY OF MEDICAL THOUGHT

Volume II of *Divided Legacy* has carried the history of medical philosophy from the sixteenth-century heirs of Paracelsus to the nineteenth-century precursors of bacteriological medicine, amplifying the thesis of Volume I that the driving force of medical speculation is provided by the tension between the Empirical and Rationalist poles of thought.

This concluding chapter will summarize the contrasts between the two medical orientations, emphasizing the holism of Empiricism and reductionism of Rationalism, demonstrating their relevance to scientific method, and showing how the psychological types they represent are affected by the socio-economic influences at work on physicians and the medical profession.

The Reassertion of Perennial Thought Patterns

The Empiric is oriented toward the outside, receptive to influences and stimuli from his surroundings. The Rationalist is oriented inward and resists external stimuli.

The outward orientation represents openness to experience. The inward orientation represents the impulse to structure experience. Both must be combined if the individual is to have a relationship with the world around him.

Hence Empiricism and Rationalism each contain a part of the other (like the Yin and Yang of Chinese philosophy). They are contrasted by the way the two elements are combined and the proportion of each in the combination.

Thus, while each allocates a place to experience and to structured knowledge, Empiricism emphasizes the former and Rationalism the latter. The Empiric assumes that the pattern of relationships forming the structure of knowledge is inherent in nature; he elicits it through his sympathetic reception of information from nature, i.e., through his experience, and assumes that the structure will change with the increasing input of such information. The Rationalist imposes on nature an *a priori* pattern or structure of ideas derived elsewhere and is less willing than the Empiric to alter this structure in the light of new experience, i.e., new information.

The relationship between the individual and his surroundings becomes, in medicine, that between the physician and his patients. The combination of Empirical and Rationalist elements in the physician's medical philosophy determines his attitude toward the patient and his success or failure as a healer.

Between the sixteenth and nineteenth centuries medical Empiricism was reasserted by Van Helmont, Stahl, Bordeu, Sydenham, Baglivi, Laennec, Pinel, Trousseau, and especially by Samuel Hahnemann, while Rationalism was represented by Sylvius, Willis, Cheyne, Boerhaave, Hoffmann, Rostan, and Bouillaud.

Methodism, a sub-category of Rationalism, also figured in the history of this period, being represented by Descartes, Cullen, Brown, Broussais, Magendie, Virchow, and Bernard.

The perennial opposition between Empiricism and Rationalism/Methodism is thus exemplified in the conflict between Hahnemann and Bernard.

As we have stated repeatedly above, the two orientations proceed from differing assumptions about the nature of the organism, the nature of man's knowledge of the organism, and the meaning of a "scientific" therapeutics.

The Empirics are vitalists, assuming the existence of a living force in the organism which reacts purposively to external stimuli and maintains equilibrium with the environment.

Acceptance of a vital force, whether called the *physis,* the *Archeus,* or the *Anima sensitiva,* leads to a particular interpretation of the organism.

The symptoms are seen as generated by this force and thus prior to any material change in the body. Symptoms precede pathology.

The organism reacts in a specific and purposive way to each specific stimulus, even responding differently at different times to the same type of stimulus. Therefore, the reaction cannot be predicted *a priori.* Knowledge of internal causal processes is unattainable.

But such knowledge is, in any case, not needed for medical practice: "as it is clearly impossible that a physician should discover those causes of disease that are not cognizable by the senses, so it is unnecessary that he should attempt it."[1] The symptoms themselves are an accurate picture of the changes in the vital force.[a] Being evidence of the body's reaction to a morbific stimulus, they must be intrinsically beneficial—reflecting the striving for health.[2] And if each such reaction is a response to a specific morbific influence, the *propria* (representing the specificity of the reaction) must take precedence over the *communia* (the symptoms common to many reactive processes).[3]

[a]Stahl, like Paracelsus, justified this on religious grounds: God is manifested in His works (Blondin, *Oeuvres de Stahl,* VI 68; *Divided Legacy,* I, 462). Hahnemann placed on the title page of the first edition of the *Organon* the following passage from the poet, Christian Gellert (1715-1769):

> Die Wahrheit die wir alle noethig haben,
> Die uns als Menschen gluecklich macht,
> Wird von der weisen Hand die sie uns zugedacht,
> Nur leicht verdeckt, nicht tief vergraben.

(S. Hahnemann, *Organon der rationellen Heilkunde* [1810], Title Page).

Treatment is guided by the body's reaction and aims to intensify it (even where, as with Hahnemann, Empirics thought to improve on this reaction). If the illness is not treated in this way, its natural course is perverted, it metastasizes into chronic disease, and the patient becomes difficult or impossible to cure.[4]

To assist the body's reaction Empirics in ancient times used "similars" or "furthering remedies" (*secunda remedia*). Paracelsus introduced the "specific," and Hahnemann demonstrated the specific to be merely an instance of the operation of similars. His "provings" gave the ancient principle of similarity a new content which it has retained ever since.

Practice comes before theory, and in several different senses.

The Empirics are more concerned with practical healing than with theoretical speculation: "Who wants as his physician a man who can explain everything and who (like so many professors whose doctrines are now forgotten) commences every treatise on medicine with a long discourse on the elements and an enumeration of the parts of the body?"[5] "The moderns shine . . . only in their books."[6]

In the second place, the practice of the *physis* is the source of the physician's theory.[7] Theory is only a "way of viewing the facts."[8] The true theory is the "faithful echo of practice."[9]

Bordeu's pulse theory was founded "solely on practice . . . a history of the observed facts."[10]

And practice has primacy over theory in the final sense that the only proof of the accuracy of theory is the patient's recovery:

> The pomp and dignity of the medical art is less seen in neat and elegant formulas than in the cure of diseases.[11]

> The whole philosophy of medicine consists in working out the histories of diseases and applying remedies which may dispel them; and experience is the only guide.[12]

Stahl held his theory to be the "one and only truth" in medicine because it yielded better results, experience showing all others to be erroneous.[13] Hahnemann insisted that homoeopathy be judged by the results:

> "Refute," I cry to my contemporaries, "refute these truths if you can, by pointing out a still more efficacious, sure, and agreeable mode of treatment than mine—and do not combat them with mere words, of which we have already too many."[14]

> The doctrine appeals not only chiefly, but solely, to the verdict of experience—"repeat the experiments," it cries aloud, "repeat them carefully and accurately, and you will find the doctrine confirmed at every step"—And it does what no medical doctrine, no system of physic, no so-called therapeutics ever did or could do, it *insists* upon being "judged by the result."[15]

> Is it really credible that in these illumined times a work of experience like my *Organon of Rational Healing,* springing purely from experience, referable only to experience, and confirmable or refutable only by counter-experience and counter-experiments, was put on one side by several reviewers merely with empty words and expressions from the Old School? In similar manner they tried of old to refute Copernicus' proof of the movement of the earth around its axis and around the sun with Ptolemaic statements, and Harvey's proof of the greater blood circulation with Galenical quotations.[16]

Thus the Empirics comprehend the pattern of the body's reactions not *a priori* but *a posteriori*—through attentive examination of its specific acts.[17] Stahl called this a process of induction:

> The mind is as incapable of arriving *a priori* at precise notions of the relations which physiological facts have with one another as it is capable of grasping *a posteriori* their sequence and the consequence of their succession.[18]

> We have always, in all our works, endeavored first to present the principal phenomena of morbid affections and then to derive from them the principal inductions, rather than first to establish general propositions which need ultimately to be confirmed by practical examples.[19]

He quotes the Hippocratic/Empirical writing, *Precepts,* which censures the Rationalist School for attempting to fit the phenomena into an *a priori* theory rather than adjusting the theory to the phenomena themselves.[20 b]

Even the most unusual and apparently abnormal phenomena have their place in the generation of theory. "Rare cases" help to refine the physician's understanding of the movements of the physis.[21]

The *ratio* is implicit in the events, and the physician's *ratio* must always be subordinate to observation, since the materials of *ratio* are provided only by observation.[22] The *physis* possesses its own *ratio,* and each of the body's organs, in turn, possesses an *organica ratio atque proportio* guiding the performance of its functions.[23]

By his practice the physician comes to understand this *ratio*—the "order, time, succession, and perfect harmony which govern the vital movements."[24 c]

The structure of the Rationalist therapeutic philosophy is quite different.

It is anti-vitalist, rejecting the existence of an autonomous and purposive force in the organism:

> Vitalistic ideas . . . are just a kind of medical superstition, a belief in the supernatural. Now, in medicine, belief in occult causes, whether it is called vitalism or is otherwise named, encourages ignorance and gives birth to a sort of unintentional quackery—that is to say, belief in an inborn indefinable science.[25]

[b]On *Precepts* see *Divided Legacy,* I, 241-244.

[c]Hahnemann's first title for the *Organon*—the *Organon of Rational Healing*—reveals the same concept of *ratio.* Otherwise he was scornful of physicians' claims to act "rationally" (Hahnemann, *Lesser Writings,* 736, 752).

Stahl and the Empirics attributed priority to the body's *movements,* being the mode of expression of the autonomous *physis.*[26] The Rationalists, however, reduce movement, hence the body's vitality, to a mere attribute of its material structure: "the conjunct power of all these actions of the body for preserving its own health, which arises from the wonderful structure of its parts, is what Hippocrates calls NATURE."[27] [d]

Far from viewing the organism as a *sui generis* and dynamic entity, the laws of whose intrinsic movements remain to be discovered, these thinkers see it only as a material object governed by the laws applicable to other material objects: "to claim that the phenomena of life are entirely distinct from the phenomena of nature generally would be to profess a serious error, to be opposed to the further progress of science."[28]

> Certainly a special force in living beings, not met with elsewhere, presides over their organization; but the existence of this force cannot in any way change our idea of the properties of organic matter—matter which, when once created, is endowed with fixed and determinate, physico-chemical properties. Vital force is, therefore, an organizing and nutritive force; but it does not in any way determine the manifestations of the properties of living matter. In a word, physiologists and physicians must seek to reduce vital properties to physico-chemical properties, and not physico-chemical properties to vital properties.[29]

The material changes in the body are regarded as in every way prior to the dynamic (vital, symptomatic) changes—being the "proximate causes" of these latter changes. The first are concrete and real, the second unstable and ephemeral. A disease and its symptoms always proceed from a

[d]Bacon had written: "A greater evil arises from the contemplation and investigation rather of the stationary principles of things from which, than of the active by which, things themselves are created. For the former only serve for discussion, the latter for practice" (*Novum Organum,* I, Aph. LXVI).

material or physico-chemical lesion, and if a lesion cannot be observed, it must still be assumed present. There is no lesion of the vital force, no dynamic lesion without a material basis.[30]

Symptoms are important only as signs of an underlying material alteration:

> A sign in physic is termed an appearance perceptible to the senses, from which the physician discovers something different from the sign itself, and which he could only discover by its appearance.[31]

> The effects or symptoms manifest the nature of their causes, the diseases themselves; and as these effects are evident to the senses, they afford great light toward discovering . . . disease in itself.[32]

> Now what we call the immediate cause of a phenomenon is nothing but the physical and material condition in which it exists or appears. The object of the experimental method . . . is, therefore, the same for living bodies as for inorganic bodies; it consists in finding the relations which connect any phenomenon with its immediate cause, or, putting it differently, it consists in defining the conditions necessary to the appearance of the phenomenon.[33]

The symptoms of greatest interest to Rationalism are the *communia,* those "common to a great number of very different disorders," since they indicate the most general–consequently, the most important–material causes at work in the organism.[34] The *propria* are reduced to the status of "supervening" or "incidental" symptoms, "symptoms of symptoms," etc.

> If the appearance proceeds from some other antecedent symptom as its cause, it is called a symptomatic symptom or a symptom of a symptom. But such an appearance as happens in the course of a disease from a different cause or origin, distinct from the disease itself, its cause or symptoms, may be more properly denominated a supervening or incidental symptom.[35]

> Such are properly termed accidental symptoms as do not arise from the disease itself, but from some alteration of air or error in the patient or his attendants.[36]

Boerhaave wrote extensively on the extrapolation from symptoms to invisible causal process in the organism. An alkaline disorder, for instance, is marked by a "fetid cadaverous smell either in the whole, or in some particular part of the body; a taste in the mouth like that of putrid flesh or urine, an ash-colored, leaden, or blackish erosion of the skin . . . intense thirst . . . loss of appetite . . . looseness of the feces," etc.[37] In an acid disorder there is "an acid smell in the breath and taste in the mouth, a pale color in the face, in the corners of the eyes, lips, mouth, gums, and fauces . . . a strong inclination to eat earthy and absorbent matters, gripings in the bowels, attended with a paleness and coldness of the body, green griping stools of an acid smell, urine acrid."[38] In general, chemistry tells the physician "the true disposition of the water, salt, oil, and earth in the urine, and consequently in the blood at that time; and hence . . . the intimate disorders of the humors, which are otherwise out of our reach."[39] Where William Harvey had ascribed a rapid pulse to "the more frequent reception of the vital blood from the veins into the heart, and the expulsion of it thence into the arteries," chemistry gives a more profound explanation of fever and of the rapid pulse:

> that by this increase of heat from the celerity of the pulse, the more fluid parts of the humors must necessarily be dissipated, and the remainder inspissated; that the oils will be dissolved and mixed with the blood, and by the attrition they suffer in the course of circulation, will become acrid, volatile, and putrid, and in this condition, being strongly pressed against the fine vessels of the brain, will of consequence wonderfully disturb it, nor will be easily again disengaged from their union with blood; that the salts of the humors will lose their natural ineptitude to motion, and become almost volatile; from an innocent, mild disposition, will grow vastly acrimoni-

ous and change their soft saponaceous quality into a fiery corrosive one, and become, as some have asserted, a perfect alkali. By this means, therefore, the chemist comes to a right understanding of the sign, and at the same time explains to us the use of it.[40]

Boerhaave made a specialty of diagnosis from the urine. Excess amounts of this fluid indicate "an imperfect mixture of the blood, whence the watery parts easily recede from the rest."[41] Scanty urine portends "future repletions, heaviness, stupidity, sleepiness, convulsive tremblings."[42] Thin inodorous urine indicates "that the renal ducts are much contracted, while the humors in the meantime are violently agitated by too swift a circulation. That there is too strict a cohesion of the oils, salt, and earth in the substance of the urine, a tenacity of the humors, and a difficulty of intermixing watery liquors with them . . . that the viscera are incapable of concocting the alimentary humors, whence crudities, phlegm, and coldness of habit . . ." etc., etc.[43]

He warns against the danger of faulty diagnosis:

> Even the most skilful physician may be imposed upon, so as to think the urine presages ill if the patient sups upon asparagus, and afterwards in the night takes a bolus of cassia with rhubarb; for by this means the urine will be rendered black and very fetid, so that the physician, though skilful, being ignorant of what the patient has took, might pronounce that the owner of the urine must in a little time perish by a gangrene of the internal parts, when the very next day the patient, being very well, will deride the physician. Even urine of almost any color may be discharged either yellow, green, or red, only by taking inoffensive and simple medicines. Turmeric being taken inwardly tinges the urine as in a jaundice, and saffron renders the urine like that of a person in an ardent fever, etc. By these artifices I saw two professors of this university imposed upon, who, having well considered the urine, without being acquainted with what the patient had taken, pronounced their judgment according to the rules of art.[44]

And the practitioner must avoid presaging from the urine any condition other than the patient's disease:

> Much less can anyone determine whether the person to whom the urine belonged was a virgin, a married woman, or with child; all which pretensions deserve only to be laughed at. I remember two professors many years ago in this city of Leyden who were egregiously deceived in their uromancy, when, according to the rules of their art, they denied a certain noble lady was with child, till the birth of the infant silenced the prophets. I have known the principal urine judgers of this republic to have been guilty of such egregious and glaring errors, that if they had the least shame or merit, they would have never after appeared in that character.[45]

Another source of causal knowledge is the autopsy.[46] "Hippocrates was the best observer concerning the phenomena during life, [but] those made the greatest contribution to the art of medicine who investigated bodies after death."[47] [e] "While clinical observation teaches [the physician] to know the form and course of diseases, it cannot suffice to make him understand their nature; to this end he must penetrate into the body, to find which of the internal parts are injured in their functions."[48]

> It is not enough for physiologists to know empirically the normal and abnormal phenomena of living nature, but, like physicists and chemists, they mean to go back to the immediate causes of phenomena, i.e., to their necessary conditions.[49]

The nineteenth-century allopaths criticized homoeopathy as irrational and unscientific for concentrating exclusively on symptoms and ignoring the findings of pathological anatomy.[50]

[e]Contrast this with Stahl's advice that the physician avoid excessive anatomical detail which only loads the mind with prejudices and wrong ideas (Stahl, *Theoria Medica Vera,* I, 68-69).

Physics and chemistry are also acceptable techniques for establishing a causal relation between symptoms and anatomical changes: "a physician may, and ought, to furnish himself with, and reason from, such things as are demonstrated to be true in anatomy, chemistry, and mechanics, with natural and experimental philosophy, provided he confines his reasoning within the bounds of truth and simple experiment."[51]

When physiology in the nineteenth century shifted emphasis to "functional disturbances" rather than anatomical changes,[f] vivisection took precedence over autopsy:

> I consider that the most complex of all sciences, physiology, cannot be completely explained by anatomy.[52]

> The anatomy of corpses cannot and does not teach anything. All our knowledge on this subject must necessarily come from experiment or from observation of the living.[53]

> For pathology we must therefore establish pathological vivisection, that is to say, we must create diseases in animals and sacrifice them at various stages of these diseases . . . When the animal dies, we must make an autopsy immediately after death, just as if we were dealing with one of those instantaneous diseases called poisoning . . . In a word, a physician should not hold to anatomical pathology alone, to explain the disease.[54]

But symptomatic alterations were still regarded as posterior to some, not always clearly defined, physico-chemical alteration occurring inside the body: "some histological unit has lost its physiological properties, a loss which has brought on the disruption of vital phenomena."[55]

> I shall not admit that cells or fibers of tissues are always primarily attacked; a morbid physico-chemical change in

[f]The concept of physiological "function" was by no means new, as Boerhaave had discussed it extensively (*Academical Lectures,* V, 255-277).

the organic environment being able, in itself, to lead to the morbid phenomena, in the manner of a toxic symptom which occurs, without primary lesion of the tissues, through mere change in the environment.[56]

Whichever discipline is used, the conclusions reached in it are extrapolated into the diseased organism, and this is the work of *ratio.* The pattern of causal relations is drawn from some area of knowledge external to the diseased organism—from chemical and physical experiments, from the observation of corpses, from the vivisection of animals. And these relations are projected into the body by *ratio.* The physician reasons about the invisible by analogy with the visible.[57] He "above all stands in need of just reasoning to assist him in the discovery of many things of the human body."[58] "We may by a slow and solid judgment determine the latent causes of diseases."[59] "Our real eyes are inside the head, and the eyes of the spirit show us what the eyes of the body do not."[60] [g]

The organism is knowable *a priori,* and Boerhaave rejects Hippocrates' opinion that "we are altogether ignorant of what is performed within the body of the living patient."[61]

When the diagnosis has been made, the physician endeavors to act upon the "proximate cause" of the disease: "we never act on the essence of natural phenomena, but only on their determining causes."[62] And the appropriate medicine is the "contrary." Just as the thrust of Empirical philosophy leads to the use of similars, so *ratio*-based Rationalism necessarily issues in the concept of cure through contrariety.[h]

Since diagnosis is based on the *communia,* Rationalist theory has no space for unusual, irregular, or "abnormal"

[g] "The wise man's eyes are in his head" (*Ecclesiastes* II: 14).

[h] Cure by "contraries" stems from Aristotle's "principle of contradiction"—"it is impossible for anyone to believe the same thing to be and not to be" (*Divided Legacy,* I, 131).

phenomena, and these are interpreted as chance departures from a standard of "normality."[i]

The relationship between theory and practice is the reverse of that obtaining in Empiricism: theory is first and is the basis of practice, while practice only supplies the raw material of theory:[63]

> A physician ought to be furnished with a just notion of all diseases before he ventures upon the practice, that when he comes to a patient he may readily discover his known disorders by their proper signs.[64]

> The cure of diseases is chiefly, and almost unavoidably, founded in the knowledge of their proximate causes. This requires an acquaintance with the Institutions of Medicine; that is, the knowledge of the structure, action, and functions of the human body.[65]

> At almost all times the practice has been, and still is, with every person, founded more or less upon certain principles established by reasoning.[66]

This is sometimes described as the primacy of science over art, or of the general over the particular:

> The theoretical part of physic may be termed a science, but the practice of it is to be reckoned among the arts.[67]

> Mechanical laws are eternally the same, and must remain perpetually true; though in our application of them to bodies not sufficiently known we are frequently deceived.[68]

> There are indeed some who affirm physic to be wholly conjectural, which is false; it has this in common with all other arts, that it is imperfect, but that imperfection is the default of the artist, which is generally greater in the professors of this, than of other arts.[69]

[i]For Aristotle chance was a separate category of causation, unincorporated in the substance of his philosophy (*Divided Legacy,* I, 131).

> Practice . . . requires knowledge of particulars . . . generalization leads to the law of phenomena and is the true scientific goal.[70]

While theory is scientific, a variety of factors prevent it from always being scientifically applied:[j]

> A remedy which is often remarkably helpful to one or even many is very harmful to another if not properly and skilfully administered.[71]

> It is quite familiar in practice that remedies lose or retain their powers or acquire new powers according to the nature and activity of the disease and the various conditions under which the remedies are administered.[72]

> A certain active principle inheres in drugs but widespread observations indicate that the effect may be impaired, set aside, or changed, because of differences in the patients.[73]

The Rationalist physician imagines himself a skilled artist who adjusts a scientific theory to the specific practical features of the case before him.[k]

The orientation toward *communia* vs. that toward *propria* determines the nosologies of the two doctrines. Where Rationalism classifies diseases in terms of their *communia* and associated pathology, Empiricism (especially in its homoeopathic form) classifies according to the *propria* of the curative remedy.

Nosological classification in Rationalism is a necessary preface to treatment. Since Empiricism classifies in terms of

[j]At times Boerhaave was unwilling to admit that practice was unscientific: "there are other reasons why [practice] should rather be called a science . . . because its theory is put into practice not by simple imitation, but by the knowledge of causes" (*Academical Lectures,* I, 55).

[k]Bacon denied that this was possible: "For though one might speciously pretend that a learned physician should rather suit his medicines occasionally, as the constitution of the patient, his age, customs, the seasons, etc. require, than rest upon any certain prescriptions; yet this is a fallacious opinion that underrates experience and overrates human judgment" (*Adv. of Learning,* VI, cap. II).

the curative remedy, i.e., after treatment has been completed, the need for a nosology disappears. Empiricism renounces classification in favor of the individualization of treatment.

The two doctrines may be contrasted in terms of their respective theories of causation.

Rationalism hypothesizes the existence of an infinite series of material or efficient causes culminating in the "proximate cause" of the disease. While these anterior causes (and final causes as well) are unknown to the physician, they are unimportant for practice.[74]

> We may also affirm that the primary physical causes, in what manner, and the [final] metaphysical causes, for what end, the most general appearances are in a determinate manner effected, are neither possible, useful, nor necessary to be investigated by a physician.[75]

> First causes are outside the realm of science.[76]

Hoffmann explains this as follows: the growth of plants is caused by light, heat, and rain, and the gardener manipulates these to promote better growth, but he is not interested in what causes the light, heat, and rain themselves.[77] Bernard discusses it in terms of the "how" and "why" of phenomena: "in medicine it is . . . absurd to concern oneself with the question 'why'."[78]

> Men of science who carry experimental analysis to the point of relatively determining a phenomenon doubtless see clearly their own ignorance of the phenomenon in its primary cause; but they have become its master; the instrument at work is unknown, but they can use it.[79]

To Stahl Rationalism is illogical in hoping to affect the (material) "proximate cause" without affecting the chain of preexisting material causes. He considers this an unpromising avenue of investigation and discards material causes as appropriate only to mechanics and hydraulics. The cause of interest to the physician is the formal cause represented by the

Anima sensitiva.[80] Being autonomous and self-determined, the *Anima* is not dependent on any preexisting cause, and it can—with perfect doctrinal consistency—be acted upon by the physician. The cause of the *Anima*'s actions lies in the future, not in the past; it is a final (teleological) cause—God's will that man enjoy long life. All efforts by the physician in the patient's behalf are necessarily in harmony with this final cause.[l]

While God, in Boerhaave's system, is the efficient cause of the material changes which lead up to the proximate cause of disease, in Stahl's system He is the goal toward whom the universe and its inhabitants are tending.[81]

Holism vs. Reductionism

The necessary corollary of Empiricism's outward orientation is holism: since the world of nature is a whole, the doctrine which seeks to represent it must be holistic. Rationalism, by the same token, is reductionist: guided by an *a priori* idea, it cuts into the living phenomena to seek security in some subsurface abstraction.

In the eighteenth century the dispute between holism and reductionism was over the validity of the "formal cause," brought into medicine by Paracelsus and taken up by Van Helmont, Sydenham, Baglivi, and Stahl.[82] [m] Boerhaave refused to accept this "seminal principle which so determines the structure of vegetable bodies in their growth that they can appear in such a particular form and no other."[83] Hoffmann was even more to the point: "there are no substantial forms, but all of these represent accidents with respect to matter . . . Hence all forms are material [*mate-*

[l]Stahl observes that since man does not possess comprehensive knowledge of God's plans for the world, medicine is based upon uncertain causal knowledge (*Theoria Medica Vera,* I, 125).

[m]See *Divided Legacy,* I, 409-410 and above, pp. 34, 57, 200, 236.

riales] and can be transformed into one another. They are produced in mechanical fashion."[84]

Virchow wrote in 1849: "it is a pity that not a few people suppose that when processes are considered as a whole, something peculiar and individual always remains . . ."[85] Bernard realized that holism was a necessary corollary of the vitalism which he rejected:

> Many physicians and speculative physiologists . . . assume a vital force in opposition to physico-chemical forces, dominating all the phenomena of life, subjecting them to entirely separate laws, and making the organism an organized whole which the experimenter may not touch without destroying the quality of life itself . . . Cuvier, who shares this opinion and thinks that physiology should be a science of observation and of deductive anatomy, expresses himself thus, "All parts of a living body are interrelated; they can act only insofar as they act all together; trying to separate one from the whole means transferring it to the realm of dead substances; it means entirely changing its essence."
>
> If the above objections were well founded, we should either have to recognize that determinism is impossible in the phenomena of life, and this would be simply denying biological science; or else we should have to acknowledge that vital force must be studied by special methods, and that the science of life must rest on different principles from the science of inorganic bodies.[86]

Physiology's answer to the holistic challenge was the cell: thereafter researchers could penetrate into the body at will without trespassing on holistic ground provided they remained above the cellular level.

> Physiologists, indeed, have only to take apart the living machine . . . with the help of tools and processes borrowed from physics and chemistry.[87]

It is doubtless correct to say that the constituent parts of an organism are physiologically inseparable one from

> another, and that they all contribute to a common vital result; but we may not conclude from this that the living machine must not be analyzed as we analyze a crude machine whose parts also have their role to play in a whole.[88]

The holism of Empiricism and reductionism of Rationalism lead them to opposed interpretations of certain critical elements of medical doctrine.

For example, the Empirics have no difficulty accepting the "idiosyncrasy"—as merely another instance of the inaccessibility of biological causes to the human mind. Describing disease and health in symptomatic terms, they can fit idiosyncrasy into their method. But Bernard sees idiosyncrasy as a potential methodological obstacle, its acceptance meaning that medicine, "in contrast to the other sciences, should be established more and more on particulars. This opinion is incorrect . . . for in all sciences generalization leads to the law of the phenomena and the true scientific goal . . ."[89] He reduces idiosyncrasy to "the degree of organic sensitivity, which can be varied to infinity."[90] "I will show that if these differences were essential [*differences de nature*], rather than merely of degree, the science [of medicine] would be an impossibility."[91]

On the meaning of "sickness" itself the two traditions diverge.

Empirics look upon sickness and health as a continuum, since the organism interacts with the environment in both.[n] The dictum, "Man is always sick," attributed to Hippocrates by Stahl, best characterizes this viewpoint.[92]

Therefore, Empiricism does not distinguish between physiology and pathology.[93]

Rationalism, on the contrary, draws a line between physiology, the science of the "normal," and pathology, the

[n]The healthy organism's "idiosyncrasy" is, *inter alia,* a predisposition to certain types of sickness, being converted into sickness if carried to an extreme. Homoeopathic experience has shown that the symptoms of the sick patient are often only an intensification of the symptoms he manifests in a state of health.

science of the "abnormal."[94] The physician must understand the "normal" in order to comprehend the "abnormal."[95] [o] Sicknesses are *"res contra naturam,* things preternatural or contrary to nature."[96]

The Methodists also assimilate sickness and health but, in contrast to Empiricism, view the organism as always healthy—sickness being normal physiology under altered conditions. Pathology is absorbed by physiology: "general physiology is the basic biological science toward which all others converge."[97] "Pathology . . . is no longer merely applied physiology; it has become physiology itself."[98]

Where the Empirical assimilation of health to sickness is holistic, based on an interpretation of man's place in the universe, the Methodist assimilation of sickness to health is reductionism in its ultimate form—the logical consequence of a cellular or corpuscular theory of the organism.

Their differing interpretations of sickness lead the Empirics, Rationalists, and Methodists to different positions with respect to the number of symptoms significant for treatment and the number of diseases in the world.

To the Empirics the number of morbific stimuli, as exciting causes of sickness, is infinite; hence the number of possible reactions to these stimuli must also be infinite, and there is an infinity of diseases (or sicknesses) in the world—each, *in each individual patient,* distinguished from all others by its own *propria.*

The Rationalists look not to the exciting cause in the environment but to the "proximate cause" inside the organism and limit the number of significant symptoms to those which seem clearly related to this cause. And for psychological reasons—the inability of the human mind to imagine an infinity of abstract processes inside the body—they hold the number of diseases to be finite, not infinite.

[o]Lordat of Montpellier criticized Magendie for asserting that knowledge of the normal organism is needed to treat correctly (Lordat, *De la Necessite de Creer dans Chaque Faculte de Medecine une Chaire de Philosophie Naturelle Inductive,* 35).

Boerhaave provides many examples of this reductionist process. A large number of diseases are caused by "obstructions."[99] Again, "an irregular motion of the animal spirits differently varied may produce, maintain, and increase a great number of diseases, with various symptoms."[100] Or, "hysterical women often become paralytic or apoplectic from slight passions . . . all these disorders lie in the same humor."[101] He holds that pathological changes generally can be reduced to alterations in the humors or in the connections among the component parts: "from this consideration only, an infinite number of kinds of disease may be banished."[102] In short, many different symptom patterns can be ascribed to "one and the same simple, material, and efficient cause, if it is applied after a different manner to different parts of the body."[103]

Even the theory of coction, the key to the natural variety of diseases in Empiricism, becomes a reductionist technique with Boerhaave:

> The concoctions are as various as the crudities themselves, and these again as various as their proximate causes; from thence proceeds that infinite variety in the method of healing. Yet in general is this matter comprised in a few heads which are simple enough; for all that Nature does by concoction is to attenuate the humors inspissated, to obtund those which are acrid, relax the fibers and vessels which are rigid, etc.[104]

Reductionism is carried to an extreme in Methodism. This school in ancient times reduced the classes of disease to three, Brown limited them to two, and Broussais cut them down to only one. Not to be outdone, Bernard seems to reduce the number of diseases to zero when he states that "disease does not exist, in the sense that it is only a special case of a general physiological law,"[105] and he was strongly opposed to what he viewed as the "nosology" or "ontology" of Empiricism: "the modern physiologist wants to destroy pathology as a distinct science and thereby to destroy nosologies."[106] Diseases are no longer to be considered, as in

Hippocratic medicine, "entities, beings which develop, live, and die as individuals."[107] They disappear, being absorbed by the three physiological functions which Bernard recognizes: the blood, the nervous system, and the connective tissue.[108] [p]

Hence, although individual differences among patients introduce an element of "frightful complexity" into medicine, this should not "terrify" the physician.[109] "No two patients are ever exactly alike, their age, sex, temperament, and any number of other circumstances involve differences."[110] But the variety is only apparent and can be reduced ultimately to a finite number of underlying mechanisms: "the real and effective cause of a disease must be *constant* and *determined,* that is, unique; anything else would be a denial of science in medicine."[111] "Science consists in subordinating the particular to the general, understanding all varieties in terms of a unitary type."[112] [q]

> A poison or a morbid condition, acting on a definite histological unit, should attack it in like circumstances in all animals furnished with it; otherwise these units would cease to be of like nature; and if we went on considering as of like nature units reacting in different or opposite ways under the influence of normal or pathological vital reagents, we should not only deny science in general, but also bring into zoology confusion and darkness that would absolutely block its advance.[113]

Rationalism is so convinced of the truth and accuracy of its disease categories that it denies legitimacy to those which

[p]He did not even admit that syphilis is a specific disease, while measles and scarlet fever are only functional disorders of the skin (*Principes,* 140-141).

[q]Knud Faber wrote about Bernard: "He had not the slightest comprehension of the continual growth, the continual scientific development, and transformation of conceptions of disease which takes place in clinical medicine. A similar point of view is still sometimes taken by physiologists and experimental pathologists who have received their training far from the bedside" (Faber, "Nosography in Modern Internal Medicine," 27).

fall outside the classification. Galen spoke of "illegitimate" fevers and fevers with "extra" symptoms.[114] Boerhaave divides diseases into "original" ("idiopathic") and "symptomatic" ("deuteropathic"), these latter "being themselves a symptom or consequence of another disorder, as, for example, a peripneumonia arising from a pleurisy is a symptomatic disorder."[115]

Curtailing the number of possible diseases, Rationalism also curtails the number of remedies needed: "many diseases are often removed by one remedy."[116]

> As from one humor all others are derived, it may be granted, say the chemists, that one medicine may cure them all. Thus the same medicines which taken inwardly will remove an inflammation in the finger, will likewise remove an equal degree of inflammation in the kidneys, pleura and other internal parts.[117]

Booerhaave treated all "obstructions" with mercury and "diluent" medicines,[118] all "irregular motions" of the animal spirits with opium.[119] And the diseases associated with coction were also subjected to the same kinds of therapy:

> If Nature excites too much motion in the humors, they are to be quieted; if an inflammatory spissitude offends, the vessels are to be relaxed, and the humors to be attenuated that they may freely circulate.[120]

Hoffmann, referring all diseases to the systole and diastole of the heart, states: "having noted how few are the sources of diseases and how simple the causes which derange the economy of the body, it is not surprising that I maintain that there are only a few remedies for curing them."[121] "We should realize that no sort of remedy is effective in single cases only. Hence, unless effectiveness is properly observed in all cases of the remedy . . . you will not gain your desired goal."[122]

While to Empiricism, and especially to homoeopathy, each remedy is specific to a given diseased state, Rationalist doctrine has no metaphysical space for a theory of specific remedies. Such remedies were used because quinine and mercury, for example, were staples of practice, but Cullen's and Brown's remarks about "specifics" show graphically the Rationalist/Methodist distrust of medicines which could not be doctrinally explained.[r]

The preference of Rationalists and Methodists for more "general" remedies which acted according to known principles and could be used in a variety of different diseased states is seen in Virchow's remark that the use of "specifics" reflects the "ontological standpoint" in therapy–rightly attacked by Broussais and represented, above all, by homoeopathy:

> As soon as one is convinced that disease entities do not exist, one must also understand that therapeutic entities cannot be opposed to them, or, to speak in the style of Hahnemann, that a battle between two instances of the same entity cannot be engendered in the same body. This question has been adequately disposed of in scientific medicine. If disease is only an orderly manifestation of certain phenomena of life, normal in themselves, that occur under abnormal conditions, with deviations that are merely quantitative, then all treatment must be directed essentially against the altered conditions . . . Thus a rational interpretation of specific remedies must concern itself only with the question of whether a definite, particular, and specific therapeutic procedure . . . ought to be set up for a definite phase of a disease.[123]

And Rationalists not only give preference to "proximate causes" inside the body over exciting causes in the environment, they reduce the latter to the status of the former,

[r]See above, pp. 296-297.

bringing exciting causes inside the body and thereby rupturing the holistic tie between organism and environment.

Rationalists view exciting causes as difficult to define (Sydenham's "constitutions" being the most notorious), hence resistant to incorporation in a logically structured doctrine. They project them into the body where they can be analyzed better.

Boerhaave defines the "proximate cause" as the product of the "remote cause" and the "accessory cause."[124] The "remote cause," which "so changes the body that it becomes disposed or inclined to receive the disorder," can be outside the body, but also *inside* it—where it is termed the "proegumenal or predisposing cause; and such, for example, is the temperature, or constitution, a plethora, or cacochymia."[125] Other typical "remote causes" are "internal morbid dispositions of the body, of so general a nature that a great number of diseases may derive their causes from thence."[126] And the "accessory cause," also called by Boerhaave the "exciting cause," is "sometimes internal and sometimes external"—food, the movements of the body, the state of the *retenta* and *excreta,* baths, ointments, environmental influences, etc.[127]

What Boerhaave hesitantly commences Bernard's *milieu interieur* takes to a triumphant conclusion—pulling the whole external environment into the body, with all its exciting causes: Hippocrates thought that the external environment plays the major role in the development of disease, but physiology shows that the internal environment—the blood and the nervous system—are more important still.[128]

Only vegetables and the lower animals are dependent upon the external environment; as organisms evolve, they develop an internal environment which largely isolates them from external influences.[129] These latter can no longer affect the organism directly, so to speak, but only by passing first through the *milieu interieur.*[130]

> In the case of the complex higher organisms, physiologists and physicians must study the stimuli of vital

> phenomena, not in the relations of the whole organism with the general cosmic environment, but rather in the organic conditions of the inner environment. Considered in the general cosmic environment, the functions of man and of the higher animals seem to us, indeed, free and independent of the physico-chemical conditions of the environment, because its actual stimuli are found in an inner, organic, liquid environment. What we see from the outside is merely the result of physico-chemical stimuli from the inner environment; that is where physiologists must build up the real determinism of vital functions.[131]

The organism in the world of nature has been converted into a cell in the *milieu interieur.* When Bernard states "phenomena exhibiting life, like physico-chemical phenomena, result from contact between an active body and the environment in which it acts," he has in mind no longer a human body but an "anatomical unit" or "cell" in the *milieu interieur.*[132]

The exciting cause now acts only through building up in the individual a "predisposition"—a modification in the structure or properties of the *milieu interieur* and similar to the idiosyncrasy.[133] If the exciting cause were the principal factor, for instance, in pneumonia, everyone exposed to cold would come down with this disease, whereas only an occasional case of chill turns into pneumonia.[134] Unless the subject is predisposed, the most powerful causes (venoms, viruses) will have no effect on him.[135] Predisposition is the "pivot of all experimental physiology" and the real cause of most diseases.[136] In fact, only epidemic diseases have their causes in the external environment; all others have their locus, cause, and origin in the *milieu interieur.*[137]

An understanding of the Rationalist interpretation of disease and the exciting cause clarifies the development of the concept of the specific disease and Rationalism's acceptance of the germ theory of disease.

The "specific disease" concept was developed and expanded in the early nineteenth century by such Empirical

Paris thinkers as Bretonneau, Pariset, and Louis. Its reluctant acceptance by the Rationalist majority of the profession was a concession—a fusion of the finite Rationalist disease categories with the Empirical *divinum quid* or unknowable essence of disease.

The Empirical "sickness" of the individual person, unknowable in its essence, became the "disease" common to many which was also unknowable in its essence.

By the middle of the century thinkers had defined and isolated such attributes of the specific disease as materiality, contagiousness, and immunity. All that was lacking was a proximate cause.

Rationalism could not rest easy with its concession to Empiricism and was anxious to fill the gap in knowledge represented by the admission of a *divinum quid.* At the same time, causal speculation was tending to move the exciting cause out of the environment into the organism itself. So the causal factor needed to round out the theory of specific diseases was one which could exist in the external environment as well as in the human body: the "exciting cause" had to be convertible into a "proximate cause." The microorganisms of Pasteur and other researchers completely met this need and for that reason were at once accepted by the medical profession.

Like other Rationalists in history, those of the late nineteenth century thought that the discovery and definition of this new "cause" had made medical practice scientific. A truly rational causal therapy seemed at hand.

But, in fact, this doctrinal development only created a source of confusion in Rationalist medicine which persists to this day, i.e., the failure to distinguish between germs as possible causal agents in the environment and as causal factors (maintaining and supporting the disease) inside the body. The corollary of the realization that some diseases are generated by microorganisms in the environment seemed to be that cure is effected by eradicating or neutralizing these same microorganisms inside the body.

Virchow was wiser than most of his contemporaries in remarking that the bacterium in the environment may be the exciting cause of the disease, but it cannot be the disease itself when in the body, since the same microorganisms (of diphtheria, for instance) are also found in healthy persons.[138]

The tendency to seek "magic bullets" for each microorganism in the body was, of course, stimulated by the great success of preventive medicine in the latter decades of the nineteenth century. The reduced incidence of many epidemic and infectious diseases–due to better sanitation and nutrition–was ascribed to improved therapy.

The homoeopathic attitude toward the germ theory of disease resembles Virchow's. Hahnemann accepted the full variety of exciting causes in the environment and would have had no difficulty accepting microorganisms if he had lived in the bacteriological era. He did, after all, ascribe the 1832 cholera epidemic to a "brood of . . . excessively minute, invisible, living creatures."[139]

But homoeopathy also considers microorganisms as disease products in many cases, not causes. And it does not agree that diseases caused by microorganisms are cured by killing the microorganism inside the body. The vital energy reacts against miasmatic diseases and their exciting causes just as it does against other exciting causes, and the physician must support this reaction.

Hahnemann gave camphor in the early stages of cholera for its curative effect but also as a disinfectant–because it would "destroy the miasm [i.e., the microorganisms] about the patient."[140] Later stages of the disease, however, when the miasm or microorganisms had been internalized by the patient, were to be treated only with remedies directed at sustaining the vital force.[141]

His attitude toward microorganisms was identical with his attitude toward the treatment of worms. He held the presence of tapeworm to be the consequence of the patient's predisposition ("a general taint of the constitution"), and the remedy was not directed against the tapeworm itself. Rather it aimed to correct the patient's predisposition:

> so that the ill health of the patient, which causes this parasitic animal to be restless, is thereby for the time removed; the tapeworm then feels at ease, and lives on quietly in the excrement of the bowels without particularly distressing the patient or his intestines, until the antipsoric treatment is so far advanced that the worm, after the eradication of the psora, finds the contents of the bowels no longer suitable for its support, and therefore spontaneously disappears for ever from the now cured patient, without the least purgative medicine.[142] [s]

Scientific Medicine

Scientific method is a set of procedures for investigating nature to discover new knowledge. Its three stages are: (1) observation of the phenomena, (2) formulation of a hypothesis or hypotheses elucidating the laws and patterns of the observed phenomena, and (3) experimental verification of the hypothesis or hypotheses for accuracy and completeness.

When Empiricism and Rationalism are contrasted in terms of the requirements of scientific method, the former is seen to be congruent with this method, while the latter is alien, both in spirit and structure, to the scientific method of investigation.

Empiricism's assumption that the explicatory pattern of laws and relationships lies concealed beneath the surface of nature orients this school toward the discovery of new knowledge. Van Helmont wrote:

> Things not known before are properly discovered or found out, even as things not had, nor possessed, are gotten by discovery [*inventio*] or gift. For when any one showeth me *lapis Calaminaris,* the preparing of Cadmia or brass ore, the content of, or what is contained in, copper,

[s]This may be contrasted with Bernard's views on the treatment of scabies (above, p. 644).

> the mixture and uses of *Aurichalcum*, or copper and gold, which things I knew not before, he teacheth, demonstrateth, and giveth the knowledge of that which before there was ignorance of. But such like things logic never taught. Therefore, logical discovery is a mere retaking of that which was known before . . . which thing, indeed, is not the inventive office of sciences . . .[143]

Sydenham and Baglivi, quoting Bacon, repeatedly emphasize the importance of discovering new knowledge: "we have not to imagine, or to think out, but to find out, what nature does or promises."[144] "True medicine consists in the discovery of the real indications."[145]

Hence the Empirics are aware of the dichotomy between the external world of nature and the internal world of man's ideas, while the Rationalists are unaware of this or underemphasize it.

The distinction between the two schools in this respect was most pronounced in the ancient world where Rationalism read into natural processes the categories of formal logic, interpreting sickness and health as the interplay of the Aristotelian hot, cold, wet, and dry. But the same division was perpetuated in post-Renaissance medicine when Rationalism projected into the human physiology relationships derived from physics, chemistry, and hydraulics. Empirical physicians decried this also as illegitimate: however valuable physical, chemical, or hydraulic research may have been for the advancement of these disciplines, their results were as alien to medicine as the productions of formal logic. In both cases it meant extrapolating a rational construction of ideas into the human organism. Hence Sydenham calls Rationalism the "art of talking rather than the art of healing."[146] Baglivi urges the physician to proceed, not by disputation, but by experiments to "torment nature" and elicit the meaning of her secrets.[147] "Since all these [operations of the *physis*] are accomplished not by the work of the [physician's] mind, but independently of his mind, subtle and arcane disputation will not be of any use to us, but repeated and diligent observation of those things which occur in the individual patient."[148] Stahl, quoting Seneca, accuses Boerhaave of ignoring the distinction between how to dispute and how to live.[149]

And not only are the Empirics concerned to make discoveries, they do so by applying a method. "I was wholly absorbed in the grand operation of forging a Delphic sword in the shape of some *methodus medendi* which should meet all cases from amidst the multiformities and versatilities of nature."[150] "By a long continuance and frequent repetition of his experiments [the physician] may lay down and prescribe for himself a *methodus medendi* from which, in the cure of this or that disease, he need not deviate a single hair's breadth."[151]

Such a method is necessarily laborious and time-consuming:

> The reducing these rules and methods to a certainty, on the practice whereof the ease and recovery of sick men depends . . . whosoever shall think to compass it alone will find himself engaged in a business too large for any one man's comprehension and too great for his own single endeavors.[152]

> Ten men, succeeding each other through ten lifetimes, would not do it—not even though they had, each and all, unrivalled genius, unwearied industry, and the skill arising from long and manifold practice.[153]

> Medicine is the daughter of time, not of the human mind.[154]

The work involved in constructing the science is only a corollary of that required to cure the individual patient: "the laborious, sometimes very laborious, search for and selection of the homoeopathic remedy most suitable in every respect to each morbid state, is an operation which demands . . . a great amount of circumspection and serious deliberation . . . a laborious, care-demanding task . . ."[155]

Finally, they want the knowledge discovered to be *useful.*

> All speculations on this subject, however curious or refined, or seeming profound and solid, if they teach not their followers to do something either better or in a shorter and easier way than otherwise they could, or else lead them to the discovery of some new and useful invention, deserve not the name of knowledge.[156]

Bacon was the first to realize that practical utility is the goal of scientific endeavor–a feeling which motivated the scientific investigators of the seventeenth century and after: "the point in view is not only the contemplative happiness, but the whole fortunes, and affairs, and powers, and works of man."[157]

In order to discover this pattern concealed in nature the Empirics commence by developing the faculty of observation.[158] Sydenham is typical in holding that "true practice consists in the observations of nature; these are finer than any speculations."[159] Baglivi even urges the physician to provide a description of the method of observation employed.[160] Hahnemann's fanatically accurate observation of symptoms was only the culmination of an established tradition.

These observations give rise to a primary hypothesis–that cure is by the intrinsic healing power of the organism–the *physis*–assisted when necessary by the physician.[t]

Prior to the seventeenth century these thinkers used the word, "theory," not "hypothesis"; later the word, "hypothesis," was also used.[u] This hypothesis or theory, of course, itself emerged from centuries of experience which brought home to these physicians the important role played by the body's recuperative powers in healing.

Since the *physis* cures through coction, crisis, and evacuation, Empirical physicians endeavor to promote and

[t]See *Divided Legacy,* I, 10-33 and 68-88.

[u]Baglivi observes that the astronomers use various "hypotheses" to explain the movements of the stars and planets (*De Praxi Medica,* 108).

assist this natural process. When an Empiric treats a patient in this way, he is testing the validity of the hypothesis that cure is by the *physis*.

But prior to Hahnemann this method was relatively crude. His discovery of the proving and his new formulation of the principle of similars refined the Empirical technique of diagnosis and prescribing.[v]

Hahnemann asked himself the following questions:

I. How is the physician to ascertain what is necessary to be known in order to cure the disease?

II. How is he to gain a knowledge of the instruments adapted for the cure of the natural disease, the pathogenetic powers of the medicines?

III. What is the most suitable method of employing these artificial morbific agents (medicines) for the cure of natural diseases?[161]

The provings gave answers to questions I and II. The symptom-pattern of each drug revealed its pathogenetic (i.e., its therapeutic) powers. And this same symptom-pattern, as perceived in the patient, was "what is necessary to be known in order to cure the disease."

Furthermore, it was now possible to distinguish methodically between *propria* and *communia*—in the symptom-patterns of drugs as in those of the patients.[w]

[v]However, many of Hahnemann's pharmacological insights had already been prefigured in Van Helmont: that very small doses are effective (*Oriatrike*, 595), that poisons are remedies (*ibid.*, 465), that medicines act more strongly on the sick person (*ibid.*, 593), that "quality" is more important in a medicine than "quantity" (*ibid.*, 594), that medicines can transfer their "quality" to a neutral medium (*ibid.*, 576, 585), that unity of the disease presupposes unity of the remedy (i.e., the single remedy) (*ibid.*, 574), etc.

[w]In this way homoeopathy solves the problem posed by William Windelband of combining "idiographic" and "nomothetic" knowledge (see *Divided Legacy*, I, Introduction). The law of similars and the provings made possible the generation of a large number of idiographic "drug pictures" which at the same time serve as standards of identity for an equal (or greater) number of diseased states. And yet they are all tied together in an intellectual and scientific structure by the law of similars.

Question III was answered by the law of similars—Hahnemann's new hypothesis which was auxiliary to the traditional Empirical hypothesis that cure is by the *physis.*

Like this traditional hypothesis, Hahnemann's law of similars itself emerged from experience—Hahnemann's testing, on himself and his family, of substances for their pure pharmacological effects.[x]

From the point of view of scientific method the law of similars is seen to have refined the traditional hypothesis of cure by the *physis,* to have made possible its elaboration into a series of far more precise hypotheses—each relating to the use of a given medicinal substance in a given diseased state as defined by its symptoms.

Hahnemann revalued the Empirical concepts, "observation" and "experience." "Observation" henceforth meant observation of the pure symptoms developed by healthy persons during the proving of remedies. "Experience" meant practice guided by the hypothesis that cure is by similars.

Empirics prior to Hahnemann had realized that all experience is not equally valid. They had a sophisticated understanding of the relationship between the "facts" observed, i.e., the "experience," and the "theory" or "hypothesis" generating these "facts" and "experience." Stahl, for instance, states that only those facts are valid which emerge during the course of treatment based upon a correct understanding of final causes (i.e., of the *Anima sensitiva*).[162] All others corrupt medical thought and engender dangerous therapeutic procedures.[163] Boerhaave's "facts," in particular, are selected arbitrarily—hence fallacious: he invents new diseases and confuses the cases he has before him.[164]

Bordeu exclaims: "every purblind person today says 'I have seen this, done that, observed the other thing,' " but

[x]The homoeopathic school called attention to the fact that these were the first pure pharmacological experiments in the history of medicine (*Arch. de la Medecine Homoeopathique* I [1834], 91-108).

what is significant is the role which theory allocates to these observations and this experience; useful observations must be distinguished from useless ones.[165]

Hahnemann also knew that all "experience" is not equally valid. Physicians invariably invoke it to justify their preferred procedures, but "experience" is meaningless in the absence of the correct method and the necessary controls:

> Occasionally a regular brother practitioner stumbles by a lucky hit upon a cure which astonishes half the world about him, and not less himself; but among the many medicines he employed he is by no means sure which did good. Not less frequently does the neck-or-nothing practitioner, without a degree, whom the world calls a quack, make as great and wonderful a cure. But neither he nor yet his worshipful brother practitioner with a diploma knows how to isolate the evident and fruitful truth which the cure contains. Neither can separate and record the medicine which certainly was of use out of the mass of useless and obstructing ones they employed; neither precisely indicates the case in which it did good and in which it will certainly benefit again. Neither knows how to abstract a truth which will hold good in all future time, an appropriate, certain, unfailing remedy for every such case that may occur hereafter. His experience in this case, remarkable though it seemed, will almost never be of service to him in any other.[166]

> I do not mean that sort of experience of which the ordinary practitioners of the Old School boast, after they have for years worked away with a lot of complex prescriptions on a number of diseases which they never carefully investigated, but which, faithful to the tenets of their school, they considered as already described in works of systematic pathology, and dreamed that they could detect in them some imaginary morbific matter, or ascribed to them some other hypothetical internal abnormality. They always saw something in them, but knew not what it was they saw, and they got results, from the

> complex forces acting on an unknown object, that no human being but only a God could have unravelled—*results from which nothing can be learned, no experience gained.* Fifty years' experience of this sort is like fifty years of looking into a kaleidoscope filled with unknown colored objects, and perpetually turning around; thousands of ever-changing figures and no accounting for them.[167]

Successes obtained in this way teach the physician nothing; they are like winning a lottery by playing the same number every day.[168]

To acquire genuine experience the physician must be guided by a hypothesis:

> "Surely the physician," I fancy I hear one exclaim, "requires a theory at once for a clue, a thread upon which to string his ideas and systematic practice, and a line to direct him at the sick-bed. Every artist who is not a mere mechanic must desire to have some connection of ideas in his mind as he works, concerning the character of the object on which he is to labor and the condition into which he is to mold it."
>
> "True," I reply, "but this clue must neither be a flimsy cobweb nor a false guide, for then it were worse than none."[169]

Experience in the absence of a hypothesis Hahnemann calls "parempiricism," that acquired by applying the hypothesis of similars "empiricism": *"parempiricism* may stand for the evil demon, *empiricism* for the good genius of experience."[170] [y]

Hahnemann defined homoeopathy as the "science of experience."[171] Because its method was scientific, homoeo-

[y]By coining this new word Hahnemann solved the problem of how to distinguish the Empiric (an adherent of the Empirical tradition) from the "empiric" (an uneducated physician). The latter denotation was presumably introduced by the ancient Rationalists who regarded their competitors, the Empirics, as uneducated (see *Divided Legacy,* I, 321).

pathy in the nineteenth century was able to revise, restructure, and revolutionize the greater part of existing pharmacology, developing hundreds of new applications of medicines of which many were adopted by allopathy.[z] This body of pharmacological knowledge is still in use today by homoeopathic practitioners in most countries of the world.[a] It has not had to undergo the periodic upheavals to which Rationalism is subject because this knowledge, generated by a valid method, remains valid.[b]

A method which relies on symptomatic description and eschews speculation about internal physiology and pathology is able to sidestep the perennial reformulations of physiological and pathological theory which are the hallmark of Rationalism. The symptoms themselves, after all, do not change. Provings made 150 years ago remain valid and useful today, and the same is true for many of the homoeopathic case histories.[c]

The stability of homoeopathy—today nearly 200 years old and unchanged in any essential respect from its original

[z]See Coulter, *Homoeopathic Influences in Nineteenth-Century Allopathic Therapeutics.* This was the heart of nineteenth-century medicine, but it has been slighted by historians who seem to write principally about the discovery of ether (betokening their unconsciousness of the real issues). The contemptuous dismissal of homoeopathic pharmacology reflects the assumption that "truly effective" drug therapy commenced in the early twentieth century with the synthesis of acetanalide by the German petrochemical industry. The argument that most or all of the existing pharmacological agents were impotent was initially advanced by William Osler as part of his campaign against homoeopathy (*Divided Legacy,* III, 250, 448-449). The ambiguous attitude of historians to nineteenth-century pharmacology is perhaps a subconscious reaction to the dominant role played by homoeopathy.

[a]It is, of course, ignored by allopathy and remains buried in the libraries and basements of medical schools, subject only to the gnawing criticism of the mice.

[b]The stability of the homoeopathic method is interpreted by Rationalism as a sign of stagnation.

[c]Carroll Dunham, a leader of American nineteenth-century homoeopathy, defined a scientific medicine as one possessing the "capability of infinite progress in each of its elements without detriment to its integrity as a whole" (*Homoeopathy, the Science of Therapeutics* [Philadelphia: Boericke, 1885], 13).

formulation by Hahnemann—is thus evidence of its scientific nature.[d]

Another characteristic of scientific knowledge is precision. Hahnemann thought that homoeopathy, relying on the *propria* rather than on the *communia,* would make medicine as precise as mathematics.[172] And he held his followers to this standard of precision: "He who does not walk on exactly the same line with me, who diverges, if it be but the breadth of a straw, to the right or the left, is an apostate and a traitor, and with him I will have nothing to do."[173] [e]

Finally, a scientific medicine is concise—reflecting Bacon's dictum: "Once fashioned into methods, the science no longer grows in bulk."[174] Since new knowledge can be assimilated into the existing corpus, the essentials of homoeopathy can be compressed into a handful of books. The whole science becomes manageable by the individual practitioner.

Rationalist theory has a different purpose and function—consequently, a different structure. Whereas Empirical "theory" is a set of rules for medical practice, Rationalist "theory" is a metaphysic of the human physiology. While, in Empiricism, observation, hypothesis, and experience are directed at elaborating the doctrine of cure by the *physis*—i.e., of developing a therapeutic method—these same ingredients in Rationalism are employed to develop a theory of how the sick and healthy organism functions. Healing

[d]The impact of homoeopathy on world medicine may be judged from the number of editions of the *Organon* published to date: 115 editions in 16 languages, published in 18 different countries of Europe, Asia, and North and South America (J. Baur, M.D., *Petite Histoire de l'Organon et de ses Metamorphoses* [privately printed, 1975], 159).

[e]While welcomed by the patients, this precision (a necessary attribute of any scientific endeavor) created serious difficulties for the homoeopathic physicians. The conflict between those who urged precision and those who attempted to evade it seriously weakened American homoeopathy in the late nineteenth and early twentieth centuries (*Divided Legacy,* III, Chapter VI). Even the homoeopathic physician was unwilling to have his practice held up to an objective standard.

practice is derived from this theory of the organism by applying an auxiliary hypothesis—that cure is by "contraries."

The most comprehensive Rationalist (or Rationalist/ Methodist) medical theory of modern times, that of Claude Bernard, is still regarded as a model for physicians in the twentieth century.[f]

The most striking characteristic of his writings on medicine and physiology is the pervasive assumption that the organism is material and functions in a physico-chemical fashion—meaning that it obeys the laws of physics and chemistry and that the movements of the organism are determined *a priori* by the laws of these disciplines. "Determinism in the conditions of vital phenomena should be one of the axioms of experimenting physicians."[175] "It is precisely the recognition of determinism that characterizes true men of science."[176]

This determinist hypothesis was never examined, but merely taken on faith:

> The absolute determinism of phenomena, of which we are conscious *a priori,* is the only criterion or principle which directs and supports us.[177]
>
> If [physicians] are fully imbued with the truth of this principle, they will exclude all supernatural intervention from their explanations; they will have unshaken faith in the idea that fixed laws govern biological science.[178]

George Cheyne, in a more believing era, had also taken this hypothesis on faith:

> We must not think that the beneficent Author of nature has left men to chance, casualty, or blind fate, in the

[f]"At once the reader obtains a clear and penetrating view of the nature of science and an insight into the growth of the ideas of one of the greatest of all men of science" (from the 1957 Foreword to the Dover edition of Bernard's *Experimental Medicine*). Twentieth-century physicians have been conspicuously reluctant to discuss the theoretical bases of what is called "scientific medicine" (understandably, in view of the tremendous economic interests involved), leaving Bernard's formulation unchanged.

> conduct of their life and health. There are in physic, as in the natural and moral world, general laws, universal propositions, and a perpetual analogy that runs through the world of science for that end.[179]

Thus Rationalism equates physico-chemical or mechanistic determinism with biological "science."

> We must acknowledge as an experimental axiom that in living beings as well as in inorganic bodies the necessary conditions of every phenomenon are absolutely determined . . . Negation of this proposition would be nothing less than the negation of science itself.[180]

> Real science exists, then, only from the moment when a phenomenon is accurately defined as to its nature and rigorously determined in relation to its material conditions, that is, when its law is known.[181]

Determinism had strong emotional roots in Bernard—who devoted his life to biology: "absolute determinism exists indeed in every vital phenomenon; hence biological science exists also; and consequently the studies to which we are devoting ourselves *will not all be useless.*"[182]

Since medical science must exist, and science is determinism, medical determinism must exist also.[g]

Like Descartes, Bernard advocates invincible distrust of every idea except the one at the root of his own philosophy:

> The first condition to be fulfilled by men of science, applying themselves to the investigation of natural phenomena, is to maintain absolute freedom of mind, based on philosophic doubt. Yet we must not be in the least sceptical; we must believe in science, i.e., in determinism . . .[183]

While doubting is good, "scepticism" is harmful: "the sceptic disbelieves in science and believes in himself . . . The doubter

[g]Bernard's way of reasoning resembles Louis' holding that patients must fall into discrete pathological-anatomical classes because medical science so requires (above, p. 519).

is a true man of science; he doubts only himself and his interpretations [*sic*], but he believes in science; in the experimental sciences he even accepts a criterion or absolute scientific principle. This principle is the determinism of phenomena which is as absolute in the phenomena of living bodies as in those of inorganic matter."[184h]

Just as Empiricism is permeated by the assumption of the organism's vitality, Rationalism is permeated by a mechanistic determinism.

The effects of the two assumptions, however, are quite different. Whereas the vitalist assumption encourages observation and reliance on experience–since knowledge of the spontaneous and autonomous *physis* can be discovered only in this way–the determinist assumption has the opposite effect, vitiating and denaturing observation and experience.

For a determinist approach to biology is equivalent to assuming that the requisite knowledge of the organism is already available. Nothing really new remains to be discovered, since the causal relations are already known in principle and only need elaboration. Observation and experience are directed to the detailed working out of known relationships–not to the discovery of new knowledge.

Rationalist thinkers had always mistrusted observation and experience.[i] The final vitiation and evisceration of these concepts was the work of Claude Bernard.

He mistrusts pure observation–appropriate only to the "sciences of observation" or "empirical sciences" which are to be transformed into "experimental sciences."[185]

[h]Magendie also prided himself on his philosophic "doubt": "Doubt, and I am not talking here of that scepticism which questions even that which has been proved, doubt as applied only to facts not yet clarified and to suppositions devoid of proof–this doubt, I say, is the seal of true knowledge" (*Systeme Nerveux,* I, 17).

[i]Cullen had written, for instance: "when the physician cannot establish a system of practice chiefly founded on the doctrine of proximate causes . . . [he] will have recourse to experience alone, always, however, aware of the hitherto incomplete and fallacious state of Empiricism" (*First Lines of the Practice of Physic,* I, 54).

In the "observational sciences," of which astronomy is the best example, the scientist can observe events but does not know their causes and cannot affect their progress and outcome; in the "experimental sciences" the scientist knows the causes and can participate in bringing about certain results: "in this power of the investigator to act on phenomena, precisely here is the difference separating the so-called sciences of experimentation from those of observation."[186] [j]

Hence, in experimental science the observation is only a starting-point which must be developed by adding to it a knowledge of the causal mechanism: "an observation made, a comparison established, and a judgment rendered."[187] Observation without an explanation of what has been observed is worthless:

> If I were planning a treatise on experimental medicine, I should go to work by invariably making observation of disease the basis of every experimental analysis. I should then proceed with my explanations, symptom by symptom, until I had exhausted all the information obtainable from present experimental physiology, and the result of all of this would be medical observation reduced to its simplest terms.[188]

Or, in short, "to make a good medical observation it is not only necessary to have an observing mind, but also to be a physiologist."[189]

This brings Bernard to the next stage, the hypothesis. His dominant hypothesis is the mechanistic determinism of vital functions, but he calls this an "axiom," a "criterion," or a "principle," rather than a hypothesis.[190] What he calls "hypothesis" is an anticipative idea or feeling that some observed phenomenon is generated by a particular causal

[j]But "from the point of view of philosophic method there is no essential difference between sciences of observation and sciences of experimentation" (Bernard, *Experimental Medicine,* 18).

mechanism: "Feeling gives rise to the experimental idea or hypothesis, i.e., the previsioned interpretation of natural phenomena."[191]

> The mind of man cannot conceive an effect without a cause, so that the sight of a phenomenon always awakens an idea of causation. All human knowledge is limited to working back from observed effects to their cause. Following an observation, an idea connected with the cause of the observed phenomenon presents itself to the mind. We then inject this anticipative idea into a train of reasoning by virtue of which we make experiments to verify it.[192]

> The goal which the experimental method sets itself is everywhere the same; it consists in connecting natural phenomena with their necessary conditions or with their immediate causes.[193]

Experiment serves only to verify the correctness of the scientist's assumption of a particular causal mechanism at work: "to reason experimentally we must usually have an idea and afterwards induce or produce facts, i.e., observations, to verify our preconceived idea."[194]

The outcome or product of such experiments is a series of "facts":

> The experimenter . . . makes suppositions about the cause of actions taking place before his eyes; and to learn whether the hypothesis which serves as groundwork for his interpretation is correct he takes measures to make facts appear which in the realm of logic may be either the confirmation or the negation of the idea which he has conceived.[195]

These "facts" exist independently and eternally, regardless of the method used to investigate and elucidate them: "the relation of a phenomenon to a definite cause is necessary and independent of experiment; it is necessarily mathematical and absolute."[196] "If a hypothesis is not verified and disappears, the facts which it has enabled us to find are nonetheless acquired as indestructible materials for science."[197] Before their causation is known, they are "crude facts"; afterwards they become "scientific facts"—"facts are necessary materials, but their working up by experimental reasoning, i.e., by theory, is what establishes and really builds up the science."[198]

Bernard thus views the organism as a piece of clockwork which can operate in only one direction. However it is set moving, it always goes the same way: "there is nothing disturbed or abnormal in nature; everything happens according to laws which are absolute, i.e., always normal and determined . . ."[199] Just about any sort of "experiment" has some value. One he frequently employed involved "a variation or disturbance that an investigator brings into the conditions of natural phenomena . . . we suppress an organ in the living body by a section or ablation, and from the disturbance produced in the whole organism or in a special function we deduce the function of the missing organ."[200] He called these "experiments by destruction," and they had an ancient lineage:

> Galen performed almost no other kind of experiment than that which we call disturbing experiments, which consist in wounding, destroying, or removing a part, so as to judge its function by the disturbance caused by its removal . . . Since Galen at long intervals in the midst of medical systems, eminent vivisectors have appeared.[201]

He even followed Magendie in suggesting "fishing in troubled waters," meaning cutting at random into the body of a live animal to see what would happen: "such groping experiments . . . may be called *experiments to see,* because they are intended to make a first observation emerge, unforeseen and undetermined in advance, but whose appearance may suggest an experimental idea and open a path for research."[202] [k]

Bernard took his definition of "fact" from Magendie, the uneducated primitive who knew nothing of medical histo-

[k] These seem to be patterned on Bacon's "experiments for light"!! See above, p. 90*c*.

ry,[203] refused to discuss theory,[l] and was convinced that all "facts" (especially his own) were equally valid. He called himself a "ragpicker, with my spiked stick in my hand and a basket on my back, wandering over the field of science and picking up whatever I find."[204] [m] "The facts are no different in Paris than in Montpellier."[205]

The definition of "fact" given by Bernard and Magendie should be contrasted with Stahl's—meaning what is revealed during the course of cure when treatment is based on the true theory.[n]

Bernard's "experimental medicine" is a major effort to come to grips with the concept of medical "experience." By reducing observation and experience to "experiment," "experiment" to "fact," and "fact" to *ratio*, he brings all medical experience under the sway of the experimental physiologist's reasoning power.[o,p]

[l]Bernard wrote that Magendie had a "truly extraordinary revulsion for systematic thought. Whenever one spoke to him of medical doctrine or theory, he instinctively manifested a feeling of horror. On him this produced the effect which a false note produces on the trained ear of a musician. He always answered in the same way: 'All this,' he would say, 'is only words.' " To show his contempt for theoretical explanations (other than his own) Magendie liked to assert that he had "eyes but no ears" (Claude Bernard, *Francois Magendie: Lecon d'Ouverture du Cours de Medecine du College de France (29 Fevrier, 1856)* [Paris: Bailliere, 1856], 8, 25, 28).

[m]Magendie held that medical science progresses by assimilating more and more "facts." In its primitive "systematic" form, the facts are selected according to the fancy of the investigator; in its advanced, "theoretical," form all the "facts" have been incorporated (Magendie, *Precis Elementaire de Physiologie,* I, i).

[n]See above, p. 685.

[o]A small side-effect of Bernard's doctrine is that animals, devoid of *ratio,* are incapable of acquiring experience: "man alone is capable of gaining experience and perfecting himself by it" (*Experimental Medicine,* 11). While this may have been an advance over Descartes, who had denied that animals are even alive, the zoological realm in general seems to fare poorly in Rationalism.

[p]Paracelsus contrasted "experience" (*erfahrenheit*) with "experiment" (*experimentum*), using the latter word pejoratively (with the same meaning as Hahnemann's "parempiricism") (*Divided Legacy*, I, 468-469). Boissier de Sauvages

> Experience may be gained by empirical and unconscious reasoning, but the obscure and spontaneous movement of the mind has been raised by men of science into a clear and reasoned method . . . Such is the experimental method in the sciences by which experience is always gained by virtue of precise reasoning based on an idea born of observation and controlled by experiment.[206]

> Considered in itself, the experimental method is nothing but reasoning by whose help we methodically submit our ideas to experience—the experience of facts.[207]

> Experience is the fruit of exact reasoning applied to the interpretation of facts. It follows from this that we can gain experience without making experiments, solely by reasoning appropriately about well-established facts.[208]

> Outside of experimental reasoning observation and experiment no longer exist in this abstract sense; there are only concrete facts in each.[209]

In a word, "experience . . . is the privilege of reason."[210]

In this way Bernard expropriated the physician's right to independent experience: "the experimental method is characterized by being dependent only on itself, because it includes within itself its criterion—experience."[211] "Now, I repeat, only this logical verification can teach him and give him experience."[212]

Bernard's mechanist/determinist hypothesis thus cannot be disproved by any other therapeutic "facts," observations, or experience. If such a "fact," by some mischance, emerges, it must be rejected:

> If a phenomenon in an experiment had such a contradictory appearance that it did not necessarily connect itself with determinate causes, then reason should reject the

altered the meaning of "experiment": "experience" is what happens to the physician, "experiment" is what he helps bring about (*Nosologie Methodique,* I, 5).

> fact as non-scientific . . . to accept a fact without a cause, that is, indeterminate in its necessary conditions, is neither more nor less than the negation of science.[213]

> Of course I admit that facts are the only realities that can give form to the experimental idea and at the same time serve as its control; but this is on condition that reason accepts them. I think that blind belief in fact, which dares to silence reason, is as dangerous to the experimental sciences as the beliefs of feeling or of faith which also force silence on reason. In a word, in the experimental method as in everything else, the only real criterion is reason.[214]

Only the "empirics" attribute such great importance to "facts." They have an "exclusive cult of the fact" which is as deleterious for science as an exclusive cult of theory.[215]

No mere "fact" can stand in the way of all-conquering *ratio:*

> Indeed, while an experimenter must submit his ideas to the criterion of facts, I do not acknowledge that he must submit his reason; for then he would extinguish the torch of his inner criterion and would necessarily fall into the realm of the indeterminable.[216]

At most, such a "fact" should be held in abeyance until its cause has been ascertained:

> A crude fact is not scientific, and a fact whose causation is irrational should thus be ejected from science . . . In science many crude facts are doubtless still incomprehensible; I do not mean to conclude that we should wilfully reject all these facts. I wish simply to say that they should be held in reserve for a time as crude facts, and not introduced into science, i.e., into experimental reasoning, until their necessary conditions are defined in terms of rational determinism.[217]

The contrast between Rationalism and Empiricism as scientific disciplines can be summarized in terms of how they handle the hypothesis. Empiricism derives its hypothesis of the *physis* from observation and experience with the living organism (just as Hahnemann derived his subsidiary hypothesis of cure through similars by observing himself and his patients). The hypothesis originates in experience. And it is continually tested by experience—the physician's day-to-day treatment of his patients. But Bernard's mechanist/determinist physiological hypothesis is *a priori,* not derived from experience but taken on faith and imposed on experience. Nor can it be tested in practice, since all practice, observation, and experience have been reinterpreted in terms of this very hypothesis. The nature of the Rationalist theory and method prevents the mechanist/determinist hypothesis from being disproved.

Hence Empiricism must be considered a scientific discipline, while Rationalism, in both structure and purpose, is unscientific.

In fact, it is only a restatement of scholasticism. Bernard was a great scholastic thinker, in the debased Aristotelian tradition of Galen and Boerhaave.[q] The syllogism is the only true investigative technique: "[man] always proceeds instinctively from a principle, acquired or invented by hypothesis; but he can never go forward in reasoning otherwise than by syllogism, that is, by proceeding from the general to the particular."[218] He rejects induction and favors deduction, disparages Bacon while extolling Descartes.[219]

He alludes to the "joy of discovery which is certainly the liveliest that the mind of man can ever feel" but by this only means the joy of discovering another link in the causal chain proving the correctness of his mechanist/determinist hypothesis.[220] Such knowledge is not "new," in the Empirical sense of a new and permanent acquisition for science, because it is immediately vitiated by the elucidation of more

[q]His philosophy of medicine is patterned on Johan Georg Zimmermann's *Traite de l'Experience en General, et en Particulier dans l'Art de Guerir* (Paris: Vincent, 1774) which itself is entirely Galenic. See Bernard, *Principes,* 32.

distant links in the causal chain: "the joy of discovery, so sought and hoped for, vanishes as soon as found. It is but a flash whose gleam discovers for us fresh horizons toward which our insatiate curiosity repairs with still more ardor. Thus, even in science itself, the known loses its attraction, while the unknown is always full of charm."[221]

He is the best example of the type of scientist he criticized, the "scholastics or systematizers" who "never question their starting-point, to which they seek to refer everything; who have a proud and intolerant mind and do not accept contradiction, since they do not admit that their starting-point may change."[222] "Systematic and doctrinal physicians . . . take pure hypotheses, or else the facts taught them by empiricism, and join them together with the help of an ideal system from which they later deduce their line of medical conduct."[223] "Men who have excessive faith in their theories or ideas are not only ill prepared for making discoveries, they also make very poor observations. Of necessity they start with a preconceived idea, and when they devise an experiment, they can see in its results only a confirmation of their theory."[224] "Man is by nature metaphysical and proud. He has gone so far as to think that the idealistic creations of his mind, which correspond to his feelings, also represent reality."[225]

We have stated that Empiricism, and especially homoeopathy, is a stable doctrine, precise in its details, and compact in size.[r] By proceeding only on the basis of the known, i.e., the symptoms which are visible to the senses, homoeopathy remains on stable ground, and by relying on the *propria,* rather than the *communia,* it permits precise, hence effective, treatment.

The contrast with Rationalism is very great, for the latter is imprecise in detail, doctrinally unstable, and vast in amplitude.

[r]See above, pp. 688-689.

Imprecision is built into the structure of Rationalism, a consequence of its reliance on the *communia,* not the *propria.* When diagnosis and treatment are based upon the *communia,* representing the least common denominators of a variety of patients (differing to some extent among themselves), each individual patient must deviate from the norm. Hence there is no definition of the individual patient in Rationalism, only a statistical mean, and when this mean is applied by the physician to his patient, it can fit only approximately.[s]

The instability of Rationalism also stems from reliance on the *communia,* and in two ways:

(1) the *communia* are thought to represent an underlying causal entity, and Rationalist theory is made up of these causes. With every change in physiological theory, therefore, medical practice based upon the *communia* must also change.

(2) medicines developed to treat diseases defined by their *communia* must be sufficiently powerful to possess an impact over the range of slightly different conditions comprehended under each single *commune.* The consequence is an ever-increasing incidence of untoward effects (known as "side effects").[t]

Attention has been directed to this last point by Rene Dubos, a leading twentieth-century physiologist:

> Most of biological, physiological, and biochemical research has been focused so far on the study of the phenomena which are common to all living things . . . While this so-called fundamental approach has been immensely fruitful for the discovery of the structures and

[s]See *Divided Legacy,* III, 478-484.

[t]The expression, "side effects," is a misnomer, since, however undesired by the physician or patient, these are as much the "direct" effects of the drug as are the desired effects.

> reactions which are *common* to all forms of life, it has almost completely failed to provide information concerning the structures and reactions which determine the *peculiarities* of each organ and function . . . Powerful metabolic inhibitors have been synthesized on the basis of this knowledge, but in general they lack selectivity. Being directed against fundamental processes, they affect many different biological functions and are therefore likely to exhibit various forms of toxicity which sharply limit their usefulness.
>
> It is obvious that the sharper the selectivity of a biologically active substance, the greater the probability that it will be innocuous for cells and functions other than the one for which it has been designed. In other words, a substance is more likely to be therapeutically useful if it acts almost uniquely against a structure or an activity peculiar to the organism or function to be affected. Unfortunately, the physiological or chemical definition of these specific structures and activities is an aspect of biology which is grossly neglected at the present time.[226]

As each of these non-selective medicines comes into wider and wider use, the "side-effects" become more and more evident—leading to the medicine's eventual abandonment and supersession by others which, being equally non-specific, suffer the same fate.

This stream of new drugs is called medical "progress."

While the instability of Rationalism is thought to reflect strength and dynamism, it is actually the consequence of methodological weakness.

And these two factors together, imprecision and doctrinal instability, give rise to the third characteristic of Rationalism—its tremendous bulk. The thousands of textbooks and periodicals, requiring the computerization of knowledge and retrieval systems, the proliferating specialties and sub-specialties—are all the result of Rationalism's refusal to base medical thought on the known. When the only available data are statistical abstractions, the precise comparisons needed for a scientific medicine become impossible, writers rely on changing sets of assumptions, and much of the literature is incommensurable with itself. This generates renewed attempts at synthesis, but the weakness of the method, while increasing the bulk of the material, condemns such efforts to failure.

The Sociology of Medical Knowledge

Rationalism is clearly an unscientific doctrine, while Empiricism is scientific, but, as far as can be determined from the evidence, Rationalists have always been in the majority, while Empiricism has been a minority form of practice.

This is certainly the case for twentieth-century medicine in industrialized societies, and it seems paradoxical, since Empiricism—as a scientific form of medicine—must in every period of history have been more therapeutically effective than Rationalism.

This paradox can be unravelled only by examining the relations between the two doctrines and the socio-economic needs of the medical profession.

For the practice of medicine in a social setting involves much more than merely healing sick persons. The physician wants to do this, indeed, but he has other desiderata also. In particular, he wants to earn a respectable living from this activity and, in an undertaking so fraught with uncertainty, he may at times desire protection from the objects of his services.

Medical doctrines, or "ideologies," as they may be called,[u] appeal to physicians not only by their therapeutic

[u] "We refer to the ideology of an age or of a concrete historico-social group . . . when we are concerned with the characteristics and composition of the total structure of the mind of this epoch or of this group" (Karl Mannheim, *Ideology and Utopia* [London: Routledge and Kegan Paul, 1960], 49-50).

potential but also by their ability to: (1) bind the medical profession together in a group which can resist social pressure, (2) create psychological distance between the physician and the patient, and (3) enable the physician to earn a satisfactory living.

Only a sense of these other services of a medical ideology will clarify the reasons for the relative professional positions of Rationalism and Empiricism and, at the same time, yield solutions to some of the problems of medical practice in the twentieth century.

Ideologies as Instruments of Professional Cohesion

A major function of an ideology is to bind its adherents together for struggle against the supporters of rival ideologies and against society as a whole. An examination of the structures of Empiricism and Rationalism shows that the former is an inadequate instrument of professional cohesion, while the latter fulfills this function very well.

As already mentioned, the "theory" of Empiricism is a set of rules for practice, sufficiently detailed to be readily applicable to individual cases of sickness. But the clarity which such a set of rules introduces into practice can only have the effect of sowing discord among its adherents, since differences between one physician and another become immediately apparent.[v]

Rationalist theory, being abstract, has the opposite effect. Application of theory to the individual case is left to the physician's judgment, while all pay lip-service to the abstract theory itself. Such a theory, "explaining" the phenomena in language accepted by all, unifies its adherents instead of fragmenting them.

The role of the two "theories" can be viewed from a different perspective.

[v]This can be seen from the history of nineteenth-century homoeopathy (*Divided Legacy,* III, Chapter VI).

The concreteness of Empirical "theory" and its "outward" orientation direct the physician's attention to the sick patient. The "inward" orientation of Rationalism and its abstractness direct the physician's attention away from the patient and concentrate it on the body of cause-and-effect relationships which make up the Rationalist physiological metaphysic. But since this body of relationships, this "theory," is incorporated in the group of persons owing allegiance to it, the Rationalist physician's attention is directed, above all, to the needs and interests of the medical profession.

An important corollary of Empirical concreteness and Rationalist abstraction is the former's reliance on the past as a source of knowledge vs. the latter's reliance on the future.

Empiricism is permeated with an awareness of history. Disease itself is a historical process, as is the emergence of therapeutic doctrine. Empirical thinkers have been aware of, and respectful toward, the great figures of their tradition—regarding them not as mere relics but as continuing sources of valuable therapeutic assistance and information.[w]

Rationalists, on the contrary, have seen their discipline as analytical rather than historical and for that reason have slighted past thinkers and the history of medicine generally. Instead, they have looked to the future as the proper source of knowledge.

Boerhaave states that doubtful issues can be left "to be solved by our posterity," and this tendency of Rationalism was exacerbated by the fixation of society on "progress" in

[w]See *Divided Legacy,* I, 267-268. Stahl calls even physiology the *genealogia rerum,* since it is a *history* of the *Anima* (*Theoria Medica Vera,* I, 123, 152, 485).

While Hahnemann did not lavish praise on his predecessors, he refers to "the later sects of the empirics—worthy of all respect" and "the honorable Stahl" (*Lesser Writings,* 420; *Defence of the Organon,* 70). He also mentions Van Helmont quite favorably: "one of these sects, and that not the worst, expressed this in some degree special life and the peculiarities and particular actions of each individual organ, by the figurative name of an *Archeus* . . ." (*Lesser Writings,* 536). But he disapproved of Paracelsus and the alchemical tradition (*Lesser Writings,* 421, 502, 546. Haehl, *Hahnemann,* I, 274).

the nineteenth century.[227] Andral,[228] Darbefeuille,[229] Magendie,[230] and others all came to feel that medicine was in its infancy and destined to make a precipitate advance. Bernard wrote: "it is a progressive medicine that I am recommending . . . I am destroying nothing, I am proposing nothing, I am only calling attention to the scientific evolution going on around us."[231] When critics told him that vivisection was a defective technique, he answered that it must then be improved: "science would never progress if we thought ourselves justified in renouncing scientific methods because they were imperfect; in this case the only thing to do is to perfect the methods."[232]

He was not much interested in old books: "the experimental physician's library is the physiological laboratory."[233] [x]

> A man of science must, of course, know and deal with his predecessors' work. But he must be thoroughly convinced that this work is merely a support from which to go farther, and that new scientific truths are not to be found in study of the past, but rather in studies made anew on nature, i.e., in the laboratory . . . what use can we find in exhuming worm-eaten theories or observations made without proper means of investigation . . . I deem it highly important to guide the minds of students early toward active experimental science, by making them understand that it develops in laboratories, instead of leading them to believe that it awaits them in books or in the interpretations of ancient writings.[234]

With the triumph of Methodist doctrines in the latter part of the century all interest in medical history came to an end.[y] It

[x]In a parallel to the mystic's "withdrawal" into his own soul, and Van Helmont's "withdrawal" to Vilvoorde, Bernard urges the physician to "withdraw" into his laboratory (*Experimental Medicine,* 140). See above, pp. 6 and 17.

[y]The ancient Methodists themselves had felt contempt for the history of their predecessors, calling Hippocratic medicine the "management of death" (*Divided*

was no longer taught in the medical schools and became, in effect, an abandoned discipline.[235] This was perfectly natural from the Rationalist/Methodist viewpoint, since an analytical medicine must be considered to incorporate in itself all that is useful from the past.

Any hope for improvement, therefore, could come only from the future, and late nineteenth-century medicine became increasingly fixated on the future, as directed by Claude Bernard:

> For the moment . . . the prudent and reasonable thing to do is to explain all that we can explain in a disease by physiology and leave what is still inexplicable to the future progress of biological science.[236]

> We are doubtless far from the time when all medicine will be scientific, but this need not prevent our conceiving it possible and making every effort to strive toward it.[237]

> Of course we shall not see scientific medicine blossoming in our day, but that is man's lot.[238]

> In spite of our efforts, we are still very far from this absolute truth, and it is probable, especially in the biological sciences, that it will never be given to us to see it in its nakedness. But this need not discourage us, for we are constantly nearing it.[239]

These different orientations of Empiricism and Rationalism reflect the holism of one and reductionism of the other. What could be more holistic than incorporating into a medical doctrine the whole history of this doctrine? And what could be more reductionist and abstract than the future—which does not exist and may never come into being?

The Empirical orientation toward the past, however, contributes to the fissiparous nature of this doctrine,

Legacy, I, 199). The effects of late nineteenth-century Rationalism's contempt for medical history are felt to this day in medical education, few schools offering courses in this discipline and few students evincing an interest in it.

perpetually raising the question of the correct understanding and interpretation of the past. The homoeopathic profession has never ceased quarreling over the precise meaning of Hahnemannism. And the Rationalist orientation toward the future reinforces professional solidarity: all agree that medical theory is approaching perfection.

Rationalism's fixation on the future smooths out yet another source of possible professional disunity—the internal confusion and contradictions of this doctrine. For, although priding itself on logical consistency, Rationalism is steadily incapable of providing precise definitions of its guiding concepts.

For instance, while "disease," "cause," and "symptom" are essential elements of Rationalist theory, neither Boerhaave nor Bernard can give them satisfactory definitions. Boerhaave tries to define them in terms of each other and ends in confusion. Disease is: "any state of the living body which impairs or destroys the faculty of exercising [a] function,"[240] "the injury of some function,"[241] "some action of life changed or injured,"[242] "an effect resulting from its cause . . . a distinct, physical, and created entity or being,"[243] etc. The "cause" is a "latent entity,"[244] "all that which occasions the whole present indisposition which it constitutes . . . almost the same thing with the entire disease itself,"[245] "the physical cause of the disease differs not in the least from all the conjunct effects taken together,"[246] "almost constantly some real or physical thing, corporally present . . . which in a manner is the distemper itself,"[247] etc. The symptom is "part of the disease, and all the symptoms together make up the whole disease,"[248] it "flows from the distemper as its cause, yet so as to be distinguishable from the disease itself and from its proximate cause,"[249] "curing all the symptoms together is almost curing the whole disease."[250]

Claude Bernard, by the same token, defines "disease" as a "mechanism, not an entity," "life under other conditions," "disturbed function," a poisoning process, a deviation of "functional irritability," an "exaltation of irritability," an "exaggeration of life,"[251] etc. His philosophy cannot distinguish among "facts," "causes," "laws," and "material conditions."[252]

None of this should be of concern to the Rationalist physician, however, since confidence in the future means that no medical truth is permanent; the doctrine accepted today differs from that prevailing tomorrow, and all inconsistencies will merge in the higher synthesis of the future: "theories are never absolute truths; they may always be improved and so are always mobile."[253] "In science the best precept is to alter and exchange our ideas as fast as science moves ahead."[254]

This position benefits the physician in his social role. Vis-a-vis the patient he can assert his doctrine as "scientific," and hence above criticism, while vis-a-vis himself he can maintain the changeableness of medical "science" and its tendency to ever-greater perfection. Failures of theory and practice are forgiven the physician by the merciful future.

No wonder this abstraction of abstractions, the future, is one of the strongest ties binding together the members of the Rationalist profession.

Finally, Rationalist theory unifies its adherents by relieving them of responsibility—through its expropriation of therapeutic experience:[z] "the diagnosis and prognosis of the physician are based on the experiments [*die Erfahrungen*] of the pathological anatomist and the physiologist."[255] Theory, and with it responsibility for the outcome of practice, is no longer the province of the physician: "practical medicine is never the same thing as scientific medicine but rather, even in the hands of the greatest master, an application of it."[256] Bernard even refused the physician the right to determine whether or not his treatment was effective:

[z]See above, pp. 696-698.

> Where is the work of art by which the medical artist is to be judged? Is it the cure of the disease? . . . The criterion evidently disappears, because no physician's ability can be judged by the number of patients he says he has cured; he must first of all prove scientifically that it was he who cured them, and not nature.[257]

The inherent urge of Rationalism to expropriate the practitioner's therapeutic experience became especially pronounced with the emergence of physiology:

> Clinics are not the foundation of scientific medicine; physiology is the foundation of scientific medicine because it must yield the explanation of morbid phenomena by showing their relations in the normal state.[258]

> Now the science that gives man means of analyzing and experimentally mastering phenomena is the furthest advanced. It must necessarily be the last established . . . Physiology . . . is the highest and most difficult science of human beings . . . The very evolution of human knowledge means that experimental science must be the goal.[259]

Clinical experience is important in the primitive, "observational," stage of a science but is superseded by "experiment" in the stage of "experimental science."[260]

Just as the Rationalist physician asserts his knowledge of causes and monopoly of experience against the layman, so Bernard and the physiological school made the same claim against physicians. In either case the aim was to deprive the opponent of the right to competing experience.

Bernard liked to maintain that this was only substituting an objective criterion, scientific truth, for the authority of some individual.[261] Medical "tact" would disappear before the objective authority of "science."[262] But it was no secret that he was the foremost physiologist in the world at that time, writing in his notebooks "I am the director of the modern physiological movement" and "I am physiology."[263] So his efforts to establish an "objective" criterion could have been interpreted as simply a drive to assert his authority over the medical profession.

This suspicion, together with Bernard's well-known antipathy toward physicians, made physiology an unpopular subject with physicians and a neglected one by medical students. Many considered it a "luxury" which could easily be dispensed with. Even at the end of Bernard's career his lectures were largely deserted. Physicians objected to his using the Chair of Medicine to expound physiology, and they wanted the course to be entitled experimental "physiology."[264] Bernard complained that "the progress or modification of physiological theories exercises for the most part only an uncertain influence on the art of healing, and we even see a great number of practitioners isolating themselves completely from physiology as if it were useless and even dangerous to follow its various fluctuations."[265]

After his death, however, medical resistance to physiology collapsed, and Bernard's teachings came into the kingdom he had prepared—the *fons et origo* of Rationalist medicine, a metaphysic unifying all who professed Rationalist therapeutics.

Ideologies as Creators of Psychological Distance

By welding its adherents together into professional unity Rationalism deflects their attention from the patient. It creates psychological distance between physician and patient, alienating one from the other. Empiricism does the opposite—orienting its adherents away from the medical profession to the needs and interests of the patient, minimizing the psychological distance between physician and layman, and maximizing professional disunity.

As noted above, this egalitarian orientation of Empiricism has usually been allied with Pietism, Mysticism, or some other variety of religious belief stressing the equality of the faithful before God and the need for charity toward one's fellow humans.[a] A corollary has been the willingness of

[a]See above, pp. 61-62, 64-66, 92, 230-232.

Empiricism to recognize the medical contributions of the lay public.

Paracelsus is the most famous example of Empirical alienation from the medical profession combined with sympathy for the patient, but Van Helmont was also estranged from his profession while carrying on a free practice among the poor.[b] Like Paracelsus, he investigated the diseases of miners and metal-workers, noting that "diggers, melters of metals, separators . . . artificers of *aqua regis,* cerusse, red-lead, verdigris," etc. are subject to asthma from breathing the fumes, but the schools have ignored these diseases like the "Levites passing by in Jericho."[266] Sydenham had serious difficulties with his profession, being "fretted by the sneers and insults of pretenders."[267] His biographer wrote:

> The great Sydenham, for all his labors, only gained the sad and unjust recompense of calumny and ignominy; and that from emulation of some of his collegiate brethren and others, whose indignation at length arose to that height that they endeavored to banish him, as guilty of medicinal heresy, out of [the Royal College of Physicians] ; and by the whispering of others was balked the employment of the royal family, where before he was called among the first physicians.[268]

Hahnemann was ostracized by his allopathic colleagues, and had rather poor relations with his own followers,[c] but was open to knowledge from lay sources and recognized that most of the valuable medicines in use were taken originally from lay and domestic practice.[269]

> The humiliating confession must be made that most of the virtues of medicinal bodies were discovered by

[b]See above, pp. 17-18.

[c]He stated in the end of his life that, although thousands accounted themselves his followers, he recognized fewer than could be numbered on the fingers of both hands (*Divided Legacy,* III, 334). On this see Haehl, *Hahnemann,* I, 184 ff.

> *accidental, empirical* experience, by *chance;* often first observed by non-medical persons. Bold, often over-bold physicians, then gradually made use of them.[270]

> If some of the common people had not, at their own risk, undertaken experiments, and communicated the results of these, we should not have known even the little we do at present about the action of most medicines.[271]

He even wrote a commendatory account of the therapeutic efforts of the peasant women who were the only sources of medical knowledge in many of the German villages of his time.[272]

But Rationalism not only binds physicians together, thus setting their interests against those of the patient and of society, it acts even more directly to elevate the status of the physician over that of the patient.

This is a major function of the doctrine of "proximate causes." The learned physician is privy to knowledge denied the uninitiated. His social status depends upon the claim to understand invisible physiological processes. By his ability to "explain" them he acquires ascendancy over the patient.

Boerhaave illuminates this aspect of the psychology of Rationalism in noting that the ancients had insufficient knowledge of physiology to reach a scientific conclusion about the source of the heart's heat, but did so anyway:

> Who would have suspended their judgment on this affair, from the time of Hippocrates down to our own day, the space of 2000 years? That would have been declaring himself ignorant in one of the most considerable articles of his profession, yet is it what ought to have been done.[273]

Since Galen's time, and probably before,[d] Rationalists have treasured this metaphysical knowledge as a source of prestige, because it sets them apart from laymen. Magendie wrote,

[d]*Divided Legacy,* I, 324-327.

"what immense resources are provided by a profound study of [alterations in the blood] to the physician anxious to take as guide a healthy theory rather than a blind and shameful empiricism!"[274] [e]

> The true physician is not always the one who claims to have seen much and observed much. Just because for several years you have listened to the heartbeat and the rales in the chest are you any further along than the mechanic who listens every day and every minute to the clang of the rocker-beam and the hum of the wheels?[275]

Unless he studies physics and chemistry the physician is condemned to a "blind routine."[276] "The man who cleans up in the laboratory, with a little training, becomes competent to pass on these crude surface appearances. Physicians! You are called to a more honorable role. By studying the cause of these morbid extravasations, of these modifications of the fluids and of their conduits, you will elevate yourself to the true dignity of your art."[277]

> At the bedside what is the difference between the physician and a nurse? Suppose he is called for a case of smallpox. During his studies he will have attended clinics, he knows the symptoms and the course of this disease: it commences with general phenomena, it is an eruption of a particular kind which lasts a certain time, then the pustules dry out, and finally the skin comes off. Well, do you think that the nurse (if she has had even a little experience at her job) does not know all of this as well as he does? Then does he know any better than she why this smallpox will be benign or confluent; or why, all of a sudden, taking on a different form (*purpura*), it carries off the patient in a few hours? No, the most skilful and experienced physician is ignorant of all these things; he is

[e]His practice was "not more unfortunate than theirs" (i.e., that of the "empirics") even though "infinitely more circumspect" (*Systeme Nerveux,* I, 9).

> the spectator, ignorant and too often impotent before these serious modifications of the initial disease. He will prescribe the same things which, if need be, the nurse could prescribe as well.
>
> You will ask: is this the sort of superiority to which the physician can aspire? In the present state of the science, I will not hesitate to answer: It is the only one. Let us then, through serious study directed toward a truly useful and logical goal, cast off the almost humiliating role which our ancestors have left us. Let us create pathology instead of the simple and sterile notation of the symptoms of diseases. Let us create experimental medicine which will doubtless reveal to us the mechanism of the morbid alterations, and then we will be able to attack vigorously the causes of these changes, to modify them, and perhaps even to prevent them. This is my approach to our studies, and I don't think that in any epoch it has been formulated more rationally.[278]

This knowledge of causal theory enables the physician to tell the patient that his disease is incurable, that medical science can do nothing for him:

> We cannot deny that in treatment the heavens sometimes interpose a certain force, so that, however the physician strives and with whatever art, he nevertheless may fail to achieve a successful outcome.[279]

The physician's knowledge of causes is a "compensation for the painful setbacks which we often encounter at the sickbed."[280] While it is "afflicting to us as physicians to be unable to arrest the frightful symptoms of diseases," it is "satisfying for us as men of science to be able to some extent to predict their course, ravages, and outcome . . . sad certainty of knowing that at such and such a time, and in such and such a way, death is inevitable."[281] [f]

[f]Cf. Hahnemann: " 'Yes,' I hear the medical school whisper with a seemingly compassionate shrug, 'Yes, these are notoriously incurable evils; our books tell us they are incurable.' As if it could comfort the millions of sufferers to be told of

The explanatory function of Rationalism even takes precedence over the curative: "first of all, we must inspire young men with the scientific spirit and initiate them into the ideas and tendencies of modern science."[282] Then the healing role of the physician is derided: "the requirements of medical practice . . . help keep medicine in the personal realm and thus oppose the experimental development."[283] "In our faculties of medicine we must not limit ourselves to making empirical healers; that would degrade medicine and reduce it to the level of a business."[284]

Hahnemann's envenomed eye perceived this aspect of Rationalism very well:

> They acted, as we see, like other sects, quite arbitrarily, but obviously with an endeavor (not indeed to cure, that would be vulgar, no!) to give to their arbitrary procedures the highest possible coloring of rationality.[285]

Healing, the practical part of medicine, is regarded by Rationalism as less worthy than pursuing the abstractions of "science." It is less dignified for the same reason that Empiricism itself is less dignified—because it involves an element of practical skill.[g]

Thus the allopaths criticized the homoeopaths in the nineteenth century for reducing medicine to the level of a trade or occupation, healing for money, *"l'industrialisme medical."*[286] [h]

And, indeed, the Empirics were vulnerable on this count. Their theory did little or nothing to elevate the physician's status over that of the layman. He could impress the patient only by his therapeutic skill—which, because the physician's contribution to cure is rarely clearcut or unambiguous, confers less prestige than the ability to explain the invisible.

the vain impotence of our art! As if the Creator of these sufferers had not provided remedies for them also!" (*Lesser Writings,* 415).

[g]The physician is called a "craftsman" (*kheirotekhnes*) in *Ancient Medicine,* the leading Empirical writing of the Hippocratic Corpus (*Divided Legacy,* I, 85).

[h]See, also, *Divided Legacy,* III, 174-179.

Another Rationalist technique for alienating physician from patient is the use of Latin- and Greek-derived polysyllables to describe its assumed physiological processes. Not only does it hypostatize invisible entities within the organism, it gives them long names which are unintelligible to those without the requisite training.

This may be contrasted with the Empirical use of non-technical language because diseases are described in symptomatic terms, i.e., in the language of the patient.[i]

A final way in which Rationalism elevates the physician above the patient is by denigrating the vital force.

Acceptance of the *physis* is repugnant to Rationalism for two reasons: (1) it seems to introduce confusion into disease descriptions, thus detracting from the physician's dignity, and (2) it sets up a source of healing potential in competition with the physician's own efforts.

Baglivi writes that "persons of more delicate taste [*delicatioris palati*]"—meaning his Iatromechanist confreres object to his use of the word, *Natura,* "as if this should be a refuge for ignorance."[287] Hoffmann criticizes Stahl's *Anima sensitiva* as a metaphysical principle which cannot be defined and cannot explain the functioning of the organism. Stahl does not assign a "real cause, one susceptible of demonstration, and gives no explanation which one can grasp."[288]

> If we referred everything to the [*Anima*], we would only upset at one blow everything which is certain in medicine, the certainty of the effectiveness of remedies, all doctrines based on reason, and, in a word, all application of physics and anatomy.[289]

[i]Note Stahl's interjection of the German expressions used by his patients into the text of his Latin treatise (above, p. 377*g*).

Chinese traditional medicine, which is Empirical in structure, also employs a formalized lay language (relying on sensory data) to describe physiological and pathological phenomena.

By ignoring any consideration of the *physis* Hoffmann hoped to

> give to medicine that certainty which has been so long desired . . . to reduce all of medicine to a rational system, so that the principles follow one another in the most natural way and can be used to explain a series of phenomena.[290]

Cullen writes:

> Although the *vis medicatrix naturae* must unavoidably be received as a fact, yet wherever it is admitted, it throws an obscurity upon our system; and it is only where the importance of our art is very manifest and considerable that we ought to admit of it in practice.[291]

He tried to avoid "hypotheses" and "theories," of which the principal one was the Hippocratic theory of coction,[292] relying only on "proximate causes":

> I have, indeed, endeavored to establish many general doctrines, both physiological and pathological, but I trust that these are only a generalization of facts, or conclusions from a cautious and full induction . . . I have myself [tried to prove] that the proximate causes which I have assigned are true in fact as well as deductions from any reasoning that I may seem to have employed.[293]

Magendie also inveighed against the supposed vagueness of vitalism.[294] Vitalist explanations are a "cloak for laziness."[295] "Any physician with a severely critical mind must henceforth renounce these pretended explanations provided by the vital properties."[296]

> Their essential character is that they cannot be interpreted. They escape our analyses; they escape our reasoning; often they even escape our experimental research; their realm is that of doubt and conjecture; ours at the present time should be that of the real and positive.[297]

He protested against Bichat's preference for a degree of indeterminacy in physiological explanations:

> We must then despair of the future of our art; we would be condemned never to leave this humiliating rut of uncertainty and error. Really! is a fact to be proscribed from physiology merely because it is authentic, merely because it is rigorously demonstrated? No, gentlemen, this is not the destiny of our science. We will protest by our words, we will protest above all by our acts, against such strange maxims whose inevitable result would be to keep us forever plunged in the shadows of ignorance.[298]

Bernard calls the *physis* only a "hypothesis" whose correctness remains to be proven.[299] He calls, instead, for "unshaken faith" in determinism which will give the physician a "reliable criterion for judging the often variable and contradictory appearance of vital phenomena."[300]

Acceptance of the *physis*, however, impaired the physician's authority in yet another way: to the extent that he recognizes its efficacy, or even its existence, he restricts his own freedom of action in the treatment of disease. Recognition of the *physis* means respect for its capacities and subordination of the physician's efforts to those of the *physis*.

But this reduces the physician to the level of the patient and is thus intolerable to Rationalism which wants to be guided by a "healthy theory," not by the wishes of the patient or the needs of the *physis*.

Subservience to the *physis* means interpreting disease as a process with its necessary stages, to which the physician must subjugate himself.[j] It also suggests the use of *secunda*

[j]In Methodism, where the physician's activism was most pronounced, the *physis* was completely dissolved in the corpuscles. Mannheim writes that in politics "the groups oriented toward the left intend to make something new out of the world as it is given, and therefore they divert their glance from things as they are, they become abstract and atomize the given situation into its component elements in order to recombine them anew" (*Ideology and Utopia*, 246).

remedia, the furthering remedies or similars which assist the *physis* along the path it has chosen—rather than the powerful "contraries" which are themselves an assertion of the physician's authority.

Recognition of the *physis* thus detracts from the physician's self-image as an active agent in the therapeutic process and places him in a position of insupportable subordination to the patient. Hoffmann states that his theory is the key to a "certain, safe, and facile practice," enabling the physician to "act promptly."[301] Cullen's theory permitted a "more scientific and decided method of cure," and he criticized the Stahlians who, "following the general principles of their system, always mysterious, have introduced archeal remedies, and many of them a superstitious and inert kind; while at the same time, trusting to the *autokrateia,* they have opposed and rejected some medicines of the most powerful nature."[302] "The operations of nature are very precarious, and not so well understood as to enable us to regulate them properly. It appears to me that trusting to these operations has often given occasion to a negligent and inert practice; and there is reason to believe that an attention to the operations of nature may often be superseded by art."[303]

> It appears to me that the general doctrine of *Nature curing diseases,* the so much vaunted *Hippocratic* method of curing, has often had a very baneful influence on the practice of physic; as either leading physicians into, or continuing them in, a weak and feeble practice, and at the same time superseding or discouraging all the attempts of art . . . even in the hands of Sydenham it had this effect. Although it may sometimes avoid the mischiefs of bold and rash practitioners, yet it certainly produces that caution and timidity which have ever opposed the introduction of new and efficacious remedies.[304]

In Magendie this activism was carried to sadistic lengths in the name of "science." Bichat had noted that living membranes will resist the passage of a liquid harmful to the organism;

Magendie states with satisfaction that harmful liquids can be forced through a living membrane.[305] When asked by his students the purpose of an experiment injecting a particle of starch into the vein of a laboratory animal to block the capillaries of the lung, he replied:

> These experiments, it will be said, may be very curious but where is their practical utility? One never injects starch into the blood. Gentlemen! there are circumstances when it has been attempted to inject various liquids and medicinal agents into the circulation of man himself. I myself have performed such experiments several times. Medicine does not always consist of giving prescriptions or formulating run-of-the-mill directions for the patient. In emergencies it must be less timid. One must know how to dare. What would be only blameworthy temerity in the blind Empiric is, in the educated and conscientious man, the proof of a noble ambition and an enlightened philanthropy.[306] [k]

This same activist orientation led Bernard to insist that medicine must pass from the "observational" to the "experimental" stage:

> The observational sciences are expectant and passive; the experimental sciences are conquering and powerful, powerfully active by their own initiative.[307]

> In sciences of experimentation man observes, but in addition he acts on matter, analyzes its properties, and to his own advantage brings about the appearance of phenomena . . . in conditions which nature often has not yet achieved. With the help of these active experimental sciences man becomes an inventor of phenomena, a real foreman of creation, and under this head we cannot set

[k]In the light of this comment, Magendie's refusal to accept any appointment which compelled him to relinquish ward practice in a hospital seems a little sinister (Flourens, *Eloge Historique de M. Magendie,* 40).

> limits to the power he may gain over nature through future progress in the experimental sciences.[308]

The *milieu interieur*, bringing environmental (exciting) causes inside the organism, catered to the physician's urge to feel in control of all possible causes: "physiologists and physicians gain mastery over the phenomena of life by learning which conditions, in this inner environment, are normal and which abnormal . . ."[309]

The Economic Function of Medical Ideologies

Finally, Empiricism and Rationalism differ in their economic potential.

The physician has a limited number of hours in the day, and his income is maximized by seeing the largest possible number of patients during these hours. A doctrine which facilitates rapid diagnosis and treatment is bound to have preference over one which delays them.

It can be seen that the Rationalist "proximate cause," which was often disclosed by the mere application of *ratio*, made diagnosis easier than the Empirical reliance on symptomatic description. And, by the same token, the prescription of a "contrary" medicine which nullified or removed this "proximate cause" was a more rapid therapeutic technique than following the disease through its stages and assisting it along with "furthering remedies" or similars.

Thus a final reason for Rationalist rejection of the *physis* was that its recognition made medical practice less rapid, i.e., less gainful.

These matters are discussed in detail in the following volume.[1]

* * * *

The problems inherent to the practice of medicine in a social setting stem from the conflicting demands upon the

[1]*Divided Legacy,* III, 119-124, 210-211, 376-382, 418-419.

physician: he must engage in a scientific activity and at the same time earn a living. The conflict between Empiricism and Rationalism is a conflict between the need to practice scientifically and the need to achieve a standard of living deemed respectable.

There is no reason why these two requirements should be in harmony, and, in fact, they are not. They must be reconciled and adjusted to one another, and each physician selects his own balance between them.[m]

Empiricism is the ideology which best meets the needs of the physician oriented toward the scientific practice of medicine, but at the same time it is excessively difficult to practice and has never enlisted the allegiance of more than a minority of the profession.[n] Rationalism meets the social, economic, and organizational needs of physicians by holding up a false ideal as "scientific."[o]

Being a scientific endeavor, Empiricism has been the agent of medical discovery. The role of Rationalism has been to trim and adjust new knowledge to the institutional and socio-economic needs of the profession. Galen's therapeutics was a Rationalization of the Hippocratic teachings about the *physis,* a reinterpretation of the theory of coction in Aristotelian terms. Iatrochemistry was a similar reinterpretation, in the language of laboratory chemistry, of the therapeutic insights of Paracelsus and Van Helmont. Iatromechanism was a restatement, in the language of hydraulics, of Harvey's discovery of the circulation. Haller's sensitivity and irritability—consequently, the Methodist doctrines of

[m]As mentioned by us earlier, the ordinary physician practices an "eclectic and inconsistent mixture of the two bodies of doctrine" (*Divided Legacy,* I, xiii).

[n]Even in the homoeopathic movement only a minority practiced pure Hahnemannism (*Divided Legacy,* III, 334).

[o]A malicious person could carry the argument so far as to suggest that the smaller the scientific content of a therapeutic doctrine, the greater the need for professional consolidation. In this case the components of Rationalism could be seen as self-reinforcing.

Cullen and Brown—were provoked by the need to account for Stahl's autonomous and spontaneous *Anima sensitiva.* The experiments with poisons on animals done by Magendie, Buchheim, Mitscherlich, and Bernard were an attempt to Rationalize the insights offered by Hahnemann's provings.

Even the nineteenth-century shift of Rationalism from pathological anatomy to physiology as the principal source of medical knowledge may have been essentially a reaction to Hahnemann's dynamic theory of the organism.

Often the Rationalist has to introduce gratuitous and unfounded assumptions to accommodate Empiricism to his own needs. Boerhaave, for instance, arbitrarily divides symptoms into those relating to the "proximate cause" and others supposedly arising from the "life remaining."[310] Mitscherlich distinguishes the "physiologic effect" of a drug on the body from its "symptomatic effect."[p] Bernard limits the role of the vital force to creation and repair, denying that it controls the functions; he states that depressing (suffocating) the diseased organism has no effect on the reparative effort of the vital force, etc. etc.[q]

Of similar nature was the assumption, by Sauvages and Barthez, of a dichotomy in the body between the "animate" and "inanimate" forces—an effort to adjust Stahlian doctrine to the proto-Rationalist form Empiricism was taking at their hands.[r]

Rationalists even, at times, accept certain Empirical principles which are in contradiction with their own system. Bernard, for instance, in several passages extols the holism of the organism, although this is incompatible with the structure of his doctrine.[311]

[p]See above, p. 635.

[q]See above, pp. 624, 642.

[r]See above, pp. 238, 245.

None of these inconsistencies or admissions weakens the Rationalist's adherence to his own principles, however, since this has a firm basis in emotion—his feeling of vulnerability to socio-economic forces and need to protect himself against them.

Thus one should not be surprised that Empiricism, although scientific and hence a more effective medicine, has never been adopted by a majority of the profession. The patient's desire to be healed *tuto, cito, et jucunde*[s] does not prevail over the Rationalist preferences of most physicians. The majority of the profession always imposes an unscientific therapeutics on society,[t] and in the late twentieth century physicians' organizations are more powerful than ever.

Instead of advancing to a "scientific" millenium, majority medicine in industrialized society is condemned to an endless cycle of progress in some areas and regress in others. As was stated four centuries ago by the insightful Van Helmont:

> The art of medicine alone, if it hath not gone backwards, at leastwise hath stood at a stay and whirled around the same deceitful point.[312]

The promise of "breakthroughs" (financed largely out of public funds) must be seen as a fairy tale of medical politicians. It also reflects Rationalism's perennial faith in the future for solutions to its problems—whereas the problems are here and now, a function of the organization of medicine and the medical profession.

[s]"Safely, quickly, and agreeably."

[t]This lends point to Bacon's warning against relying on majority views in scientific matters: "Even if it were a real and extensive unanimity, so far from being esteemed a true and solid confirmation, it should even lead to a violent presumption to the contrary. For there is no worse augury in intellectual matters than that derived from unanimity . . . For nothing pleases the multitude unless it strike the imagination or bind down the understanding . . . with the shackles of vulgar notions . . . Men should immediately examine what error or fault they have committed when the multitude concurs with and applauds them. This . . . is one of the most unfavorable signs" (*Novum Organum,* I, Aph. LXXVII).

Even though public opinion cannot prevail against the majority of the medical profession, however, its role should not be discounted entirely. By voicing its preferences it can ameliorate some of the excesses of majority medicine:

> It is only by the discretion of the patients themselves that physicians can ultimately be improved.[313]

Empiricism, despite its socio-economic and organizational weakness, has maintained its position over the centuries through public support. Once exposed to Empiricism, the layman feels instinctively at home with it—for its reliance on sensory data, its sympathy with the lay contribution to medicine, and, not least of all, for its therapeutic efficacy.

The history of public support for Empiricism in the nineteenth and early twentieth centuries is detailed in Volume III of *Divided Legacy.*

NOTES

[1] Baglivi, *De Praxi Medica,* 8, 211-214, 219.
[2] Blondin, *Oeuvres de Stahl,* II, 713-714.
[3] Stahl, *Theoria Medica Vera,* I, 152, 156-157, 478-479.
[4] Baglivi, *De Praxi Medica,* 254-255.
[5] *Oeuvres de Bordeu,* II, 600.
[6] *Ibid.,* II, 800.
[7] Blondin, *Oeuvres de Stahl,* II, 715. Stahl, *Theoria Medica Vera,* I, 150, 157, 490-491. See also Baglivi, *De Praxi Medica,* 95.
[8] Barthez, *Nouveaux Elements,* II, 23.
[9] Blondin, *Oeuvres de Stahl,* II, 595. Stahl, *Theoria Medica Vera,* I, 78.
[10] *Oeuvres de Bordeu,* I, 421.
[11] *The Works of Thomas Sydenham,* II, 181.
[12] *Ibid.,* II, 182.
[13] Blondin, *Oeuvres de Stahl,* II, 595, 715. Stahl, *Theoria Medica Vera,* I, 50. See also Baglivi, *De Praxi Medica,* 109.
[14] Hahnemann, *Lesser Writings,* 521.
[15] *Ibid.,* 661.
[16] Haehl, *Hahnemann,* I, 93.
[17] Stahl, *Theoria Medica Vera,* I, 152.
[18] *Ibid.,* I, 136. See, also, Blondin, *Oeuvres de Stahl,* VI, 183-184.
[19] Blondin, *Oeuvres de Stahl,* II, 711.
[20] *Ibid.,* II, 155. See, also, Stahl, *Theoria Medica Vera,* I, 131, 224.
[21] Stahl, *Theoria Medica Vera,* I, 478; II, 53 ff.
[22] Baglivi, *De Praxi Medica,* 3, 6, 8, 238.
[23] Stahl, *Theoria Medica Vera,* I, 476-477.
[24] *Ibid.,* I, 477.
[25] Bernard, *Experimental Medicine,* 68.
[26] Stahl, *Theoria Medica Vera,* II, 112-113.
[27] Boerhaave, *Academical Lectures,* I, 8.
[28] Magendie, *Phenomenes Physiques de la Vie,* I, 6.
[29] Bernard, *Experimental Medicine,* 202.
[30] Bernard, *Principes,* 167-168.
[31] Boerhaave, *Academical Lectures,* VI, 113.
[32] *Ibid.,* VI, 115-116.
[33] Bernard, *Experimental Medicine,* 65-66.
[34] Boerhaave, *Academical Lectures,* V, 363.
[35] *Ibid.,* VI, 1.
[36] *Ibid.,* VI, 2.
[37] *Ibid.,* VI, 152.

[38] *Ibid.*, VI, 155.
[39] Boerhaave, *Elements of Chemistry*, I, 54.
[40] *Loc. cit.*
[41] *Ibid.*, VI, 217.
[42] *Ibid.*, VI, 219.
[43] *Ibid.*, VI, 220.
[44] *Ibid.*, VI, 216.
[45] *Ibid.*, VI, 235-236.
[46] *Ibid.*, I, 57, 59.
[47] Boerhaave, quoted in John Baptist Morgagni, *The Seats and Causes of Disease Investigated by Anatomy* (New York: Academy of Medicine, 1960), I, xxx.
[48] Bernard, *Experimental Medicine*, 140.
[49] *Ibid.*, 209.
[50] Ameke, *History of Homoeopathy*, 181.
[51] Boerhaave, *Academical Lectures*, I, 74. See, also, Hoffmann, *Medicinae Rationalis*, 5, 12.
[52] Bernard, *Experimental Medicine*, 107.
[53] *Ibid.*, 107-108.
[54] *Ibid.*, 114-115.
[55] *Ibid.*, 114. See, also, *ibid.*, 157.
[56] *Ibid.*, 113-114.
[57] Boerhaave, *Academical Lectures*, I, 58.
[58] *Ibid.*, I, 60.
[59] *Ibid.*, I, 61.
[60] Bernard, *Principes*, 167.
[61] Boerhaave, *Academical Lectures*, VI, 167.
[62] Bernard, *Experimental Medicine*, 219.
[63] Bernard, *Principes*, 8.
[64] Boerhaave, *Academical Lectures*, I, 2.
[65] Cullen, *First Lines of the Practice of Physic*, I, 53.
[66] *Ibid.*, I, 6.
[67] Boerhaave, *Academical Lectures*, I, 55. See, also, *ibid.*, VI, 279 and Bernard, *Principes*, 31, 175.
[68] Boerhaave, *Academical Lectures*, I, 44.
[69] *Ibid.*, I, 48.
[70] Bernard, *Experimental Medicine*, 92.
[71] Hoffmann, *Fundamenta Medicinae*, 118.
[72] *Ibid.*, 119.
[73] *Ibid.*, 118.
[74] Boerhaave, *Academical Lectures*, I, 7, 10. Hoffmann, *Medicinae Rationalis*, 44. Bernard, *Principes*, 11, 124.
[75] Boerhaave, *Academical Lectures*, I, 71.
[76] Bernard, *Experimental Medicine*, 66.
[77] Hoffmann, *Medicinae Rationalis*, c-3, 44-45.
[78] Bernard, *Experimental Medicine*, 80.
[79] *Ibid.*, 82.
[80] Blondin, *Oeuvres de Stahl*, VI, 67. Stahl, *Theoria Medica Vera*, I, 34; II, 3.
[81] Boerhaave, *Academical Lectures*, I, 71. Blondin, *Oeuvres de Stahl*, VI, 16, 18.

[82] Baglivi, *De Praxi Medica,* 108-109. Boerhaave, *Academical Lectures,* I, 71.
[83] Boerhaave, *Academical Lectures,* I, 73.
[84] Hoffmann, *Fundamenta Medicinae,* 7.
[85] Virchow, *Disease, Life, and Man,* 47.
[86] Bernard, *Experimental Medicine,* 60.
[87] *Ibid.,* 94.
[88] *Ibid.,* 89.
[89] Bernard, *Experimental Medicine,* 92-93.
[90] Bernard, *Principes,* 157.
[91] *Ibid.,* 232.
[92] Stahl, *Theoria Medica Vera,* II, 7-8.
[93] *Ibid.,* II, 4-5.
[94] Boerhaave, *Academical Lectures,* V, 257, 268, 276.
[95] *Ibid.,* V, 273. Bernard, *Experimental Medicine,* 76.
[96] Boerhaave, *Academical Lectures,* I, 77-78.
[97] Bernard, *Experimental Medicine,* 65.
[98] Virchow, *Post-Mortem Examinations,* 129.
[99] Boerhaave, *Academical Lectures,* VI, 377.
[100] *Loc. cit.*
[101] *Ibid.,* VI, 379.
[102] *Ibid.,* V, 293.
[103] *Ibid.,* VI, 377.
[104] *Ibid.,* VI, 375.
[105] Bernard, *Experimental Medicine,* 92.
[106] Bernard, *Principes,* 98-99. See, also, *ibid.,* 128.
[107] *Ibid.,* 15.
[108] *Ibid.,* 170.
[109] *Ibid.,* 145. *Experimental Medicine,* 65.
[110] Bernard, *Experimental Medicine,* 136.
[111] *Ibid.,* 83.
[112] Bernard, *Principes,* 142.
[113] Bernard, *Experimental Medicine,* 124.
[114] *Divided Legacy,* I, 228, 232.
[115] Boerhaave, *Academical Lectures,* V, 364-365.
[116] *Ibid.,* VI, 379.
[117] *Loc. cit.*
[118] *Ibid.,* VI, 361, 376, 379.
[119] *Ibid.,* VI, 379.
[120] *Ibid.,* VI, 375.
[121] Hoffmann, *Medicinae Rationalis, c.*
[122] Hoffmann, *Fundamenta Medicinae,* 116.
[123] Virchow, *Disease, Life, and Man,* 59.
[124] Boerhaave, *Academical Lectures,* V, 379.
[125] *Ibid.,* V, 379-380.
[126] *Ibid.,* V, 466.
[127] *Ibid.,* V, 381-382.
[128] Bernard, *Principes,* 130.
[129] Bernard, *Experimental Medicine,* 64, 97-98.
[130] *Loc. cit.* and *Principes,* 303-304.

[131] Bernard, *Experimental Medicine,* 79.
[132] *Ibid.,* 76.
[133] *Ibid.,* 126. *Principes,* 162.
[134] Bernard, *Principes,* 161.
[135] *Ibid.,* 163.
[136] *Ibid.,* 160-161.
[137] Bernard, *Experimental Medicine,* 215.
[138] Virchow, *Disease, Life, and Man,* 210.
[139] Hahnemann, *Lesser Writings,* 758.
[140] *Ibid.,* 758, 761.
[141] *Ibid.,* 753-756.
[142] Hahnemann, *Organon,* Introduction, 50, note 13.
[143] Van Helmont, *Oriatrike,* 40.
[144] Thomas Sydenham, *Tractatus de Podagra et Hydrope* (London: Kittleby, 1683), Title Page (*Novum Organum,* II, Aph. X). Baglivi, *De Praxi Medica,* 1, 91.
[145] *The Works of Thomas Sydenham,* I, 24.
[146] *Ibid.,* I, 18.
[147] Baglivi, *De Praxi Medica,* 40, 92.
[148] *Ibid.,* 7.
[149] Blondin, *Oeuvres de Stahl,* II, 154.
[150] *Works of Thomas Sydenham,* I, 4. See, also, *Ibid.,* I, 18.
[151] *Ibid.,* I, 17.
[152] Dewhurst, *Dr. Thomas Sydenham,* 79.
[153] *Works of Thomas Sydenham,* II, 31.
[154] Baglivi, *De Praxi Medica,* 3.
[155] Hahnemann, *Organon,* Sec. 148, note 108.
[156] Dewhurst, *Dr. Thomas Sydenham,* 83. See, also, Baglivi, *De Praxi Medica,* 2, 7 and Stahl, *Theoria Medica Vera,* I, 58, 73, 476.
[157] *The Physical and Metaphysical Works of Lord Bacon,* 20 (*The Great Instauration,* Distribution of the Work).
[158] *The Works of Thomas Sydenham,* I, 12. Baglivi, *De Praxi Medica,* 11, 214-215.
[159] *The Works of Thomas Sydenham,* II, 22.
[160] Baglivi, *De Praxi Medica,* 157, 164, 174.
[161] Hahnemann, *Organon,* Sec. 71.
[162] Blondin, *Oeuvres de Stahl,* II, 711; VI, 16, 18. Stahl, *Theoria Medica Vera,* III, 393.
[163] Stahl, *Theoria Medica Vera,* III, 393-394.
[164] *Ibid.,* I, 15, 59-62, 72-73, 134, 152; II, 3. Blondin, *Oeuvres de Stahl,* II, 640.
[165] *Oeuvres de Bordeu,* I, 251.
[166] Hahnemann, *Lesser Writings,* 417.
[167] Hahnemann, *Organon,* Sec. 25, note 13 (stress added).
[168] Hahnemann, *Lesser Writings,* 532.
[169] *Ibid.,* 491.
[170] *Ibid.,* 522, note 2.
[171] Hahnemann, *Lesser Writings,* 439.
[172] Hahnemann, *Organon,* Sec. 145, note 106.
[173] Quoted in R. E. Dudgeon, *Lectures on the Theory and Practice of Homoeopathy* (London: Leath and Ross, 1854), xlii.

[174] *The Physical and Metaphysical Works of Lord Bacon,* 51 (*Adv. of Learning,* Bk. I).

[175] Bernard, *Experimental Medicine,* 69.

[176] *Ibid.,* 55.

[177] Bernard, *Experimental Medicine,* 54.

[178] *Ibid.,* 69.

[179] Cheyne, *The Natural Method of Curing,* 46.

[180] Bernard, *Experimental Medicine,* 67-68.

[181] *Ibid.,* 74.

[182] *Ibid.,* 65 (stress added).

[183] *Ibid.,* 35.

[184] *Ibid.,* 52.

[185] *Ibid.,* 15-19, 140.

[186] *Ibid.,* 18, 205-218.

[187] *Ibid.,* 12-13.

[188] *Ibid.,* 200.

[189] *Ibid.,* 191.

[190] *Ibid.,* 54, 69.

[191] *Ibid.,* 32.

[192] *Ibid.,* 33.

[193] *Ibid.,* 60.

[194] *Ibid.,* 20.

[195] *Ibid.,* 32.

[196] *Ibid.,* 54.

[197] *Ibid.,* 24.

[198] *Ibid.,* 26.

[199] *Ibid.,* 10.

[200] *Ibid.,* 8-9.

[201] *Ibid.,* 100-101.

[202] *Ibid.,* 21.

[203] Dubois, "Eloge de Magendie," xxii.

[204] L. Deloyers, *Francois Magendie, 1783-1855. Precurseur de la Medecine Experimentale* (Bruxelles: Presses Universitaires de Bruxelles, 1970), 252.

[205] C. Bernard, *Francois Magendie: Lecon d'Ouverture du Cours de Medecine du College de France (29 Fevrier, 1856)* (Paris: Bailliere, 1856), 9.

[206] Bernard, *Experimental Medicine,* 12.

[207] *Ibid.,* 2.

[208] *Ibid.,* 11.

[209] *Ibid.,* 13.

[210] *Ibid.,* 12.

[211] *Ibid.,* 40.

[212] *Ibid.,* 32.

[213] *Ibid.,* 54.

[214] *Ibid.,* 53.

[215] Bernard, *Principes,* 75.

[216] Bernard, *Experimental Medicine,* 178.

[217] *Ibid.,* 178-179.

[218] *Ibid.,* 47.

[219] *Ibid.,* 51-52. *Principes,* 210.

[220] *Ibid.,* 222.

[221] *Loc. cit.*
[222] *Ibid.*, 50.
[223] *Ibid.*, 211.
[224] *Ibid.*, 38.
[225] *Ibid.*, 27.
[226] Paul Talalay, ed., *Drugs in Our Society* (Baltimore: Johns Hopkins, 1964), 39.
[227] Boerhaave, *Academical Lectures,* I, 50.
[228] Andral, *Clinique Medicale,* Third Edition, I, vi.
[229] Darbefeuille, *Propositions sur la Medecine,* vi.
[230] Magendie, *Phenomenes Physiques de la Vie,* I, 6.
[231] Bernard, *Principes,* 112-113.
[232] Bernard, *Experimental Medicine,* 126.
[233] *Ibid.*, 141.
[234] *Ibid.*, 145.
[235] Owsei Temkin, "An Essay on the Usefulness of Medical History for Medicine," *Bulletin of the History of Medicine* XIX (1946), 9-47, at 34.
[236] Bernard, *Experimental Medicine,* 199.
[237] *Ibid.*, 214.
[238] *Ibid.*, 216.
[239] *Ibid.*, 54.
[240] Boerhaave, *Academical Lectures,* V, 268.
[241] *Loc. cit.*
[242] *Ibid.*, V, 276.
[243] *Ibid.*, VI, 113.
[244] *Ibid.*, VI, 167.
[245] *Ibid.*, V, 377.
[246] *Ibid.*, VI, 433.
[247] *Ibid.*, V, 371.
[248] *Ibid.*, VI, 114.
[249] *Ibid.*, VI, 1.
[250] *Ibid.*, VI, 433.
[251] Bernard, *Principes,* 7, 15, 99, 131, 139, 150, 156, 159. *Experimental Medicine,* 76.
[252] Bernard, *Experimental Medicine,* 57, 74, 209, 219.
[253] *Ibid.*, 219.
[254] *Ibid.*, 41.
[255] Virchow, *Disease, Life, and Man,* 149.
[256] *Ibid.*, 27.
[257] Bernard, *Experimental Medicine,* 204.
[258] *Ibid.*, 146.
[259] *Ibid.*, 144.
[260] *Ibid.*, 140.
[261] *Ibid.*, 40, 218.
[262] *Ibid.*, 204.
[263] Bernard, *Cahier de Notes, 1850-1860,* 9, 19.
[264] J. M. D. Olmsted, *Claude Bernard, Physiologist* (New York: Harper and Brothers, 1938), 70.
[265] *Ibid.*, 71.
[266] Van Helmont, *Oriatrike,* 363, 617-618.

[267]*The Works of Thomas Sydenham,* I, 5.
[268]*Ibid.,* I, xliii.
[269]Hahnemann, *Organon,* Introduction, 82. *Lesser Writings,* 637, 646.
[270]Hahnemann, *Lesser Writings,* 258.
[271]*Ibid.,* 427.
[272]*Ibid.,* 175-176.
[273]Boerhaave, *Academical Lectures,* I, 50.
[274]Magendie, *Phenomenes Physiques,* I, 142.
[275]Magendie, *Systeme Nerveux,* I, 4.
[276]Magendie, *Phenomenes Physiques,* I, 7.
[277]*Ibid.,* II, 176.
[278]*Ibid.,* IV, 5-6.
[279]Hoffmann, *Fundamenta Medicinae,* 118.
[280]Magendie, *Systeme Nerveux,* I, 4.
[281]*Ibid.,* I, 9.
[282]Bernard, *Experimental Medicine,* 212.
[283]*Ibid.,* 215.
[284]*Ibid.,* 212.
[285]Hahnemann, *Lesser Writings,* 538.
[286]Paul Andral, *La Medecine Traditionnelle et l'Homoeopathie,* 41. Requin, *Homoeopathie,* 15. *Bulletin General de Therapeutique* IX [1835], 298.
[287]Baglivi, *De Praxi Medica,* 154. See, also, *ibid.,* 215.
[288]Hoffmann, *Medicinae Rationalis,* c-3, 21.
[289]*Ibid.,* c-3.
[290]*Ibid.,* a.
[291]Cullen, *First Lines of the Practice of Physic,* I, 17.
[292]*Ibid.,* I, 45.
[293]*Ibid.,* I, 43.
[294]Magendie, "Quelques Idees Generales sur les Phenomenes Particuliers aux Corps Vivants," 146.
[295]Magendie, *Phenomenes Physiques,* IV, 37-38.
[296]*Ibid.,* II, 47.
[297]*Ibid.,* II, 129.
[298]*Ibid.,* II, 130.
[299]Bernard, *Experimental Medicine,* 208.
[300]*Ibid.,* 69.
[301]Hoffmann, *Medicinae Rationalis,* 11.
[302]Cullen, *First Lines of the Practice of Physic,* I, 45. *Treatise of the Materia Medica* I, 29.
[303]Cullen, *First Lines of the Practice of Physic,* I, 166.
[304]*Ibid.,* I, 16.
[305]Magendie, *Phenomenes Physiques,* I, 20.
[306]*Ibid.,* II, 188.
[307]Bernard, *Principes,* 2.
[308]Bernard, *Experimental Medicine,* 18.
[309]*Ibid.,* 76.
[310]Boerhaave, *Academical Lectures,* VI, 176-180.
[311]Bernard, *Experimental Medicine,* 90-91. *Principes,* 69.
[312]Van Helmont, *Oriatrike,* 534.
[313]Hahnemann, *Lesser Writings,* 658.

BIBLIOGRAPHY

(a) Books and Articles

Ackerknecht, Erwin H. "Anticontagionism between 1821 and 1867." *Bulletin of the History of Medicine* XXII (1948), 562-593.

__________. "Aspects of the History of Therapeutics." *Bulletin of the History of Medicine* XXXVI (1962), 389-419.

__________. "Broussais, or a Forgotten Medical Revolution." *Bulletin of the History of Medicine* XXVII (1953), 320-343.

__________. "Laennec und sein Vorlesungsmanuskript von 1822." *Gesnerus* XXI (1964), 142-153.

__________. *Medicine at the Paris Hospital.* Baltimore: Johns Hopkins, 1967.

__________. "Die Therapie der Pariser Kliniker zwischen 1795 und 1840." *Gesnerus* XV (1958), 151-163.

__________. *Rudolf Virchow, Doctor, Statesman, Anthropologist.* Madison: University of Wisconsin Press, 1953.

Albury, William R. "Physiological Explanation in Magendie's Manifesto of 1809." *Bulletin of the History of Medicine* XLVIII (1974), 90-99.

Alibert, J. L. M. "Dartres." *Dictionnaire des Sciences Medicales.*

__________. *Nouveaux Elements de Therapeutique et de Matiere Medicale.* Paris: Crapart, Caille, and Ravier, *an* XII [1804]. Two Volumes.

__________. Fifth Edition, Paris: Bechet Jeune, 1826. Three Volumes.

Amber, Reuben B. and Babey-Brooke, Anna. *The Pulse in East and West.* New York: Santa Barbara Press, 1966.

Ameke, Wilhelm. *History of Homoeopathy.* London: Gould, 1885.

American Institute of Homoeopathy. *Pharmacopoeia of the American Institute of Homoeopathy.* Boston: Otis Clapp, 1897.

Anderson, F. H. *The Philosophy of Francis Bacon.* Chicago: University of Chicago Press, 1948.

Andral, G. *An Antiquorum Doctrina de Crisibus et Diebus Criticis Admittenda? an in Curandis Morbos et Praesertim Acutis Observanda?* Paris Dissertation, 1824.

__________. *Clinique Medicale, ou Choix d'Observations Receuillies a la Clinique de M. Lerminier.* Paris: Gabon, 1823-1827. Four Volumes.

__________. Third Edition. Paris: Deville Cavellin; Montpellier: Louis Castel, 1834. Five Volumes.

__________. *Cours de Pathologie Interne Professe a la Faculte de Medecine de Paris par M. Andral.* Second Edition. Paris: Bailliere, 1848. Three Volumes.

__________. *Essai d'Hematologie Pathologique.* Paris: Fortin, Masson, 1843.

————. *Precis d'Anatomie Pathologique.* Paris: Gabon, 1829. Three Volumes in Two.

————. Second Edition. Bruxelles: Societe Typographique Belge, 1837. Two Volumes.

————. *Recherches sur l'Expectoration dans les Differentes Maladies de Poitrine.* Paris Dissertation, 1821.

"Andral." *Gazette des Hopitaux Civils et Militaires* XLIX (1876), 185-188.

Apert, E. "Bretonneau et la Specificite des Maladies," *Bulletin Medical* XXXVI (1922), 1083-1085.

Aristotle. *Metaphysics. Parts of Animals.*

Auenbrugger, Leopold. *Nouvelle Methode pour Reconnaitre les Maladies Internes de la Poitrine par la Percussion de cette Cavite.* Translated from the Latin with comments by Jean-Nicolas Corvisart. Paris: Migneret, 1808.

Autenrieth, J. H. F. *Versuche fuer die praktische Heilkunde aus den clinischen Anstalten von Tuebingen.* Tuebingen: Cotta, 1807-1808. Volume One (parts I and II).

Baas, Johann Hermann. *Grundriss der Geschichte der Medicin und des heilenden Standes.* Stuttgart: Enke, 1876.

————. *Outlines of the History of Medicine and the Medical Profession.* New York: J. H. Vail and Co., 1889.

Bacon, Francis. *The Physical and Metaphysical Works of Lord Bacon.* Edited by John Devey. London: Henry G. Bohn, 1853.

————. *The Works of Francis Bacon.* Edited by James Spedding, Robert Leslie Ellis, and Douglas Denon Heath. London: Longmans, 1858-1874. Fourteen Volumes.

Baglivi, G. *De l'Accroissement de la Medicine Pratique.* Paris: Labe, 1851.

————. *Opera Omnia Medico-Practica et Anatomica.* Edited by Philippe Pinel. Paris: Duplain, 1788.

————. *De praxi medica ad priscam observandi rationem revocanda.* Romae: Typis Domenici Antonii Herculis sumptibus Caesaretti, 1696. Two Volumes.

Barbier (d'Amiens), J. G. *Traite Elementaire de Matiere Medicale.* Second Edition. Paris: Mequignon-Marvis, 1824. Two Volumes.

Barral, Georges. *Claude Bernard.* Ververs: Gilon, 1889.

Barthez, Paul-Joseph. *Memoires sur le Traitement Methodique des Fluxions et sur les Coliques Iliaques qui sont Essentiellement Nerveuses.* Montpellier: Sevalle, 1816.

————. *Nouveaux Elements de la Science de l'Homme.* Second Edition. Paris: Goujon, 1806. Two Volumes.

————. Third Edition. Paris: Bailliere, 1858. Two Volumes.

————. *Traite des Maladies Goutteuses.* Paris: Deterville, 1802. Two Volumes.

Bartholow, Roberts. *A Practical Treatise on Materia Medica and Therapeutics.* New York: Appleton, 1876.

————. Eleventh Edition. New York: Appleton, 1904.

————. *A Treatise on the Practice of Medicine.* New York: Appleton, 1880.

————. Eighth Edition. New York: Appleton, 1895.

Baur, J. *Petite Histoire de l'Organon et de ses Metamorphoses.* Privately Printed, 1975.

Bayle, A. L. J. *Bibliotheque de Therapeutique.* Paris: Gabon, 1828-1837. Four Volumes.

Bayle, G. L. "Anatomie Pathologique (Considerations Generales sur les Secours que l'Anatomie Pathologique peut Fournir a la Medecine)." *Dictionnaire des Sciences Medicales.*

____________. *Considerations sur la Nosologie, la Medecine d'Observation, et la Medecine Pratique.* Paris Dissertation, *an* X [1802].

____________. "Idee Generale de la Therapeutique" in Corvisart, J. N., *Essai sur les Maladies et les Lesions Organiques du Coeur.* Paris: Delahaye, 1855.

____________. *Recherches sur la Phthisie Pulmonaire.* Paris: Gabon, 1810.

Becker, G. W. "Heilung einer dreijaehrigen Paralyse der untern Extremitaeten." *Journal der practischen Heilkunde* XXVII (1808), *st.* III, 83-101.

Beclard, J. "Trousseau," *Gazette Medicale de Paris* XXV (1870), 25-30, 37-44.

Bell, Benjamin. *A System of Surgery.* Third Edition. Edinburgh: Elliot, 1789-1790. Six Volumes.

Bell, Charles. *The Nervous System of the Human Body.* London: Longman, 1830.

Bernard, Claude. *Cahier de Notes: 1850-1860.* Edited by Mirko Drazen Grmek. Paris: Gallimard, 1965.

____________. *Francois Magendie: Lecon d'Ouverture du Cours de Medecine du College de France (29 Fevrier, 1856).* Paris: Bailliere, 1856.

____________. *An Introduction to the Study of Experimental Medicine.* New York: Dover, 1957.

____________. *Principes de Medecine Experimentale.* With Introduction and notes by Leon Delhoume. Paris: Presses Universitaires de France, 1947.

Bichat, Xavier, *Anatomie Generale, Appliquee a la Physiologie et a la Medecine.* Paris: Brosson, Gabon, *an* X [1801]. Four Volumes in Two.

____________. *Recherches Physiologiques sur la Vie et la Mort.* Paris: Brosson, *an* VIII [1800].

____________. *Traite des Membranes en General et de Diverses Membranes en Particulier.* Paris: Richard, Caille, and Ravier, *an* VIII [1800].

____________. New Edition. Edited by Francois Magendie, Paris: Gabon, 1827.

Blakney, R. B. *Meister Eckhart: A Modern Translation.* New York: Harper, 1941.

Blankard, Etienne. *Traite de la Verole, Gonorrhee, Chancres, Bubes Veneriens, & de leurs Accidens.* Amsterdam: Corneille Blankard, 1688.

Boeckel, Theodore. *Exposition de la Doctrine Homoiopathique* [*sic*] *du Dr. Hahnemann et Reflexions sur Cette Doctrine.* Strasburg Dissertation, 1826.

von Boenninghausen, C. *Die Aphorismen des Hippokrates nebst den Glossen eines Homoeopathen.* Leipzig: Willmar Schwabe, 1863.

Boerhaave, Hermann. *Academical Lectures on the Theory of Physic: Being a Genuine Translation of his Institutes and Explanatory Comment, Collated and Adjusted to Each Other as They Were Dictated to his Students at the University of Leyden.* London: W. Innys, 1742-1746. Six Volumes.

____________. *Elements of Chemistry.* Translated by Timothy Dallowe. London: Pemberton, 1735. Two Volumes in One.

Boissier de Sauvages de la Croix, Francois. *Nosologie Methodique dans laquelle les Maladies sont Rangees par Classe suivant le Systeme de Sydenham et l'Ordre des Botanistes.* Paris: Herissant, 1770-1771. Three Volumes.

____________. *Nouvelles Classes de Maladies.* Avignon: B. d'Avanville, [1731].

Bordeu, Theophile. *Dissertatio Physiologica de Sensu Generice Considerato.* Montpellier: Rochard, 1742.

____________. *Lettres Contenant des Essais sur l'Histoire des Eaux Minerales du*

Bearn et de Quelques Cures. Amsterdam: Les Freres Poppe, 1746.

____________. *Oeuvres.* Paris: Caille and Ravier, 1818. Two Volumes.

Bouchut, E. *Histoire de la Medecine et des Doctrines Medicales.* Paris: Bailliere, 1873. Two Volumes.

Bouillaud, J. B. *Essai sur la Philosophie Medicale et les Generalites de la Clinique Medicale.* Paris: De Just, Rouvier, and Le Bouvier, 1836.

____________. *Nouvelles Recherches sur le Rhumatisme Articulaire Aigu en General.* Paris: Bailliere, 1836.

____________. *Traite Clinique et Experimental des Fievres dites Essentielles.* Paris: Bailliere, 1826.

____________. *Traite Pratique, Theorique, et Statistique du Cholera-Morbus de Paris.* Paris: Bailliere, 1832.

Boyd, Linn J. *A Study of the Simile in Medicine.* Philadelphia: Boericke and Tafel, 1936.

Boyle, R. *Of the Reconcileableness of Specifick Medicines to the Corpuscular Philosophy.* London: S. Smith, 1685.

Boym, Michael. *Clavis Medica ad Chinarum Doctrinam de Pulsibus.* Nuernburg: Andreas Cleyerus, 1686.

Bretonneau, Pierre-Fidele. *Des Inflammations Speciales du Tissu Muqueux et en particulier de la Diphtherite ou Inflammation Pelliculaire.* Paris: Crevot, 1826.

Bricheteau, Isidore. "Discours sur Philippe Pinel, son Ecole, et l'Influence qu'Elle a Exerce en Medecine," *Journal Complementaire des Sciences Medicales* XXIX (1824), 289-304.

Broussais, F. J. V. *Examen de la Doctrine Medicale Generalement Adoptee et des Systemes Modernes de Nosologie.* Paris: Mequignon-Marvis, 1816.

____________. Second Edition. Paris: Mequignon-Marvis, 1821. Two Volumes.

____________. *Histoire des Phlegmasies ou Inflammations Chroniques, Fondee sur de Nouvelles Observations de Clinique et d'Anatomie Pathologique.* Paris: Gabon, 1808. Two Volumes.

____________. *De l'Irritation et de la Folie.* Paris: Delauney, 1828.

____________. *Recherches sur la Fievre Hectique Consideree comme Dependante d'une Lesion d'Action des Differentes Systemes, sans Vice Organique.* Paris Dissertation, *an* XI [1803].

____________. *Traite de Physiologie Applique a la Pathologie.* Paris: Delauney, 1822-1823. Two Volumes.

Brown, John. *The Elements of Medicine.* Portsmouth, New Hampshire: Treadwell, 1804.

von Brunn, W. L. "Homoeopathie als Medizingeschichtliches Problem," *Sudhoffs Archiv* XLVIII (1964), 137-156.

Bruppacher-Cellier, Marianne. *Rudolph Buchheim (1820-1879) und die Entwicklung einer experimentellen Pharmakologie.* Zuercher Medizingeschichtliche Abhandlungen. Neue Reihe, #88. Zuerich: Juris Druck, 1971.

Buchheim, Rudolph. *Lehrbuch der Arzneimittellehre.* Third Edition. Leipzig: Leopold Voss, 1878.

Cabanes, A. "Le Scepticisme Therapeutique de Jean-Jacques Rousseau." *Bulletin General de Therapeutique* CLVIII (1909), 33-48.

Cabanis, Pierre Jean-Georges. *Oeuvres Completes.* Paris: Bossange Freres, 1823-1825. Five Volumes.

Caelius Aurelianus. *On Acute Diseases and on Chronic Diseases.* Translated by I. E. Drabkin. Chicago: University of Chicago Press, 1950.

Castaigna, Gaston. *Etude sur Bordeu.* Montpellier Dissertation, 1878.

Celsus, *De Medicina.* Translated by W. G. Spencer. Loeb Classical Library. Three Volumes.

Chambers, E. *Cyclopedia: or an Universal Dictionary of Arts and Sciences.* Fifth Edition. London: D. Midwinter, 1741-1743. Two Volumes.

Chauffard, Paul E. *Andral: la Medecine Francaise de 1820 a 1830.* Paris: Bailliere, 1877.

Chaussier, Francois. *Table Synoptique des Proprietes Caracteristiques et des Principaux Phenomenes de la Force Vitale.* Paris: Barrois, [1815].

Chauvet, N. M. *L'Avenir de la Homoeopathie. Lettres a M. le Docteur Bretonneau.* Tours: Ladeveze and Gilland-Verger, 1859.

Cheyne, George. *The English Malady: or, a Treatise of Nervous Diseases of all Kinds, as Spleen, Vapours, Lowness of Spirits, Hypochondriacal and Hysterical Distempers, etc. in Three Parts.* London: G. Strahan and J. Leake, 1733.

__________. *The Natural Method of Curing the Diseases of the Body and the Disorders of the Mind Depending on the Body.* Third Edition. London: Strahan and Knapton, 1742.

__________. *A New Theory of Acute and Slow Continued Fevers. To Which is Prefixed an Essay Concerning the Improvements of the Theory of Medicine.* Seventh Edition, Corrected. London: Browne, 1753.

Chirac, Pierre. *Traite des Fievres Malignes, Pestilentielles, et Autres.* Paris: Vincent, 1742. Two Volumes.

Chomel, Auguste Francois. *Des Fievres et des Maladies Pestilentielles.* Paris: Crochard, 1821.

__________. *Elements de Pathologie Generale.* Second Edition. Paris: Crochard, 1824.

__________. *Lecons de Clinique Medicale Faites a l'Hotel-Dieu de Paris.* Paris: Bailliere, 1834-1840. Three Volumes.

Chortet, J. F. *Traite de Pharmacologie (Matiere Medicale) Base sur la Theorie de Brown Suivi d'un Nouvel Essai sur l'Art de Formuler.* Luxembourg: Lamort, 1806.

Christison, Robert. *A Treatise on Poisons.* Edinburgh: Adam Black, 1829.

Cleyer, Andreas. *Specimen Medicinae Sinicae, sive Opuscula Medica ad Mentem Sinensium.* Frankfurt-am-Main, 1692.

Condillac, Etienne, Baron de. *Traite des Sensations.*

Coquerelle, Jules. *Bretonneau (1778-1862): La Doctrine Specifique.* Paris Dissertation, 1892.

Corvisart, Jean-Nicolas. *Aphorismes de Medecine Clinique.* Paris: Masson, 1929.

__________. *Essai sur les Maladies et les Lesions Organiques Du Coeur.* Paris: Delahaye, 1855.

Coulter, Harris L. *Divided Legacy: A History of the Schism in Medical Thought. Volume I. The Patterns Emerge: Hippocrates to Paracelsus.* Washington, D.C.: Wehawken Book Co., 1975. *Volume III. Science and Ethics in American Medicine.* Washington, D.C. Wehawken Book Co., 1973.

__________. *Homoeopathic Influences in Nineteenth-Century Allopathic Therapeutics.* Washington, D.C.: American Institute of Homoeopathy, 1973.

Crosland, M. P. *Science in France in the Revolutionary Era.* Cambridge and London: MIT Press and the Society for the History of Technology, 1969.

Cruveilhier, Jean. *Essai sur l'Anatomie Pathologique en General et sur les Transformations et Productions Organiques en Particulier.* Paris: Crochard, 1816. Two Volumes.

__________. *Medecine Pratique Eclairee par l'Anatomie et la Physiologie Pathologiques.* Paris: Igonette, 1821.

__________. "Phlebite." *Dictionnaire de Medecine et de Chirurgie Pratique,* Vol. II (Paris, 1834), 637-681.

__________. *Traite d'Anatomie Pathologique Generale.* Paris: Bailliere, 1849-1864. Five Volumes.

Cullen, William. *First Lines of the Practice of Physick.* Edinburgh: Bell and Bradfute, 1796. Four Volumes.

__________. *Institutions of Medicine: Part I. Physiology.* Fourth Edition. Edinburgh and Boston: Norman, 1788.

__________. *Lectures on the Materia Medica.* Philadelphia: Robert Bell, 1775.

__________. *A Synopsis of Methodical Nosology in Which the Genera of the Disorders are Particularly Defined and the Species Added, with the Synonimous of Those from Sauvages.* Translated from the Fourth Edition by Henry Wilkins, M.D. Philadelphia: Parry Hall, 1793.

__________. *A Treatise of the Materia Medica.* Edinburgh: Charles Elliot, 1789. Two Volumes.

__________. *William Cullen's Abhandlung ueber die Materia Medica nach der nunmehr von dem Verfasser selbst ausgearbeiteten Originalausgabe, uebersezt und mit Anmerkungen von Samuel Hahnemann der Arzneikunde Doktor.* Leipzig: im Schwickertschen Verlage, 1790. Two Volumes.

Daniel, Christian Frid. *Systema aegritudinum conditum per nosologiam, pathologiam, tam generalem, quam specialem, et symptomatologiam, aetiologiae.* Lipsiae: Boehm, 1781. Two Volumes in One.

Darbefeuille, A. *Propositions sur la Medecine.* Paris Dissertation, 1808.

Debre, Robert. *Discours. Institut de France, Academie des Sciences. Celebration du Centenaire de la Mort de Pierre-Fidele Bretonneau, a Tours, dimanche, 18 Fevrier, 1962.*

Debus, Allen G. "Guintherius, Libavius, and Sennert: the Chemical Compromise in Early Modern Medicine," in Allen Debus, *Science, Medicine and Society in the Renaissance: Essays to Honor Walter Pagel.* Science History Publications. A Division of Neale Watson Academic Publications. New York, 1972. Two Volumes.

Deichgraeber, Karl. *Die Griechische Empirikerschule.* Berlin: Weidmann, 1930. Reprinted Berlin/Zurich: Weidmannsche Verlagsbuchhandlung, 1965.

De la Caze, Louis. *Idee de l'Homme, Physique et Moral, Pour Servir d'Introduction a un Traite de Medecine.* Paris: Guerin and Delatour, 1755.

Delauney, Paul. "Un Medecin Broussaisien: le Docteur Beunaiche la Corbiere." *Bulletin de la Societe Francaise d'Histoire de la Medecine* XX (1926), 397-428.

Deloyers, L. *Francois Magendie, 1783-1855. Precurseur de la Medecine Experimentale.* Bruxelles: Presses Universitaires de Bruxelles, 1970.

Desault, Ph. J. *Cours Theorique et Pratique de Clinique Externe.* Paris: Delaplace, 1803. Two Volumes.

Desault, P. J. *Oeuvres Chirurgicales, ou Expose de la Doctrine et de la Pratique de P. J. Desault, par Xavier Bichat.* Third Edition. Paris: Bailliere, 1830. Three Volumes.

Descartes, Rene. *Oeuvres.* Edited by Charles Adam and Paul Tannery. Paris: Leopold Cerf, 1897-1913. Thirteen Volumes.

__________. *Rene Descartes: Treatise of Man.* Translated and Annotated by Thomas S. Hall. Cambridge: Harvard University Press, 1972.

Des Essartz, Jean-Charles. "Eloge de Bordeu," *Memoires de la Faculte de Medecine de Montpellier* XIV (1777).

Desportes, Eugene-Henri. *De la Noix Vomique.* Paris Dissertation, 1808.

Dewhurst, Kenneth. *Dr. Thomas Sydenham (1624-1689). His Life and Original Writings.* Berkeley and Los Angeles: University of California Press, 1966.

__________. *Thomas Willis as a Physician.* Williams Andrews Clark Memorial Library. University of California, Los Angeles, 1964.

Dictionnaire des Sciences Medicales. Paris: Rapart, 1812-1822. Sixty Volumes.

Dictionnaire Encyclopedique des Sciences Medicales. Paris: Masson, 1869-1889. 100 Volumes.

Double, F. J. *Semeiologie Generale, ou Traite des Signes et de leur Valeur dans les Maladies.* Paris: Croullebois, 1811, 1817. Two Volumes.

Dubois, F. "Eloge de Magendie. Academie de Medecine de Paris. 15 decembre, 1857." *Memoires de l'Academie Imperiale de Medecine* XXII (1858).

Dudgeon, R. E. *The Homoeopathic Treatment and Prevention of the Asiatic Cholera.* London: Bowron, 1847.

__________. *Lectures on the Theory and Practice of Homoeopathy.* London: Leath and Ross, 1854.

Dunham, Carroll. *Homoeopathy, the Science of Therapeutics.* Philadelphia: Boericke, 1885.

Dupuytren, Guillaume. "Observations sur la Note Relative aux Alterations Organiques Publiee par M. Laennec dans le Dernier Numero du *Journal de Medecine.*" *Journal de Medecine, Chirurgie, Pharmacie* IX (1804-1805), 441-446.

"Eloge de Broussais." *Archives Generales de Medecine* VI (1839), 510-516.

Encyclopedie, ou Dictionnaire Raisonne des Sciences, des Arts, et des Metiers. Par une Societe de Gens de Lettres. Lausanne and Berne: chez les Societes Typographiques, 1780-1782. Thirty-Six Volumes.

Faber, Knud. "Nosography in Modern Internal Medicine." *Annals of Medical History* IV (1922), 1-73.

Fabre, Pierre. *Essais sur Differents Points de Physiologie, de Pathologie, et de Therapeutique.* Paris: Didot, 1770.

Fauconneau-Dufresne. "Souvenirs des Commencements de la Carriere du Professeur Andral." *L'Union Medicale* XXIII (1877), 921-927.

Flourens, P. *Eloge Historique de M. Magendie.* Paris: Garnier, 1858.

Floyer, John. *The Physician's Pulse-Watch. To Explain the Art of Feeling the Pulse and to Empire it by the Pulse-Watch.* London: Smith and Walford, 1707, 1710. Two Volumes.

Foissac, M. P. *Rapports et Discussion de l'Academie de Medecine sur le Magnetisme Animal.* Paris: Bailliere, 1833.

Fonssagrives, J. B. *Traite de Matiere Medicale, ou Pharmacographie, Physiologie, et Technique des Agents Medicamentaux.* Paris: Delahaye and Lecrosnier, 1885.

Foster, M. *Lectures on the History of Physiology.* Cambridge: at the University Press, 1901.

Foucault, Michel. *Naissance de la Clinique: Une Archeologie du Regard Medical.* Paris: Presses Universitaires de France, 1963.

Frick, Melchior. *Tractatus Medicus de Virtute Veneniorum Medica.* Ulm, 1701.

Friedell, Egon. *A Cultural History of the Modern Age.* New York: Knopf, 1953. Three Volumes.

Galdston, Iago. "The Concept of the Specific in Medicine." *Transactions of the College of Physicians of Philadelphia* IX (1941-1942), 25-34.

Garrison, F. H. *An Introduction to the History of Medicine.* Philadelphia: Saunders, 1913.

____________. Third Edition. Philadelphia: Saunders, 1922.

Gendron. "Recherches sur les Epidemies des Petites Localites." *Journal des Connaissances Medico-Chirurgicales* I (1833-1834), 193-198, 225-232, 295-302.

Gibson, A. G. *The Physician's Art.* Oxford; at the University Press, 1933.

Gouraud, Henri. *Eloge de M. Recamier.* Paris: Douniol, 1853.

Grimaud, Jean Charles Marguerite. *Cours de Fievres.* Montpellier: Picot, 1815-1816. Four Volumes.

Gross, Samuel David. "Brunonianism, Toddism, and Other Isms." *North American Medico-Chirurgical Review* V (1861), 66-83.

Guerard, Alphonse. *Des Indications que la Therapeutique peut Tirer de l'Action Physiologique des Medicaments.* These pour le Concours pour le Chaire de Matiere Medicale. Paris: Faculté de Medecine, 1839.

Haehl, Richard. *Samuel Hahnemann, His Life and Work.* London: Homoeopathic Publishing Company, 1922. Two Volumes.

Haeser, Heinrich. *Lehrbuch der Geschichte der Medicin und der epidemischen Krankheiten. Erster Band: Geschichte der Medicin.* Second Edition. Jena: Mauke's Verlag, 1868.

Hahnemann, S. *Anleitung alte Schaeden und faeule Geschwuere gruendlich zu heilen.* Leipzig, 1784.

____________. *Die chronischen Krankheiten, ihre eigenthuemliche Natur und homoeopathische Heilung.* Dresden: Arnold, 1828, 1830. Four Volumes.

____________. Second Edition. Duesseldorf: Schaub, 1835-1839. Five Volumes.

____________. *The Chronic Diseases, their Peculiar Nature and their Homoeopathic Cure.* Translated from the second enlarged German edition of 1835 by Professor Louis H. Tafel. Philadelphia: Boericke and Tafel, 1904.

____________. *Doctrine et Traitement homoeopathique des Maladies Chroniques.* Translated by A. J. L. Jourdan. Paris: Bailliere, 1832. Two Volumes.

[S. Hahnemann]. *Defence of the Organon.* Philadelphia: Boericke and Tafel, 1896.

____________. *Dissertatio historico-medica de helleborismo veterum.* Leipzig Dissertation, 1812.

____________. *Fragmenta de viribus medicamentorum positivis sive in sano corpore observatis.* Leipzig: Barth, 1805. Two Volumes in One.

____________. *The Lesser Writings of Samuel Hahnemann.* Collected and Translated by R. E. Dudgeon. New York: Radde, 1852.

____________. *Materia Medica Pura.* Translated from the German by Ernst Stapf. Dresden: Arnold, 1826, 1828. Two Volumes.

____________. *Organon der rationellen Heilkunde.* Dresden: Arnold, 1810.

____________. Second Edition. *Organon der Heilkunst.* Dresden: Arnold, 1819.

____________. Third Edition. Dresden: Arnold, 1824.

____________. *The Organon of Medicine.* Sixth Edition. Translated with preface by William Boericke, M.D., and Introduction by James Krauss, M.D. Calcutta: Roysingh and Co., 1962.

____________. *The Homoeopathic Medical Doctrine or "Organon of the Healing Art"; a New System of Physic, translated from the German of S. Hahnemann by Charles H. Devrient, esq.* Dublin: W. F. Wakeman, 1833.

____________. *Reine Arzneimittellehre.* Dresden: Arnold, 1811-1821. Six Volumes in Four.

____________. Second Edition. Dresden: Arnold, 1822-1827. Six Volumes.

____________. Third Edition. Dresden: Arnold, 1830-1833. Two Volumes in One.

____________. "Was sind Giften, was sind Arzneien?" *Journal der practischen Heilkunde* XXIV (1806), st. III, 40-57.

Hall, Thomas S. *Ideas of Life and Matter: Studies in the History of General Physiology, 600 B.C.-1900 A.D.* Chicago: University of Chicago Press, 1969. Two Volumes.

von Haller, Albert. *A Dissertation on the Sensible and Irritable Parts of Animals.* London: J. Nourse, 1755. Reprinted, with an Introduction by Owsei Temkin, Baltimore: Johns Hopkins University Press, 1936.

____________. *First Lines of Physiology.* Translated from the Latin by William Cullen. Troy, N.Y.: Obadiah Penniman, 1803.

____________. *Memoires sur les Parties Sensibles et Irritables du Corps Animal.* Lausanne, 1760. Four Volumes.

____________. *Primae lineae physiologiae.* Gottingae: A. Vandenhoeck, 1747.

Harvey, Gideon. *The Art of Curing Diseases by Expectation: with Remarks on a Supposed Great Case of Apoplectick Fits.* London: Partridge, 1689.

Harvey, William. *Lectures on the Whole of Anatomy.* Edited by C. D. O'Malley, F. N. L. Poynter, and K. F. Russell. Berkeley and Los Angeles: University of California Press, 1961.

____________. *The Works of William Harvey.* Translated from the Latin, with a life of the author, by Robert Willis. London: The Sydenham Society, 1847.

Heckel, E. *Histoire Medicale et Pharmaceutique des Principaux Agents Medicamenteux Introduits en Therapeutique depuis ces dix Dernieres Annees.* Bruxelles: Manceaux, 1874.

Hecquet, Philippe. *Observations sur la Saignee du Pied et sur la Purgation. Raisons de Doute contre l'Inoculation de la Petite Verole.* Paris: Cavelier, 1724.

Van Helmont, J. B. *Oriatrike, or Physick Refined.* Translated by J. Chandler. London, 1662.

____________. *Supplementum de spadanis fontibus.* Leodii, 1624.

Hering, Constantine. *Analytical Therapeutics.* New York and Philadelphia: Boericke and Tafel, 1875. Volume One (no more published).

____________. *The Guiding Symptoms of Our Materia Medica.* Philadelphia: The American Homoeopathic Publishing Society, 1879-1891. Ten Volumes.

____________. "Hahnemann's Three Rules Concerning the Rank of Symptoms." *Hahnemannian Monthly* I (1865), 5-12.

Hippocrates. *Works.* Translated by W. H. S. Jones. Loeb Classical Library. Four Volumes.

Hirschel, Bernhard. *Geschichte des Brown'schen Systems und der Erregungstheorie.* Leipzig: Arnold, 1850.

Hoffmann, Friedrich. *Fundamenta Medicinae.* Translated by Lester Snow King. London: Macdonald. New York: Elsevier, 1971.

____________. *Medicinae rationalis systematicae tomus primus-quartus. Venetiis: ex typographia Balleoniana, 1737-1741.* Four Volumes in Three.

____________. *Medicinae rationalis systematicae tomus prior quo philosophia corporis humani vivi et sani ex solidis mechanicis et anatomicis principiis methodo plane demonstrativa per certa theoremata ac scholia traditur et pathologiae ac praxi medicae clinicae ceu verum fundamentum praemittitur in usum docentium et discentium.* Halae magdeburgica, 1718.

____________. *La Medecine Raisonnee.* Translated by Jacques-Jean Bruhier. Paris: Briasson, 1738. Two Volumes.

____________. *Opera Omnia Physico-Medica.* Geneva: Fratres de Tournes, 1740. Six Volumes.

L'Homoeopathie dans les Hopitaux. Memoire a Propos de la Petition des Ouvriers de Paris et de la Discussion au Senat (Seance du Premier Juillet, 1865). Paris: Bailliere, 1865.

Hufeland, C. W. "Homoeopathy." *British Journal of Homoeopathy* XVI (1858), 177-198.

Hughes, Richard. *A Manual of Pharmacodynamics.* Sixth Edition. London: Leath and Ross, 1893.

Hunter, John. *Observations on the Inflammation of the Internal Coats of Veins.* Transactions of a Society for the Improvement of Medical and Chirurgical Knowledge. London: J. Johnson, 1793.

____________. *Works.* London: Longman, 1837. Four Volumes.

Imbert-Gourbeyre, Antoine. "Memoire sur les Proprietes Antinevralgiques de l'Aconit." *Gazette Medicale de Paris* IX (1854), 704-720.

"In Memoriam J. Ev. Purkyne, 1787-1937," in *Purkynova Spolecnost.* Prague, 1937.

d'Irsay, Stephen. *Albrecht von Haller: Eine Studie zur Geistesgeschichte der Aufklaerung.* Leipzig: Georg Thieme, 1930.

Isler, H. *Thomas Willis, 1621-1675.* New York and London: Hafner, 1968.

Jaumes, F. A. *Essai de Pharmacologie Therapeutique Generale.* Montpellier: Castel, 1847.

____________. *Traite de Pathologie et de Therapeutique Generales.* Paris: Masson, 1869.

Joerg, Johann. *Materialien zu einer kuenftigen Heilmittellehre durch Versuche der Arzneyen an gesunden Menschen.* Leipzig: Carl Cnobloch, 1825. Volume One (no more published).

"Johann Joerg," *Monatsschrift fuer Geburtskunde* XI (1858), 439-441.

Kentish, Edward. *A Second Essay on Burns, in Which an Attempt is Made to Refute the Opinions of Mr. Earle and Sir W. Farquhar, Lately Advanced, on the Supposed Benefit of the Application of Ice in Such Accidents.* Newcastle on Tyne: Walker, 1800.

King, Lester Snow. *The Growth of Medical Thought.* Chicago: University of Chicago Press, 1963.

____________. *The Medical World of the 18th Century.* Chicago: University of Chicago Press, 1958.

Kratzmann, Emil. *Die neuere Medizin in Frankreich nach Theorie und Praxis.* Leipzig: Brockhaus, 1846.

Kunzli, Jean. *Essai Critique sur l'Homoeopathie.* Paris: Bailliere, 1840.

Laennec, Rene T. H. "Anatomie Pathologique." *Dictionnaire des Sciences Medicales.*

____________. *Laennec, 1781-1826. Documents Inedits Publies a l'Occasion de son Centenaire.* Paris: Masson, 1926.

____________. "Extrait du Discours Prononce par M. Laennec a l'Ouverture de son Cours de Medecine au College Royale de France." *Archives Generales de Medecine* I (1823), v-xx.

____________. "Note sur l'Anatomie Pathologique." *Journal de Medecine, Chirurgie, Pharmacie* IX (1804-1805), 360-378.

————. *Propositions sur la Doctrine d'Hippocrate Relativement a la Medecine Pratique.* Paris Dissertation, *an* XII [1804].

————. *De l'Auscultation Mediate; ou, Traite du Diagnostique des Maladies des Poumons et du Coeur.* Paris: Brosson and Chaude, 1819. Two Volumes.

————. Second Edition. *Traite de l'Auscultation Mediate et des Maladies des Poumons et du Coeur.* Paris: Chaude, 1826. Two Volumes.

————. Third Edition, with notes by Meriadec Laennec. Paris: Chaude, 1831. Two Volumes.

————. Fourth Edition, considerably expanded by M. Andral. Paris: Chaude, 1837. Two Volumes.

————. *Traite Inedit sur l'Anatomie Pathologique.* Paris: Alcan, 1884.

Laignel-Lavastine. "La Source des Idees Medicales de Jean-Jacques Rousseau: Desessartz et *L'Emile." Chronique Medicale* XXVI (1919), 227-234.

de Lamure, Francois. *Nouveaux Elements de Matiere Medicale.* Montpellier: Tournel, 1784.

Landre-Beauvais, Augustin Jacob. *Semeiotique: ou Traite des Signes des Maladies.* Paris: Brosson, 1809.

Langley, J. N. "Sketch of the Progress of Discovery in the Eighteenth Century As Regards the Autonomic Nervous System." *Journal of Physiology* L (1916), 225-258.

Lebert, Hermann. *Physiologie Pathologique, ou Recherches Cliniques, Experimentales, et Microscopiques sur l'Inflammation, la Tuberculisation, les Tumeurs, la Formation du Cal.* Paris: Bailliere, 1845. Two Volumes.

Lechler, W. H. *Philippe Pinel, seine Familie, seine Jugund- und Studienjahre, 1745-1778.* Munich, 1959 (privately printed).

Legallois, Julien Jean Cesar. *Oeuvres.* Paris: LeRouge, 1824. Two Volumes.

Lemoine, Albert. *Le Vitalisme et l'Animisme de Stahl.* Paris: Bailliere, 1864.

Lepelletier de la Sarthe, Almire. *Histoire de la Revolution Medicale du XIX Siecle.* Paris: Bailliere, 1854.

Lettres Edifiantes et Curieuses Ecrites des Missions Etrangeres par Quelques Missionaires de la Compagnie de Jesus. Volume XXI (Paris, 1731).

Liebig, Justus. *Animal Chemistry, or Organic Chemistry in its Application to Physiology and Pathology.* Second Edition. Cambridge, Mass.: Owen, 1843.

Lieutaud, Joseph. *Synopsis of the Universal Practice of Medicine. Exhibiting a Concise View of all Diseases, both Internal and External: Illustrated with Complete Commentaries.* Philadelphia: Parker, 1816.

von Lippmann, Edmund O. *Beitraege zur Geschichte der Naturwissenschaften und der Technik.* Weinheim: Verlag Chimie, GMBH, 1953. Two Volumes.

Locke, John. *An Essay Concerning Human Understanding.*

Lordat, Jacques. *Essai d'une Caracteristique de l'Enseignement Medical de Montpellier.* Montpellier: Castel, 1843.

————. *Exposition de la Doctrine Medicale de Paul-Joseph Barthez et Memoires sur la Vie de ce Medecin.* Paris: Gabon, 1818.

————. *De la Necessite de Creer dans Chaque Faculte de Medecine une Chaire de Philosophie Naturelle Inductive.* Montpellier: Castel, 1846.

————. *Premiere Lecon du Cours de Physiologie de 1838-1839 sur la Necessite d'Etudier les Cas Rares.* Montpellier: Martel, 1840.

Louis, Pierre Charles Alexandre. *An Essay on Clinical Instruction.* London: Highley, 1834.

____________. *Examen de l'Examen de M. Broussais Relativement a la Phthisie et l'Affection Typhoide.* Paris: Bailliere, 1834.

____________. *Recherches Anatomico-Pathologiques sur la Phthisie.* Paris: Gabon, 1825.

____________. Second Edition. *Recherches Anatomiques, Pathologiques, et Therapeutiques sur la Phthisie.* Paris: Bailliere, 1843.

____________. *Recherches Anatomiques, Pathologiques, et Therapeutiques sur la Maladie Connue sous les Noms de Gastro-Enterite, Fievre Putride, Adynamique, Ataxique, Typhoide, etc.* Paris: Bailliere, 1829. Two Volumes.

____________. Second Edition. *Recherches Anatomiques, Pathologiques, et Therapeutiques sur la Maladie Connue sous les Noms de Fievre Typhoide, Putride, Adynamique, Ataxique.* Paris: Bailliere, 1841. Two Volumes.

____________. *Recherches sur les Effets de la Saignee dans Quelques Maladies Inflammatoires et sur l'Action de l'Emetique et des Vesicatoires dans la Pneumonie.* Paris: Bailliere, 1835.

Lovett, Beatrice R. "Pierre-Fidele Bretonneau." *Bulletin of the Society of Medical History of Chicago* IV (1928-1935), 54-70.

Lux, Johan Joseph Wilhelm. *Die Isopathik der Contagionen.* Leipzig: Kollmann, 1833.

Mabit, J. *Observations sur l'Homoeopathie.* Bordeaux: Gassiot, 1835.

Magendie, Francois. "Examen de l'Action de Quelques Vegetaux sur la Moelle Epiniere. Avril, 1809." *Bibliotheque Medicale* XXV (1809), 3-22.

____________. *Formulaire pour la Preparation et l'Emploi de Plusieurs Nouveaux Medicaments.* Third Edition. Paris: Mequignon-Marvis, 1822.

____________. *Lecons sur le Cholera Morbus.* Paris: Mequignon-Marvis, 1832.

____________. *Lecons sur les Fonctions et les Maladies du Systeme Nerveux.* Paris: Ebrard, 1839. Two Volumes.

____________. *Phenomenes Physiques de la Vie. Lecons Professees au College de France.* Paris: Bailliere, 1842. Four Volumes.

____________. *Precis Elementaire de Physiologie.* Paris: Mequignon-Marvis, 1816. Two Volumes.

____________. "Quelques Idees Generales sur les Phenomenes Particuliers aux Corps Vivants." *Bulletin des Sciences Medicales* IV (1809), 145-170.

____________. *Recherches Physiologiques et Medicales sur les Causes, les Symptomes, et le Traitement de la Gravelle.* Paris: Mequignon-Marvis, 1818.

Malpart, Michel. *Un Medecin Romantique: Eusebe de Salles (1796-1873).* Paris Dissertation, 1928.

Mannheim, Karl. *Ideology and Utopia.* London: Routledge and Kegan Paul, 1960.

Marandel, J. *Considerations Generales sur les Irritations.* Paris Dissertation, 1807.

Mercier, Raoul. "L'Extraordinaire Vie de Pierre-Fidele Bretonneau." *Progres Medical* XIV (1937), I, *Supplement,* 1-8.

Meyer, Alfred and Hierons, Raymond. "On Thomas Willis's Concepts of Neurophysiology." *Medical History* IX (1965), 1-15, 142-155.

Mitchell, G. Ruthven. *Homoeopathy: the First Authoritative Study of its Place in Medicine Today.* London: W. H. Allen, 1975.

Mitscherlich, C. G. *Lehrbuch der Arzneimittellehre.* Second Edition. Berlin: G. Bethge, 1847-1851. Three Volumes.

Moers, Ellen. *The Dandy: Brummell to Beerbohm.* New York: Viking Press, 1960.

Moliere. *L'Amour Medecin.*

Morgagni, G. B. *De sedibus et causis morborum per anatomen indagatis libri quinque.* Venice, 1761.

____________. *The Seats and Causes of Diseases Investigated by Anatomy*. In Five Books. Translated from the Latin of John Baptist Mergagni by Banjamin Alexander, M.D. Published under the auspices of the Library of the New York Academy of Medicine by Hafner Publishing Co., New York, 1960. Three Volumes (facsimile of the London, 1769 edition).

Multhauf, R. P. "Medical Chemistry and 'The Paracelsians.'" *Bulletin of the History of Medicine* XXVIII (1954), 101-126.

Neve de Mevergnies, Paul. *Jean-Baptiste van Helmont, Philosophe par le Feu.* Liege: E. Droz, 1935.

Nihell, James. *New and Extraordinary Observations Concerning the Prediction of Various Crises by the Pulse.* London: Society of Booksellers for Promoting Learning, 1741.

"Notice Necrologique sur Laennec." *Archives Genèrales de Medecine* XIII (1827), 620-623.

"Notice Necrologique sur Pinel." *Archives Generales de Medecine* XIII (1827), 625-628.

Olmsted, J. M. D. *Claude Bernard, Physiologist.* New York and London: Harper and Brothers, 1938.

____________. *Claude Bernard and the Experimental Method in Medicine.* New York: Schuman, 1952.

____________. *Francois Magendie: Pioneer in Experimental Physiology and Scientific Medicine in XIX Century France.* New York: Schuman, 1944.

Orfila, M. P. *Traite des Poisons tires des Regnes Mineral, Vegetal, et Animal, ou Toxicologie Generale.* Paris: Crochard, 1815. Two Volumes.

Osler, William. *The Principles and Practice of Medicine.* New York: Appleton, 1893.

____________. Eighth Edition. New York: Appleton, 1912.

Pagel, Walter. "Harvey and Glisson on Irritability with a Note on Van Helmont." *Bulletin of the History of Medicine* XLI (1967), 497-514.

____________. *J. B. Van Helmont: Einfuehrung in die Philosophische Medizin des Barock.* Berlin: Springer, 1930.

____________. *The Religious and Philosophical Aspects of Van Helmont's Science and Medicine.* Supplement No. 2 to the Bulletin of the History of Medicine. Baltimore: Johns Hopkins University Press, 1944.

Paracelsus. *Paracelsus: Selected Writings.* Edited with an Introduction, Jolande Jacobi. Translated by Norbert Guterman. Second Edition. New York: Pantheon Books, Bollingen Series XXVIII, 1958.

____________. *Theophrastus von Hohenheim, genannt Paracelsus: Saemtliche Werke. I. Abteilung. Medizinische, naturwissenschaftliche, und philosophische Schriften.* Ed. Karl Sudhoff. Vols. VI-IX. Munich: O. W. Barth, 1922-1925; I-V, X-XIV. Munich, Berlin: R. Oldenbourg, 1928-1933.

Pariset, Etienne. "Coction." *Dictionnaire des Sciences Medicales.*

____________. "Diathese." *Dictionnaire des Sciences Medicales.*

____________. "Eloge de Pinel." *Revue Medicale* XXVI (1827), 520-533.

____________. *Memoire sur les Causes de la Peste et sur les Moyens de la Detruire.* Paris: Bailliere, 1837.

____________ and Mazet, A. *Observations sur la Fievre Jaune a Cadix en 1819.* Paris: Audot, 1820.

Parseval, Ludovic de. *Homoeopathie et Allopathie.* Paris: Bailliere, 1856.

Partington, J. R. *A History of Chemistry.* Volumes II-IV. London: Macmillan, 1961-1964.

Perdrix, M. C. *Notices Historiques et Biographiques sur Ambroise Pare et Guillaume Dupuytren.* Paris: Crapelet, 1836.

Pereira, Jonathan. *The Elements of Materia Medica and Therapeutics.* London: Longman, 1839, 1840. Two Volumes.

————. Fourth Edition. London: Longman, 1854. Two Volumes.

————. *Handbuch der Heilmittellehre nach dem Standpunkte der Deutschen Medizin. Bearbeitet von Rudolph Buchheim.* Leipzig: Voss, 1846, 1848. Two Volumes.

Petit, Marc-Antoine. *Eloge de Pierre-Joseph Desault.* Lyon: l'Imprimerie des Halles de la Grenette, *an* IV [1795].

————. *Essai sur la Medecine du Coeur.* Lyon: Garnier, 1806.

Phillips, C. D. F. *Materia Medica and Therapeutics. The Vegetable Kingdom.* London: J. and A. Churchill, 1874.

————. *Materia Medica and Therapeutics of the Vegetable Kingdom.* Edited and adapted to the U.S. Pharmacopoeia by Henry G. Piffard. New York: W. Wood and Co., 1879.

————. *Materia Medica and Therapeutics. Organic Compounds. Animal Kingdom.* London: J. and A. Churchill, 1886. Philadelphia: Blakiston, 1886.

Pidoux, H. "Trousseau. Eloge Prononce a la Societe de Therapeutique, dans sa Seance du 5 Mars, 1869." *L'Union Medicale* VII (1869), 349-356, 369-376.

Pinel, C. "Biography of Pinel." *Journal of Psychological Medicine* XIII (1860), 184-205.

Pinel, P. "Agissante (Medecine)." *Dictionnaire des Sciences Medicales.*

————. "Alienation." *Dictionnaire des Sciences Medicales.*

————. "Analyse Appliquee a la Medecine." *Dictionnaire des Sciences Medicales.*

————. "Chronique (Maladies Chroniques)." *Dictionnaire des Sciences Medicales.*

————. "Classification des Maladies Internes." *Dictionnaire des Sciences Medicales.*

————. "Clinique." *Dictionnaire des Sciences Medicales.*

————. "Expectation." *Dictionnaire des Sciences Medicales.*

————. "Experience en Medecine Consideree d'une Maniere Generale." *Dictionnaire des Sciences Medicales.*

————. *La Medecine Clinique Rendue plus Precise et plus Exacte par l'Application de l'Analyse.* Paris: Brosson, *an* X [1802].

————. Second Edition. Paris: Brosson, *an* XII [1804].

————. Third Edition. Paris: Brosson, 1815.

————. *Nosographie Philosophique, ou la Methode de l'Analyse Appliquee a la Medecine.* Second Edition. Paris: Brosson, *an* XI [1802-1803]. Three Volumes.

————. Sixth Edition. Paris: Brosson, 1818. Three Volumes.

———— and Bricheteau, I. "Medecine." *Dictionnaire des Sciences Medicales.*

———— and Bricheteau, I. "Nosographie." *Dictionnaire des Sciences Medicales.*

Plan General de l'Enseignement dans l'Ecole de Sante de Paris: Imprime par Ordre du Comite d'Instruction Publique de la Convention Nationale. An III de la Republique [1795].

Plato. *Timaeus.*

Pomme. *Refutation de la Doctrine Medicale du Docteur Brown.* Paris: Cussac, 1808.

Potter, Samuel O. L. *A Handbook of Materia Medica, Pharmacy, and Therapeutics.* Philadelphia: Blakiston, 1887.

____________. Eighth Edition. Philadelphia: Blakiston, 1901.

Poullain, J. B. Isidore. *Des Medecins Physiologistes et de leur Doctrine.* Paris Dissertation, 1826.

Prost, P. A. *Medecine Eclairee par l'Observation et l'Ouverture des Corps.* Paris: Demonville, *an* XII [1804]. Two Volumes.

Purkyne, Jan Ev. "Einige Beitraege zur physiologischen Pharmacologie." *Neue Breslauer Sammlungen aus dem Gebiete der Heilkunde* I (1829), 423-444.

____________. "Rozprava o tom jak rozlicne veci lekarske na svem tele zkousel." *Casopis lekaruv Ceskych* V (1866), 12-14.

Puschmann, T. *Handbuch der Geschichte der Medizin.* Jena: Gustav Fischer, 1905. Three Volumes.

____________. *History of Medical Education.* New York and London: Hafner, 1966.

Quin, F. H. F. *Du Traitement Homoeopathique du Cholera.* Paris: Bailliere, 1832.

Quissac, J. *De la Doctrine des Elements et de son Application a la Medecine Pratique.* Montpellier: Sevalle, 1850. Two Volumes.

Raffenau-Delile, Alire. *Dissertation sur les Effets d'un Poison de Java appele Upas Tieute.* Paris Dissertation, 1809.

Rapou, Auguste. *Histoire de la Doctrine Medicale Homoeopathique.* Paris: Bailliere, 1847. Two Volumes.

Regnault, J. B. *Considerations sur l'Etat de Medecine en France Depuis la Revolution jusqu'a nos Jours.* Paris: Mequignon-Marvis, 1819.

Reil, J. C. *Entwurf einer allgemeinen Pathologie.* Halle: Curt, 1816. Three Volumes.

Requin, Achille-Pierre. *Homoeopathie.* Paris: Martinet, 1851.

Richerand, A. *Nouveaux Elements de Physiologie.* Second Edition. Paris: Crapard, 1802. Two Volumes.

Ricord, Philippe. *Traite Pratique des Maladies Veneriennes, ou Recherches Critiques et Experimentales sur l'Inoculation Appliquee a l'Etude de ces Maladies.* Bruxelles: Societe Typographique Belge, 1838.

Ringer, Sydney. *Handbook of Therapeutics.* New York: W. Wood, 1870.

____________. Sixth Edition. New York: W. Wood, 1878.

____________. Thirteenth Edition. New York: W. Wood, 1897.

Risueno de Amador. *Des Decouvertes en Medecine.* Montpellier: Boehm, 1843.

____________. "Memoire sur l'Action des Agents Imperceptibles sur le Corps Vivant." *Bulletin de la Societe Medicale Homoeopathique de Paris* II (1846), 131-164.

Rolleston, J. D. "Bretonneau: His Life and Work." *Proc. Royal Society of Medicine* XVIII (1924-1925), History of Medicine Section, 1-12.

Rommelaere, Willem. *Etudes sur J. B. Van Helmont.* Bruxelles: Manceaux, 1868.

Rostan, Leon. *Cours de Medecine Clinique ou sont Exposes les Principes de la Medecine Organique.* Second Edition. Paris: Bechet Jeune, 1830. Three Volumes.

____________. *Exposition des Principes de l'Organicisme Precedee de Reflexions sur l'Incredulite en Matiere de Medecine.* Second Edition. Paris: Labe, 1846.

Rousseau, Jean-Jacques. *L'Emile. Les Confessions.*

Rousset, M. "Notice sur M. le Professeur Risueno d'Amador." *Academie des Sciences de Montpellier, Section de Medecine. Memoires* I (1849-1853).

Sauve, Louis. *Le Docteur Recamier.* Paris: Spes, 1938.

Schwilgue, C. J. A. *Dissertation sur le Croup Aigu des Enfants.* Paris Dissertation, *an* X [1802].

____________. *Traite de Matiere Medicale.* Paris: Brosson, *an* XIII [1805]. Two Volumes.

____________. Second Edition. Paris: Brosson, 1809. Two Volumes.

Semelaigne, R. "Jean-Jacques Rousseau Juge par Pinel." *Chronique Medicale* XIX (1912), 627-628.

Societe Royale de Medecine. *Nouveau Plan de Constitution pour la Medecine en France, Presente a l'Assemblee Nationale par la Societe Royale de Medecine, 1790.*

Solano de Luques, F. *Idioma de la Naturaleza, con el qual Ensena al Medico como ha de Curar con Acierto los Morbos Agudos.* Cadiz: Geronymo de Peralta, 1737.

Soules, Henri. *Essai d'un Examen de la Doctrine Homoeopathique de Hahnemann.* Montpellier Dissertation, 1858.

Sprengel, Curt. *Histoire de la Medecine.* Paris: Deterville, 1815-1822. Ten Volumes.

Stahl, Georg Ernst. *Ars Curandi cum Expectatione, Opposita Arti Curandi Nuda Expectatione. Satyra Harveana Castigata.* Paris: Horth-hemels, 1730.

____________. *Oeuvres Medico-Philosophiques et Pratiques.* Edited by T. Blondin. Paris: Bailliere, 1859-1864. Volumes II to VI.

____________. *Theoria Medica Vera. Physiologiam et Pathologiam tanquam Doctrinae Medicae Partes vere Contemplativas e Naturae et Artis veris Fundamentis Intaminata Ratione et Inconcussa Experientia Sistens.* Leipzig: Choulant, 1831-1833. Three Volumes.

Stille, Alfred. *Therapeutics and Materia Medica.* Philadelphia: Blanchard and Lea, 1860. Two Volumes.

____________ and Maisch, John M. *The National Dispensatory.* Philadelphia: Lea, 1879.

____________. Fifth Edition. Philadelphia and New York: Lea, 1896.

Storck, Anton. *Etudes de Therapie Experimentale: Stramoine, Jusquiame, Aconit, Fraxinelle, Pulsatille.* Translated and edited by H. Piedvache. Paris: Bailliere, 1887.

____________. *Libellus quo demonstratur: stramonium, hyosciamum, aconitum non solum tuto posse exhiberi usu interno hominibus, verum et ea esse remedia in multis morbis maxime salutifera.* Vienna: Trattner, 1761.

Sudhoff, K. *Kurzes Handbuch der Geschichte der Medizin.* Berlin: Karger, 1922.

Sydenham, Thomas. *Tractatus de podagra et hydrope.* London: Walter Kittleby, 1683.

____________. *The Works of Thomas Sydenham,* London: The Sydenham Society, 1848-1850. Two Volumes.

Sylvius, Franciscus de le Boe. *A New Idea of the Practice of Physic. The First Book.* Translated faithfully by Richard Gower. London: Brabazon Aylmer, 1675.

____________. *Opera Omnia.* Amsterdam: Elsevir, 1679.

____________. *Praxeos Medicae Idea Nova. Liber Primus de Affectibus Naturales Hominis Functiones Laesis vel Constituentibus, vel Producentibus, vel

Consequentibus. Lugduni batavorum: Joannis le Carpentier, 1671.

Talalay, Paul, ed. *Drugs in Our Society*. Baltimore: Johns Hopkins Press, 1964.

Taton, Rene. *Enseignement et Diffusion des Sciences en France au XVIII Siecle*. Paris: Hermann, 1964.

Temkin, Owsei. "The Classical Roots of Glisson's Doctrine of Irritation." *Bulletin of the History of Medicine* XXXVIII (1964), 297-328.

———. "An Essay on the Usefulness of Medical History for Medicine." *Bulletin of the History of Medicine* XIX (1946), 9-47.

———. *Galenism: Rise and Decline of a Medical Philosophy*. Ithaca and London: Cornell University Press, 1973.

———. "Galen's Pneumatology." *Gesnerus* VIII (1950), 180-189.

———. "The Philosophical Background of Magendie's Physiology." *Bulletin of the History of Medicine* XX (1946), 10-35.

———. "The Role of Surgery in the Rise of Modern Medical Thought." *Bulletin of the History of Medicine* XXV (1951), 248-259.

———. *Soranus' Gynecology*. Baltimore: Johns Hopkins Press, 1956.

Tessier, Jean-Paul. *De la Medecine Homoeopathique, suivi d'un Releve Comparatif des Malades Traites a l'Hopital Sainte Marguerite par la Methode de Hahnemann et par la Methode Ordinaire Pendant les Annees 1849, 1850, 1851; Reponse a la Lettre de Fredault*. Paris: Bailliere, 1852.

———. "Les Precurseurs de M. Pasteur." *Bulletin de la Societe Medicale Homoeopathique de France* XXVI (1884-1885), 97-107, 177-192.

Tischner, Rudolf. *Geschichte der Homoeopathie. Erster Teil: Die Vorlauefer der Homoeopathie. Zweiter Teil: Hahnemann, Leben und Werk. Dritter Teil: Ausbreitung der Homoeopathie (bis 1850). Vierter Teil: Die Homoeopathie seit 1850*. Leipzig: Dr. W. Schwabe, 1932-1939.

Triaire, Paul. *Bretonneau et ses Correspondants*. Paris: Alcan, 1892. Two Volumes.

———. *Recamier et ses Contemporains, 1774-1852*. Paris: Bailliere, 1899.

Trousseau, Armand. *Clinique Medicale de l'Hotel Dieu de Paris*. Paris: Bailliere, 1861. Three Volumes.

———. Seventh Edition. Paris: Bailliere, 1885. Three Volumes.

———. Twelfth Edition. Paris: Bailliere, 1931. Three Volumes.

———. *Conferences sur l'Empirisme*. Paris: Delahaye, 1862.

———. "De la Maladie a laquelle M. Bretonneau, medecin de l'Hopital de Tours, a Donne le Nom de Dothinenterie ou Dothinenterite." *Archives Generales de Medecine* X (1826), 67-78, 169-216.

———. *Dissertation sur les Generalites de la Physiologie*. Paris: Fournier, 1831.

——— and Pidoux, H. *Traite de Therapeutique et de Matiere Medicale*. Paris: Bechet Jeune, 1836-1839. Two Volumes.

———. Sixth Edition. Paris: Bechet Jeune, 1858. Two Volumes.

———. Eighth Edition. Paris: Bechet Jeune, 1868. Two Volumes.

———. *Treatise on Therapeutics*. Translated from the ninth edition. New York: W. Wood, 1880. Three Volumes.

Velpeau, A. "Note sur l'Emploi des Caustiques, comme Moyen d'Arreter l'Eruption Varioleuse." *Archives Generales de Medecine* VIII (1825), 427-436.

Vess, David. *Medical Revolution in France.* Gainesville: Florida University Press, 1975.

Virchow, Rudolf. *Die Cellularpathologie in ihrer Begruendung auf physiologische und pathologische Gewebelehre. Zwanzig Vorlesungen gehalten waehrend der Monate Februar, Maerze, und April, 1858, im pathologischen Institute zu Berlin.* Berlin: August Hirschwald, 1858.

____________. *Disease, Life, and Man: Selected Essays Translated and with Introduction by Lelland J. Rather.* Stanford, Cal.: Stanford University Press, 1958.

____________. *Handbuch der speciellen Pathologie und Therapie. Erster Band. Allgemeine Stoerungen der Ernaehrung und des Blutes. Krankheiten des Bewegungsapparates.* Erlangen: Enke, 1854.

____________. "Die Naturwissenschaftliche Methode und die Standpunkte in der Therapie." *Archiv fuer pathologische Anatomie und Physiologie und fuer klinische Medicin* II (1849), 3-37.

____________. *Post-Mortem Examinations and the Position of Pathology among Biological Studies.* New York Academy of Medicine, History of Medicine Series, No. 37. Metuchen, N.J.: Scarecrow Reprint Corp., 1973.

Weber, Georg Adolph. *Der Milzbrand, eine unter dem Rindviehe, den Pferden, und Schweinen haeufig herrschende Seuche, und deren sicherstes Heilmittel.* Leipzig: Reclam, 1836.

Wedel, Georg Wolfgang. *Introduction to the Whole Practice of Physick, Showing the Natures and Faculties of Medicine.* London: Thackery and Teate, 1685.

____________. *De medicamentorum facultatibus cognoscendis et applicandis libri duo.* Jena: J. Bielck, 1678.

Wesley, John. *Primitive Physick, or an Easy and Natural Method of Curing Most Diseases.* Dublin: Nelson, 1752.

Wichmann, Johann Ernst. *Aetiologie der Kraetze.* Second Edition. Hannover: Koenigliche Hofbuchhandlung, 1791.

Willis, Thomas. *Dr. Willis's Practice of Physick, Being the Whole Works of that Renowned and Famous Physician.* London: T. Dring, C. Harper, and J. Leigh, 1684.

____________. *Pharmaceutice Rationalis. Sive, Diatriba de Medicamentorum Operationibus in Humano Corpore.* Two Parts. Sheldonian Theater, 1674, 1675.

Windelband, William. *A History of Philosophy.* New York: Harpers, 1958. Two Volumes.

Wood, Horatio C. *The Dispensatory of the United States of America.* Fourteenth Edition. Philadelphia: Lippincott, 1877.

____________. Nineteenth Edition. Philadelphia: Lippincott, 1907.

____________. *A Treatise on Therapeutics Comprising Materia Medica and Toxicology.* Philadelphia: Lippincott, 1874.

____________. Twelfth Edition. Philadelphia: Lippincott, 1905.

Wunderlich, Carl. *Wien und Paris.* Stuttgart: Ebner and Seubert, 1841.

Zimmermann, Johan Georg. *Traite de l'Experience en General, et en Particulier dans l'Art de Guerir.* Paris: Vincent, 1774. Three Volumes.

(b) Periodicals Consulted

Allgemeine homoeopathische Zeitung XXVI (1844)
Annalen der gesammten Medicin II (1810)
Archives de la Medecine Homoeopathique I-VIII (1834-1838)
Archives Generales de Medecine V (1824)
Bibliotheque Homoeopathique I-VIII (1832-1837)
Bibliotheque Medicale XXV (1809), LIII (1816)
Boston Medical and Surgical Journal LI (1854-1855)
British and Foreign Medico-Chirurgical Review (1872)
British Journal of Homoeopathy VII (1849), XII (1854), XXVI (1868)
Bulletin de l'Academie Royale de Medecine I (1836-1837)
Bulletin de la Societe Medicale Homoeopathique de Paris II (1846)
Bulletin General de Therapeutique V-IX (1833-1835)
France Medicale XXIII (1876)
Gazette des Hopitaux VIII (1835), IX (1835)
Gazette Medicale de Paris II (1834), III (1835)
Homoeopathic World XVI (1881)
Hygeia IV (1836)
Journal de Medecine Pratique I (1835)
Journal de Medecine, Chirurgie, Pharmacie XLII (1774), XLVII (1777), I (1801)
Journal der Pharmacie II (1794)
Journal der practischen Heilkunde XLIX (1819)
Journal des Connaissances Medico-Chirurgicales I (1833-1834)
Moniteur, an III (1794-1795)
Montpellier Medical II (1859)
Philadelphia Journal of Homoeopathy III (1854-1855)
Physisch-Medicinisches Journal II (1801)
The Practitioner XIII (1874)
Revue Medicale Francaise et Etrangere I (1834), II (1835)
L'Union Medicale III (1849), V (1851), VI (1852), VII (1853)

INDEX

This volume of **Divided Legacy** was first published with the title: *Progress and Regress: J.B. Van Helmont to Claude Bernard.*

ISBN 0-916386-00-7 (Volumes I-III)
0-916386-01-5 (Volume I)
0-916386-03-1 (Volume III)

Wehawken Book Co.
4221 45th St., N.W.
Washington, D.C. 20016
(202) 364-0898

North Atlantic Books
2320 Blake St.
Berkeley, CA 94704
(415) 540-7934